Praise for *Yoga Therapy*

"A deep bow to Mark Stephens for this substantial contribution to the growing field of yoga therapy! Thoroughly grounded in yoga's historical and philosophical foundations, this book balances well-researched, practical information with heart-felt wisdom. From the insightful section on "Healing and Curing" to the practical applications of yoga therapy for a wide range of conditions, Stephens skillfully conveys the truly integrative nature of yoga therapy. An essential resource for yoga therapists, clinicians, and educators in the field!"

—JANICE GATES, past president, International Association of Yoga Therapists (IAYT), author of *Yogini: The Power of Women in Yoga* and founder/director of Marin Yoga Therapy and Somatic Yoga Therapy Programs

"Yoga therapy is a big field, encompassing the entirety of yoga and its many practices along with aspects of Western medicine, ayurveda, physiology, physical therapy, kinesiology, psychology, philosophy, spiritual development, and more. No single volume can do it full justice, but Mark Stephens has done a yeoman's job to assemble much of the background information aspiring yoga therapists will need to understand. This book is smart, thoughtful, and well researched and doesn't shy away from presenting a strong—and sometimes provocative—point of view. I recommended it highly."

—TIMOTHY MCCALL, MD, author of *Yoga As Medicine,* coeditor of *The Principles and Practice of Yoga in Health Care,* and medical editor of *Yoga Journal*

"Mark Stephens' capacity for conveying both the depth and the breadth of the yogic sciences is all the more powerful because of his commitment to practice. His works to date on teaching, sequencing, and adjustments have already established him as one of the foremost authorities in yoga education. With the emergence of yoga therapy in recent years as a powerful form of integrative healing, Stephens now brings his scholar's mind and practitioner's wisdom to the field. A boon for all!"

—MICAH MORTALI, director of The Kripalu Schools (School of Integrative Yoga Therapy, School of Yoga, School of Ayurveda), Kripalu Center for Yoga and Health

"Going back to the time of the Buddha, yoga practitioners have been divided into two groups: Experimentalists who know yoga through their bodies and Speculatives who know yoga through its philosophical teachings. Mark Stephens' *Yoga Therapy* is proof that he has mastered both paths."

—DAVID GORDON WHITE, author of *Sinister Yogis* and *The Yoga Sutra of Patanjali: A Biography*

"*Yoga Therapy*, a thorough and comprehensive landmark book, offers illuminating insight into yoga, yoga therapy, and the interface with Western medicine. Along with Stephens' generous offering of practical information, he espouses the attributes of kindness and compassion in yoga therapy practice, which although often overlooked are indeed the very heart of yoga itself. An essential read for every yoga therapist!"

> —NISCHALA JOY DEVI, yoga teacher and therapist and author of *The Healing Path of Yoga* and *The Secret Power of Yoga*

"The next great yoga therapy book from an excellent teacher and author. Highly recommended for yoga teachers, health professionals, and students."

> —LARRY PAYNE, coauthor of *Yoga Therapy & Integrative Medicine, Yoga Rx,* and *Yoga for Dummies* and founding director of Yoga Therapy Rx & Prime of Life Yoga Programs, Loyola Marymount University

"Mark Stephens' *Yoga Therapy* is a complete guide to anyone who wants thorough information on subtle as well as gross anatomy, ayurvedic principles, and insight into the many intricacies of the human body and spirit as it relates to yoga and healing. The scope of this book is clearly a labor of devotion and knowledge."

> —JO ANN STAUGAARD-JONES, author of *The Vital Psoas Muscle* and *Concise Book of Yoga Anatomy*

"Prolific author Mark Stephens offers a comprehensive primer on yoga therapy and his synthesis of theories, practices, and remedies for a host of ailments."

> —GANGA WHITE, author of *Yoga Beyond Belief* and codirector of White Lotus Foundation

"This comprehensive textbook for yoga therapists offers an original synthesis of yoga practices with the insights of Western medicine."

> —BARBARA DOSSEY, PhD, RN, AHN-BC, FAAN, HWNC-BC, author of *Holistic Nursing* and codirector of International Nurse Coach Association

"Mark Stephens' sober but optimistic assessment of the potential for yoga therapy inside the Western medical model is a welcome addition. My hope is that the field will follow his well-informed guidance in the attempt to responsibly integrate these two models of healthcare that have so much to offer each other because, ultimately, it is the patients that will benefit."

> —DAVID EMERSON, author of *Trauma-Sensitive Yoga in Therapy* and director of Yoga Service, The Trauma Center at Justice Resource Institute

Yoga
Therapy

FOUNDATIONS, METHODS, AND
PRACTICES FOR COMMON AILMENTS

MARK STEPHENS

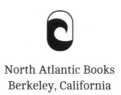

North Atlantic Books
Berkeley, California

Published by
North Atlantic Books
Berkeley, California

Cover photo by: iStock/MotoEd
Cover design by Nicole Hayward
Book design by Maureen Forys, Happenstance Type-O-Rama
Printed in the United States of America

Yoga Therapy: Foundations, Methods, and Practices for Common Ailments is sponsored and published by the Society for the Study of Native Arts and Sciences (dba North Atlantic Books), an educational nonprofit based in Berkeley, California, that collaborates with partners to develop cross-cultural perspectives, nurture holistic views of art, science, the humanities, and healing, and seed personal and global transformation by publishing work on the relationship of body, spirit, and nature.

MEDICAL DISCLAIMER: The following information is intended for general information purposes only. Individuals should always see their health care provider before administering any suggestions made in this book. Any application of the material set forth in the following pages is at the reader's discretion and is his or her sole responsibility.

North Atlantic Books' publications are available through most bookstores. For further information, visit our website at www.northatlanticbooks.com or call 800-733-3000.

LIBRARY OF CONGRESS CATALOGING-IN-PUBLICATION DATA

Names: Stephens, Mark, 1958– author.
Title: Yoga therapy: foundations, methods, and practices for common ailments / Mark Stephens.
Description: Berkeley, California: North Atlantic Books, [2017]
Identifiers: LCCN 2017006387 (print) | LCCN 2017010318 (ebook) | ISBN 9781623171063 (paperback) | ISBN 9781623171070 (ebook)
Subjects: LCSH: Hatha yoga. | Medicine, Ayurvedic. | Mind and body. | BISAC: HEALTH & FITNESS / Yoga. | BODY, MIND & SPIRIT / Healing / General. | HEALTH & FITNESS / Healing.
Classification: LCC RA781.7 .S7278 2017 (print) | LCC RA781.7 (ebook) | DDC 613.7/046—dc23
LC record available at https://lccn.loc.gov/2017006387

1 2 3 4 5 6 7 8 9 UNITED 17 18 19 20 21

Printed on recycled paper

North Atlantic Books is committed to the protection of our environment. We partner with FSC-certified printers using soy-based inks and print on recycled paper whenever possible.

TO ROYAL SARAH STEPHENS

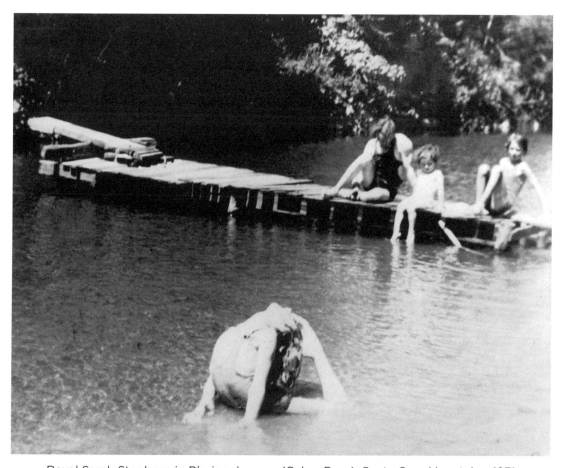

Royal Sarah Stephens in Bhujanghasana (Cobra Pose), Santa Cruz Mountains, 1931

Contents

PART III: Helping Others Heal with Yoga

PART IV: Yoga Therapy Practices

PART V: Healing Common Conditions

PART VI: Epilogue: The Promising Future of Yoga Therapy

Preface

QUESTIONS OF HEALTH AND HEALING first come to us in the earliest childhood experiences of sickness and injury. I grew up in the mountains surrounding Santa Cruz, California, with two older siblings who had me running through the wild woods and climbing redwood trees before I entered kindergarten. With a sense of wholeness in the beauty of nature, it seems that nearly every day we nevertheless came into an intense bodily experience: sprained ankles, poison oak, bee stings, thorn punctures, cuts, and bruises. We also brought playful competitive energy into many of our adventures—whether in sports or in playing chess—with the injuries or challenges to our bodyminds often overshadowed by the joy of being in the mix of it all.

Meanwhile, we experienced the ordinary illnesses children typically contract in their early development. Each illness was met with certain forms of care that our mother, a nurse, thought to be the best treatment. In infancy I developed an acute pneumonia, and with it, life-threatening dehydration that, after hospital care, my mother ultimately addressed with teaspoon after teaspoon of hand fed water. She had a deep understanding of medical science yet often went with the folk medicine she had learned from her own mother and grandmother, as well as experience she got as a nurse on a Hoopa Indian Reservation. Whether it was influenzas, measles, or so-called common colds, all were met with a variety of natural and medical treatments. In these experiences she gave us a sense that pain and suffering are part of life yet can be relieved or experienced in ways that are not self-defeating, but she gave us little sense of how to prevent them beyond healthy food, exercise, rest, and a positive outlook on life.

One can choose a life that dramatically reduces the risk of being hurt by living like the paranoid hypochondriac as depicted by Woody Allen in his film *Manhattan*. I, on the other hand, have chosen a somewhat adventurous life, replete as it is with both awe and pain in the natural experience of it all. At age four I tore open the palm of my hand on a rusty nail while fearlessly climbing a tree, leading to my first tetanus shot and several stitches. My sports injuries were mostly minor, although I fractured my right elbow playing football when I was nine years old. At fourteen I weighed about 125 pounds, yet while hanging out with friends, I pressed a 120-pound barbell overhead, only to lose my balance and fall backward, simultaneously breaking one wrist and severely spraining the other. At sixteen I crashed my road-racing motorcycle into the side of a car that pulled out in front of me, dislocating my left shoulder for the first of many times. A few years later I dislocated the other shoulder while tumbling 40 feet off the highly exposed East Face of Mount Whitney in the Sierra Nevada Mountains of California. At twenty-five I experienced a concussion after landing on my head in a mountain bike crash. These various injuries gave me an abundant and humbling appreciation of human frailty (and foolishness and folly).

This inherent human frailty also showed up in doing yoga. Although I tended to be very cautious with the asanas during my first year of consistent practice, my ego soon propelled me to do everything as strongly as possible, with little sense of balance between effort and ease. While progressing deeply into the Ashtanga Vinyasa practice, I strained my hamstrings, knees, lower back, shoulders, and wrists more times than I can remember. It would be many years before I came to appreciate the benefits of a sustainable practice over one focused on attainments. We can call these *aparigraha* issues: being covetous of deeper asana expressions, I would have rather foregone *ahimsa* (nonhurting) and *satya* (truth, starting with being true to my bodymind's pleas to take it easier) than to have held back from anything.

The pain and suffering I experienced in my childhood and youthful exuberance pales in impact to what I experienced at age ten when my mother was diagnosed with breast cancer. My mother was a healer who lived a very healthy lifestyle—with wholesome foods, close friends and family, lots of laughter, focused work, creative projects, and community work—all inspired and enriched by her deep and abiding Christian faith and practices. Well trained and practiced in the medical sciences, she was terrified—mostly for her three children and her husband—when she learned that she had what today is described as stage IV (metastatic) breast cancer. Despite a radical mastectomy, lymphadenectomy, and radiation treatments, it took a mere six months for the cancer to enter her brain and end her life.

My mother's death was both traumatizing and awakening. I was very close to her and wonder to this day how my life would have been different had she lived longer. Her absence was my first experience of profound loss and sadness. Her illness was my first observation of the aggressive potential of biological infection, the delicate fragility of the human organism, the somewhat tenuous nature of a human life, and how the loss of any one life can be a loss to many others.

Yet it also taught me about resilience and fortitude, love and relationship, hope and prayer. Odd as it may sound, in dying my mother gave me a second birthing, opening me to more richly sensing the vitality of life and how in every moment we can make choices to live our lives in more awakened ways, regardless of our circumstances. I think this is an important part of the path that led me to begin exploring the nature of life and consciousness in my early teen years, foregoing high school in favor of my own ways of learning in the world, and that eventually brought me to yoga at age seventeen (inspired in large part by Alan Watts) while I was living in a culturally desolate crossroads hamlet in the dusty Mojave Desert of southern California.

These early years of my yoga practice were all about the mind and spiritual exploration, even when the practices involved asanas and pranayama. I was curious about how we think and feel, why we think and feel in the ways we do, why we react to things as we do, the power of mental and emotional habit, and the possibility of a clearer mind and a more open heart. I read books that made fantastic promises about human potential, from Herbert Marcuse and Aldous Huxley to Carl Rogers and Fritz Perls to Joseph Campbell and Anaïs Nin, and I committed to daily meditation using what limited insights I could find in books and in Watts's radio broadcasts. I sat, breathed, did asanas, breathed more, and sat longer.

While in this practice I was also interested in other things, especially outdoor adventure and what was becoming a strong and lifelong commitment to trying to make the world a better place in our social and ecological relationships. For many years I went deeply into academic and activist work, all the while backpacking, skiing, surfing, rock climbing, doing triathlons, lifting weights, and exploring all I could in the realm of physical culture. Although earlier questions about being and consciousness were still there, they were increasingly folded into my academic work in comparative and historical sociology and my activist work in community organizing and other efforts to promote progressive social change. The more deeply I went into it—especially during my seven years of doctoral studies at UCLA—the further I drifted from the core curiosities that first led me to explore with yoga. In a sense, I lost my way. Fully engrossed in my work, I became increasingly stressed out; then I remembered yoga.

I came back to yoga in 1991 and have practiced ever since. Some of my first classes were with the light-hearted, yet spiritually inspiring Steve Ross, whose seemingly natural joy made the practice delightfully contagious. I soon met Erich Schiffmann and studied with him intensively for a few years, learning techniques for going more deeply inside and for guiding one's own asana practice. To this day I think back on these two teachers with profound fondness and gratitude for the gifts they conveyed to me. Both are healers in their unique ways who perhaps unknowingly helped point me toward a sustainable yoga path, a path with joy and spontaneity, even amid the detailed minutia of the practice I was soon to explore more deeply.

As I went more deeply into yoga practice in the mid-1990s—committing to Ashtanga Vinyasa (eventually completing the third series), studying extensively with numerous Iyengar teachers, apprenticing with the brilliantly insightful yoga and physical therapist Jasmine Lieb, enjoying creative flow with Shiva Rea, and more and more coming to a personal home practice—I made a fortuitous and formative connection that would change how I approach teaching all yoga practices: yoga outside of the mainstream studio. I had worked for many years with young gangsters on the streets and in the institutions of incarceration in Los Angeles County—this at the height of the LA gang wars in which thousands of youth were killed year after year in internecine street battles and another 40,000 were locked in juvenile prisons every year (there were and are nineteen juvenile prisons in Los Angeles County).

In one of many projects, when I was working with Barry Bryant's Samaya Foundation, we gained the Dalai Lama's blessing to bring six Tibetan monks from Dharmsala to teach meditation in juvenile prisons. The experiment of teaching meditation to incarcerated youth proved very effective in helping them gain a healthier perspective on their lives and a sense that they could make changes for the better starting in the present moment. As this project came to an end, it inspired me to bring yoga into similar institutions, which in 1997 led me to create Yoga Inside Foundation as a vehicle for bringing yoga into over 300 prisons, schools, drug and alcohol treatment centers, veterans' homes, homeless shelters, and other exceptional settings across North America.

What we discovered while teaching yoga in these settings was very insightful because of the highly pronounced physical, emotional, and mental challenges of those we served—conditions that fell far from the mainstream students we were trained to teach in basic and advanced yoga teacher training. It was very clear that we needed better adaptive approaches to yoga practices, including adaptations to better support healing and well-being in the physical, mental, emotional, and spiritual realms of experience. Among the clearest insights is that these "realms" (physical, mental, etc.) are part of the whole of one's being, and that healing and self-transformation are about regaining a healthy sense of this wholeness, even as there are insights and methods associated with each realm. Exploring with this sensibility, we worked closely with a plethora of volunteer professionals—yoga teachers, psychotherapists, physical therapists, spiritual guides, and others—to explore a variety of alternative ways of tapping into yoga and other healing arts to adapt the practices for our students. In my teaching and writing since then, I have continued to tap and expand upon these insights to teach yoga as an adaptive, integrative, and transformative practice, whether I'm working with special students in alternative settings or students in regular classes anywhere in the world, all of whom are uniquely special and deserving of individualized guidance.

The primary (beginning) series of Ashtanga Vinyasa is called *yoga chikitsa*, meaning "yoga therapy." I now understand that this form of yoga therapy is largely about deep self-purification, opening the flow of pranic energy throughout the bodymind, and gaining some sense of a quieter, clearer, and calmer mind on the path toward the second series. In my experience, this practice holds great promise in each of those ways and more, but only for those whose bodyminds allow such vigorous, acrobatic, and contortionist forms of asana practice. Even the ostensibly beginning level primary series is inaccessible and even contraindicated for all but a small and physically blessed portion of humanity. There are other approaches to *yoga chikitsa*.

The longer one practices, the more one tends to evolve in how he or she practices. My own practice has changed over the past quarter century. In the early years it was about trying to figure out basic things at the level of physical strength, flexibility, and balance; then gradually it became about refinement, making it all simpler and thereby deeper. My youthful competitive tendencies often came into play, and it was mostly then that I pushed myself into usually mild injuries. About fifteen years ago I jumped off the Ashtanga Vinyasa and other vigorous flow trains to go with what for me is a more open-minded and intuitive practice. In doing so, I more fully let go of an attainment mentality and found the portals of energy and awareness more gracefully opening in dedicated pranayama and meditation. Today my asana practice feels more in balance; it helps me maintain my health, open to deeper pranayama, and more easily go into quieter meditation and clearer awareness, all with a sense of *aparigraha*, nongrasping, simply letting it come to me as I show up in it. It is, in a sense, my own form of yoga self-therapy, all on the path of the healthiest possible life.

It is from this cumulative and ongoing set of personal experiences in life and yoga practices that I now attempt to share insights that might help make others' lives healthier and better.

About This Book

MANY PEOPLE COME TO YOGA classes with acute or chronic conditions of compromised health, or ordinary conditions such as pregnancy, that indicate the value of a specialized or adapted practice. In any given large yoga class there are usually students who have at least some minor ache or condition that suggests modification of postural and breathing practices. What are those modifications? How might you best communicate with, assess, and guide students with any one (or more) of many different conditions? How can yoga be part of healing? How can it support a feeling of wholeness and greater vibrancy in one's life? How can you go further in offering yoga as a therapeutic tool—*yoga chikitsa*—as a yoga therapist working with private clients?

These are a few of the motivating questions at the heart of this book. To most fully explore them, we will look deeply into the ancient wisdom, modern practices, and most contemporary insights of yoga and related disciplines available today. One of the challenges we have in sorting through the libraries, compendiums, and other sources of transmitted knowledge is that much of the source material arrives through approaches that contradict each other. At the broadest level, we must appreciate the fundamentally different approaches of evidence-based scientific medicine and divinely inspired, intuited, or otherwise received insights of yoga and ayurveda. Although we see considerable progress in their integration, for some practitioners these approaches will always be mutually exclusive, each rejecting the other as fundamentally flawed in its basic assumptions and methods. Here we will look to unravel some of these tensions to distill methods that make practical sense in teaching yoga therapeutically and offering services as a yoga therapist.

In Part I, "The Origins and Sources of Yoga Therapy," we present what at first glance seem to be conflicting paradigms of human life and health given by ancient-to-modern yoga and ayurveda and by largely Western medical sources before we discuss treatment methods that tap into both views with integrative intention.

Part II, "The Human Bodymind's Major Systems," provides a layperson's introduction to the structure, function, and common pathologies of our major systems, with Chapters 5–8 and 10–16 covering skin, bones, muscles, nerves, movement, the heart and blood, lymph, breathing, hormones, digestion, elimination, and reproduction. We also look closely (in Chapter 9) at the biomechanics and kinesiology of movement, thus giving closer attention to the neuromuscular system and how we move in space with relative stability and ease or instability and difficulty.

Part III, "Helping Others Heal with Yoga," first explores the meaning of yoga therapy and attempts to more clearly define a yoga therapy scope of practice in ways that differentiate it from other healing modalities and offer greater clarity about the work of the yoga therapist; then discusses the qualities of communication and interaction in therapeutic relationships; and finally provides guidance on assessing clients and planning uniquely adapted yoga practices to support them in their healing.

Part IV, "Yoga Therapy Practices," discusses the essential elements and basic yoga therapy tools of asana, pranayama, and meditation, with a chapter on each of these core yoga practices.

Part V, "Healing Common Conditions," applies yoga practices to healing a variety of human ailments and conditions. In doing so, the focus is on musculoskeletal complaints, mental health conditions, and reproduction system issues. Scores of physiological ailments are beyond the scope of this already large book; where there is clear evidence for yoga in healing them, we offer references to these best-known practices.

Part VI, "Epilogue: The Promising Future of Yoga Therapy," offers some reflections on the future of yoga therapy.

Acknowledgments

AS WITH ALL WRITING, the writer is fortunate for whatever life experiences have shaped his or her bodymind. In writing this book, I am particularly fortunate for everyone I have experienced on the yoga path, especially my students, who are my best teachers. They have taught me to listen, to honor that they know themselves better than anyone else ever can, and to offer them guidance in the spirit of sharing in the gems I have been lucky to gather in my personal yoga practice and studies.

Students in my open yoga classes have allowed me to explore with them the various ailments that have come their way, ranging from minor repetitive stress injuries and bouts of melancholy to chronic depression and terminal cancer. Students in Yoga Inside Foundation classes—in prisons, drug rehabs, shelters, and schools—have given me the opportunity to share yoga with them in ways that allowed me to discover that yoga can make everyone's life better so long as we open our hearts to this truth. Students in my workshops and teacher trainings have helped me deepen my understanding of asana, pranayama, and meditation practices in part by tolerating my passion for learning and my intensity in striving to give them all I can.

In researching this book, I did my best to find the most relevant and insightful sources on every topic. There are many sources that might be surprising, including from a newer generation of thinkers and doers in the realms of yoga and the healing arts whose names might not appear among those of the esteemed faculty of professional yoga conferences and institutions. My only criteria for inclusion are relevance and insight, with both considered through the prisms of accuracy and veracity rather than relying on a source's ostensibly authoritative assertion. I apologize to those who might feel slighted and invite their substantive commentary and open conversation for future editions.

Deep bows of gratitude to Tim McKee, Emily Boyd and Vanessa Ta at North Atlantic Books for affirming that the present book was the one to write and for their gracious patience in its research and composition. Louis Swaim kindly and expertly guided the process of converting the manuscript and artwork into this finished book. Rebecca Rider thoroughly read, edited and refined the entire manuscript. Suzanne Albertson's compelling cover design and Maureen Forys of Happenstance Type-O-Rama's clean and clear interior design—transforming the manuscript into a book—speak for themselves.

Melinda Stephens-Bukey, a lifelong teacher (and the best sister one can imagine), encouraged me to do the deeper study involved in this project. My brother, Michael

Stephens, provided vital support in matters of home, hearth, and levity amidst the rigors of writing and traveling. Scores of students in my Advanced Yoga Training programs did independent study projects with me related to yoga and healing that helped me to better navigate the massive array of sources on every health condition. Michael Lerner devoted precious time walking the bluffs around Commonweal to engage in conversation about the ultimate sources of healing that reside in the heart. Janice Gates hiked with me on Mt. Tamalpais to share her insights into yoga and healing that are rooted in years of her yoga therapy practice and leadership with the International Association of Yoga Therapists (IAYT), including as its former president. Nischala Joy Devi reminded me that the greatest healing arises in loving communication. Anne Tharpe engaged in innumerable conversations with me on many of the topics covered in this book and assisted in the compilation and creation of the book's images. Jennifer Stanley, MD, an open-minded explorer of all things human, spiritual, and mysterious, was unrelenting in subjecting my ideas to scrutiny, all the while giving me the support of her friendship; she also patiently sat and posed for many of the asana photographs. Reema Prasad provided helpful research assistance, and both she and J. K. Hopper were supportive in sitting for asana photographs. Kyla Roessler assisted with the bibliography. Mike Rotkin continued his over thirty-five years of mentoring me in how taking conscious action in the world is all that ever makes the world a better place to live, this while consistently showing up as a friend. Throughout this project, Dagmar Stuhr nurtured my spirit and inspired me to balance disciplined intellectual work with a healthy daily rhythm filled with abundant laughter, and to more consciously live, work, and share from the truth, wisdom, and love emanating from the heart.

In my earlier writings on yoga I have emphasized that the best teacher one will ever have is inside, and that much of the practice is about learning to listen to and honor one's inner teacher. This idea is wisely amplified with respect to yoga therapy. The outer healer has a role. But in the practice of yoga in which we are sometimes helping others to heal, the most important healer is the student or client. Our role as yoga teachers and yoga therapists is to guide and support our students and clients with the best of our knowledge, skills, and loving compassion.

Introduction:
Yoga for Healing and Wholeness

YOGA OFFERS A RICH ARRAY of resources for living healthier and better lives. The asana, pranayama, and meditation practices of yoga are well-honed tools for cultivating an abiding sense of wholeness in our lives and for opening to a more expansive appreciation of life itself as part of the sublime nature of human existence. They can also be applied in uniquely customized yoga practices to help us heal common injuries and ailments, including those that can arise when practicing yoga.

From the earliest times of yogic exploration in India's Vedic period (circa 1500 BCE), seers, sadhus, and various seekers have sought to make life better by reducing or eliminating suffering. This is the leitmotif of yoga. For some yogis, suffering is an inherent part of the human condition that is ultimately addressed on the path of ritualistic self-transcendent practices, while for others, yoga offers a path for living a healthier and more joyful life in the present moment regardless of one's conditions or circumstances. Here we take more of the latter path, exploring how best to heal and have greater joy in the here and now.

Throughout the ages and up to the present, we can see tremendous progress in understanding human health, with many advances leading to letting go of what in earlier times was considered most efficacious or beneficial. Many ancient yogis and their healing arts peers, especially the pioneers of ayurveda, did their best in using speculation (or, as many assert, divine transmission) and experimentation to understand the nature of human nature and how best to live in the healthiest ways. Although we can find some healthy yoga practices in the ancient mists of early Indian civilization, our deepening understanding of the human organism in the modern world is generating more refined and effective tools for healing, even as some modern developments are the cause of great disease. In the light of our greater knowledge we can recognize some earlier practices as beneficial even as others are ineffective or even harmful, this while considering innovative methods and techniques that are developing to the present day.

As an evolving practice for self-cultivation and self-awakening, yoga invites us to go beyond the practices given by the ancients. It is thus, in the spirit of yoga as a living and evolving tradition, that this book attempts to offer insights drawn from ancient-to-modern yoga, ayurveda, and what is often called modern scientific medicine in addressing practices for healing what ails us on and off the yoga mat.

According to the most recent cross-national survey of yoga students in the United States,[1] doing yoga on a regular basis makes people feel better—calmer amid stressful conditions, more positive in outlook, and more self-accepting. With these benefits, yoga typically leads to taking better care of oneself, with better diet, sleep, and balanced exercise. With self-improvement we also find social benefits, with clearer communication, deeper appreciation of human diversity, and better care for others and the planet.

Every physiological system is affected in doing yoga. There is a growing body of evidence that yoga practices can have specific effects on these systems, including in healing a variety of increasingly common health conditions and offering potential cures for some maladies that remain largely mysterious to modern medical science. There are also many mysteries in how yoga works in the human organism, especially as there is a vast array of different practices called yoga and an even greater diversity of conditions and intentions of those who do these practices.[2] As we move further into the twenty-first century, we have a growing body of research revealing how various yoga practices are sources of harm, health, or sometimes both.[3]

We can also find insights into health and healing in the annals of modern medical science, even as many mainstream medical practices are anathema to some adherents of yoga and alternative medicine and sometimes cause harm. Here we will open to insights into healing regardless of their source—Eastern, Western, allopathic, ayurveda, integrative, or complementary—thereby allowing us to tap into yoga, ayurveda, and scientific medicine for all they offer in healing our ailments.

Being Healthy Human Beings

Yoga is now part of the zeitgeist of most Western societies just as these societies are undergoing tremendous challenges to advances in health, well-being, and life expectancy. Amid fast-paced lives and increasing socioeconomic pressure, stress is a leading cause of illness and a leading motivator for doing yoga. We also live in a global environment beset by rapid climate change, resistant infectious organisms, and social dislocation and alienation that reflect and are exacerbated by the very globalizations in which most of us actively participate. Yet human beings are naturally healthy. According to the World Health Organization (WHO), being healthy is "a state of complete physical, mental, and social well-being and not merely the absence of disease or infirmity."[4] The alternative definition given by Andrew Weil, MD, as "a dynamic and harmonious equilibrium of all of the elements and forces making up and surrounding a human being," gives similar emphasis to wholeness, which is the basic idea at the etymological root of the term *health*.[5]

Our natural tendency is to live with all the strength and vitality with which we are endowed by our nature. We promote and maintain our health by taking care of ourselves and one another with food, exercise, sleep, love, ritual, and optimism. We go further in cultivating healthy lives by ensuring access to adequate housing, education, and health care services; sharing in social relationships and spaces that are safe and supportive of living life to our fullest potential; striving for a healthy planet that can sustain healthy lives; and opening ourselves to the greater powers manifest in the universe in ways that give deeper meaning to our lives.

Still, our health can be challenged by our genetics, lifestyle, and environment. The traits we inherit from our parents play a significant role in our lives, predisposing us to certain diseases, conditions, and behavioral habits, all akin to what the ancient yogis called *samskaras*. The physical and social conditions of our natural and built environment can introduce toxicity that we experience as disease. Our way of life—including our values, beliefs, relationships, hygiene, physical activities, and diet—can lead to stress, anxiety, depression, and greater susceptibility to injury or disease. Taken together, these factors affect our homeostasis, the balanced regulation and stabilization of our whole being.

We can take a snapshot of global health conditions with these annual data from the WHO 2016 World Health Statitics:[6]

- 1.1 billion people smoke tobacco.
- 156 million children under five years old are stunted, and 42 million children under five are overweight.
- 1.8 billion people drink contaminated water, and 946 million people defecate in the open.
- 303,000 women die due to complications of pregnancy and childbirth.
- 5.9 million children die before their fifth birthday.
- 2 million people are newly infected with HIV, and there are 9.6 million new TB cases and 214 million (range 148–304 million) malaria cases.
- 1.7 billion people need treatment for neglected tropical diseases.
- More than 10 million people die before the age of 70 due to cardiovascular diseases and cancer.
- 800,000 people commit suicide.
- 1.25 million people die from road traffic injuries.
- 4.3 million people die due to air pollution caused by cooking fuels.
- 3 million people die due to outdoor pollution.
- 475,000 people are murdered, 80% of them men.

The conditions of health and well-being in the world today give definite cause for pause in considering how we live our lives and share in it all with one another as citizens of the planet. The data on world health make clear the patterned relationships between levels of economic development, access to health care, and qualities of health and life. Although life expectancy worldwide increased by five years from 2000 to 2015, there is a vast discrepancy in life expectancy related to economic conditions.

Table I.1: Life Expectancy, Top and Bottom Five Countries, 2015

TOP FIVE	BOTTOM FIVE
Japan 83.7	Cote d'Ivoire 53.3
Switzerland 83.4	Chad 53.1
Singapore 83.1	Central African Republic 52.5
Australia 82.8	Angola 52.4
Iceland 82.7	Sierra Leone 50.1

With the quality of life in the balance, we have a range of defenses to ward off attacks on the bodymind originating from inside or outside and to thereby optimize our health.[7] When attacked from the outside by living microbes, toxins, or chemicals, the skin, mucous membranes, cilia, and saliva provide crucial physical barriers and filters. When harmful pathogens get inside, our finely tuned immune system brilliantly distinguishes friend and foe, generating more than 100 million types of antibodies that can quite effectively ensure our survival. Add our natural tendency to cough and sneeze for immediate rejection of irritants, to produce interferon to ward off tumors, and to become inflamed to kill bacteria or heal traumatized tissues, and we are pretty well protected.

The bodymind knows all of this in its inner workings, even if we tend to forget it in our mental wondering, wandering, and worrying. In forgetting—in losing conscious awareness of ourselves as beings that are naturally healthy—we tend to diminish our defense mechanisms. When experiencing an infection or injury, we tend to say to ourselves, "I'm sick" or "I'm hurt," defining ourselves in self-deflating reductionist terms, rather than saying, "I'm a healthy person living with or healing from this condition that makes me feel unhealthy." In habitually thinking we are unhealthy, we tend to become so, compromising our natural healing resonance as we degenerate into irrational neuroses and unhealthy activities.

Such neuroses can become more palpable when we consider our mortality. Realizing that our health in this bodymind is temporary, we tend toward fear, denial, and adherence to comforting beliefs that may or may not have any basis in reality. Every culture offers up at least one belief system, most commonly a religion that explains everything from birth to death (and in many religions rebirth, transcendence, or even transmutation). If we agree to follow certain prescriptions—believe this, not that; do this, not that—we are guaranteed ultimate liberation from suffering and possibly even everlasting life in what often amounts to something of a Faustian bargain.

These matters are experienced in every culture and civilization across human history, all of which have used what means they have to try to make life better. This meliorative project of humanity finds expression in ritual, prayer, meditation, and scientific experimentation and application. As a result, there is now a vast accumulation of techniques thought or proven to promote and maintain health. One of these is yoga, the primary source of insight into healing offered in this book, while in ayurveda and scientific medicine we can find some wonderfully complementary practices.

The Promise of Yoga in Healing

Yoga makes life better. We know this from direct experience. It is why most people do yoga. At the most superficial level, it makes our bodies healthier—stronger, more flexible, and more supple, with all of our systems better integrated and functioning. It helps us keep our energy more in balance and more sustainable. It can help settle the mind and the emotions, opening us to clearer self-awareness and better interaction with others. For many it is also a spiritual practice, opening us to a greater sense of the world within and far beyond us, bringing deeper meaning into our everyday lives.

In each of these ways and more, yoga offers the promise of personal growth and transformation to everybody in the world, regardless of one's age or condition. Yet for the benefits of yoga to best manifest in anyone's life, it is important for each of us to find the yoga path that is right for us. By this we mean that the yoga one does should make sense in relation to one's existing conditions and intentions, with our conditions informing our intentions.

The vast diversity of conditions and intentions we see across the landscape of humanity calls upon yoga teachers to suggest and guide yoga practices along yoga paths that make sense for unique individuals based upon the existing realities of their lives. Although many yoga styles, brands, and gurus promote their approach as the right one for everybody, the reality is that we are organic human beings whose individual uniqueness suggests doing somewhat or entirely different yoga practices—or doing similar practices in different ways.[8] Aspects of our uniqueness will point to the practices that are appropriate for us and to others that are not. A healthy athlete, a young child, a pregnant woman, an elderly person with advanced osteoporosis, a war veteran with posttraumatic stress disorder (PTSD), and someone undergoing chemo-therapy will most likely benefit from different practices. Yet most yoga instruction today is in a class setting in which every student is given mostly the same guidance, including suggestions for modification, use of props, and exploration of variations. In some styles the asanas, sequences, pace, and overall guidance is the same for every-body, with prescripted sequences and narrative overlays, which perhaps makes sense only if everyone in the class has the same condition and the class is designed and taught in a way that is appropriate for that condition—which is unlikely.

Yoga in general is a healing practice when done sensibly, meaning in keeping with one's actual conditions. With yoga as a healing practice, we look to more fully adapt yoga practices to support healing and wholeness in unique individuals, whether individual students in classes or one's private clients, and to address problems with health in a far more specific way than we do in general yoga practices. This approach, sometimes called "yoga therapy" (rooted in the ancient concept of *yoga chikitsa*, which is also the title given to the extremely vigorous and often injurious primary series of Ashtanga Vinyasa Yoga), is defined by the IAYT as "the process of empowering individuals to progress toward improved health and well-being through the application of the teachings and practices of yoga."[9] Its many applications are helpful in many situations, including guiding students who are injured, pregnant, ill (physically or mentally, which are always intertwined), or experiencing any of a myriad of debilitating or otherwise challenging conditions.

The adaptive nature of yoga as a healing modality thus invites us to make the existing conditions of a student's life the starting point in offering him or her a guided yoga practice. Given that most yoga is taught in classes and that yoga teachers often encounter students with injuries and other special conditions, it is important that yoga teachers have the knowledge and skills with which to guide students with appropriate adaptations and similarly important for students to develop this knowledge base in using yoga for self-healing. To do this well, teachers and students must tap into the deepest wells of learning and experience, exploring the asanas, pranayamas, meditations, and other practices that allow us to heal, feel better, and live the best lives possible. This book offers resources for doing this—for learning more about how the bodymind functions, dysfunctions, and can be healed in doing adaptive yoga.

THE SEVEN GOALS OF YOGA THERAPY

1. Eliminate, reduce, or manage symptoms that cause suffering.

2. Improve function.

3. Help to prevent the occurrence or reoccurrence of underlying causes of illness.

4. Move toward improved health and well-being.

5. Change our relationship to and identification with unhealthy conditions.

6. Empower people to be their own best teacher and healer.

7. Teach, share, and guide yoga in ways that support and inspire others to be as awake, vibrant, and filled with awe in every moment of life.

Adapted from The International Association of Yoga Therapists (IAYT)

Part I

The Origins and Sources of Yoga Therapy

THE YOGIC FRAMEWORK FOR HEALTH is typically rooted in philosophical notions of spiritual being in which the condition of any human being is seen as a manifestation of larger forces in the universe. Just what these forces are and how they manifest is given widely varied descriptions across the landscape of the yoga literature and practices, with literally thousands of philosophical, psychological, and spiritual concepts and terms. We often find numerous terms for essentially the same thing; the differences often amounting more to variation in mood or emphasis than substantive variance or disagreement. We also find vast differences in fundamental ideas, including with respect to yoga itself and the very concept of life. Part of the challenge in clearly discussing therapeutic yoga practices arises from the differences in underlying philosophy and even the language of discourse. What we attempt here is a synthesis and summary of the most salient and significant concepts that allow us to articulate a coherent and practical yogic view of human life, health, and healing.

In a contemporary yoga scene in which new brands and styles are launched nearly every day, it might seem as if yoga therapy is another such recent innovation. Add recent definitive scholarship showing modern postural yoga practices most fully developing only in the past century—this in contrast to many yoga styles that claim pure uninterrupted lineage to ostensibly ancient forms and methods—and we find ourselves questioning the historical and philosophical foundations of yoga.[1] Although we can now confidently say that the last one hundred years is perhaps the greatest watershed in the development of yoga practices and techniques, including in yoga therapy, there is a deep well of healing wisdom found in ancient, classical, and modern sources from which contemporary yoga draws in various ways.

When anyone in the contemporary yoga culture begins discussing topics of history and philosophy, it is very easy for myth and mystery to blend with fact and rationality. These ends of one philosophical continuum continue to manifest today when considering any aspect of yoga. As with yoga generally, some claim there is an original source of all yoga and that yoga has come to us in the present without interruption, even if diluted by those who would change certain of its elements. Others claim there is an original source, that yoga has evolved from this source over the millennia through various innovations, and that the true essence of the original yoga remains at the heart of certain practices (usually one's own style or brand). In a yoga culture in which truth is put forth as a central moral value, the persistence of such claims despite overwhelming evidence to the contrary is ironic, if not concerning.

These tensions are evident in the realm of yoga therapy and can easily cloud and confuse its history—as with all of yoga, we should more accurately say "histories"—as well as any principles and techniques put forth. Meanwhile, the histories of healing with yoga are often inextricably intertwined with those of ayurveda and scientific medicine. Here we will attempt to reveal these relationships by surveying yoga, ayurveda, and scientific medicine from their earliest expressions in the ancient world to today before distilling and exploring the received wisdom, concepts, and practices that might best inform yoga therapy in the twenty-first century.

1

Yoga Sources

Yoga is an art and science of living.
—INDRA DEVI

What Is Yoga?

We start with a simple question, the answers to which are potentially vast: What is yoga? In exploring it, we will move gradually to the other question implied by the title of this book: What is healing? This way of beginning is for the sake of clarity, which is at the heart of yoga: a basic aim in doing yoga is to relieve suffering through clearer awareness and healthy actions, an intention we find in the ancient-to-modern yoga literature as well as in what can naturally come to us doing asana, pranayama, and meditation practices today.[1]

Some also maintain that in writing about any topic, it is important to be clear in our use of words. Dictionaries give definitions that allow us to share words with one another in ways that are mutually understandable. Even though different dictionaries give slightly different definitions of some of the same words, they are generally in agreement. Imagine the confusion if there were fifty different definitions of the term *vocabulary*, which fortunately there are not: it generally means "the words that make up a language."[2]

Yet with yoga the definitions are anything but clear or consistent, which creates problems in attempting to clearly present the essential tenets of yoga as a healing practice. Yoga is many different things to different people. From all we can gather in excavating ancient-to-modern sources, it has always been this way, and by all appearances it is becoming more and more diverse. As we shall see, there is beauty in this diversity and ambiguity, even as it makes some discussions such as we are in here more complicated. Indeed, here we begin with many areas of confusion and attempt to move steadily toward greater understanding, mirroring what for many is the path of yoga practice itself.

A "philosophy of yoga" is a relatively coherent, systematic, and comprehensive approach to practices referred to as yoga. Just as there appears always to have been many different yoga practices, so too there appears always to have been many different philosophies of yoga. Thus, the phrase "traditional yogic philosophy" is sensibly pluralized. Contrary to some common misunderstandings, we even find confusion with the term "traditional," which for some connotes a relatively certain time period while for others it pertains to a particular tradition of yoga (and in some cases both). In the former, we find references to the "pre-Vedic period," or the "period of Classical Yoga," and so on, while in the latter we find "Vedanta," "Tantric," "Hatha," and a seemingly infinite array of others.[3]

When we attempt to discover the meaning of yoga as it developed over the millennia, we first come to concepts that have little to do with what one might recognize as yoga today.[4] What we find is the Sanskrit term *yuj*. The earliest use of this term is in the *Rigveda*, probably from around 1500 BCE, where the meaning is "to yoke or join or fasten or harness horses or a chariot," as well as the chariot itself. In the *Ramayana* (around 200 BCE to 200 CE), the term is used variously to mean to make ready, to prepare, arrange, fit out, apply, or to equip an army. There are vastly different meanings found in the *Mahabharata*, the earliest verses of which (there are over 200,000 lines, from around 300 BCE to 300 CE) date from the Vedic period: to put arrows on a bow string, to be united in marriage, to set snares, to embrace, and to wish to appoint or institute, among many, many others.[5]

A common thread in many of these and other early writings on yoga is the chariot as a vehicle for transporting oneself to heaven. In the great Mahabharata War, a great injustice has occurred in the kingdom as the rightful leaders have been usurped and have escaped to the jungle. It falls to Prince Arjuna to lead in restoring justice and harmony. He rides a chariot into battle at Kurukshetra, with his charioteer, Krishna, conversing with him about *maya* (illusion), correct perception, and *dharma* (one's purposeful, even dutiful path in life). The practical and deeply spiritual point is about not confusing the *maya* of immediate experience with the truth of divine being, living, and even transcendence. Just as the gods above ride chariots, symbolizing being in or being transported to God consciousness, so too the yogi rides the chariot of practices to overcome illusion and thereby attain salvation from suffering in this world. Krishna also points out that there is not just a single yoga path, but at least three, giving us the first yoga styles: *bhakti* yoga (the yoga of devotion), *jnana* yoga (the yoga of knowledge), and *karma* yoga (the yoga of service).[6]

The widely varied Vedic uses of the term *yuj* gradually give way to concepts more familiar to today's yoga culture, starting with the third century BCE *Kathaka Upanishad*, which gives us some of the key elements that will appear in much of the further development of yoga and yoga therapy practices across the next several hundred years: a yogic physiology, identification of the individual self or soul with the universal self (*brahman*), and a dualistic mind-body system that reflects Samkhya philosophy (one of the six main branches of Indian philosophy).[7] All involve rising to higher states of consciousness, many come to prescribe mantra as an essential practice (especially chanting *Aum*, the sound of brahman), and most are increasingly systematized with specific *kriyas* (actions) said to bring one to *moksha* (liberation from illusion and thereby from suffering).

Asana is rarely mentioned in these early years of yoga, appearing in only two of the 195 aphorisms that comprise the early fourth century common era *Yoga Sutra of Patanjali* and not at all in the *Bhagavad Gita,* the two most oft-cited books on yoga in the modern era. What we find instead is yoga as a means of salvation one attains by reorienting one's cognitive faculties to accurately perceive reality, primarily through self-disciplined meditation, sometimes accompanied by *pranayamas* (specific breathing techniques). In the *Yoga Sutra*, we are offered what in the late nineteenth century Swami Vivekananda would coin as *raja* yoga ("royal" or "king" yoga), a synthesis of certain strands of yoga extant at the time (to which Vivekananda liberally and creatively added from various sources, especially elements taken from Theosophy).[8]

The purpose of yoga is given in the second aphorism as *chitta vritti nirodha*, which we can translate as "to still the fluctuations of the mind." From this starting point, Patanjali presents an intricate yogic psychology—including *samskaras* (inherited mental tendencies and habits), *kleshas* (mental afflictions), and *avidya* (ignorance, the overarching klesha)—along with disciplined contemplative methods one can undertake to reduce or overcome these conditions. That is all in Chapter 1, where he presents his methodical path. In Chapter 2 he gives an alternative to this difficult approach: the persevering yet nonattached practice of *ashtanga* yoga (eight-limbed yoga), to which we will return later. Going further, one can gain supernatural powers, gain omniscience (Chapter 3), and even attain such high and expanded consciousness as to transcend the mortal realm altogether (Chapter 4).[9]

Although many other ideas about yoga would persist to the present, within a few hundred years after Patanjali's *Yoga Sutra,* we find broad recognition of yoga being primarily about salvation through correct perception and clear mental functioning, with meditation and mantra as the primary forms of practice. As White puts it, "Gnosis—transcendent, immediate, nonconventional knowledge of ultimate reality, of the reality behind appearances—is the key to salvation in these soteriologies, as well as in India's major philosophical schools, many of which developed in the centuries around the beginning of the Common Era."[10] It is also about expanded pranayama, increasingly seen as an indispensable part of the practice. Later, we see this elaborated in tantric writings, with the cultivation of *prana,* an essential element of the subtle energetic physiology that brings one into a sense of being part of the whole of the universe and attaining immortality. Some take it much further, to omniscience and supernatural powers.

We noted earlier that there are many different claims made about the history of yoga as well, even fully developed myths that persist despite overwhelming evidence that they are fictional. A common tendency is to assert that one's modern-day yoga practice style is somehow the most pure, true, or original of all yoga practices, with some claiming that other approaches deviate from the true path of yoga. We find what for some in the yoga culture is perhaps a comforting yet no less mythical romantic notion that there is one yoga, meaning that all the various practices are in their essence part of an original act, impulse, or thought. Some claim that this one yoga is today as it has always been, and that anything that deviates from this original, supposedly true yoga is not yoga.[11] On yoga itself, innumerable writers and teachers make the common mythical assertion of the practice going back over 5,000 years, and further, that it is one of the few spiritual traditions that has maintained an unbroken development throughout history, assertions that are undermined by a considerable body of scholarship that reveals historical discontinuities as well as innovations from the earliest times to the present day. The quaint and false idea of one yoga has been repeated *mutatis mutandu, ad infinitum* for many years, becoming perhaps the greatest urban yoga myth that is typically accepted as conventional wisdom (or put differently, a classic case of ideological hegemony in yoga).[12] Nonetheless, it is myth.

Others claim that there is an original yoga but that it has developed (rather than remaining the same) over the millennia and continues to develop today,[13] often along with the bold yet unfounded assertion that their approach is somehow uniquely rooted in or evolved from an original and ancient source, as we find in claims about Ashtanga Vinyasa, Bikram, Sivananda, and numerous other styles.[14] We find this assertion in much of the Krishnamacharya lineage, starting with Krishnamacharya himself asserting that the methods of yoga he taught came directly to him through divine transmission from the ninth century CE sage Nathamuni and were adapted to meet modern needs.[15]

This complex web of assertions, claims, and critiques can make the head swirl. To gain clarity, we will back up and ask a deceptively simple question: What is yoga?

As a preview, answering this question points to the vastness of yoga, the diversity of approaches, the uniqueness of many techniques, and the benefits of some elements of each approach for many students' health conditions and practice intentions. With respect to yoga therapy, this vastness is a beautiful thing as it suggests that there is a similarly vast array of possibilities for how you might best work with unique students in your classes and clients in treatment sessions in support of their healing.

A Very Brief History of Yoga

Yoga comes from a wide and deep river of ancient traditions.[16] Its many currents flow from a complex history of spiritual exploration, philosophical reflection, scientific experimentation, and spontaneous creative expression. Arising primarily from the diverse and evolving cultures of India, often moored to and conditioned by Hinduism, Buddhism, Jainism, and other religions, the philosophies, teachings, and practices of yoga are as richly varied as the innumerable tributaries of the vastness of yoga in all its manifestations. What we know of the origins and development of yoga comes to us from a variety of sources, including ancient texts, oral transmission through certain yogic or spiritual lineages, iconography, dances, and songs.

Although the history of yoga may be a few thousand years old, as noted earlier, the earliest known writings on yoga are found in ancient Hindu spiritual texts known as the Vedas, the oldest being the *Rigveda*.[17] Though scholars debate the exact date and origins of the Vedas (1700–1100 BCE), most agree that the 1,028 hymns that make up the *Rigveda*, considered by many to be of divine origin, are the original written source on yoga.[18] Composed as poems by spiritual leaders (seers) in a culture where most spiritual practices connected directly and immediately with nature in the quest for meaning and well-being, these hymns reflect the mystical exploration of consciousness, being, and connection with the divine. It is here that yoga is first mentioned in writing and given one of its many meanings, "to yolk." The principle spiritual yoking is that of one's mind and the divine, a self-transcendent quality creating a pure state of consciousness in which the awareness of "I" disappears into a sense of divine essence, and with it one is liberated from the existential suffering of human life.

At the later end of the Vedic period, another set of ancient writings on yoga appeared in India. Considered by some to be part of the Vedas, thirteen original Upanishads were written in the first millennium BCE as part of a spiritual movement in which reliance on elaborate and secretive rituals gave way to more purely internal practices in which an individual takes action, this in contrast to participating in rituals in which priests were the principle actors. Here we first find thorough explanations of yoga practice, although they are still focused on meditation. Considered the essence and final word of the Vedas, they became known as the philosophy of *Vedanta* ("the end of the Vedas").[19]

As an expression of Hindu religious philosophy, these classical Upanishads hold forth the belief in a universal spirit, brahman, and an individual soul, atman. Brahman is the absolute infinite, all that ever was and all that will ever be. Atman, or the inner self, is the self we experience in our limited awareness, in which we are said to experience ourselves as alienated from the true self: the absolute, or brahman. The ritualistic and contemplative practices described in the Upanishads aim to unite—yoke—atman and brahman by attaining release from the worldly constraints and limited consciousness that keep us from realizing the true state of oneness. As Georg Feuerstein notes, "The transcendental ground of the world is identical with the ultimate core of the human being. That supreme Reality, which is pure, formless Consciousness, cannot be adequately described or defined. It must simply be realized."[20] The pathway to this self-realization includes inner reflection on the mind that brings one to a place of pure wisdom.

The Upanishads are also the earliest written source describing what is referred to today as the traditional yogic anatomy of the subtle body.[21] The concept of the three-part body (causal, subtle, and physical) and *koshas* (or "five sheaths") is found in the oldest Upanishads, including the *Taittiriya Upanishad* (2.1–9) and throughout the *Kathaka Upanishad*, and is also an integral concept in ayurveda. *Prana*, or "life force," is found in several Upanishads. A passage in the *Kaushitaki Upanishad* (3.2) gives one of the most familiar descriptions of prana today: "Life is prana, prana is life. So long as prana remains in the body, so long is there life. Through prana, one obtains, even in this world, immortality."

In the later Upanishads, written through the fifteenth century, we begin to see evidence of experimentation in various yogic practices utilizing breath and sound as tools of healing and physical transformation. Much of this exploration was associated with the rise of tantra and created the groundwork for the future development of Hatha yoga. This culminates in the fifteenth century *Darshana Upanishad*'s description of specific asanas, all but one of which are sitting positions in which the essential practice is pranayama.[22]

Thought to be part of the early Upanishadic movement, the *Bhagavad Gita*, or Song of God, explores the mystery of the mind, providing a set of guiding principles for a life of conscious action.[23] Though it may be based on a historical event, the symbolism of the *Bhagavad-Gita* is a guide to spiritual liberation. The flame of desire and manifestations of ego create inner conflicts that keep us in a state of confusion and suffering. The practices described in the *Bhagavad Gita* offer different pathways to self-realization and liberation through connection with the divine: the three yogic paths corresponding to the dharmas associated with the varied natures of people—*karma yoga*, the yoga of service; *jnana yoga*, the yoga of knowledge; and *bhakti yoga*, the yoga of devotion.

Most people who study yoga philosophy have read excerpts from Patanjali's *Yoga Sutra*. Composed around 325 CE, this is the systematic and succinct presentation of what Vivekananda would later come to call *raja yoga*,[24] or "royal" yoga, and contains one of the earliest references to a practice involving asana and pranayama as part of the yogic path. Patanjali begins with a simple question: "What is yoga?" His answer makes clear that the practice described here is centered around mental experience: "*chitta vritti nirodha*," he writes, meaning, "to calm the fluctuations of the mind" or "to steady the mind."[25]

Considered by many to be the basic philosophical text on yoga, the *Yoga Sutra* explains how to cultivate one's path to *samadhi*, a blissful state where the practitioner is absorbed into oneness with the divine by releasing the ego. With the constant ego-centered activity of the mind always at work, our prejudices, desires, and passions bring us into the abyss of confusion, pain, and suffering. Yoga offers liberation from this suffering. Patanjali gives nuanced guidance on practices for stilling the mind and eradicating the mental afflictions that cause suffering in the world, including the eight-limbed path, or ashtanga yoga: yama, niyama, asana, pranayama, pratyahara, dharana, dhyana, and samadhi. We will look at how to apply these principles of yoga philosophy and practice as tools for healing in Chapter 4.

Although the historical origins and philosophical foundations of Hatha yoga mark a departure from many of the tenets of Patanjali's meditative yoga, many of today's yoga styles or lineages still pay considerable or primary homage to the *Yoga Sutra*. This is particularly strong in the Krishnamacharya lineage.

The paths from the Vedas, Upanishads, and *Yoga Sutra* to the modern and well-known contemporary practices of Hatha yoga are typically described as a series of straight evolutionary lines. This is not correct. Rather, Hatha yoga arises from the formative influence of tantra, a fact shrouded in veils of illusion cast by many Hatha adherents who passionately reject tantra as being antithetical to their spiritual and social worldview. The tantra movement in India, arising from the influence of Mahayana Buddhism in the opening centuries of the first millennium, was in part a reaction against the dualistic and renunciative practices taught in the Vedas and Upanishads and further codified in the *Yoga Sutra*. The essential idea of tantra—that everything in the universe is an expression of the divine and thus can be tapped as a source of divine consciousness and being—is a marked departure from traditional Vedic and Upanishadic teachings that would put the devoted yogi in an isolated cave and insist that normal human experiences such as desire or sexuality prevent or at least limit true happiness or enlightened being. In some of the Upanishads—particularly the nondual *Svetasvatara Upanishad*—we can find an opening to the idea of fully living here and now in a state of self-realization and liberation—*jivan mukti*—but it is still largely situated within a dualistic perspective that separates the individual and his or her experiences from the whole of the natural order and spiritual being.[26]

From the root word *tan*, meaning "expansive" or "whole," tantra recognizes the entire fabric of existence as an expression of the divine feminine, or Shakti energy. The idea is to open up to a sense of the divine within any experience. The philosophy of tantra identifies the path of freedom not through renunciation of human desire and experience, but indeed largely through it:

> *Tantra is that Asian body of beliefs and practices which, working from the principle that the universe we experience is nothing other than the concrete manifestation of the divine energy of the God-head that creates and maintains that universe, seeks to ritually appropriate and channel that energy, within the human microcosm, in creative and emancipatory ways.*[27]

Tantra offers an integrative approach to yoga in which we tap into every aspect of internal and external experience as a source of conscious awakening to divine energy, the omnipotent, omniscient, and omnipresent primordial creative force of the universe. This has a profound impact on how we think about the body and yoga practice. Since everything is a manifestation of the divine, yet different in its energetic expression, there are infinite possibilities for being in or having a sense of the divine, even amid what might seem entirely mundane activity. Tantric practitioners will go to what may seem the extremes of human experience, seeking energetic intensity to experience the purest awareness of being fully awake in one's divine being.

There are myriad so-called traditional forms of tantric practice, sometimes referred to as initiations and usually said to require the intimate guidance of a guru. Three common practices are:

Mantra: This practice takes the practitioner into the divine vibrating energy of sound through repeated chanting of hymns or words, many found in the Vedas (such as the Gayatri Mantra), in concert, with a rich set of rituals involving meditation, sacred space purification, and imagination of a protective wall of fire.

Yantra: As the intimacy between practitioner and mantric energy grows, the practice extends into meditation on a yantra, a visible vibratory expression of the divine feminine represented in geometrical form. As a map of the mantric world, this embodies the forces of Shakti energy—intensity, radiance, delight, pleasure, desire, yantra speed, illumination, being, and *vighna vinashini*, the power that destroys resistance. Yantra practice involves an array of rituals, visualization, meditation, chanting, and offerings.

Puja: In contrast to the "right-hand" tantric path of mantra and yantra, the "left-hand" path moves from esoteric internal practices to fully living in the world, embracing with intense concentration the most powerful expression of Shakti energy in the strongest sensual experiences. In puja practice, one is cultivating self-mastery, the union of sensuous pleasure and divine ecstasy, in the most intense of acts, aiming to "bring spirituality into day-to-day existence, and vice versa."[28]

At the heart of tantra is the idea, born of experience rather than grand philosophical speculation, that there is continuity between what seems the ordinary realm of human life and the infinite. Instead of transcending the material reality of human experience, going more intensely into it is the path to enlightenment and happiness. Arising from ordinary people among the lower castes of India's highly stratified society, this approach opened up the fullness of spiritual practice to anyone.[29] As Georg Feuerstein emphasizes, these people "were responding to a widely felt need for a more practical orientation that would integrate the lofty metaphysical ideals of nondualism with down-to-earth procedures for living a sanctified life without necessarily abandoning one's belief in the local deities and the age-old rituals for worshipping them."[30]

As tantra grew in influence, its essence was distorted by the reactions to some of its rituals, particularly those involving sex. Speaking of tantra in the West usually evokes notions of "sacred sex," thus rendering tantra as little more than "spiritual sexuality." Although sexual relationship is part of tantra, the spiritual philosophy and practices of tantra are deeper and more subtle. This is perhaps most richly expressed in the form of tantra that took root in Kashmir in the ninth century, known as Kashmir Shaivism, poetically expressed in the *Spanda Karika*.[31] The main idea of the *Spanda Karika* is to take all of existence as one and not divide it into pure or impure. This is the central idea of tantra, the kernels of which were found in the most ancient Vedas and Upanishads, but largely lost or discarded in the *Bhagavad-Gita* and in yoga as described by Patanjali.

The idea of yoga in the tantric perspective is to be without separation, to reconcile the body, breath, mind, and emotion as one, without distinction, without anything considered impure or profane. Most of the tantric texts state that Shiva and Shakti, or divine masculine and feminine energy, are one—one in the body, one in the mind, one in the heart of emotional being. In this expression of being we are embracing the fullness of all of our energy, to be this one thing, not to be in distinction, not to be anything but the space where everything is alive. As we go into this practice, we find liberation from the ego, from dualistic thinking, experiencing and viscerally comprehending that we are this beautiful space, this amazing wholeness.[32]

Hatha Yoga

The first substantial writing on Hatha yoga, the well-known *Hatha Yoga Pradipika*, was written in the fifteenth century by the Indian sage Swami Swatmarama. A vast text, the *Pradipika* looks in detail at asana, shatkarma, pranayama, mudra, bandha, and samadhi, giving very specific guidance on each of these interrelated practices. (We will look at these elements in a moment.) The *Shiva Samhita*, written sometime between the fifteenth and seventeenth centuries, shows more clearly than the *Pradipika* the influence of Buddhism and tantra in the development of Hatha yoga. Although only four asanas are described in detail, the *Shiva Samhita* provides an elaborate explanation of *nadis* (the energy channels through which prana flows), the nature of prana or "life force," and the many obstacles faced in practice and how to overcome them through a variety of techniques. These techniques include dristana (conscious gazing), silent mantra, and tantric practices for awakening and moving kundalini energy. The *Gheranda Samhita*, written in the late seventeenth century, reflects the diminishing influence of tantra, particularly anything involving sexual interaction. Seven chapters describe the seven means to perfecting oneself on the yogic path: shatkarmas for purification, asanas for strength, mudras for steadiness, pratyahara for calmness, pranayama for lightness, dhyana for realization, and samadhi for bliss.

According to the original texts, there are three purposes of Hatha yoga: (1) the total purification of the body, (2) the complete balancing of the physical, mental, and energetic fields, and (3) the awakening of purer consciousness through which one ultimately connects with the divine by engaging in practices rooted in the physical body. Hatha yoga uses all of who we are—physically, mentally, emotionally, our most subtle and elusive inner nature—as the raw material for learning, seeing, and integrating our entire being, opening us to our fullest imagination, intelligence, enthusiasm, energy, and awareness of spiritual life. Hatha yoga offers a way to experience this integration along a path involving very specific practices that purify the body, calm the mind, and open the heart.

Shatkarma—Purification Practices

Shatkarma, from *shat*, meaning "six," and *karma*, meaning "action," are set forth as essential Hatha yoga practices. They are designed to purify the body in a way that allows the greater benefit of asana, pranayama, and other Hatha practices. As with many other seemingly esoteric yoga practices, the ancient texts describe these as secret techniques to be learned only from an experienced and qualified teacher. Each of the six cleansing techniques—*dhauti* (internal cleansing), *basti* (yogic enema), *neti* (nasal cleansing), *trataka* (concentrated gazing), *nauli* (abdominal massage), *kapalabhati* (brain cleansing)—has a variety of practices, described most fully in the *Gheranda Samhita* and the *Hatha Yoga Pradipika*.[33]

Asana—Taking One Seat and Then Some

At the beginning of most yoga classes, there is often a moment of sitting, getting an initial sense of calm, and typically a greeting of *namaste* followed by a brief bow. We find the roots of this ritual in the *Pradipika*, with Swami Swatmarama offering just such salutations and prostrations to his guru, Adinath. It is an act of humility, symbolizing the release of the ego and the opening to something far greater, to a higher force. The *Pradipika* then departs from raja yoga by prescribing a practice that begins with shatkarmas and asanas, with asana now involving a variety of specific bodily positions that help to open the nadis (energy channels) and chakras (psychic centers) of the subtle body. The ultimate aim is the same as in raja yoga: to come into a state of samadhi. So why start with asanas?

The Hatha yogis discovered that through the practice of asanas, one attains a delicate balance of body, mind, and spirit. Following the shatkarma purification practices, asanas further cleanse the body by creating the inner fire to burn out impurities. They stimulate increased circulation, revitalize all the organs of the body, tone the muscles and ligaments, stabilize the joints, create ease in the nerves, and promote the improved functioning of all the body's systems. In the *Pradipika*'s first verse on asana, it is said, "having done asana one gets steadiness of body and mind, diseaselessness and lightness of the limbs."[34] By deeply purifying the body and cultivating steadiness, prana moves more freely, nourishing, healing, and integrating the body and mind. As in the *Yoga Sutra*, the *Pradipika* instructs opening and steadying the body through asana practice before commencing with pranayama. This is echoed by B. K. S. Iyengar, who says, "If a novice attends to the perfection of the postures, he cannot concentrate on breathing. He loses balance and the depth of the asanas. Attain steadiness and stillness in asanas before introducing rhythmic breathing techniques."[35]

In verse 33 of the *Pradipika*, Swatmarama tells us "eighty-four asanas were taught by Lord Shiva." Only fifteen asanas are described in the *Pradipika*. The *Gheranda Samhita* tells us that Shiva taught 8,400,000 asanas, "as many asanas as there are species of living beings." The point is that asana is infinite, underlining a practice that is about process rather than the attainment of some preconceived perfect form. The *Gheranda Samhita* describes seventeen asanas, in addition to the fifteen found in the *Pradipika*. Several of these are very slight variations on one another (such as a change in hand position or gaze). Even though asanas have the same names as some found in the *Pradipika*, several have slight variations in the *Gheranda Samhita*. Throughout the continued development of Hatha yoga, the specific description and form of the asanas would change, with the same name often being given to very different physical positions.

Neither of these writings offers detailed instruction on asana techniques. Four asanas are mentioned in the *Pradipika* as the "important ones." Of these, Padmasana (Lotus Pose) receives by far the most detailed explanation, which by today's standards is surprisingly brief: "Place the right foot on the left thigh and the left foot on the right thigh, cross the hands behind the back and firmly hold the toes. Press the chin against the chest and look at the tip of the nose." A few verses later we are told that "ordinary people cannot achieve this posture, only the few wise ones on this earth can."[36] Although wisdom is probably not what most determines who can or cannot do certain asanas, the intricacy of asana technique and clarity of instruction in the more recent development of Hatha yoga has certainly made this pose and others accessible to a constantly expanding world of practitioners, wise or not. Still, it would not be until the mid-twentieth century that the process of practicing asanas would be described in any greater detail than during the fifteenth century. In Chapter 20 we look at asana practice in that greater detail.

Pranayama—Cultivating and Balancing Energy

In contrast to their sparse discussion of asana, both the *Gheranda Samhita* and the *Pradipika* provide very detailed guidance on pranayama practice, beginning with statements on how prana and the mind are inextricably linked: "When prana moves, chitta (the mental faculty) moves. When prana is without movement, chitta is without movement. By this the yogi attains steadiness and should thus restrain the vayu (air)."[37] Specific techniques are explained, including setting, season, location, pace, rhythm, retention, various alternate nostril methods, and use of bandhas and mudras. We explore these practices in Chapter 21, offering safe and effective methods for teaching pranayama in different yoga class environments and to different levels of students.

Mudra and Bandha—Conscious Awakening Practices

> As the serpent upholds the earth and its mountains, so kundalini is the support of all the yoga practices. By guru's grace, this sleeping kundalini is awakened, then all the lotuses (chakras) and knots (nadis) are opened. Then sushumna (the central energetic channel through the spine) becomes the pathway of prana, mind is free of all connections, and death is averted.

Thus begins the *Pradipika*'s explanation of mudra and bandha. The energy that was unleashed in creation, kundalini, lies coiled and sleeping at the base of the spine. With the help of tantric practices described hundreds of years earlier in the *Kanka-malinitantra* and other sources, it is the purpose of Hatha yoga to arouse this cosmic energy, causing it to rise back up through the increasingly subtler chakras until union with God is achieved in the sahasrara chakra at the crown of the head. Mudras are the specific body positions, including precise placement of the fingers and gaze, that direct the pranic energy generated in asana and pranayama practice to flow in balance through the subtle body. Bandhas are "energy locks" that further generate and accumulate prana in the physical and subtle bodies. Mudras and bandhas are explored in Chapter 21 in conjunction with other elements of subtle energy.

In these early writings on yoga, we begin to see at least two clearly divergent and often conflicting pathways of practice: one renunciant and ostensibly rooted in

Samkhya philosophy and Patanjali's *Yoga Sutra*, and the other influenced by the tantric movement. The development of Hatha yoga in the centuries after the appearance of the *Hatha Yoga Pradipika* reflected these polarities of philosophical, practical, and spiritual orientation. The distinctions between these tendencies often became blurred as lineages, schools, and teachers of yoga brought their own creative expression to the evolution of yoga philosophy and practice. Yet as with all forms of evolution, even in those instances of great leaps, the colorful ancient threads of wisdom and practice can still be seen in the modern fabric of yoga and yoga therapy, rooting even the most innovative contemporary teachings in the wisdom first articulated by yogis in India thousands of years ago.

2

Ayurvedic Sources

When life is lost, everything is lost.
—CARAKA

THE TRADITIONAL SCIENCE OF MEDICINE found in India is called *ayurveda*, from the root words *ayur*, meaning "life," and *veda*, meaning "knowledge," which first appeared as a word in the epic *Mahabharata*. The basic aim of ayurveda is the balanced integration of body, mind, and consciousness in keeping with the larger balance of qualities that constitute the universe. It is often offered as an alternative to scientific medicine, which is said to emphasize symptomatic diagnosis and expensive intervention, this in contrast to ayurveda's focus on the whole person and the cultivation of a healthy lifestyle in keeping with one's unique nature. We are offered what seems like a beautiful, fragrant flower in contrast to the harsh lights, x-rays, drugs, and surgery of Western medicine. One might like to leave it at that, breathing and sharing in the light of ayurveda's sweet promise, if only because when we look more and closely at the fibers and cells of the flower its beauty and sweetness can assume other qualities.

Like with yoga, the holism, beauty, and power of ayurveda practices inspire the sense that this must be something of the gods or that it arises from the ancient mists of existence; it is something that carries the promise of the healthiest life in the here, now, and beyond. Indeed, much like the histories of yoga in which we find inspired claims of ancient Indian lineage or source, many writers and practitioners of ayurveda make the imaginative or spurious claim that Indian approaches to healing and wellness, ayurveda in particular, are already developed in ancient writings and practices dating from "over 5,000 years ago," and they go on to present it in ways that are sometimes quite at odds with the earliest known and available sources on Indian medicine and ayurveda.[1]

The Origins, Sources, and Development of Ayurveda

Although the term *veda* may tempt one to assign ayurveda to the Vedic period, there is no traditional ayurveda text dating back 3,500 years ago to the Vedic age. There are four vedas: *Rigveda, Yajuveda, Samaveda,* and *Atharvaveda.* Of these, only the *Atharvaveda*, from around 1200 BCE, discusses medicine in ancient India, albeit in clearly pre-ayurveda terms in that it does not offer a science of health and well-being.[2]

It is tempting to read classical pseudoscientific concepts of ayurveda such as *doshas* into the *Atharvaveda*'s delineation of disease as produced by qualities of air, wind, and dry, but this is in error. Rather, what we find in the *Atharvaveda* is the mystical medicine of prehistoric India wherein disease is a religious, not a natural, condition rooted in possession by evil spirits, malevolent deities, or the sorcery of enemies—just as we find in ancient approaches to medicine in Egypt, Greece, Europe, and China. Without distinguishing natural disease from demonic forces, the prescriptions for various disorders in the Vedic period are primarily sacrifice, magic spells, potions, incantations, and prayer, some of which prefigure certain aspects of ayurveda.[3] To be sure, many of these notions are put forth today as though they were part of the earliest ayurvedic practices, but as we shall see, this is quite at odds with how ayurveda actually developed in its definitive theories and practices.

Some readers will likely object to the implicit suggestion here that ayurveda and yoga are distinctive practices, much like the proverbial ships passing in the night, which a close reading of the history reveals. Nonetheless, leading exemplars of today's popular ayurveda movement assert—without reference or citation—that "yoga and ayurveda are sister sciences that developed together and repeatedly influenced each other throughout history."[4] As Wujastyk points out, "the traditional ayurveda body differs strikingly from the body revealed in the gaze of tantric adepts or yogic practitioners. Their magico-religious body is the universe in miniature, and a conduit for mystical energies that awaken consciousness in the chakras. None of these concepts is present or prominent in the ayurveda view of the body...."[5]

Developed together and repeatedly influenced by each other? Let us explore. As we continue surveying the development of yoga and healing, we want to be clear that in attempting to clarify its lines of development we are introducing the context that allows us later in this book to more clearly identify the essential concepts and principles of early Indian medicine that can inform a significant part of yoga as a healing modality today. Rather than an academic exercise, this exploration is undertaken for practical purposes.

In the next several hundred years we finally begin to find sources of rational medicine based on at least some semblance of ayurveda's scientific method for observing, identifying, and treating disease. Again, there are terms and concepts in the ancient writings, including in the Brahmanas and early Upanishads from between 800 and 600 BCE, that appear in the later ayurveda literature, often with reference to the *Atharvaveda*, yet they are still characterized by pre-ayurveda demonology.[6] To be sure, we find that many of the more ancient prescriptions, such as bloodletting and the use of heavy metals, persist not only into early ayurveda; rather, they are given in present-day practices, often with claims of legitimacy made through casual reference to the ancient sources, as though such assertions automatically confer truth, value, or efficacy.

In the post-Vedic *samhitas* (meaning "compilation of knowledge") we finally come to the two primary historical sources of ayurveda: the *Caraka Samhitā* and *Sushruta Samhitā* (meaning the samhitas written by Caraka and Sushruta, respectively, although one must note that the actual writers are probably many).[7] Indeed, these writings are compendiums of extant medical knowledge and technique that were developed, revised, and expanded from around the third century BCE to the fifth century CE.[8] They also appear to tap into the earliest reference to practices that prefigure ayurveda, found in the Buddha's teachings from around 250 BCE. In discussing factors in disease, it is reported that the Buddha listed "bile, phlegm, wind, and their pathological combination, changes of the seasons, the stress of unusual activities, external agency, as well as the ripening of bad karma,"—eight causes that appear in various ways in later ayurveda writings.[9]

It is Caraka who initially develops and explicates ayurveda as such in *Caraka Samhitaā*, including with this broad definition:

> *It is called "ayurveda" because it tells us which substances, qualities, and actions are life-enhancing and which are not.*
> —CARAKA (1.30.23)

Caraka then elaborates this practice in 120 chapters presented in eight sections of his samhita devoted to general principles (*sutra*), pathology (*nidana*), diagnostics (*vimana*), anatomy (*sarira*), sensory diagnosis and prognosis (*indriya*), therapy (*chikitsa*), pharmacology (*kalpa*), and purifying treatments (*siddhi*). In his chapter on the nature of the human being, he describes practices that reflect primarily Buddhist rather than Samkhya philosophy, emphasizing the mindfulness meditation of *satipatthana* (referred to today as *vipassana*).

In contrast to the broad scope of the *Caraka Samhitā*, the *Sushruta Samhitā* (probably from around the fifth century CE) is an extraordinarily detailed encyclopedic compendium of medical technique. Largely in common with the *Caraka Samhitā*, its major sections include concepts and principles (*sutra*), pathology (*nidana*), anatomy (*sarira*), therapy (*chikitsa*), pharmacology (*kalpa*), and a last set of chapters covering multiple topics (*uttara*). In contrast to the *Caraka Samhitā*, all are far more developed in offering what was then the definitive work on professionalized Indian medical practices. However, as Wujastyk shows, the specific surgical practices given by Sushruta were soon largely superseded by further developments in medical knowledge and method.[10] Nonetheless, Sushruta introduces several concepts that remain at the heart of ayurveda approaches to health and wellness, including the centrality of food (*rasa*), wind/breath (*vata*), and the five divisions of wind (*prana, udana, samana, vyana, apana*, what in yoga are described as *prana-vayus*).

A third and fundamental source on ayurveda appears in the sixth century CE writings of Vagbhata, most clearly and concisely in his syncretic *Ashtangahrdayasamhita* ("Heart of Medicine"), which surpasses the *Caraka Samhitā* and *Sushruta Samhitā* in depth and precision.[11] Here we are given the eight principal areas of ayurveda: internal medicine, surgery, obstetrics and pediatrics, restorative therapy, aphrodisiac therapy, toxicology, psychiatry, and ear/nose/throat. With Vagbhata, who was profoundly influenced by close study of Caraka's and Sushruta's compendiums and critically synthesized them, we receive a coherent presentation of the diagnostic and therapeutic techniques at the heart of Indian medicine, starting with ayurvedic theory (in Chapter 1, "Survey of Medicine"), seasonal adaptations, the categories of substances, the science of humors (*doshas*), which guide how to cultivate optimum balance of energy (*ojas*), the role of lethal points (*marmans*), and considerably more, as we explore in the following pages. This classic work would soon be translated into multiple Asian languages and influence medical practices across Asia and the Middle East.[12]

In what appears to be a largely derivative work from around the thirteenth century CE, *Sarngadhara's Compendium* offers a far more succinct presentation of ayurveda than is found in earlier literature, "devised," as its author put it, "to give short-lived, dim-witted people the benefit of reading the entire canon."[13] It provides a practical and accessible reference manual for the medieval physician, with specific guidance on how to conduct various diagnoses and treatments. Prefiguring the contemporary interest in medical uses of marijuana, he recommends cannabis for its narcotic effect (as well as opium and other "poisons"). Sarngadhara's work also shows us how, by the Middle Ages, there is an increasing syncretism between different schools of medical thought from around the world.

Yet despite works on ayurveda increasingly incorporating insights from outside their immediate domain of inquiry and service, the magico-religious yogic and tantric views of the body, with their concepts of dormant kundalini Shakti energy, nadis and chakras, are nowhere to be found at the time in ayurvedic teachings, even though these teachings still betray tethering to other ancient esoteric notions. We also find a deeper curiosity—one that likely arises from the admonition on dissection—a profound ignorance of the significance of major organs, particularly the brain, heart, and lungs, which although not unique in the world at the time, is more pronounced than in other medical treatises of the time (as well as in most ancient-to-modern yoga literature).[14] The brain makes no appearance, the heart is posited as the proximate locale of thought and emotion, and the lungs (*kloman*)—despite the centrality of breath—are conspicuous only in their virtual absence (there is no left lung even for Sarngadhara in the thirteenth century).

Here we must appreciate that the received wisdom and insight to this stage in the development of yoga and ayurveda practices proceeds primarily by way of intuition (which some consider to be divine transmission), introspection, and speculation, not dissection, chemical analysis, and other basic methods of modern medical research. We should not be surprised at the persistence of archaic pronouncements about human structure and function except insofar as we find this tendency manifesting today in claims that rest upon what are often quaint yet antiquated, outdated, and invalidated ideas. To wit, we find in the work of Sarngadhara further understanding of the body's physical components, yet still profound ignorance, as revealed in this passage that repeats the earlier thinking of Caraka, which is commonly repeated in just this way in most contemporary ayurveda texts: "Blood comes from chyle [digested food], and from it comes flesh; from flesh is generated fat; from fat, bone; from that marrow; and from marrow, semen is created."[15]

If in even these most advanced theories and descriptions offered by ayurveda we find such profound ignorance of the basic structure and function of human tissues, organs, and their interrelations, what confidence can we have in the efficacy of their prescribed treatments? The more immediately relevant question is this: How has this changed since the thirteenth century?

Here it behooves us to note that some prescribed ayurveda practices are not merely archaic; rather, some lack efficacy or are even potentially dangerous due to toxicity. The prime ayurvedic suspects in toxicity are in the use of heavy metals such as arsenic, lead, and mercury, which are put in many treatment tinctures. Even though some of the foundational ayurvedic texts note the toxic pharmacology of some substances and formulations, these and even credible contemporary sources on toxicity are often ignored at the peril of the patient. Many ayurvedic doctors still prescribe bloodletting—a practice now widely regarded as quackery based on pseudoscience—for a wide range of conditions (and a practice not to be confused with using phlebotomy to treat two specific blood disorders, hemochromatosis and polycythemia).

We find very little further development of ayurveda in the next few centuries before British imperial authorities arrive in India and largely quash it while introducing Western medicine. (However, there is no question that many Indians continued to use ayurvedic practices for health and healing throughout this period and indeed to the present day.) Much as with the development of yoga, we see a resurgence of ayurveda

in India only as part of the late nineteenth- and early twentieth-century social, cultural, and political movements against British rule and the concomitant rise in Indian
national pride in which many traditional Indian cultural practices reemerged. In the
wake of Indian independence, ayurveda has been woven into the Indian health care
system, where today it is among the world's leading examples of complementary and
integrated medicine.[16]

Ayurveda's Underlying Philosophy and Principles

The ayurvedic framework for health is rooted in philosophical notions of spiritual
being in which the condition of any human being is seen as a manifestation of larger
forces in the universe. Just what these forces are and how they manifest varies across
the landscape of ayurvedic literature, with literally thousands of philosophical, psychological, and spiritual concepts and terms often used in different ways. We often
find numerous terms for essentially the same thing, the differences often amounting
more to variations in mood or emphasis rather than substantive variance or disagreement, although there are fundamental disagreements over even basic concepts (such
as the relationship between *agni* [the principal of fire and heat] and *pitta* [the fundamental fiery bodily element], one of the three doshas). We also find vast differences in
fundamental ideas about yoga and the very concept of life. Part of our challenge in
giving clear explication to this framework arises from the differences in underlying
philosophy, which is often glossed over in presenting yoga and ayurveda as though
there is broad consensus on their respective principles and concepts. What we attempt
here is an inclusive yet carefully considered critical synthesis and summary of the most
salient and significant concepts that allow us to articulate a coherent and practical
yogic view of human life, health, and healing.

The Samkhya Philosophy of Consciousness and Constitution

Ayurvedic theory and practice are rooted in the rational and dualist *Samkhya* (meaning "enumeration") philosophy, the oldest of six systems of ancient Indian philosophy
and the one from which ayurveda elaborates a set of principles that explain everything
about human nature, health, and disease. The general aim of Samkhya is a quality of
salvation in which one is liberated from what is thought to be the suffering nature
of existence through the isolation of consciousness from all other aspects of being,
what in Sanskrit is called *kaivalya*.[17] This concept is presented contemporaneously
by Isvarakrisha in the *Samkhya-Karika* and by Patanjali in his *Yoga Sutra*, with the
latter offering yoga as practice for this attainment.[18] Samkhya presents the underlying
theory as a set of twenty-four core principles (*tattvas*) that, much like modern physics,

involves a stream of properties from the most subtle elements of the universe to the gross materiality of this lived existence, all discerned through the direct inner perception of sages as there is no other way to arrive at such understanding.[19]

Samkhya begins with the perception that our universe of experience consists of two separate and irreducible principles that are omnipresent and eternal: pure, transcendental consciousness or spirit, called *purusha*, and unconscious primordial matter, called *prakriti*. We can also appreciate purusha as the seer, the witness to all that is seen, with all that is seen appreciated as prakriti. Their connection, as we shall see, is the source of every further manifestation, including the interrelated components of ayurveda anatomy at the gross level of functioning life forms, including complete human beings.

The concept of purusha has evolved over time and remains subject to an array of definitions rooted in different transliterations of the *Rigveda* versus later Upanishadic writings. The earlier Vedic view has purusha as a being ("cosmic man") who is sacrificed by the gods for the creation of the universe and all life forms. In the Upanishads, purusha is spirit or the universal principle, an eternal, pervasive, and unchanging (*aksara*) essence. It is the source of all consciousness, including human consciousness, and is the causal principle that manifests in everything and everywhere. It is, yet is neither created nor creates, and thus sometimes it is not counted as among the principles (material realities) of the universe (*tattvas*). Purusha is a "content-less, non-intentional presence incapable of performing any activity" and "accompanies every particular life form."[20] Thus, rather than a single spirit or consciousness, purusha is infinitely plural in its potential manifestation of consciousness in every living being.[21]

The Tattvas

Prakriti is the primordial material reality and the cause of everything except purusha, the first principle of the universe. Put differently, everything in the physical universe, including the mind, is a manifestation of prakriti, the second principle. However, left to itself—that is, not connected to purusha and thus unconscious—it is unmanifest, just as purusha is unmanifest when not connected to prakriti. Purusha and prakriti are thus mutually dependent in the manifestation of life as we experience it; indeed, they come together to give us the greater creation of everything.

As the primal material and motive force of the universe, prakriti is thus the first material *tattva* (principle). It consists of three essential and universal qualities, or *gunatraya*, which in their unmanifest state rest in dynamic equilibrium. Note that the gunas are not tattvas, but rather in their various interactions and balances they create tattvas.

Sattva: The quality of goodness, light, balance, and essential being.[22] Sattva also describes a calm and clear state of mind, a sense of being complete and fulfilled.

Filled with this sense of levity, clarity, and tranquility, we are more kind and thoughtful toward others and ourselves. We can thereby act in the world with greater ease because our mental balance is in a natural contentment, without dependence on something external.

Rajas: The quality of passion, activity, motion, and variation.[23] Rajas involves a sense of intense dynamism, stimulating us to act in the world with excitement and passion, the mind always imbued with anxiety or expectation about how things might turn out. Driven by desire, rajas thus revolves around the feeling of needing or losing something, even to the point of becoming obsessed by it. If we do not act, we fear losing what we feel we need. If successful in attaining whatever is driving our desire, then the mind will return to a balanced state of awareness (or potentially flip into fear of loss).

Tamas: The quality of heaviness, dullness, resistance, and darkness.[24] Tamas reflects a confused state of mind that leads to indecision, lethargy, and inaction. This is the feeling of not knowing what we are feeling or what we want or need. Caught in this tendency, our behavior can become self-destructive or harmful to others. Yet tamas allows us to calm down, relax, or restore our energy through rest and sleep.

There is a tendency to feel drawn to sattva or to idealize oneself as composed of just that quality. However, each of the gunas depends upon one another. In the *Mandukya Upanishad* we are offered the metaphor of a lamp in which the heavy structure of its base (tamas) contains the ignitable fuel (rajas) that can potentially manifest a flame through the white wick (sattva). Only together do they give us the flame of life experience. As we shall see, part of the path of yoga is very much one of moving into the clarity and purity of sattvic awareness, yet it is a journey that requires the energy of rajas and the stability of tamas, even as those qualities are sources of difficulty along the way.

When connected with consciousness, prakriti becomes unbalanced and manifest, creating the manifest universe. In this manifestation, we find the interactions of the gunas giving us the unique and specific expressions of material life forms. The disequilibrium of the gunas gives us the further evolution of the universe, and more specifically, the new tattvas of our material experience and existence (the third, fourth, and fifth tattvas) that are constituted by the gunas when they are no longer in symmetry. The relative dominance or presence of the three gunas gives us not only parinama-vada—the constancy of change—but also the emergent sequence of principles, starting with *mahat*:

Mahat: Literally "the great one" (also called *buddhi*) and largely consisting of sattva with some presence of rajas, this is the principle of intellect, of knowing, that gives intelligence to all life forms (think not of the intelligence of the thinking mind, but the creative intelligence that manifests even in the interactions of cells in the physical body). It is predominantly sattvic in quality and thus a reflector for the pure consciousness of purusha. However, it is not purusha, and this common mistaken identification of mahat with purusha creates the tattva of *ahamkara*.

Ahamkara: The stirring misidentification of mahat with purusha brings a stronger rajastic quality to the otherwise sattvic quality of awareness, giving us the principle of ego identity that creates for us our sense of individuation and willingness, the self-identification of what "I" think I am based upon my accumulated experience.

Manas: The sattvic dimension of ahamkara generates the mind, *manas*, the faculty of volitional, deliberate, and emotional cognition—even if not clear.

Here we pause to offer an excerpt from Sarngadhara's thirteenth century *Compendium* as a colorful map to what we have presented thus far on the tattvas and the tattvas that manifest from them:

THE ORIGIN OF THE HUMAN BEING

*The source of the world is motiveless and has the unique appearance of consciousness and bliss. It has an eternal Nature [*prakriti*], like the shadow cast by the sun. Although herself inert, she used the consciousness of the supreme Self [*purusha*] to create all and everything which is transient, like a piece of theatre.*

*In the beginning, Nature, the mother of all, gave birth to intellect [*mahat*], composed of desire [*rajas*] and vast in appearance [*sattva*]. Out of that came personal identity [*ahamkara*]. It was born in three divisions [*gunas*], according to the qualities of purity [*sattva*], passion [*rajas*], and darkness [*tamas*]. From the unity of purity and passion arose the ten organs [*indriyas*] and also the mind [*manas*]. The organs are: the ear, the skin, the eye, the tongue, the nose, the voice, the hands, the feet, the sex organs, and the rectum. Those with detailed understanding say that the first five are the organs of intellect, while the remaining five are the organs of action.*

*From personal identity, dominated by qualities of passion and purity, arose the set of five subtle elements [*tanmatras*]. The wise recite the names of these subtle elements as follows: sound, touch, visible form, taste, and smell.*

*Sound, touch, visible form, taste, and smell, the characteristics of the respective subtle elements, arrived at a gross condition. From these subtle elements arose five gross elements [*mahabhutas*], which are considered to be space, wind, fire, water, and earth.*

These five, sound and so forth, are thought of as the organs of intellect. Similarly, the characteristics of the organs of action are speaking, grasping, walking, orgasm, and excreting.

Nature is also known by the names "Principle," "Power," "Eternal," and "Unaltered." She is in Shiva. The wise know that the following seven items are Nature and her modifications: intellect, personal identity, and each of the five elements. Having pervaded everything, they dwell in the world.[25]

The physiological anatomy of ayurveda ultimately describes three *doshas*, or body constitutions—*vata*, *pitta*, and *kapha*—that are expressions of the tattvas and the foundation for understanding specific conditions of health and disease. They are explored in detail in the following pages. The witnessing, self-identifying, and cognitive principles of mahat, ahamkara, and manas are together considered the internal organ, or *antahkarana*, which in turn manifests ten *indriyas* (sense of action organs), five *tanmatras* (subtle elements of perception), and five *mahabhutas* (the gross elements, the combination of which define the doshas). This finally gives us the twenty-five tattvas underlying all of life and of ayurveda (again, the science of life).

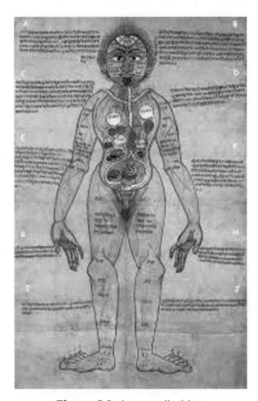

Figure 2.1: Ayurvedic Man

THE INDRIYAS: THE TEN SENSE AND ACTION ORGANS

The term *indriya* first appears in the Vedic-era *Atharvaveda* as meaning "faculty of sense," "sense," and "organ and sense." Created through the interaction of sattva and rajas, the indriyas consist of *jnanendriya* (some sources refer to this as *buddhindriyani*), sense organs, and *karmendriya*, action organs.

Jnanendriya—The Sense Organs

- Eyes for seeing
- Ears for hearing
- Nose for smelling
- Tongue for tasting
- Skin for feeling

In the Nyaya philosophy, another of the six main branches in Indian philosophy, we find each of these organs connected to an element: nose and earth, tongue and water, eyes and fire (or light), skin and air, and the ears and ether.

Karmendriya—The Action Organs

- Larynx for speaking
- Hands for grasping
- Feet for moving
- Anus for excreting
- Genitals for procreating

This ayurvedic framework explains the dynamic process of transformation from the initial connection of purusha and prakriti through the subsequent manifestations of prakriti's constituent gunas, giving us the entirety of the material universe down to the level of living human beings. As Larson and Bhattacharya put it, "The subtle body generates and then, as it were, becomes nested in a gross body (*sthulasarira*) made up of the five gross elements … The entire manifest world, 'from Brahma down to a blade of grass'(see *Samkhyakarika* LIV) is a single material continuum."[26]

THE TANMATRAS: THE FIVE SUBTLE ELEMENTS AS OBJECTS OF PERCEPTION

The interaction of tamas and rajas give us the tanmatras, objects of perception that are named after the sensory perceptions to which they correspond. They are subtle elements, from which the gross elements are produced.

- Shabda (sound)
- Sparsha (touch)
- Rupa (sight)
- Rasa (taste)
- Gandha (smell)

THE MAHABHUTA: THE FIVE GROSS ELEMENTS

The continuous interaction of tamas and rajas gives rise to the gross elements.

- *Akash* (ether) arises from the *shabda tanmatras* (sound).
- *Vayu* (air) arises from the *shabda* and *sparsha tanmatras* (sound and touch).
- *Agni* (fire) arises from the *shabda, sparsha,* and *rupa tanmatras* (sound, touch, and sight).
- *Apas* (water) arises from the *shabda, sparsha, rupa,* and *rasa tanmatras* (sound, touch, sight, and taste).
- *Prithvi* (earth) arises from the *shabda, sparsha, rupa, rasa,* and *gandhatanmatras* (sound, touch, sight, taste, and smell).

Just as the creation and interactions of the five great elements occur through the qualities of the gunas, so the gunas come to manifest the greater specificity of our physical existence through the elements they have created. The constitution of the gross elements as they manifest in a specific person brings us to the humors (*doshas*), body tissues (*dhatus*), and waste products (*malas*)—the elements and interactions of which are the foundation of ayurvedic health practices. As the five elements conglomerate to form bodily tissues and the complete living organism, their proper proportions, which are constantly in flux, allow the body to function in a healthy way.

THE SEVEN DHATUS

The *dhatus* (our tissues), which we look at more closely in a moment, are formed by food. In the fire of digestion, ingested food is first converted into *rasa* (food juice), *raksa* (blood), *mamsa* (flesh), *medas* (fat), *asthi* (bone), and *sukra* (semen). (These are only very general, provisional translations; the more refined expressions are discussed later.) The digestive and larger dhatu waste products (mala), as described by Caraka, consist of urine, sweat, feces, vata, pitta, and kapha, with vata, pitta, and kapha responsible for all pathologies and morbidities.[27] Although the malas produce the doshas of vata, pitta, and kapha, the doshas also vitiate the tissues, leading Sushruta to state that the doshas are the primary and most essential factor constituting the human organism. Food, as we shall see, is thus the very foundation of ayurvedic treatment.

Tridosha: The Three Constitutions

The theory or doctrine of *tridosha* posits that the three essential humors—wind (*vata*), bile (*pitta*), and phlegm (*kapha*)—are determined by the interactions of the gross elements:

- Ether + Air = Vata
- Fire + Water = Pitta
- Water + Earth = Kapha

Ayurveda teaches us that the relative balance of the humors, which finally express themselves as semifluid substances, constitutes anyone's physical nature and directly affects their temperament and health. The relative balance of the doshas—how each dosha interacts with the body's seven constituent tissues (*dhatus*, discussed momentarily) and waste products (*malas*, also discussed in a moment)—determines one's unique constitution. The doshas "are considered as the basic functional units of the body."[28] Thus, tridosha is the foundation of ayurvedic diagnosis, pathology, and healing. Sarngadhara writes that the humors themselves "are also considered to be body tissues (*dhatu*), because each one supports the body (*dharana*), as well as impurities. In that sense they are divided into five types. (Wind, choler, and phlegm are known as humors [*dosa*] because they corrupt [*dusana*] the body; as body tissues [*dhatu*] because they hold the body up; and as impurities [*mala*] because they foul it [*malinakara*].)"[29] It is precisely in the balance of the doshas that we come to our general and specific conditions, as the doshas "bind the five elements in living flesh." [30] Yet only air, fire, and water, as the active and changing elements, are primary in the principle of tridosha, with ether and earth, respectively, serving as the space and supporting foundation for the tridoshic whole.

Before further exploring the doshas, dhatus, and malas, consider the earlier statement that the doshas corrupt the body. Recall that everything in the manifest universe consists of the constituent elements of prakriti—the gunas of sattva, rajas, and tamas—on the journey from subtle to gross expression in a living person. Just how this manifestation occurs at the level of the unique person is determined by the balance of the doshas, which can be thought of as "that which is quick to go out of balance."[31] This implies the delicacy of health and life while also giving us a means for assessing health as a constant process of cultivating the balance of energies that constitute us in any given moment. Health is expressed in the equilibrium of our living tissues, which we maintain or lose based on the influence of the doshas: disturbance of the doshas causes disturbance of the tissues, whereas the normal state of the doshas is brought about through diet, medicine, and lifestyle.

To better appreciate how this works, we will next look closely at the three doshas and each of their five subtypes, offering various prisms to shed light on the myriad aspects of their manifestations, interactions, and effects.

THE WINDS OF VATA

Formed by the seemingly ethereal elements of air and ether (the latter either ethereal or mythological, depending on your beliefs), Sushruta tells us that vata (or breath, *prana*, *vayu*) is "free, eternal, and omnipresent, and because of this it is revered in all of the world as the Self of all creatures. It is the cause of the existence, origination, and disappearance of all creatures."[32] This primacy of vata is due to it being the "holy wind of God," which when "not irritated maintains the balance of the humours, the body tissues, and the digestive fire."[33] Its function in its normal state is to provide energy for movement, including the internal movement of the tissues. In the words of Vagbhata, it is inherently dry, light, cold, harsh, fine, and mobile. The mobility (rajas) of vata makes it the governing source of movement and communication and allows the fire of pitta in our assimilation processes, which in turn serves to balance vata and kapha.[34] For Sarngadhara the primacy of wind is made abundantly clear: "Choler (pitta) is lame, phlegm (kapha) is lame, the impurities (malas) and tissues (dhatus) are lame. They go wherever the wind takes them, just like the clouds."[35]

While each dosha is present throughout the body, each also is said to dominate in specific areas as subdoshas.[36] Vata is traditionally (i.e., in the ancient teachings) said to be most present in the colon, trunk, stomach, and heart, whereas contemporary ayurveda sources assert that it is dominant elsewhere: Lad has vata dominant in the "head, throat, diaphragm, small intestine, belly button, pelvic girdle, thighs, colon, and heart,"[37] Tiwari has vata dominant in "the lower body, pelvic region, colon, bladder, urinary tract, thighs, legs, arms, bones, and nervous system,"[38] and Pole reports that vata is "below the belly button, especially in the colon," while also in the "bladder, thighs, ears, bones, and sense of touch."[39]

The more specific manifestation of the life-force pranic energy of vata in the body occurs in five ways, what Caraka describes as the five vayus, giving us the prana-vayus, or vata subdoshas:[40]

Prana-vayu: Here the general term *prana* is applied to its specific expression as wind as it enters the body through respiration, moving downward and inward to bring life energy to the body. It regulates breathing, causes the heart to beat, sustains the flow of blood and neurological impulses, carries food through the esophagus to the stomach, and is associated with cognitive function. Thus, as wind, prana-vayu is all about movement—of the whole body, thought, feelings, emotions, sensations, and perceptions. When still, it becomes as though a mirror, a silent witness to the fullness of existence, of consciousness. When disturbed, it is said to cause anxiety, fear, and anger along with respiratory and cardiovascular ailments, joint disease, and digestive disease. Curiously, it is traditionally said to be centered in the heart, while some more recent ayurvedic thinkers[41] place its home in the brain (which is curious given that traditional ayurveda did not recognize the brain as the source of cognitive or larger neurological functions).[42]

Udana-vayu: This is the upward manifestation of vata energy, including the upward flow of energy responsible for exhalation, speech, vomiting, and memory. It is thus also associated with feeling emotionally uplifted, physically stronger, and more mentally clear. When disturbed, it interferes with clear speech (and can cause stuttering), inhibits memory, and undermines one's sense of purpose in life. As something opposed to prana-vayu, udana-vayu suggests slowing things down, being calmer, and quieting inside, thereby better sustaining the larger flow of prana and the sustained awakening of clear awareness.

Samana-vayu: As the inward movement of prana, samana-vayu stokes the digestive fire as its energy moves to the center of the body, governing digestion by stimulating the secretion of gastric juices and digestive enzymes. Lad is very specific in stating that samana-vayu in the small intestine and navel accumulates bile in the gallbladder, opens the pyloric valve, and pushes the bile into the duodenum (the segment of the gastrointestinal tract that accepts food from the stomach).[43] When disturbed, it causes indigestion, lack of nutrient absorption, and diarrhea. At a subtle level, samana-vayu is said to be associated with emotional resilience and discernment, including with respect to nutritional habits.

Vyana-vayu: The full circulation of prana is accomplished by vyana-vayu, which diffuses wind energy throughout the body. Said to be in the heart, it sustains the cardiovascular and larger circulatory systems, transporting nutrients to tissues throughout the human organism and governing movement of the muscles. When disturbed, it causes dry skin, heart disease, edema, and other circulatory issues. At a subtle level, when in balance, it makes us healthier social creatures as we more easily circulate and share energy with others.

Apana-vayu: Downward moving and most present in the pelvis, apana-vayu is said to be responsible for elimination as well as conception by regulating the urinary and reproductive systems. When impaired, it causes diarrhea or constipation, disrupts urination and menstruation, causes pain during sexual intercourse, causes premature ejaculation, and other problems, including osteoporosis and diabetes. When in balance, it allows us to more easily let go of the thoughts and things to which we might unnecessarily cling, allowing us to be nourished and cleansed.

THE FIRES OF PITTA

Pitta (or choler) arises from the combination of fire and water. Vagbhata describes choler as being "somewhat unctuous, sharp, and hot, as well as light, smelly, diffusive, and liquid."[44] Of course we think of water as dousing fire, and fire as causing water to evaporate. But here they work together as the fiery juices of passion and metabolism, their watery quality protecting the tissues from being burned in the heat of transformation, with transformation its primary function. (Think of the fiery digestive juices being sufficiently tempered by the water element to prevent them from burning through the intestinal lining.) It is said to control the heartbeat, hormones, and body temperature, along with the liver and digestion. Pitta also plays a vital role in immunity, killing bacteria in the spleen, thermal regulation, and eyesight, as certain structures of the eye are associated with pitta (lens, cornea, and cones).[45] Going further, as the digestive process leads to the nourishing of all cells, pitta is said to awaken intelligence and open us to pure consciousness. Although Caraka attributes various effects to pitta, including the powers of vision, digestion, and intelligence, he does not further classify them, as Sushruta does; Sushruta offers these five specific expressions of pitta:

Pachaka Pitta: Said to be found in the liver, gallbladder, pancreas, duodenum, and small intestine as well as the saliva and stomach, pachaka pitta is first fire.[46] A fire unto itself, pachaka pitta is also called the keeper of the flame as it supports the other expressions of pitta while relating to an alert, discriminating mind. The actions of pachaka pitta govern digestion in the stomach, duodenum, and small intestine. Once food is digested, pachaka pitta separates out nutrients from waste products. When out of balance, pachaka pitta causes indigestion and poor absorption of nutrients.

Ranjaka Pitta: The second expression of pitta, ranjaka pitta, is responsible for the formation and maintenance of blood as it acts primarily through the liver (which ayurveda has traditionally and erroneously posited as the source of blood production) and spleen. From a root word meaning "to redden" or "color," ranjaka pitta gives us our hair, skin, and eye color. Some go far beyond the understandings of traditional ayurveda theory to suggest that ranjaka pitta works in the bone marrow to produce red blood cells (which makes sense given that we now know that the liver does not produce blood). Ranjaka pitta also relates to the fiery emotions of anger and hate, helping to metabolize their expressions as they, too, are cooked in the fire of awareness.

Sadhaka Pitta: Sadhaka pitta relates to memory, self-awareness, and general mental functioning, which until recently ayurveda theory had situated in the heart. Now that ayurveda recognizes that the brain has a neurological function, sadhaka pitta is said to be in charge there as well as for all neurochemical changes. When impaired, it is the source of mental disturbance and various neuroses, including addictions.

Alochaka Pitta: Animating and governing the eyes, alochaka pitta regulates visual perception. Disturbance of the alochaka pitta, which can arise from not allowing tears to flow, interferes with vision, clouds the whites of the eyes, and stands in the way of grasping the ultimate Truth.

Bhrajaka Pitta: The fire of bhrajaka pitta gives the skin its warmth, luster, and glow. Giving us healthy skin, bhrajaka pitta helps to protect the body from pathogens while allowing the sense of touch, temperature, and pain. When disturbed, it causes various skin diseases as well as loss of tactile sensation. Its connection with emotion is revealed in blushing or becoming pale in reaction to certain types of feeling.

THE WATERS OF KAPHA

Formed by earth and water, kapha gives us structure and stability as the moisture of water binds the dry earth into shape. It is the phlegm that Vagbhata describes as "unctuous, cold, heavy, slow, smooth, slimy, and solid."[47] Kapha causes the formation of mucus and is present in the lymph, plasma, muscles, semen, connective tissue, and the white matter of the brain, where it is said to give the brain its structure.[48] Thus, it is present throughout the body, its cohesive qualities give us shape, and its fluid qualities give us the ability to taste and smell, to nourish the joints, and to protect the lining of the stomach. When in balance, it is the source of stability, strength, and endurance.[49] Again, Caraka does not specifically classify the kapha subdoshas, while Sushruta gives us five finer expressions of kapha:

Kledaka Kapha: Regarded as primary among the waters, kledaka kapha originates in the stomach and creates its protective lining, forms mucus, and aids digestion. When aggravated, it causes nausea and indigestion and may lead one to excessive eating. Its imbalance also increases anxiety, insecurity, and loneliness, which also may lead to excessive eating as one attempts to fill emotional voids. It is also said to be about the lubrication of our nature, allowing us to more easily and fluidly be in our tissues and relate to others.

Avalambaka Kapha: Sometimes called "the keeper of love," this watery quality is found in the chest and more specifically in the heart.[50] Avalambaka kapha gives vital support to the other expressions of kapha, gives the blood its plasma element, protects the lungs, and ensures the flow of energy to the limbs. When aggravated it causes laziness, respiratory disorders, and heart-related ailments.

Bodhaka Kapha: Associated with the mouth, and more specifically the tongue, bodhaka kapha sends water to the tongue to create saliva, the sensation of taste, and to prepare food for digestion. The observed qualities of the tongue (color, texture) as well as perceived taste are ayurvedic tools for assessing certain qualities of health, as we explore later. When aggravated, bodhaka kapha interferes with the natural ability to sense toxic food and contributes to eating disorders. The qualities of bodhaka kapha thus teach us about cleanliness, moderation, and self-care.

Tarpaka Kapha: Now understood to support the white matter of the brain and specifically cerebrospinal fluid, tarpaka kapha is said to nourish the brain and soothe the sense organs. When out of balance it distorts perception, causes psychological problems, and disturbs memory. It also teaches us about the lightness of being, inviting us to live more peacefully.

Slesaka Kapha: With a stickier quality of kapha, slesaka kapha is found throughout the joints of the body where it provides lubrication for easier movement. When aggravated it lends to joint diseases such as arthritis. It teaches us patience, inviting us to be clearer as we create articulations (relationships) with others along our various paths.

In these various ways, the five great elements (*mahabhutas*) combine to compose the doshas, bringing the organizing principles of prakriti closer to their full realization in the tissues of the body. The balance of the elements in each dosha gives it its character and primary functions, with the various subdoshas accomplishing more specific functions in support of the overall integration of the tissues in each unique person.

In the preceding pages, we have presented these interrelationships, functions, and effects in a very basic and general way, glossing over the fact that from ancient times to the present there have been significantly different theories and understandings that nonetheless share in the same general principles of Samkhya philosophy and the twenty-five tattvas. For example, among the ancients we find Caraka and Sushruta offering different and even conflicting views of the doshas, with Sushruta considering "the principle of blood" in combination with vata, pitta, and kapha. (Sushruta is generally more specific than Caraka, likely due to his being a surgeon.) Among contemporary ayurvedic sources, the differences are vast, as we have seen even with basic ideas such as where the doshas and subdoshas manifest in the body. Such differences persist into the understanding of the constituent tissues of the body, the dhatus: some give us all five elements, some four (earth, air, water, fire), while others (including Sushruta) give us only the three doshas as the building blocks of the body.[51]

The Dhatus—The Seven Constituent Bodily Tissues

The full manifestation of prakriti awaits the dhatus, the seven tissues that come into form and function as the complete and integrated living bodily organism, nourished and sustained through the seemingly magical dance of breath and food as they permeate the entirety of our bodymind. These are the tissues by which we live and die, tissues that, like the doshas, are formed from the interaction of ether, air, fire, water, and earth, with the transformational energy of *agni*, the essential force of transmutation. These tissues are formed in a natural order, with each a factor in the creation of the next. As quoted earlier, Sarngadhara summarizes it as follows: "They are generated from one another, being cooked in the heat of the choler. Blood comes from chyle, and from it comes flesh; from flesh is generated fat; from fat, bone; from that, marrow; and from marrow, semen is created."[52] At each level of manifestation there are two stages of transformation, from *asthayi* (unprocessed or immature) to *sthayi* (mature or processed), when it is fully nourished and stable in form and substance, with each dhatu present in the crystallization of the successive dhatus created from it. The quality of each successive manifestation is determined by the nature of the doshas and subdoshas in any person.

Rasa dhatu: The product of digested food is called *ahara rasa*, the essence of food, what Caraka and the ancients refer to as chyle. This milky, sticky, kapha-like substance is transformed by agni into *rasa dhatu*, what today we understand as plasma and what in ayurveda is the first of the seven tissues and the precursor for the other six. The transformation of ahara rasa into rasa dhatu is said to take five days (as do all dhatu manifestations, thus full manifestation of the dhatus takes thirty-five days). This and each of the subsequent manifestations require proper food, a healthy mind, and healthy prana. When these are lacking, there are disorders in rasa dhatu, which one experiences as a bad taste in the mouth, lack of faith and clarity, and nausea.

Rakta dhatu: As the agni continues its transformative (maturing) effect on the rasa, the rasa becomes *asthayi rakta*, or immature *rakta dhutu*, blood tissue. This blood tissue is seen today as purely red blood cells (separate from the plasma) that are rich in fiery ranjaka pitta. If rakta dhatu is defective, it produces excess bile. When healthy, it causes the maturation of asthayi rakta into *sthayi rakta dhatu*.

Mamsa dhatu: The further refinement of the rakta dhatu manifests *asthayimamsa dhatu*, muscle tissue that arises from the fiery force of ranjaka pitta acting in the rakta dhatu. Derived from the kapha dosha, mamsa gains shape and gives stability to the body while allowing movement. As the mamsa is nourished into its mature quality as *sthayi mamsa dhatu* it manifests as *asthayi medas dhatu*.

Medas dhatu: This is fat tissue, dominated by the water element and kledaka kapha, giving the body energy, stamina, and a sense of being grounded. Its maturation into *sthayi medas dhatu* causes the formation of the *asthayi ashti dhatu*.

Ashti dhatu: Dominated by air and space, the *ashti dhatu* is our bone and cartilage tissue as well as the source of teeth, hair, and nails. It will maturate into *asthayi majja dhatu*.

Majja dhatu: In the maturation of bone and cartilage tissues, the refined nutrients transform bone and cartilage to produce bone marrow, which matures into *sthayi majja dhatu* and the precursor of the final tissues, *asthayi shukra dhatu* or *asthayi artava dhatu*.

Shukra and artava dhatu: The most refined nutrients are formed from the matured majja dhatu, giving us our reproductive tissues: in men it is *shukra dhatu,* semen, and in women it is *artava dhatu,* ovum. The previous refinements are now manifest in their finest form, giving us their collective essences in the substances for procreation.

Etiology: The Causes of Disease in Ayurvedic Theory

We have presented the general process of tissue development without addressing the extraordinarily detailed forces that come to bear, for better or worse, in determining the specific manifestations of the successively developed tissues. In the process of manifestation, there are many things that can cause aggravation and disharmony (*dhatu-vaisamya*) in the doshas and thus in the tissues. This disharmony, or disequilibrium in the dhatus, is how Caraka defines disease. Here we will discuss general causes of disharmony.

Sushruta tells us that the production of disease is due to deranged doshas pervading the body, whereas disease itself is described as the effects on the dhatus.[53] Writing earlier, Caraka gives us three general causes of disease: 1) excessive, deficient, or wrongful use of sense objects, such as ingesting harmful substances, 2) hot and cold environments as they vary by season, and 3) the misuse of intelligence, meaning not doing the right thing at the right time with respect to sense objects (such as eating when satiated, or listening to unpleasant sounds). However, these are predisposing causes (*nidanas*), which in and of themselves do not create disease. Rather, they act on the doshas, which in turn act on the constituent bodily tissues, vitiating them—ultimately causing diseases that are classified as *nija*, meaning arising from an abnormal condition in the body. According to Caraka, disease can also be caused by accident (*agantu*)—including the acts of spirits, ingestion of poison, or violence—or by mental diseases (*manasa*) arising from conditions of the ego. In yet more refined classifications, Sushruta offers several further delineations of disease, starting with *adhyatmika* (physical, including hereditary, congenital, and dosha derangement), *adhibhautika* (caused by weapons or wild animals), and *adhidaivika* (acts of God or nature, whether seasonal, providential, or natural processes such as aging).

The nidanas act on the doshas in specific ways, possibly (but not necessarily) making them deficient or excessive, which, if aggravated, in turn causes them to vitiate the dhatus and manifest various symptoms. One can look more closely to consider how the relative deficiency or expansion of each dosha affects the other two, and how deranged doshas (and subdoshas) specifically affect each dhatu. Each affected dhatu, in its state of nourishment, affects the others in a cascading galaxy of cause and effect throughout the bodymind. This enables one to delineate cause and effect from the nidanas to every specific condition found in the body. In this we have the core practices in ayurveda diagnosis, prognosis, and prescription.

3

Modern Medical Science

Science may provide the most useful way to organize empirical, reproducible data, but its power to do so is predicated on its inability to grasp the most central aspects of human life: hope, fear, love, hate, beauty, envy, honor, weakness, striving, suffering, virtue.
—PAUL KALANITHI

THE SCIENTIFIC METHOD CLAIMS to approach health and healing with empirical evidence and a rational understanding of the human bodymind. In contrast to relatively unchanging methods of magico-religious, faith-based, and folk approaches, modern medicine attempts to build and organize medical insight in the form of replicable and verifiable explanations and predictions, seeking understanding based on facts rather than belief. This method applies sciences such as anatomy, biochemistry, epidemiology, immunology, neuroscience, pathology, and toxicology to understanding disease, trauma, and healing. In doing so, the scientific understanding of the human body rests upon systematic research in accordance with logical principles of reasoning, gradually building a storehouse of reliable methods and techniques for practical application.

The very sound of this can be deafening to those who believe in the power and efficacy of approaches such as naturopathy and faith-based healing that generally eschew methodical science in favor of congruence with spiritual faith or philosophical beliefs such as vitalism.[1] As medical anthropology shows us, ancient medicine—including animism's spirited objects and spiritualism's appeal to deities—not only makes a certain sense in various social, cultural, and historical contexts, but it can offer insights into the integration of traditional and scientific approaches.[2] Even with tremendous advances in medical science, there is still an art to healing for at least two reasons: first, there is always an element of human sensitivity or intuition in every aspect of human experience and communication; and second, the historical development of medical science arose from and retains many elements of traditional and intuitive medical arts. Put differently, the subjective or personal dimension of experience and insight on the part of both healer or physician and patient matters, with the artful ways of the doctor, therapist, or care-receiver often being of great significance.

From Mysticism to the Scientific Method

This point gains favor when we appreciate the etymology of the word *medicine* and the historical development of the medical sciences. The term medicine comes into English from the Latin *medeor*, meaning "heal" or "cure," its adjective *medicus*, "healing" or "curative," is later found in the expression *ars medicina*, "the art of healing." In the Egyptian Imhotep's third-century-BCE medical treatise, the likely source of the *Edwin Smith Papyrus*,[3] we find a commitment to systematic anatomical, physiological, and pathological observation along with hieratic—priestly—admonition and guidance. As we saw earlier, the ayurvedic surgeon Sushruta gave us detailed surgical procedures while embracing a mystical understanding of life and retaining many aspects of magico-religious technique. Even with Hippocrates, perhaps first among the so-called fathers of medicine, we find a rational approach, yet his now ubiquitous oath was then sworn on several gods. Galen, the highly accomplished Greek medical researcher and physician, who while opposing the Stoics in insisting upon the unity of bodymind was himself inspired to go into medicine rather than politics based on his father's dream that the god Aesculapius commanded it so. The mystical persists, sometimes with reason.

The development of largely Western scientific medicine from the Egyptians and Greeks forward reflects larger sociocultural, religious, and philosophical movements. Tapping into the materialist teachings of Democritus, Hippocrates (460–370 BCE) sought to align philosophy and medicine, proposing that disease arises from the environment and lifestyle, not gods or other mystical forces. More specifically, he proposed a humoral theory in which the balance of four essential bodily fluids—blood, yellow bile, black bile, and phlegm—most directly influence a person's nature.[4] Cures were to be found in rebalancing a person's humors through simple treatments involving diet,

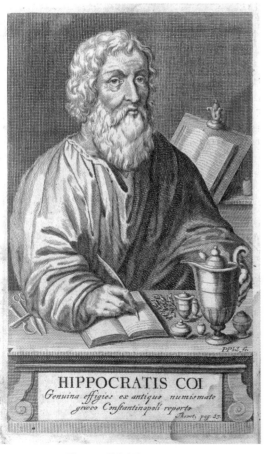

HIPPOCRATIS COI
Genuina effigies ex antiquo numismate greco Constantinopoli reperto
Thevet. pag. 27.

Figure 3.1: Hippocrates

exercise, and sleep, giving us one of the earliest expressions of a formal naturopathy. To be sure, Hippocrates went further, developing potent drugs, surgical techniques, and medical devices to improve a patient's prognosis. His humoral theory, as applied to health and medicine, became widely accepted across the span of the next 2,000 years of medicine.

Yet in the immediate wake of Hippocrates's empirical work, Aristotle, whose biological writings certainly reveal interest in empirical evidence, tended to be far more speculative, arguing that causes are found in their effects, a teleological formulation that remains common in contemporary evolutionary biology.[5] While attempting rational investigation, he retained space for the soul, albeit a "rational soul" that is expressed through the human heart (not brain), yet has an existence independent of the body while no less the animating principle of human life. It thus makes sense that Aristotle maintained the existence of a fifth element, ether, where there is space for anything one might imagine or choose to believe.

Application of humoral theory depends upon knowledge of medicinal interactions when prescribing drugs. Just as in ayurveda, the drugs of the day were primarily found in nature, not in laboratories, and had a primarily botanical basis—one that varied based on the geographical distribution of plants. The Greek physician and botanist Pedanius Dioscorides (40–90 CE) systematically researched this early form of pharmacology, producing the five-volume pharmacopeia, *De Materia Medica*. This work found translation into Latin and Arabic and was the foundation of European pharmacopeia through the nineteenth century,[6] eclipsing the Hippocratic corpus through the early modern period of medical science.

Then came Galen (129–216 CE), of Greek lineage but a Roman citizen, who built upon the work of Hippocrates (including the concept of four humors) to make vast contributions to early medical science, with significant insight into anatomy, physiology, pathology, pharmacology, and neurology.[7] His fame, suggests Guido Majno, "rests on a self-made monument of two and a half million words: twenty-two volumes … about two-thirds of what he wrote; the rest is lost."[8] This contribution to medical science "dominated medical thinking for more than a millennium."[9]

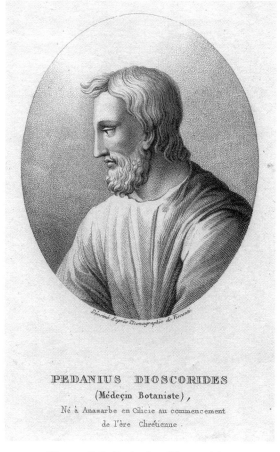

PEDANIUS DIOSCORIDES
(Médeçin Botaniste),
Né à Anazarbe en Cilicie au commencement
de l'ère Chrétienne.

Figure 3.2: Pedanius Dioscorides

He opposed the dominant Stoic paradigm that held the separation of body and mind, insisting that the organs of thought are to be found in the tissues of the body, prefiguring twentieth century somatic theory and neuroscience. He would also apply this as a theory of embodied experience in his approach to psychological problems, using what he called "talk therapy" to draw out deep mental tendencies as a curative method, thus prefiguring twentieth century psychotherapy.[10] Galen's work on physiology was particularly profound, going beyond Hippocrates's understanding of the humors to offer a detailed model of normal body functions as relying on three specific qualities of *pneuma* (air, breath) in the interactions of the lungs, heart, liver, and brain. He also deeply tapped into the *De Materia Medica* in his writings and medical practice. Yet as insightful as he was, his research, much like that of his Indian contemporaries, was limited by the religious-based prohibition against human dissection. Imagine trying to understand internal anatomy and physiology without ever peering into a body, except through wounds and natural orifices.

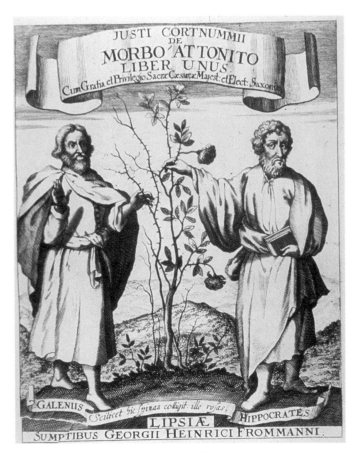

Figure 3.3: Galen

The Greeks made three major contributions to medicine, starting with the idea that disease is a natural phenomenon that can be understood as such, even if the mysteries and miseries of disease and injury were still given some explanation (and much solace) by religion and superstition. Second, the Greeks gave us a theory of humors and with it a set of principles for cultivating a healthy lifestyle based on exercise, diet, and sleep. Finally, they gave us the botanical tools for creating medicinal substances that could cause sleep, induce vomiting, heat or cool the body, and even control pain. Fortunately, much of Greek medical theory and research was translated into the Arabic and Persian languages, for medieval Islamic medical traditions would be the primary source of their transmission after the fall of the Greek and Roman empires.

The syncretic work of the Persian polymath Avicenna (980–1037 CE) during the Islamic Golden Age marks one of the most significant contributions to the early development of medical science. Tapping into the received knowledge and wisdom of Greek, Indian, Persian, and Roman medical texts, his fourteen-volume *Canon of Medicine* applies reason and logic to medicine and pharmacology in keeping with his Islamic faith. But it is his practical medical contributions that most gained traction. Avicenna (the Latin form of the Persian *Ibn Sina*) addressed anatomy and physiology, diseases and symptoms, the nature of the breath, and psychology. He discussed the preventative benefits of exercise, emphasizing self-massage, exercise, and sleep as the three pillars of health. His work clearly marks significant progress in the development of medical knowledge, and, as a complete medical textbook, the *Canon of Medicine* would go on to be the principle medical text in Europe up through the sixteenth century, including in European universities beginning in the twelfth century.

Yet we find utter stagnation in medical knowledge in Europe through the Middle Ages as religious authorities enforced their dogmas and doctrines that explained ailments in purely metaphysical and spiritual terms. It is only with the Black Death in Europe in the late fourteenth century and the emergence of the Renaissance that we find the reemergence of scientific exploration of medicine, the other side of which is the gradual dismissal of medicine based on religious authority, belief, and tradition when found to be untrue.

The second plague, a pandemic that originated in Central Asia around 1345 and killed over half of Europe's population in just a few years, hit Italy especially hard.[11] Typical prescriptions of the day were derived from the idea that the plague was God's will, making acts of repentance the primary cure. Other prescriptions included strapping live chickens around the lymph nodes, drinking potions laced with arsenic and mercury, and wearing herbal garlands to fend off the evil spirits. Historian Barbara Tuchman maintains that the horrors of the pandemic led to a greater focus on life in the here and now, including a growing openness to questioning previously held truths about nature and life, especially as the tools and ideas of open-minded thinkers provided increasingly

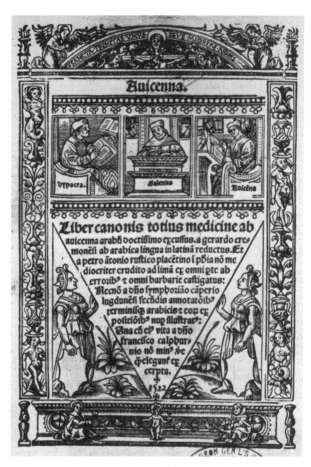

Figure 3.4: Avicenna

sound explanations for the nature of things than those prescribed by traditional authoritative sources.[12] The Copernican revolution's heliocentric model (Earth is not the center of the universe, and this planet of ours revolves around the sun, not the other way around) and multiple other discoveries—including in medicine itself—led to progressively deeper scientific study of human anatomy and physiology, the nature of disease, and methods of healing. By the sixteenth century, Avicenna's *Canon* became a standard textbook in European medical schools, even as those schools paid homage, if not fealty, to the Church.

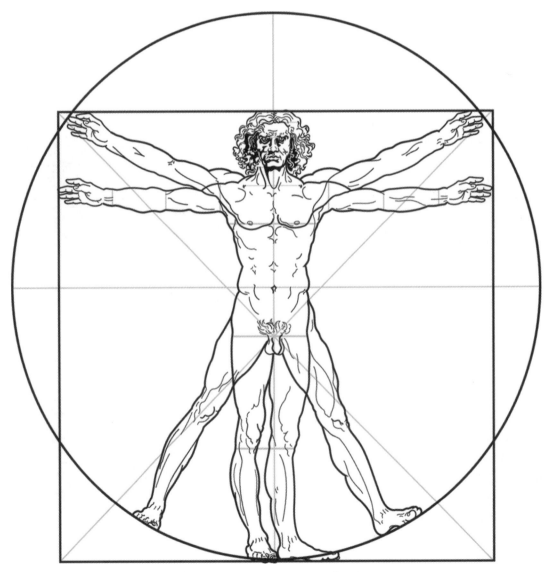

Figure 3.5: Da Vinci's *Vitruvian Man*

SCIENTIFIC DISCOVERY IN THE EARLY DEVELOPMENT OF MODERN MEDICINE

- Andreas Vesalius publishes the seven-volume *De Humani Corporis Fabrica*, 1543.

- Michael Servetus correctly describes pulmonary circulation in *Christianismi Restitutio*, 1553.

- Zacharias Janssen invents the microscope, 1590.

- William Harvey provides a complete and detailed description of the circulatory system in *Exercitatio Anatomica de Motu Cordis et Sanguinis in Animalibus*, 1628.

- Antonie van Leeuwenhoek, discovers microscopic blood cells, bacteria, and microorganisms, 1670.

Perhaps the most significant development in the early modern period of medicine came in the gradual acceptance of the practice of dissection. The first known dissection was conducted by Mondino de Liuzzi (1270–1326) in 1315, resulting in his 1316 book on anatomy, the first ever written based on looking inside a human being.[13] By the sixteenth century, dissection would become increasingly widespread, and with this insight medical science would benefit from the extraordinarily detailed anatomical drawings of Leonardo da Vinci and others. The greatest early anatomist among those others is Andreas Vesalius (1514–1564), whose *De Humani Corporis Fabrica* (1543; "On the Fabric of the Human Body") gives detailed illustrations along with medical explanations.

Scientific Advances

The insights of the anatomists would disturb and revolutionize existing medical theories and practices as they revealed actual—as opposed to imagined or deduced—structures of the human organism. This process of discovery, one that adds light to our understandings even as it casts a shadow over some of the experimental, speculative, yet comforting ideas of past ages, continues to this day with more and more refined technologies for looking inside of living human beings.

Thus, humanity learned a lot in the three hundred years of scientific exploration from the beginning of the Renaissance onward, some of which fundamentally changed our approach to disease and healing. Yet despite all we learned, we still knew very little, still embraced superstitious and faith-based methods, and still experimented (however fruitfully or morbidly), giving practical expression to Aristotle's famous quip that, "the more you know, the more you know you don't know."

In the eighteenth century Age of Enlightenment we find wide application of scientific methods to the development of medical knowledge. By utilizing increasingly powerful technological instruments such as the microscope, conducting empirical tests, measuring results, and replicating studies to verify results, scientists made life-changing discoveries. Germ theory and the larger emergent field of biochemistry helped us understand that many diseases arise from pathogens entering the body from outside. Smallpox had killed millions upon millions over the centuries due to lack of scientific understanding, including in India where it reached epidemic levels (and where the response was to worship Sitala Mata, the goddess who was thought to both cause and alleviate the condition).[14] After this point in time one could take a vaccine to acquire immunity to the disease.

SCIENTIFIC MEDICAL DISCOVERY IN THE AGE OF ENLIGHTENMENT THROUGH THE NINETEENTH CENTURY

- Louis Pasteur demonstrates the relationship between germs and disease, 1860–64.

- Charles Darwin discredits the theory of transmutation and describes the principles of natural selection in biological evolution, 1859.

- Joseph Lister publishes *Antiseptic Principle of the Practice of Surgery*, 1867.

- Robert Koch develops four postulates for isolating disease-causing organisms, 1880.

- Wilhelm Röntgen discovers x-rays, 1895.

- Alexander Fleming discovers antibiotics, 1928.

After the earliest inoculation for smallpox there were steady advances in germ theory, bacteriology, and soon immunology, including Theodor Schwann's discovery of the role of microbes in putrefaction (1837), Friedrich Henle's germ theory of disease (1840), Louis and Marie Pasteur's concept of therapeutic vaccination (1885), Heinrich Koch's demonstration of cutaneous sensitivity (1891), Paul Ehrlich's theory of antibody formation (1900), and Karl Landsteiner's identification of blood groups (1901). In human anatomy, there was already considerable pre-Enlightenment insight in the work by the Egyptians (from as early as 1600 BCE, with a school of anatomy in Alexandria by the third century BCE), the Greeks (the *Hippocratic Corpus* reveals detailed knowledge of the musculoskeletal system, followed by Galen's second-century research into anatomy), and the Belgian scientist Vesalius (his sixteenth century dissections and vivid drawings revolutionized the human anatomy). However, it pales against the precisely detailed understandings made possible by technology.

We find similarly monumental advances in every area of scientific medicine in the wake of the Enlightenment, with many informing others within the subdisciplines of medicine (for example, advances in molecular biology contributed to understanding the structure and function of glands).

Despite these advances in medical science, belief-based, pseudoscientific methods such as bloodletting (for proper balance of the humors) and trepanation persisted well into the late nineteenth century and even early twentieth century, this despite evidence at the time that they were mostly harmful. Some healers advocate these and other unfounded techniques even today.

With the arrival of the twentieth century, we had achieved relatively profound advances in science-based medical knowledge, certainly in contrast to the mostly intuition- and speculation-based understandings of earlier times. In the past one hundred years our knowledge has grown exponentially, especially with the use of technologies such as the electron microscope, magnetic

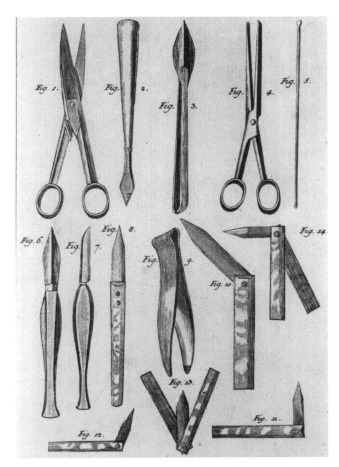

Figure 3.6: Nineteenth Century Bloodletting

resonance imaging (MRI), and more refined methods for isolating and studying the interaction of different cells. Today, we have sophisticated neonatal intensive care units (NICUs) to help newborn babies survive conditions that would have killed them just two generations ago, heart transplants are routine, and yoga students who fail to check their ego at the door and consequently blow out their knees in ill-aligned warrior poses or forced lotus poses can simply have their knees replaced in a common orthopedic procedure.

Conclusion

The advances in medical science seem to generate nearly as many questions as they answer. One question has to do with just how much—and what quality—of evidence one should apply in making health and medical decisions. In what we now call "evidence-based medicine," decisions are optimized based on the use of evidence that indicates best practices. Although this might sound perfectly rational in today's world of rationality, as we have seen, it has not been and still is not always necessarily so. Despite advances in biomedical science, traditional approaches and their underlying assumptions are very much with us today, sometimes as irrational superstition, sometimes as exhaustively considered theories and apparently beneficial practices. As we explore in Chapter 4, we might find beneficial insight in subjecting so-called alternative or nonscientific methods (chakra therapy, crystals, cupping, homeopathy, and others) to well-designed and conducted research with randomized controlled trials.[15]

We *know* there's an endocrine system; we *believe* there are nadis. We *know* there is a brain with cognitive functions shaped by our genetic endowment; we *believe* there are chakras that embody inherited mental tendencies. We *know* that the parasympathetic nervous system regulates the body's unconscious actions; we *believe* that doshic imbalance affects heart rhythm.[16] Meanwhile, much of what we know is affected by what we believe: one might "know" they have a toothache while believing it is caused by a disaffected deity, leaving open the choice of seeing a dentist versus praying to a god (or doing both). One might also so strongly believe in the power of something, say, the immune-system-strengthening effect of echinacea and golden seal, that it has the expected benefit. (This is an example of the placebo effect). Or one might know that the cartilage in her hip is nearly gone based on x-rays and MRIs, but believe that living life more lightly and gracefully is preferable to an invasive hip replacement procedure—and as a result be happier living (even while hurting) with the deteriorating hip cartilage.

Put differently, it behooves us to do our best to know all we can, to honor our beliefs and those of others in matters of life, health, and dying, and to be open to the interaction of knowledge and belief in the care we give and receive. This attitude is well expressed in much of complementary, alternative, and integrative medicine. In the following chapter we explore how we might better integrate these often antagonistic approaches to health and healing.

4

Integrating the Healing Arts and Sciences

Uncertainty is an uncomfortable position.
But certainty is an absurd one.
—VOLTAIRE

WE LIVE IN A WORLD of diverse ideas about health, wellness, and the practices that might best support living in the healthiest ways. There is similar diversity and even conflicting ideas and practices regarding the treatments for what ails us. For the purposes of initial exploration, we can usefully recognize that some of us approach matters of health and well-being with a Western medical perspective that insists on scientific evidence-based practices, while others approach health with a more holistic perspective that taps into a wide variety of what have come to be called alternative medicine and well-being practices. Whereas the former is increasingly specialized and primarily focused on finding cures and reducing specific symptoms, often very effectively, the latter is more focused on the whole being and the personal transformations that can reduce suffering and promote a sense of abiding well-being, often very effectively. Although this represents a wide continuum of typically divergent thoughts and practices, with considerable innovation in between its often opposing or conflicting ends, a basic question we face is how best to integrate various approaches in cultivating health and wellness. In order to get at this, we will look at the ends of the continuum before considering how they might be best integrated with our primary focus on healing in and with yoga.

The Efficacy and Limitations of Scientific Medicine

Since the early twentieth century, we have witnessed amazing biomedical discoveries that have revolutionized health care and led to increased life expectancy around the world. We have gained new and more accurate understandings of diseases, injuries, and other sources of disturbed well-being and how best to treat them, with new discoveries and technologies showing promise for further eradication of disease and better treatment. The burgeoning developments in medical knowledge, technology, and skill might be taken for granted if only because they are increasingly part of common experience in the modern world of medical care. But imagine not knowing that germs exist, let alone how and why they can be pathogenic. Imagine no anesthetics, vaccines, antibiotics, x-rays, insulin, sonograms, or magnetic resonance imaging (MRI). Such was the state of medicine just a century ago (and still is today in many places mired in poverty).

With this in mind, note that life expectancy in the United States, Germany, and England in 1900 was around 43 years of age (in India it was 24 years, in China 32 years),[1] with pneumonia and influenza being the leading causes of death (prior to the 1910 Spanish Flu pandemic), followed by tuberculosis, gastrointestinal infections, heart disease, and stroke. By 2010, life expectancy in the United States, England, and Germany was close to 80 years of age, with heart disease and cancer being the leading causes of death (in India life expectancy in 2010 was 65 years, in China, 76 years).[2] We have nearly doubled life expectancy globally, with the greatest advances in societies with access to clean water, sanitation, and modern health care services. Death by all causes per 100,000 of the population today is about half of what it was in 1900. The most common causes of death in 1900 are rarely causes of death today, except in places where there is a lack of access to modern scientific medicine and to clean water, sanitation, and nutritious food.

Clearly, humanity has made major progress in the quality and longevity of life with the advancement of medical education, scientific research, and treatment technique.

Advances in medical science and social and environmental conditions (especially greater social equality, clean water, and sanitation)[3] get primary credit for the improvement in global health conditions in the last century.[4] To be sure, the early twentieth century optimism that all disease would be eradicated by now was clearly faulty, especially given the current epidemic of obesity, the prevalence of diabetes, and the ongoing mysteries of cancers, all of which are most prevalent in advanced industrial and technological societies. Still, with increasing knowledge of human biology and the pathophysiological basis of disease, we have developed treatments that directly address and relieve the symptoms and underlying conditions of many illnesses, often with seemingly miraculous results. Consider that in nineteenth-century Europe one in four deaths was due to tuberculosis, at the time a condition commonly blamed on vampires, evil spirits, and other mysterious forces. Albert Calmette's and Camille Guérin's successful development of the BCG vaccine in 1906 and the later development of streptomycin finally provided an effective—seemingly miraculous—treatment and cure.[5] Medical breakthroughs with smallpox, syphilis, and tuberculosis arguably changed the world, enabling people to live better lives when they otherwise would have greatly suffered until death. In 2015, rubella—which has killed or permanently harmed millions of babies—was eliminated from the Americas.[6]

The rational scientific approach to medicine (synonymously and sometimes derisively called conventional, scientific, Western, or allopathic medicine) is giving us more and more of this type of specialized insight into disease and health, with very promising areas of further research and development in biology, chemistry, physiology, pharmacology, neurology, and technology, all of which are occurring more rapidly than ever. Much of this advancement in medical science is rooted in the 1910 Flexner Report, which addressed medical education in the United States and Canada.[7] The report highlights the importance of high standards of medical education based on adherence to the scientific method, which led to increasingly focused and specialized scientific medical discoveries—often at the expense of medical teaching and patient care.[8] Increasingly specialized medical science gives us increasingly specialized medical diagnosis and treatment, which in turn gives us increasingly specialized medical professionals with tremendous knowledge and skill in their narrow areas of specialization. If one has a special condition, for example, atrial flutter, it might be wise to see a physician who specializes in cardiac arrhythmias rather than one's primary care physician, acupuncturist, or local shaman, even though the latter might give you a greater feeling of hope, which as we shall see most definitely matters in healing and quality of life, especially with life-threatening conditions.

Yet despite what might seem like science-fictional advances in medical science and method, all is not well in the world, including in the field of medicine and with health in general. Medical care is increasingly expensive, with the highest quality care out of reach for most people. Even when one has access to the most specialized care, the experience is often more one of specialized intervention than empathetic and compassionate human caring—and *a feeling of care matters in health and healing*. Although there are significant individual exceptions, the more specialized the medical provider, the less the provider is capable of appreciating, let alone addressing, the more general conditions and needs of their patients. Unfortunately, this means that with increased specialization, we typically find decreased quality in the physician-patient relationship, moving us further away from the earliest considerations of medicine expressed in the Hippocratic Oath and the less commonly known Oath of Maimonides.

THE OATH OF MAIMONIDES

The eternal providence has appointed me to watch over the life and health of Thy creatures. May the love for my art actuate me at all time; may neither avarice nor miserliness, nor thirst for glory or for a great reputation engage my mind; for the enemies of truth and philanthropy could easily deceive me and make me forgetful of my lofty aim of doing good to Thy children.

May I never see in the patient anything but a fellow creature in pain.

Grant me the strength, time, and opportunity always to correct what I have acquired, always to extend its domain; for knowledge is immense and the spirit of man can extend indefinitely to enrich itself daily with new requirements. Today he can discover his errors of yesterday and tomorrow he can obtain a new light on what he thinks himself sure of today.

Oh, God, Thou has appointed me to watch over the life and death of Thy creatures; here am I ready for my vocation and now I turn unto my calling.

Many, if not most, physicians are motivated to study and practice medicine for its meliorative effects: they want to make people's lives better through better medical science and service, and they usually do. But from the earliest days in medical school until well into one's medical career, there are many interests at play that can compromise or altogether undermine this moral and personal commitment. One might begin by addressing the notoriously stressful conditions of medical school and residency, often rationalized as being similar to the basic training of military recruits who are steeling themselves in preparation for the battles to come.[9] Add the loss of physician autonomy in the growing world of managed care in which insurance companies and large medical corporations can veto physicians' treatment recommendations, and we are moving further and further away from the qualities of care that promote health and healing. The Oath of Maimonides is fading against the potent forces of medicine-as-business.

One could characterize this as a crisis in medical care, with rising costs, alienated medical labor, and patients choosing potentially charlatan or simply ineffective alternatives out of perceived need, confused belief, or frustration. Yet even if all were well in these areas of the medical world, we would still face the reality that despite advances in medical science and technique, many people are made worse, not better, as a direct result of some medical procedures, prescription drugs, and impersonal qualities of care.[10] This might be a significant part of explaining why more and more people are running out the doors of conventional medical institutions and turning to alternative forms of medicine. It also invites us to appreciate the term "crisis," the Mandarin Chinese character for which conveys the dual meanings of danger and opportunity. As we explore further here, we are not interested in throwing out the proverbial baby (informed and effective rational health care) with the bath water (the ill effects of many medical practices), but instead in bathing that baby in nourishing waters of care that tap the monumental insights of scientific medicine while reorienting medicine around the health and healing of whole human beings to complement the narrow focus on curing ailment or repairing injury.

The Efficacy and Limitations of Holistic Medicine

Most people want to be healthy, to experience every moment of life with the greatest sense of wholeness, balance, and well-being. When we consider health, as Andrew Weil suggests, as "a dynamic and harmonious equilibrium of all of the elements and forces making up and surrounding a human being," it opens us to appreciating a much broader perspective on well-being.[11] Rather than approaching health as simply the absence of disease and applying specialized treatment protocols to dehumanized patients, which is a tendency we find in conventional medicine, the holistic perspective on health looks at the entirety of one's life conditions and develops caring and healing (especially self-caring and self-healing) strategies tailored to the unique life of the individual.

In appreciating the whole person—(as we mentioned earlier, the very term "health" is rooted in proto-German and Old English words meaning "whole")—holistic medicine looks at everything that affects one's health and well-being, including stress, exercise, nutrition, relationships, one's sense of meaning and purpose in life, and the natural and social environments. With this expanded view of human health, the holistic health paradigm invites us to relate to health as a continuous, dynamic process of self-care in which the qualities of personal experience and social connectivity matter. In doing so, we open to understanding that our various conditions have everything to do with all we have uniquely inherited and all we have uniquely experienced in our individual lives, with this life experience involving all we have done, thought, felt, and wittingly or unwittingly ingested into our being up to the present moment. We sense that how we are presently living our lives, including our emotional states, nutrition, sleep, relationships, and qualities of meaning, is reflected in our sense balance (or imbalance) and well-being (or dis-ease). This sensibility is ancient.

The recent mantras of holism and holistic health are mere echoes of their ancient roots and long history. Holism is very much at the heart of the most ancient medical systems, whether Hippocratic, ayurveda, or traditional Chinese medicine (TCM). The entire Hippocratic Corpus—and much of ayurveda and TCM—is predicated upon fully appreciating and treating whole human beings based on the most thorough understanding of the patient's life: social and familial circumstances, environmental conditions, lifestyle, where one has traveled, and any other factors that might affect one's presenting condition.

This understanding is grounded in an underlying naturalism in which disease is seen as having natural causes that are best resolved with natural treatments, even if it is ultimately understood within a spiritual philosophy that maintains room for supernatural forces; if one is mystified by the condition, then prayer, sacrifice, or other rituals can be invoked. The humoral philosophies (both Indian and Greek) offer exhaustive explanations for how human health rests in the healing power of nature—*vix mediatrix naturae*—and/or spirit. Since disease is seen as arising from imbalance in one's humoral constitution, and restoration of balance is achieved primarily by natural forces, the purpose of medicine, treatment, or ritual is to tap into one's innate healing capacities (or to appeal to those of a deity) that allow the bodymind to heal.

Although this holistic individualism focuses on the unique needs of the individual person, there is recognition that environmental conditions and social relationships in the community are an integral component of the whole picture of human health (a view that underlies ancient-to-contemporary public health initiatives). In connecting human wellness and healing with the larger environment, ancient-to-modern holistic approaches have also looked to nature's abundant botanical diversity for medicines, leading to the various iterations of *materia medica*—compendiums of plants and herbs and their curative or palliative benefits. We also find an abiding sense of spirit amidst these naturalisms, with openness to the mysteries of life, disease, and healing that sometimes seem or are understood to be altogether magical, metaphysical, or miraculous.

Why have these sensibilities of holism, so deeply rooted in human experience and culture, not easily persisted to the present? The steady rise of scientific medicine from the Renaissance forward, particularly after the eighteenth century, gradually displaced holism with dispassionate molecular analysis of the mechanisms of disease and the related fields of specialization that collectively reduced human beings to so many seemingly disconnected parts and their interactions. Early modern scientists were surely doing their best to give better natural explanations for disease in a world in which disease was still mostly considered in various traditional and superstitious ways. As scientific researchers progressed in their medical discoveries, the intertwined rope of magic, religion, and medicine tended to unravel, despite resistance from the powerful forces of tradition, superstition, and institution. By the mid-nineteenth-century there were strong political movements in favor of scientific medicine and in opposition to what many scientists at the time (and today) considered to be unscientific medicine, some of which was ridiculously dangerous quackery, and some of which today shows efficacy or at least promise in curing disease, promoting healing, or offering hope.

It is in the early period of social and political conflict between scientific and holistic medicine that we first find the various alternatives to conventional medicine collectively referred to as alternative medicine, which covers a widely and wildly diverse array of practices of varying efficacy. The ideological hegemony of allopathic medicine as "medicine" achieved by the inestimably powerful American Medical Association (AMA), formed in 1846, makes all non-allopathic (non-AMA) approaches "alternative" by definition. Since the rise of the AMA, most developments in alternative medicine have primarily occurred outside mainstream medical institutions. This is a direct consequence of the AMA's ruthless mid-nineteenth-century campaign to discredit and marginalize what it considered unscientific medicine (particularly increasingly popular homeopathy, chiropractic, and osteopathy). Thus, whereas it appears that most approaches to medicine in ancient-to-modern times emphasized holism and connectivity—with nature, loved ones, community, and spirit—an irony of modern to contemporary scientific medicine is its tendency to minimize, mischaracterize, and dismiss the relevance of both.

This began to change in 1991 when the U.S. National Institutes of Health (NIH) established the Office of Alternative Medicine (OAM) with a mission "dedicated to exploring complementary and alternative healing practices in the context of rigorous science." The "rigorous science" element soon met resistance, including with U.S. Senator Tom Harkin, a strong advocate of alternative medicine, stating that, "It is not necessary for the scientific community to understand the process before the American public can benefit from these therapies."[12] OAM moved forward in exploring nearly the entire gamut of alternatives to mainstream medicine. One OAM board member, Barrie Cassileth, reacted to what some considered the alternative medicine free-for-all at OAM, stating that, "The degree to which nonsense has trickled down to every aspect of this office is astonishing ... It's the only place where opinions are counted as equal to facts."[13] Paul Berg, a Nobel laureate in chemistry, wrote to Congress: "Quackery will always prey on the gullible and uninformed, but we should not provide it cover from the NIH."[14] The president of the American Physical Society also wrote to Congress, complaining that OAM is "an undiscriminating advocate of unconventional medicine ... some of which violate[s] basic laws of physics and more clearly resembles witchcraft."[15]

Notwithstanding such vociferous opposition, OAM's budget increased to support clinical trials and its name was changed in 1998 to the National Center for Complementary and Alternative Medicine (NCCAM), with CAM defined as "those treatments and health care practices not taught widely in medical schools, not generally used in hospitals, and not usually reimbursed by medical insurance companies."[16] Thus, despite the AMA's and other political, scientific, and religious organizations' steadfast opposition to alternative medicine and their broad success in excluding alternative approaches from medical education, hospitals, and insurance reimbursement, alternative medicine has largely thrived.

In 2014, NCCAM again changed its name; it's now the National Center on Complementary and Integrative Health (NCCIH). Replacement of the term "alternative medicine" with "integrative health" may diminish the impression that NCCIH research, training, and outreach includes quackery, even as it supports research and education around many types of alternatives, including yoga asana, pranayama, and meditation.

The NCCIH's new mission and vision statements symbolize this opening to a more inclusive and truly complementary medicine:

> *The mission of NCCIH is to define, through rigorous scientific investigation, the usefulness and safety of complementary and integrative health interventions and their roles in improving health and health care. NCCIH's vision is that scientific evidence will inform decision-making by the public, by health care professionals, and by health policy makers regarding the use and integration of complementary and integrative health approaches.*[17]

It also defines its terms, offering what are likely to become broadly accepted distinctions. "Complementary" is where a nonmainstream practice is used together with conventional medicine; "alternative" is where a nonmainstream practice is used in place of conventional medicine; and "integrative" is where conventional and complementary approaches are coordinated with each other. NCCIH categorizes complementary health into two approaches: "natural products," including botanicals, vitamins, and minerals, and probiotics; and "mind and body practices, including yoga, chiropractic and osteopathic manipulation, meditation, massage therapy, acupuncture, relaxation techniques, tai chi, chi gong, healing touch, hypnotherapy, and movement therapies such as Feldenkrais, Alexander Technique, Pilates, Rolfing Structural Integration, and Trager psychophysical integration."[18]

Although NCCIH is the U.S. federal government's lead agency for scientific research on complementary and integrative health approaches, it is not alone in this endeavor. For example, The Bravewell Collaborative, a private foundation, chooses and manages its own integrative health initiatives, including those in partnership with the Consortium of Academic Health Centers for Integrative Medicine (CAHCIH). In 2015, CAHCIH reported over 60 major medical schools, medical centers, and research institutions across North America as members involved in significant alternative medicine research and practice, including schools of medicine at Johns Hopkins, Stanford, Harvard, all four University of California medical campuses, Yale, Duke, University of Toronto, and Universidad Autónoma Guadalajara. Kripalu Center for Yoga and

Health and the closely related Kripalu Institute for Extraordinary Living are partnering with NIH and major universities to research specific effects of yoga with children in schools and in other topical areas, including obesity and diabetes.

How will this broad societal embrace of alternative approaches play out? One can reasonably conclude from the sheer volume of current institutional commitments that alternative medicine is here to stay, including those approaches that include various elements of yoga, this despite continuing opposition to anything outside of evidence-based practices from within the medical community and among many government officials and lawmakers.

Even in the absence of mainstream involvement, two other forces continue driving the movement toward greater integration of conventional and alternative medicine: tens of millions of people are making daily choices to try alternative approaches to cures and to feeling more whole, and innumerable practitioners are offering alternative services that are making their way into the mainstream of society as more and more people choose them.[19] Taken together, these various movements show considerable promise for more widely available and better-informed health options, and for more options that connect the diverse array of yoga practices with other forms of care and therapy in order to offer therapeutic services.

Yet all is not so well in the world of alternative medicine. The many options for alternative methods of curing, healing, and living more wholly vary from some that have proven or apparent efficacy and some that plainly do not, even to the degree of being harmful. There are valid concerns raised by critics of some forms of alternative medicine, starting with some people being drawn to quack treatments over efficacious treatments and consequently worsening their condition (including their financial condition). All approaches deserve consideration in assessing their efficacy, not merely through the prism of theories of health and wellness, but through the practical prism of promoting health and wellness.

Healing and Curing: Toward an Integrative Approach

There are many adjectives modifying the concept of medicine: scientific medicine, alternative medicine, allopathic medicine, rational medicine, intuitive medicine, herbal medicine, conventional medicine, and so on. As Snyderman and Weil envision, the success of integrative initiatives will lead to dropping the adjectives in favor of the solitary term "medicine."[20] Although we are far from that occurring, especially with powerful interests, ideologies, and institutions committed to one or another preferred approach, we are closer than we might realize. We can get a clearer sense of this optimism when we appreciate what people are asking for in their lives, particularly with respect to the inevitable challenges to balance and wholeness that occur as a natural part of life, all the more so amid the intensity and complexity of modern life.

Most people want to feel good, to minimize suffering, to have their ills cured, to heal in the most natural ways, to feel whole and connected in meaningful ways, and to have an abiding sense of meaning in every part of life, including when they are ill or dying. These tendencies result in some of the most serious scientists and devoted scientific medicine doctors in the world attending yoga classes, taking non-FDA-approved herbal supplements, and exploring mindfulness meditation.[21] They also result in even the most devout alternative health advocates racing to the conventional hospital when seriously ill or injured. We all seek various forms of medicine, qualities of healing, and sources of meaning. The infinite ways that any of us can tap into the diverse resources for living better lives are primarily limited by the imagination (and access to resources), which is one reason that experience and evidence can help us in making the best choices in relating to the healing arts and sciences.

Ideally we make choices in healing that are informed by the best possible knowledge of our conditions. In writing and teaching about choices in healing and the uses of hope with respect to cancer, including how to balance scientific doubt with clinical hope, Michael Lerner offers important insights that are applicable to any condition. He points out that the term "survive" derives from the French *sur vivre*, literally "to live beyond" one's past experiences.[22] We are all, by definition, surviving (or even thriving). How we do this and the often-fateful choices we make in addressing our conditions are at the heart of integrated approaches. For example, if our condition is incurable or terminal, this points us toward palliative care and the vast range of treatment options from across the spectrum of supportive health practices that can make one's life better—more whole, fulfilling, and meaningful—amid such conditions by reducing symptoms and offering the greatest possible hope for survival.[23]

When our condition lacks clear diagnosis or prognosis, this too points toward palliative care but also curative treatments, offering hope, because hope is in itself a therapeutic tool, especially, as Bernie Siegel stresses, in the absence of certainty.[24] Even if someone has an apparently incurable disease, they can still maximize their survival by cultivating their intrinsic healing resonance, which may or may not affect the disease but that nonetheless has profound effects on other aspects of their life. Thus, it is precisely in the cultivation of wholeness that we create the greatest capacity to heal and cure, for in the absence of wholeness the bodymind's innate healing power is diminished.[25] Put differently, our emotional and mental conditions (how we "feel") are intertwined with our physical conditions (such as the course of a disease). How could they not be, given that emotion and thought arises from the same whole organism that might have a "physical" ailment? Although the focus of scientific medicine tends to be on the physiology of cure, we can enhance our curative prognosis by giving balanced attention to our larger overall state as whole human beings. Whereas alternative medicine might play a direct role in the physiology of cure, it can also play a direct and inestimably powerful role in healing and in preventative health measures.

If our intention is to live with the greatest vitality, balance, and joy possible, then we must go beyond cure to cultivate our fullest health. Even with fully curable conditions, there is much wisdom in complementing what might be considered purely curative treatments with holistic treatments. As part of this, we can offer cautionary counsel regarding potentially harmful treatments, whether allopathic or alternative, including the potential harm from impaired, incompetent, or quack practitioners. We can also look at any challenge to our health as an opportunity to learn more about ourselves and how to live in ways that best suit our conditions and enable us to be as healthy as we can be regardless of circumstance. Going further, even when fully healthy and feeling whole, we can help prevent disease and maintain wellness by utilizing the insights of holistic health in our daily lives, especially by promoting self-care in every aspect of our lifestyle.

Integrative Health in Practice

Yoga therapy, like integrative medicine, always occurs in a certain context of time, space, and culture. Where someone is in the seasons of their life and in the world shapes and conditions what is available in healing and what they might be open to exploring from all that is available. In the ideal world, every option would be available to everybody, and everybody would be open to and empowered to make whatever choices make most sense to them in healing. But this is simply not how the world is today; rather, we lived in socioeconomically stratified societies overlaid with social, cultural, and political forces that reinforce unequal access to healing resources, with the social relations of class, gender, race, and religion being the prime suspects in perpetuating this inequality. Access to mainstream medicine is beyond the means or allowances of a vast part of humanity, whereas many alternative approaches are similarly inaccessible except to the privileged few.[26]

Working in this context in making choices in healing, both yoga therapy and the larger domain of integrative health can still utilize a variety of complementary health practices that are tailored to individual needs and accessible in terms of available resources. The next chapter introduces the processes and protocols by which yoga teachers might best work with each other or with their students to choose such appropriate yoga practices, including by referring students to medical professionals and other care and therapy-givers.

Part of the challenge we face here is the powerful bias and predisposition that is at work at each end of the science-belief continuum. Some will never consider a treatment that fails to meet the highest standards of evidence-based medicine and will thus reject out of hand most alternative approaches. This has a cooling effect on those in the alternative health domain who might otherwise warm to the efficacy of conventional approaches. Others will never rule out what even the wildest imaginations might conceive as having curative power, including techniques for which there is evidence of harmful effects or that rest entirely in the supernatural realm (such as communicating with the dead or employing telekinesis, psychokinesis, or other paranormal methods). This has a cooling effect on those committed to allopathic medicine that might otherwise warm to the efficacy of many alternative approaches, including yoga practices.

The more closely one examines this apparent or potential conundrum, the more it fades when one considers one's choices through the prisms of curing and healing, thereby better appreciating what works (whether "works" is about efficacy in prevention, cure, wholeness, or hope). To better frame this analysis and find a clearer path to appropriate integrative choices and treatment guidelines, we can usefully borrow from the basic health care delivery model distinctions between primary, secondary, and tertiary levels of care, and then within each level of care, we can pose questions about efficacy, client values, conditions, and intentions that can more clearly and fully inform one's choices among the range of available treatments.

Primary Care

Although we might associate primary care with one's first point of consultation with a health professional, here we expand this concept to include one's first steps in cultivating greater health and well-being through self-care. Primary care thus involves the widest scope of practices for preventative health as well as for addressing acute and chronic health problems. It also addresses questions of access to health services, environmental factors, and lifestyle. In approaching primary care in this manner, we typically classify conditions in what are called *nosological systems*, classifications of diseases and disorders along with related treatment guidelines.

The World Health Organization's (WHO's) *International Classification of Primary Care (ICPC)*, which contains 17 categories, can help to further focus assessment of health conditions and treatment options. Category A, General and Unspecified, clearly opens the widest space for holistic approaches, yet there is an essential role for holistic methods in every category. Similarly, the *Diagnostic and Statistical Manual of Mental Disorders, Fifth Edition (DSM-5)* published by the American Psychiatric Association identifies mental health disorders and related treatment guidelines. Although these classifications and recommendations can be a source of deep insight in translating knowledge into practice, their very strengths can also be a source of weakness: the disorder orientation and narrow classification of conditions often fail to describe or fully appreciate that many conditions involve interactions across classifications or diagnostic lines, including frequent instances of dual diagnosis or comorbidity. As a result, they are limited in identifying appropriate levels of care, especially in cases in which treatment guidelines call for specific interventions without addressing the whole person and the larger therapeutic relationships involved in giving and receiving treatment. Ideally, treatment guidelines identify the maximum range of effective treatment options, thereby allowing informed and flexible decision-making in one's choices.

We thus want to give space for a continuum of primary care options, from self-care to professional health care, that can be offered based on what first brings one into contact with a service provider. Depending on the presenting condition, one's location, and availability of services, the service provider could be a yoga teacher, a health clinic, a family physician, or a medical team in a hospital emergency room, any of which might have various degrees of allopathic, alternative, or integrative approaches. In allopathic medicine, most primary care physicians are trained and skilled in family practice, pediatrics, or internal medicine, while in alternative health services, primary care can be found among a wide range of caregivers. Continuity is a key element of primary care, supporting the provision of ongoing guidance, preventative care, and the human connectivity that is essential in holistic health. Whereas acute conditions are generally referred out for secondary or tertiary care, many chronic conditions, including hypertension, depression, anxiety, diabetes, asthma, COPD (chronic obstructive pulmonary disease), back pain, and arthritis are well treated in primary care—all of which can be at least partially treated with yoga techniques.[27] Even with acute conditions, there is a vital role for ongoing primary care in conjunction with secondary or tertiary care.

Secondary Care

Many conditions indicate the need for more specialized care, which, depending upon location, the nature of the health care system, and available resources, could be provided in a variety of settings, ranging from the home to a clinic or hospital. The more focused and skilled treatments offered in secondary care typically address more acute issues as well as skilled attention during childbirth, intensive care, and ancillary treatment services. In the modern world of mostly corporate managed health care systems, secondary care typically requires referral from a primary care physician, thus inhibiting people from directly accessing secondary care. Still, many forms of secondary care, including the services of yoga teachers, physical therapists, respiratory therapists, and dieticians, can be directly accessed through self-referral.

As one gains access to secondary care, the treatment options are vast, as are the opportunities for integration across the fields of both general approach (holistic or allopathic, curative or palliative) and specific treatments. Thus, secondary care is both more specialized than primary care yet also can include the elements of primary care that support preventative care and health maintenance.

Tertiary Care

When primary and secondary caregivers are unable to adequately address a health issue, the issue indicates tertiary care, where one can receive more advanced assessment and treatment. Most cancer treatments, cardiac procedures, neurosurgery, treatment of burns, and other complex interventions are offered in tertiary care. As with secondary care, there is an important complementary role for holistic medicine in support of those undergoing tertiary treatments, even as the core of tertiary medicine remains with specialized and licensed medical professionals.

Although the levels-of-care model provides an initial framework for considering choices in healing, we can go further to explicitly address healing options that appreciate the whole person, including their internal, interpersonal, behavioral, and external conditions. In contributing to the theory of integral nursing, Barbara Dossey and Lynn Keegan utilize Ken Wilber's "great nest of being" concept of integral philosophy to offer a coherent framework for understanding and approaching complementary and integrative holistic nursing.[28] Dossey applies this model to the holistic philosophical foundations found in the British Army nurse and nursing theorist Florence Nightingale's work, which integrated care in ways that are well expressed in Wilber's model.

Here we can apply this perspective as a further refining step in making choices in healing:

Internal: The realm of one's individual personal experience, of "I," this is the space of self-care, fear, hope, and awareness. It is subjective, interpretive, and qualitative. Here our choices in healing are informed by personal intention, values, and maturity.

Interpersonal: The realm of shared experience, of "we," this is the space in which shared cultural values, including those held among caregivers, inform our choices in healing.

Behavioral: The realm of one's biological being, of "it," this is the space of our individual manifestation in the world, where objective and observable qualities inform our choices in healing.

External: The realm of the larger systems we inhabit, of "its," this is the social and environmental space that shapes and delimits our experience of organized health care, including the policies and practices of institutions and government. Here choices in healing are conditioned by laws, policies, and access to resources.

Although replete with potential philosophical dualisms amid a reality we take here as whole, we can avoid the dualist traps and limitations (and equally, materialist or idealist reductionism) by appreciating how with praxis—the realization of theory in practice—the separate realms are convenient abstractions from the ground of experience and actual decision-making. When one comes to making concrete decisions among choices in healing and curing, there will always be some degree of tension among the qualities in the four quadrants of the Wilber/Dossey model that arise from the uniqueness of one's values, conditions, place, relationships, and resources. There will also always be some degree of tension between scientific doubt and clinical hope, the resolution of which is best discovered in informed practice (praxis). As we shall see, questions of evidence or efficacy do not simplistically fall into opposing categories of so-called scientific and so-called alternative medicine, but rather they must apply equally to both.

As Dalen suggests, the primary difference between conventional and unconventional therapies is not their basis in science versus faith, but in their source of introduction: when introduced from within mainstream Western medical circles, they are considered valid by those most in or influenced by those circles, even if introduced without the benefit of scientific study (as with warfarin, heparin, and aspirin in antithrombotic therapy).[29] Similarly, when introduced from outside mainstream Western medical circles, they are considered less valid by those most in or influenced by those circles, even when presented with some semblance of scientific study—and for some in the alternative medicine circles, the findings and practices of allopathic medicine are automatically suspect while there is common deference to the claims of others in alternative medicine, whether or not their claims of efficacy are supported by valid evidence.

To the extent that we wish to offer our services as a complement or alternative to conventional approaches, it will be necessary to establish specific efficacy of yoga practices that are considered valid in conventional circles. As Mohan and Mohan remark regarding traditional knowledge and prioritizing effective methods in yoga, "The fact that knowledge has persisted or been conserved does not mean that it is valuable or effective. History documents superstitions and flawed beliefs being passed on for generations."[30]

To best inform one's decisions at any level of care, we can usefully return to the considerations given in Lerner's work on choices in healing and add recent refinements in how to assess options in promoting health, healing, and wholeness, including the emerging commitment in leading integrative medicine circles to insisting upon the same standards of evidence of efficacy for alternative treatments as applied to conventional treatments.[31] In doing so, we want to preserve the openness to practices and qualities of care that offer hope and palliative experience when one's condition appears incurable or terminal, assessing for safety (does it do no harm?) while letting go of insistence upon efficacy in curing. Integrating these evaluations of practices or interventions, we can usefully proceed by successively posing the following questions that are informed by the American Psychological Association's "Criteria for Evaluating Treatment Guidelines."[32]

WHAT IS THE SCIENTIFIC EVIDENCE FOR THE EFFICACY OF THE PRACTICE?   The basic question here is whether the practice works in relation to the practice objective (i.e., some quality of curing or healing): Is there a beneficial effect that can be demonstrated scientifically? The practice objective is ideally based on the most informed understanding of the condition and its prognosis. To more fully answer this basic efficacy question, one must answer a series of other questions:

- What does the relevant empirical literature indicate about the practice? In giving broad and close consideration to various studies, it is important to evaluate the quality of the studies themselves, particularly the integrity of their experimental design and the consideration of alternative explanations.

- What is the methodological rigor and clinical quality of research supporting the practice? Here we can identify three levels of scientific validity, from strongest to weakest:

    1. Randomized controlled experiments, including clinical trials that rule out plausible alternative explanations

    2. Systematic clinical observation, including systematized clinical case studies and clinical replication series with diverse clients who have a given condition

    3. Clinical opinion, observation, and consensus among qualified caregivers and healers

- What are the practice conditions to which specific interventions have been compared? Again, we can identify three levels of scientific validity, from strongest to weakest:

    1. Is there evidence—based on demonstrations—that the practice is more effective than other known practices?

    2. Is there evidence that the practice is effective beyond simply being in a practice? Put differently, how does the practice compare to placebo?

    3. Is there evidence that the practice is more effective than doing nothing (nontreatment)? If so, is it also harmless?

- Are the special needs of the unique person well matched to the practice, level of care, and type of setting needed for doing the practice? How have efficacy studies for a particular practice considered the special needs of the unique person?

- What is the evidence for specific outcomes in the relevant studies of the practice:

  Population Sample: How well does the method and rationale for selecting participants in the study reflect the actual population of those with the condition?

  Practice Goals: What are the varied values and goals of the student, practitioners, scientists, and others involved in assessing the practice?

  Quality of Life: How does the practice affect one's ability to function in life, including subjective feelings, freedom from symptoms, relationships with others, and larger social, occupational, and environmental interaction?

  Long-Term Consequences: What happens following termination of the practice? What are the enduring effects of the practice?

  Indirect Consequences: What are the effects of the practice beyond reduction of symptoms or prevention of disease or disorder? Does the practice choice enhance qualities of subjective feeling or have other unintended benefits?

  Side Effects: Does the practice cause other types of discomfort, disease, or disorder?

  Satisfaction: How does the person feel, irrespective of measured improvement?

WHAT IS THE PROVIDER'S CREDIBILITY? While the basic issue is competence, we want to go further, insisting upon qualities of care that are consonant with the student's values in healing and reflect a truthful representation of the teacher's qualifications. It is important to note that in most conventional medical settings, there are strong checks on training, competence, and ongoing performance, yet we still find frequent significant lapses despite those checks. There are altogether fewer and far weaker qualifications and checks in the realms of alternative treatment, with some practitioners creating impressions that exaggerate their qualifications. (For example, we find some self-anointed yoga therapists with PhDs in economics or spiritual psychology from unaccredited colleges wearing white lab coats labeled "Dr. John Doe" presenting themselves—with the medical doctor's signature stethoscope around their necks—as though they are on a medical par with trained and licensed medical doctors or other health professionals and teaching college courses on disease or injury-related therapies.) Consider posing these questions:

- What is the practitioner's training? Does he or she hold a professional credential and license in their field of stated expertise?

- What are the standards of competence in the practitioner's field? Does it appear that his or her training occurred in a school or other setting that upholds those standards?

- What claims of skill and accomplishment does the practitioner make in relation to the specific treatments one is seeking? Does the practitioner have and openly share evidence of past efficacy in providing those treatments to others with similar conditions?

- How is the practitioner viewed among his or her professional peers? Does the practitioner have evidence of reviews of his or her work?

- What is the experience of others who have sought treatment from the practitioner for similar conditions?

- Is the practitioner open about sharing the value of other approaches and making referrals for those alternatives? Does he or she tend to downplay or reject the efficacy of other treatments for which there is strong evidence of efficacy?

- Does the practitioner seem honest, trustworthy, and psychologically balanced? Does the client feel comfortable and confident with the practitioner's interpersonal manners?

WHAT IS THE QUALITY OF PRACTICE DELIVERY? Most people make choices in healing and curing in the context of limited financial resources along with whatever physical, mental, and emotional pressures are present in their condition. Consider posing these questions:

- Is the treatment reasonably priced and affordable? If the price is significantly higher than that charged by others, how does the practitioner explain this difference? Does the difference seem reasonable?

- Is the treatment provided in what seems to be a healing or curing setting? Is the setting comfortable to the client?

- What is the experience of others with the qualities of treatment provided by the practitioner?

- Does the practitioner seem open to discussing all treatment options?

- Is the practitioner accessible leading up to and following the treatment?

Essential Considerations in Health and Healing

From ancient times to the present, whether informed or guided by faith, experience, or science, people have attempted to find a greater sense of wholeness and well-being through the four interrelated cornerstones of spirituality, mental hygiene, nutrition, and physical activities (including bodymind practices such as yoga). The first, spirituality, refers to that which gives one a sense of being part of the greater reality of nature, the universe, or spirit, whether this is thought of or experienced in theological terms as given by a religion or through the immediacy of one's sense of being in the currents and mysteries of life. Matters of mental hygiene, highlighted in the first chapter of the *Yoga Sutra of Patanjali* and expressed today largely in the field of psychology, invite us to appreciate and explore the relationship between the activity of the mind and the experience of injury or disease, including how mental activity can affect one's healing. Innumerable dietary and nutritional approaches to health and healing recognize that our tissues are profoundly affected by what we eat, with vast synergistic potential for special dietary approaches offered in conjunction with various forms of treatment. Physical and psychophysiological approaches recognize the role of special forms of exercise, movement, and breathing in both curing and healing.

Yoga and ayurveda attempt to work with each of these elements in integrated ways, including ways that can be integrated with other treatment modalities. Here our primary focus is on yoga, with references to ayurveda and other potentially healing modalities where there is evidence for their complementary efficacy. We will look closely at the general methods of yoga therapy as well as specific yoga practices.

When thinking about health and healing, we are wise to always appreciate the realities of aging, the natural processes of living that lead to dying, and the limitations of medicines and treatments. Whatever one's beliefs or nonbeliefs, we were all born and we will all die—even if what happens after is either a complete mystery or a matter of faith. Living more consciously can bring us to aging more gracefully and dying more lightly, our acceptance of these realities giving us much of our character and the quality of our experience all along the path.

Part II

The Human Bodymind's Major Systems

IN THE VIEW OF THE scientific model of the human bodymind, we are, at least in part if not wholly, biological systems that nature has evolved to become as we are becoming. In this becoming we are also aware, with some modicum of consciousness, of being alive. In this life, we can become more conscious of the wholeness of our being, even to awaken consciousness throughout the entirety of our somatic selves, and live consciously in ways that relate to our own development and life experience.[1] How we do this, the very prisms through which we seek to understand ourselves and become more powerfully conscious agents of our own destinies, will go far in determining the quality of our lives.

When thinking of biological systems, many people think of plants and animals in nature, a nature that some consider somehow distinct from human beings. We think of bees drinking sweet juices from flowers, sustaining the energy demands of their rapid wing movements while helping spread pollen from flower to flower. We think of fish swimming in tidal reefs in symbiotic relationships with algae and other life. We think of ancient forests, their trees rooted deeply into soil that sustains myriad interrelated life forms. And sometimes we might even think of ourselves, especially when feeling something awry. But what we often fail to remember or simply do not appreciate is that we too are biological systems rooted just as deeply in the soil, the water, the air, the energy of the sun, and all that makes up our natural environment.

Our own biological systems are many and complex. As with all living creatures, we are made up of molecules that are organized for certain functions, which in turn give us the cellular interactions that form our various tissues, such as muscles, bones, and nerves. Our tissues combine to carry out certain functions through organs such as the heart, lungs, and kidneys. The organs are organized in a certain way that makes these functions possible and sustainable. For example, the heart is a set of muscular chambers that pulsate to pump blood through the vessels of the circulatory system.

In every instance, we find that human organ systems are integrally interrelated, even while retaining their defining features. They do not function either independently or autonomously from one another. Rather, every human body system initially gains its functionality—and we gain life as wholly integrated human organisms—through the reproductive system, where two interconnected cells develop into many more cells that are mutually supportive and develop into the entirety of the bodymind. This quality of interdependence of cells and systems is essential, not only to our existence, but to the existence of all life forms (except for single-celled organisms such as bacteria and algae), however simple or complex they may be. Consider these examples of human system interdependence:

- Without the reproductive system, there would be no systems. It is the source of all systems and the one that allows our species to continue.

- Take away the endocrine system and there would be no hormones to regulate and support reproduction, digestion, circulation, or our immunities.

- Take away the digestive or urinary system and the musculoskeletal system would not be able to obtain nutrients, gain energy, or rid itself of waste.

- The circulatory system helps with some of those same functions, starting with carrying oxygen and nutrients to every cell in the body, plus it transports white blood cells to all infections and injuries, contributing a vital element to the immune system.

- The circulatory system needs the respiratory system for gas exchange, the muscles need oxygen that is absorbed through the lungs in order to move, and the brain needs it to cogitate.

- Skeletal muscles move the skeleton, cardiac muscle allows the heart to pump, and smooth muscle is the source material of our internal organs, including all of our various tubes.

- Without a skeleton the human body would have no shape, there would be no red blood cell production, and the brain, heart, spinal cord, and other internal organs would be exposed to physical trauma.

- Without skin we would lose our first line of defense against pathogenic invasion and would be seriously challenged in maintaining heat and homeostasis. We would also dry out.

- Without the nervous system, the heart would not know when to beat, the digestive system would not know when to add enzymes, and the body would not know when to move.

This interdependence is evident in illness and injury, as we will explore more in looking at each system and also with regard to specific conditions. For now, consider these examples of interdependence and interrelationship:

- Smoking tobacco not only irritates the lungs, it destroys the macrophages of the immune system.

- If you develop AIDS, the immune system is severely challenged, increasing your likelihood of contracting pneumonia (a respiratory condition), a yeast infection (most often a reproductive system condition), or Kaposi's sarcoma (an integumentary system condition).

- An intestinal infection that causes diarrhea can result in dehydration due to fluid loss, and, although very rare, to cerebral edema (brain swelling), seizures (when electrolytes are out of balance), kidney failure (when they are no longer able to remove excess fluids and waste from the blood), and even coma and death.

Taken as a whole, our system of organs—eleven organ systems in all—gives us the wholeness of our biological existence as living and integrated human organisms, otherwise known as human beings. The complex interactions of these systems strive for homeostasis, a quality of internal self-regulation of temperature, acidity/alkalinity (pH), blood glucose levels, circadian rhythms, and other balances that maintain the stability of our whole organism in constant interaction with the natural environment. This reality, even if described with abstract concepts and turgid prose, can be a thing of profound, sublime beauty. It is the scientific prism through which we understand the human bodymind. Here we will survey these systems of the human bodymind.

5

Skin:
The Integumentary System

The finest clothing made is a person's own skin, but, of course, society demands something more than this.
—MARK TWAIN

THE SKIN—in medical terms the integument—is literally (anatomically) superficial: closest to the surface of the bodymind. The common metaphorical phrase "only skin deep" taps this superficiality. But the skin is a deeply significant part of our inner and outer relationships, serving as a porous barrier to the outside environment that protects us from infectious agents, helps maintain homeostasis through sweat glands and blood vessels, and sensitizes us to our surroundings through sensory nerve endings. Indeed, when unaffected by things, we might say someone has "thick skin." But you might want to be careful not to "play out of your skin," especially when exposed to the sun. This is because the skin's protective role, in relative combination with internal biochemistry, also subjects it to potentially injurious forces that can cause abrasion, laceration, and infection, including life-threatening melanoma and other forms of skin cancer.[1]

Although superficial and vital, the skin is also a complex organ that makes up about 15 percent of body weight, forming an envelope for the body's deeper tissues and organs. It is the outermost layer of the larger integumentary system, which is comprised of the skin itself, the subcutaneous layer, deep fascia, and integumentary derivatives such as hair and sweat glands. This surface (integument) level is comprised of three layers: the epidermis, dermis, and hypodermis, the latter also called the subcutaneous tissue or superficial fascia.

The Epidermis, Dermis, and Hypodermis

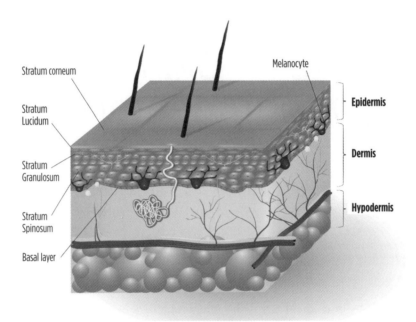

Labels on figure: Stratum corneum, Stratum Lucidum, Stratum Granulosum, Stratum Spinosum, Basal layer, Melanocyte, Epidermis, Dermis, Hypodermis

Figure 5.1: The Integument: Epidermis, Dermis, Hypodermis

The epidermis, the most superficial layer of cells in the skin, is made up of ninety percent keratinocytes, which produce keratin, the fibrous structural substance that makes skin into the protective layer it is. More technically known as a stratified squamous epithelium,[2] it is an avascular structure (i.e., it has no blood vessels—and no lymphatics) that is constantly shedding its most superficial cells while being fed new cells from below (from its lowest layer, the basal layer). It is nourished by both the vascular dermis below and oxygen in the surrounding air. The epidermis itself has a layered structure, from the superficial cornified layer to the basal (or germinal) layer, that germinates and releases keratin cells that rise to the surface, constantly creating new skin even as old skin sheds. Put differently, the basal layer is the source of the rest of the epidermis. Nerve endings rising from the subcutaneous layer through the dermis and into the epidermis give us surface-level sensitivity to touch and temperature.

The dermis is immediately below the epidermis, separated from it by a thin basement membrane; together they form the cutis, below which are the subcutaneous tissues. Interlaced collagen and elastic fibers arranged in parallel rows form the dermis layer, giving the skin its strength, tone, and wrinkle lines. (This layer in animal hides is used to make leather.) It has fingerlike projectiles that extend into the epidermis to keep the two layers from sliding over each other. Within the dermis we find sensory nerve endings as well as hair follicles, sweat and subcutaneous glands, and vessels carrying lymph and blood.

Below the dermis we find the hypodermis, also called the subcutaneous tissue or superficial fascia. Composed of fatty connective tissues, the hypodermis has varied distribution and density of fat, with very little in some places (such as the shin) and often more or less than one wishes in other places (such as around the belly or in the face). The density and distribution of fatty subcutaneous tissue is determined by one's genetics, including sex, and lifestyle, especially diet and exercise. Within this fatty tissue we find hair follicle roots (with hairs growing en route to the surface), blood vessels (en route to the dermis), lymphatic vessels (en route from the dermis), cutaneous nerves (en route to the dermis and free endings within the hypodermis), and sweat glands (en route to the surface). These integumentary derivatives (sometimes called appendages) are essential components of the larger integumentary system that are made from elements of the system itself.

Hairs: Hairs—actually, hair follicles—are formed by extension of the skin (epidermis and dermis cells) deeper into the body, sometimes into the hypodermis. The hair shaft grows out from the hair root located at the base of the hair follicle. Whereas scalp and facial hairs grow continuously, most other hairs grow to fixed lengths.

Glands: There are three types of glands in the integumentary system. Sweat glands—specifically eccrine sweat glands—are found in the skin over almost the entire expanse of the body and serve primarily to regulate body temperature by secreting water to the surface of the skin. They also serve to excrete water from the body and to protect the body from colonization of bacteria. (Apocrine sweat glands are located only in the armpits and perianal areas and produce an odor that may contain pheromones and have a role in social interaction (specifically in attraction or revulsion). Sebaceous glands, which produce an oily substance that lubricates the skin and hairs, keeping them flexible, are in all areas of the skin except the palms and soles. They are most prolific around the walls of hair follicles but are also found in areas free of hair where they rise to the surface. These glands are the source of acne, sebaceous cysts, and adenoma, a slow-growing tumor that indicates a potential for skin cancer. Mammary glands are found in adult females anterior to the chest muscles in the subcutaneous layer, providing a source of milk for newborn babies. Mature mammary glands secrete milk not from the sucking action of the infant but rather from oxytocin-induced stimulation of myoepithelial cells. Breast cancer most commonly develops in these cells and the lobules that supply the ducts with milk.

Nails: Nails, which grow continuously, are produced by the epidermis and serve to protect the ends of the thumbs, fingers, and toes. They readily reveal recent physiological imbalances, including the effects of nutrition, and have been used since ancient times (in Western and Eastern medicine) as an indicator of certain health conditions. Although we think of the nails as being hard and solid, they are in fact more permeable than skin and can thus allow the introduction of bacteria, even though the relatively common paronychia starts as a soft tissue infection, not because of bacteria coming through the nail.

Deep Fascia

Going deeper yet, we come to a thin layer of investing deep fascia, what some consider true fascia in contrast to the superficial fascia found in the subcutis of the integument. Deep fascia is dense, organized, fibrous connective tissue that surrounds and penetrates ("invests" in) deep structures such as muscles, bones, nerves, and blood vessels. (Visceral [or parietal] fascia suspends the organs within their cavities.) Like ligaments, aponeuroses, and tendons (they are all made of closely packed bundles of collagen fibers), the deep fascia is a relatively flexible structure; while flexible, the deep fascia forms compartments capable of resisting muscular tension, limiting outward expansion of muscles as they contract, and thereby contributing to pushing blood out of muscles and toward the heart (becoming a musculovenous pump).

Common Integumentary Pathologies

Although the skin is our first line of defense and a vital player in homeostasis, it is also the source of insight into a variety of imbalances or pathologies hiding deeper in the body's tissues. Much of this insight arises from understanding outward appearance and sensation, where surface-level symptoms might provide clues to underlying conditions. There are literally thousands of different skin diseases.

Rash: There are innumerable causes of skin rash, ranging from allergic reactions to food, medicines, stings, and plants such as poison oak or sumac; overexposure to sun, heat, or dry conditions; emotions such as anxiety; external chafing; and skin diseases such as eczema and acne that are caused by conditions deeper into the integument itself. Less common causes include autoimmune disorders such as psoriasis, and diseases such as Lyme disease, measles, chicken pox, scabies, and scarlet fever.

Blisters: Blisters form when serous fluid (pus) collects in between the epidermis and dermis. Like rashes, blisters have a variety of causes, mostly from external sources such as friction, pinching, crushing, extreme temperature, or chemical agents. Internal conditions such as chicken pox and measles can also result in blisters.

Athlete's Foot: This contagious skin disease is part of a larger group of fungal infection (mycoses) conditions called *tinea* (more commonly known as ringworm). *Tinea pedis* (Athlete's Foot) specifically manifests between the toes but may spread through contact to other parts of the body.

Sunburn: Like other radiation burns, sunburn damages the skin. Ultraviolet radiation causes protective inflammation (thus the reddening of the skin), direct DNA damage, and the release of melanin as a protective agent, which gives the skin a tan hue. Sunburn can increase risk of developing melanoma, a form of skin cancer.

Skin cancer: Basal cell carcinoma (rarely metastasizes), squamous cell carcinoma (more frequently metastasizes), and melanoma are the main types of skin cancer. Their primary causes are overexposure to UV radiation, smoking tobacco products, chronic nonhealing wounds, and papillomas.[3]

Acne: Technically called *acne vulgaris,* 80 percent of acne is caused by genetics and most of the remainder is caused by hormonal activity or bacterial infection. Blockages in the follicles from oil and dead skin cells prevent glandular secretions from traveling along the hair shafts and through the portals of the hair follicles to the surface of the skin. This creates a plug in the pores where bacteria can thrive, resulting in various degrees of acne.

Herpes: The herpes simplex virus causes this viral disease. There are two viruses, HSV-1, which manifests around the mouth, and HSV-2, commonly known as genital herpes, both of which cause blistering or small ulcers. Once infected, one will always carry the virus, which is highly transmittable. These viruses can decrease immune function and are sometimes associated with various cognitive disorders. They are also found together with human papillomavirus (HPV).

Psoriasis: From a Greek word meaning "itching condition," *psoriasis vulgaris* is a poorly understood chronic immune system–related systemic condition with both genetic and environmental influences. It is associated with increased risk of cancer, cardiovascular disease, and immune-mediated disorders such as Crohn's disease.

Cultivating a Healthy Integumentary System

The top seven results of a Google search for the terms "skin" and "yoga" are all about the most superficial aspect of skin: not the health of the most superficial layer of the dermis, but how it appears. We are offered "yoga for naturally glowing skin" (artofliving.org), "6 powerful yoga asanas for glowing skin" (stylecraze.com), "yoga asanas and pranayamas to get a glowing skin naturally" (healthnbodytips.com), "how to get that yoga glow: 5 yoga poses for beautiful skin" (yoga.com), "how 30 days of yoga gave me the best skin of my life" (self.com), "15 best yoga asanas and pranayama for naturally glowing skin" (thefitindian.com), and "9 yoga poses that promise beautiful and glowing skin" (indiatimes.com). The results are about the same when substituting the term "ayurveda" for "yoga." In Tara Stiles's *Yoga Cures*, we find practices for four skin conditions (acne, cellulite, dark eye circles, and wrinkles), starting with a discussion of acne that celebrates "that yoga glow."[4] She goes on to offer a few asanas for each condition. "Have acne?" she says. "Try Plank, Chataranga Dandasana, Side Plank, and Bow." She seems to be working under the theory that chemical aspects of stress cause acne and that these stressful asanas are a way to practice being calm amid stressful circumstances and can thereby help reduce acne. We appreciate the idea and indeed recognize this as a general benefit in practicing many yoga asanas, even if the development of acne follows a more nuanced course.

Here we want to emphasize that healthy skin depends primarily on a healthy diet and minimal exposure to the sun, including the routine use of sunscreen whenever outdoors. And healthy skin is deeper than the skin's most superficial layer, the appearance of which reveals deeper conditions than those addressed by the various superficial recommendations found in the preceding yoga sources.

Most studies of exercise and skin health focus on the effects of sweat on skin tissues, which is generally beneficial unless accumulated sweat is left on the surface of the skin for too long (which can lead to conditions like miliaria in which sweat glands get plugged, which causes a mild rash). We often find promotions for "yoga detox" classes in which sweating is offered as a way to both rid the body of toxins—which is pure myth except for the sweat glands in the armpits and crotch—and beautify the skin. Put differently, sweating is not a significant means of detoxification.

Skin appearance manifests from the functioning of every human physiological system. Our skin thereby reveals disease or dysfunction in most of our systems. When we are generally healthy, when all of our systems are properly functioning, and we minimize sun exposure, we tend to have healthy skin. Thus, rather than doing a specific set of asanas or pranayamas said to affect the skin, the basic yoga approach to healthy skin is to have a well-balanced and regular yoga practice that helps to ensure overall health.

In ayurveda, skin prescriptions are based on the balance of doshas. The vata person tends to have dry and thin skin, the pitta person tends to have reddish and warm skin, and the kapha person tends to have oily and thick skin. Pacifying treatments are given for each doshic constitution: if vata, drink warm water, eat sweet fruit, add oils to your diet, and receive *abhyanga* (warm oil massage); if pitta, avoid spicy food, eat sweet fruit, receive a rose (cooling) oil massage, and use cooling spices such as fennel in cooking; if kapha, avoid sweet and fried food, receive daily abhyanga, cook with warming spices such as ginger, and exercise to stimulate circulation.

Want healthy skin? Cultivate general health. And rather than doing yoga on the beach, try doing it under a tree or in a yoga studio. Enjoy the shade and you will enjoy a healthier integumentary system.

6

Bones and Joints: The Skeletal System

To live in this world you must be able to do three things: to love what is mortal; to hold it against your bones knowing your life depends on it; and, when the time comes to let it go, let it go.
—MARY OLIVER

WESTERN MEDICAL SCIENCE HAS FOUR main disciplines for studying and understanding human stability and movement. Osteology studies the bones and skeletal system, arthrology looks at joints and articulations, myology studies the muscles, and neurology considers the nervous system. Stability and movement arise from the interaction between these systems, which taken together, give us the mainstays of our neuromuscular functioning. Here we will first look at the skeletal system, including its arthrology, before we survey the muscular system that acts on the skeletal system to create stability and movement. Later we will revisit stability and movement, looking through the prism of kinesiology to consider the interactions of neuromuscular and biomechanical forces.

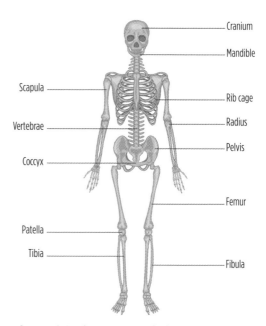

Figure 6.1: The Human Skeleton (Revealing Axial and Appendicular Parts)

Bones

The adult human skeletal system consists of two hundred and six bones, most with accompanying cartilage that allow for their smooth movement. As we will soon see, the bones come in a variety of shapes and sizes, with greater concentrations of bones in areas that require greater support and mobility. Over half of all bones in the human body are found in the hands (twenty-seven bones each) and feet (twenty-six bones each); another twenty-four are found in twelve pairs of ribs, twenty-six are in the vertebral column, and twenty-nine are in the head, leaving only twenty-one bones for the rest of the body. (The fifty-two teeth are technically part of the skeletal system, but they are not generally counted as bones.)

This internal structural framework of the body has six major functions:

Support for the Body: The basic structure of the skeleton provides general support for the body's overall shape and posture.

Protection of Vital Organs: Various bone structure protect different vital internal organs. For example, the rib cage protects the heart and lungs (with help from the spine and sternum), the skull protects the brain, the vertebrae protect the spinal cord, and the pelvis protects the lower pelvic organs.

The Mechanical Basis of Movement: Bones provide attachment points for muscles that, when stimulated by neurological impulses, cause the bones to move. This movement occurs at the intersection—joints—of different bones.

Blood Formation: Hematopoiesis, the continuous process of blood cell production from stem cells, occurs in the marrow of the femurs, humeri, vertebral bodies, and the sternum. (If necessary, extramedullary hematopoiesis—blood cell production outside the bones—can occur in the liver, thymus, and spleen, as is the case during fetal development when the bones are not yet developed.)

Mineral Production and Storage: The bones produce and store several minerals that are essential elements in bone development and larger system physiology, including calcium and phosphorus.

Endocrine System Regulation: Bone cells secrete a protein called osteocalcin that regulates insulin production and sensitivity, a relatively recent discovery that solves the mystery about the function of this protein.[1]

The skeleton can be divided into two parts, the axial skeleton and the appendicular skeleton. The axial skeleton consists of the skull, hyoid, vertebral column, thorax, and pelvis. It serves as a protective encasement for the central nervous system and many vital organs. The appendicular skeleton consists of the upper and lower extremities, including the pelvic and shoulder girdles. It serves as a means of movement in space (as in walking) and creative expression (as in whatever we do with our arms and hands). (Some anatomists classify the pelvis with the axial skeleton because of its important articulation of the spine with the lower extremities.)

Bones take many years to grow. In a newborn infant, the skeleton has over 275 different bone and cartilage structures, with the cartilage gradually ossifying into bone and some bones fusing to form larger bones. As we explore here and elsewhere, the fact that bones and their closely related structures (tendons, cartilage, and ligaments) are not fully formed until adulthood has major implications for children and youth in the practice of asanas.[2] Fully developed bones are classified in five categories:

Long Bones: Tubular in shape, long bones have a cylindrical shaft called the diaphysis that contains the medullary cavity where bone marrow is found. The diaphysis is covered with a fibrous membrane called the periosteum (as are all bones, except at the articular surfaces of long bones), where arteries enter the bones to provide vasculature. Long bones have rounded protruding heads at each end of the shaft called epiphyses, which are usually enlarged and shaped to allow articulation with the bone(s) to which they are linked. The epiphysis is covered with articular (hyaline) cartilage to allow the smooth movement where bones articulate at joints. Most bones in the limbs are long bones (thigh, lower leg, upper arm, forearm, toes and fingers).

Short Bones: Roughly cube-shaped, relatively small, and solid (they have only a thin layer of compact bone and a spongy interior), short bones are found primarily in the carpal (wrist) and tarsal (ankle/foot) structures where one function of their structure is shock absorption.

Flat Bones: Typically thin, curved, and varying from thick to thin, flat bones have two layers of compact bone that sandwich a thin layer of spongy bone. They are generally protective structures, comprising most of the bones of the skull (protecting the brain) as well as the ilia, sternum, and scapulae.

Irregular Bones: With irregular and complicated shapes other than long, short, or flat, the irregularity of these arises from either multiple

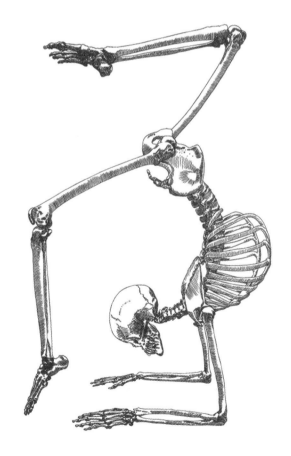

Figure 6.2: Diverse Bone Shapes

centers of ossification or boney sinuses. The vertebrae, ishium, and sphenoid bones are all irregular.

Sesamoid Bones: These small bones develop in certain tendons to provide protection (in the case of the patella) and/or greater mechanical leverage (the patella in the knee, the pisiform in the wrist).

Various markings and other external features are found on bones to serve specific functions. Markings are divided into processes and cavities. Processes are elevations or projections (such as the spinous processes of the vertebra) that either form joints (such as the articular facets of the vertebra) or provide for the attachment of tendons or ligaments. Cavities are depressions that allow for the passage of tendons, vessels, and nerves. There are many more specific markings and formations, including condyles, crests, foramen, fossa, grooves, lines, notches, protuberances, spines, trochanters, and tubercles. Each has specific characteristics that give it its unique function in the skeletal system.

Joints

Most bones in the human skeleton join with other bones to form links or segments called joints.[3] We will survey a wide variety of joints in the following pages. These articulations allow movement except where they function more exclusively for stability and protection (in the skull, sternum, and pelvis, where movement is either nonexistent or extremely minimal). As a general principle, the most stable joints are least movable (think of the skull), while the most movable are the least stable and thus vulnerable to dislocation (think of the shoulder).

There are three types of joints: cartilaginous, fibrous, and synovial. These classifications reflect how and with what substance the articulating bones are joined.[4]

Cartilaginous Joints

Cartilaginous joints are only slightly movable. They are either primary cartilaginous joints connected by hyaline cartilage, or secondary cartilaginous joints joined by fibrocartilage. Primary cartilaginous joints are temporary unions in early life that allow space for growth and eventually develop into bone. Secondary cartilaginous joints, or symphyses, are coated with hyaline cartilage and have fibrocartilage between them. Examples include the pubic symphysis and intervertebral discs. We closely consider the intervertebral discs when looking at the spine and the pubic symphysis when looking at pregnancy (related to the effects of relaxin hormone, as discussed in Chapter 25).

Fibrous Joints

Fibrous joints are sutured together by fibrous tissue. Fibrous joints of the skull (also called suture joints) and those of the teeth (gomphosis joints) are immovable. Another type of fibrous joint allows for slight movement: the syndesmosis, found in the joint of the distal tibia and fibula in the lower leg, and, with a connection through the interosseous membrane, between the ulna and radial bones in the forearm.

Synovial Joints

Synovial joints are the most common type of joint. They are freely movable (diarthrodial) and are joined by a ligamentous tissue called the articular or joint capsule that envelopes a joint cavity. Resilient hyaline cartilage coats the articulating bone surfaces, protecting the bones from wear. Aging and excessive use can cause premature or excessive wear to the cartilage and bone ends, leading to pain and limited range of motion. The fibrous joint capsule is lined with a synovial membrane that seals in viscous synovial fluid, which lubricates the cartilaginous joint surfaces and thereby further reduces friction and wear. Most synovial joints with incongruous articulating surfaces have fibrocartilaginous discs between their articular surfaces that enhance shock absorption. Examples include the menisci of the knees and glenoid labrum of the glenohumeral (shoulder) joint.

Synovial joints gain greater stability with the support of ligaments, which connect bone to bone (not to be confused with tendons, which connect muscle to bone). The ligaments can be either extrinsic or intrinsic: extrinsic ligaments are independent of the joint (but nonetheless hold together the bones comprising the joint); intrinsic ligaments are a thickening part of the joint capsule and surround it. In most people, the ligaments are naturally taut, helping to stabilize the joint within a safe range of motion. Where there is ligament laxity (a hereditary condition) or where ligaments are forcefully stretched (causing ligament laxity), the joint is less stable and consequently more vulnerable to hypermobility (moving beyond safe range of motion) or injurious dislocation.

There are six major types of synovial joints:

Ball and Socket Joints: Also called spheroidal or enarthrodial joints, ball and socket joints are highly mobile multiaxial structures that allow movement in every plane of motion (frontal, sagittal,

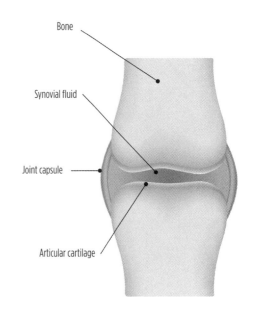

Bone

Synovial fluid

Joint capsule

Articular cartilage

Figure 6.3: Synovial Joint

transverse): flexion and extension, abduction and adduction, medial and lateral rotation, and circumduction. Here a rounded surface of one bone articulates with the socket of another bone (such as the femoral head in the acetabulum and the humeral head in the glenoid cavity).

Biaxial Ball and Socket Joints: Also called condyloidal (knuckle-like) or ellipsoidal joints, these ball and socket joints allow movement in two planes (frontal and

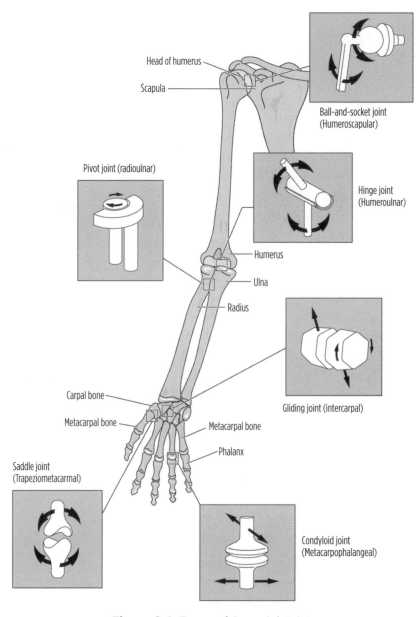

Figure 6.4: Types of Synovial Joints

sagittal) but no rotation. Examples include the radiocarpal (wrist) joints and meta-carpophalangeal (knuckle) joints.

Hinge Joints: Also called ginglymus joints, hinge joints typically have a wide range of motion but only move in one plane, allowing flexion and extension only. The hinge is stabilized by strong ligaments on the sides of the joint while its anterior and posterior sides are free of such ligamentous limitation of movement. Examples are the knees and elbows.

Pivot Joints: Also called trochoidal, rotary, or screw joints, pivot joints allow rotation along an axis. In the forearm, rotation of the proximal radius bone creates supination and pronation; rotation of the Atlas (the C1 vertebra) around the dens (odontoid process) of the Axis (the C2 vertebra) rotates the head at the atlantoaxial joint.

Plane Joints: Also called arthrodial joints, plane joints have relatively flat opposing surfaces that allow sliding or gliding movements between bones, with range of motion being limited by tight articular capsules. Examples are the carpal bones of the wrists and the acromioclavicular joint between the acromion of the scapula and the clavicle in the shoulder girdle.

Saddle Joints: Also called seller joints, saddle joints allow movement similar to biaxial ball and socket joints (flexion, extension, abduction, adduction) but no rotation. The prime example is the base of the thumb (the carpometacarpal joint, which is more prone than any other joint to arthritis), where reciprocally opposing convex and concave surfaces mutually articulate.

Joint Stability and Movement

All joints are relatively stable and relatively mobile, with these qualities typically in inverse proportion to each other: more stability generally yields more mobility and vice versa. However, this is not always true: one can have both great stability and mobility depending on the condition of their muscles and ligaments (think of the adept yogi who is capable of calmly stabilizing in fantastically open asanas, or most high-level gymnasts). We can define *stability* as the ability of a joint to move through its range of motion free of injury to the joint itself and to its stabilizing tissues (primar-ily ligaments and muscles). We find even greater stability when a joint can withstand shock from high-impact movements, such as catching a fall by placing one's hand on the ground without separating joints in the shoulder girdle. When lacking stability, one is more prone to dislocation, sprained ligaments, or undue pressure on surround-ing muscle and nerve tissues.

There are three sources of joint stability, with weakness in any compromising the support of the others and making the joint less stable:

A snug fit in the joint articulation: The glenohumeral joint of the shoulder is relatively shallow and thus not stable, whereas the hip joint—both are ball and socket structures—has a deep recession in the receiving acetabulum and is therefore more stable.

A robust and well-structured set of ligaments: The quality and quantity of ligaments surrounding the hip joint help prevent its potential dislocation, whereas ligaments around the shoulder joint are far less sufficient to prevent dislocation.

Strong muscular support: Rather than merely strong muscles, the key to the muscular stability of a joint is in the opposing forces that muscle can create to maintain the proximity of the bones comprising the joint. For example, there are four muscles in the shoulder joint that provide opposing directions of force that help maintain its stability (together they form the shoulder rotator cuff, which we explore later).

Mobility is the ability to fully and naturally move a joint without disturbing or being limited by surrounding tissues. As discussed earlier, many joints are capable of multiple movements. We define these movements as *range of motion (ROM),* a common measure of flexibility. Joint ROM ranges from hypomobility, in which different structures limit full ROM, to hypermobility, in which one can create movement beyond the joint's normal maximum extension. Whatever one's ROM in any joint, it is ultimately limited either by bony structures (one bone hits another), ligaments (which have very little elasticity), and/or muscular tension.

Although ROM in any joint varies across the landscape of humanity, kinesiologists provide us with average normal ranges of motion that are good starting points for considering generally safe ROM.[5] Although it may seem that greater flexibility is associated with weakness—and as discussed earlier flexibility is typically associated with instability—strength can be developed in tandem with flexibility to allow for greater range of stable movement. Still, moving beyond normal range of motion into hypermobility, particularly when a joint is bearing weight or other tension, can further destabilize the joint by causing injury to the supportive ligaments, muscles, and other tissues such as cartilage.

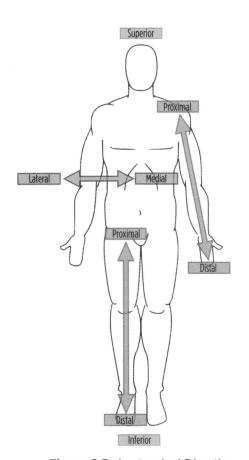

Figure 6.5: Anatomical Direction

HYPERMOBILITY AND INSTABILITY

Many people with tight muscles and limited range of motion think they can't do yoga, while many people in yoga classes are in envious awe when they behold the student who clasps her ankles with her hands in *Urdhva Dhanurasana* (Upward Bow or Wheel Pose) or the one who effortlessly brings his sternum to his shin in *Hanumanasana* (Pose of Hanuman, or Splits) before yoga class. Yet it is precisely such hypermobile students who are among our greatest concern in teaching safe yoga asana practices, whereas the tightest among us will most benefit from stretching. Let's look more closely.

Hypermobility can arise from several conditions, including bone shape at its joint articulation, connective tissue defects (such as Ehlers-Danlos syndrome) that allow lax ligaments, impaired proprioception (imagine not feeling—and thus not being aware of—knee hyperextension unless looking at the joint), and/or overly flexible (and thus inadequately toned) muscles. In people for whom the primary cause is a connective tissue defect, an inheritable disease in which gene mutations fail to properly code collagen, elastin, and tenascin, the potential harmful consequences go beyond the musculoskeletal system to include effects on the circulatory and lymphatic systems due to lax vessels. There is also a high association between hypermobility and anxiety.

The primary issue with hypermobility in yoga is joint instability, which can lead to long-term and debilitating conditions, including joint pain, sprains, bursitis, subluxations or dislocations, nerve compression, and arthritis. The presence of relaxin hormone (discussed in greater depth in Chapter 25), which is released during pregnancy to allow for the greater mobility of the pelvis required in natural childbirth, can also lead to long-term hypermobility, which is far like-lier among pregnant and postpartum women who are hypermobile prior to pregnancy.

Given these risks associated with hypermobility and the inverse relationship between mobility and stability, the hypermobile yoga student or client is at great risk of instability. Thus, we want to encourage those with hypermobility to stop stretching their excessively stretchy muscles and focus instead on strengthening those muscles using slow concentric contraction (not eccentric contraction, which further lengthens muscles).

Describing Anatomical Direction

The various terms we use to describe the human body are like the ordinal compass on a map indicating north, south, west, and east: specific terms allow clear orientation and direction. Here we give the basic terms of anatomical direction as pairs of opposites:

Superior–Inferior: Relatively above or below. *Example:* The head is superior to the pelvis (above it), and the knees are inferior to the hips (below them).

Anterior–Posterior: Relatively to the front or back. *Example:* The sternum is anterior to the spine (to the front of it), and the spine is posterior to the belly button (back from it).

Medial–Lateral: Relatively toward or away from the midline of the body (the midsagittal plane). *Example:* The sternum is medial to the shoulder joint (close to the midline of the body), and the hips are lateral to the pubis (farther out to the side of the body).

Proximal–Distal: Relatively close or far from the axial skeleton. *Example:* The wrist is distal to the elbow and shoulder (farther from the axial skeleton), and the hips are proximal to the knees and ankles (close to the axial skeleton).

Superficial–Deep: Relatively close or far from the outer surface of the body. *Example:* The skin is superficial to the bones (farther out), and the heart is deep to the rib cage (deeper in).

Supine–Prone: Lying on the belly (supine) versus lying on the back (prone).

Ipsilateral–Contralateral: On the same side versus on the opposite side.

Movement in Planes of Motion

Joint movement and position are most clearly and consistently described through the prism of imaginary planes of motion that bisect the body in different ways. In considering the planes, we begin with the body in anatomical position, which is essentially the same as Tadasana (Mountain Pose), as shown in Figure 6.6. There are three planes of the body: frontal (also called coronal), sagittal (also called medial), and transverse (also called horizontal). Although we will generally describe movements as being in one plane, our natural movements typically happen in all three planes, even if they are primarily in one.

Frontal Plane: The frontal plane bisects from side to side, dividing the body into anterior and posterior halves. Movement in this plane is described as abduction or adduction (these terms are defined in a moment). For example, moving from

Tadasana to the preparatory position of Prasarita Padottanasana (Wide Angle Forward Fold), we position our feet in a wider lateral stance (abducting our legs) while lifting our arms out level with the floor (abducting our arms). Jumping jacks occur in this plane. We also create spinal lateral flexion in this plane: arching the torso laterally.

Sagittal Plane: The sagittal plane bisects the body from front to back, dividing the body into left and right halves. Movement in this plane is described as flexion or extension (see these following definitions). For example, folding forward from Tadasana to Uttanasana (Standing Forward Fold Pose) is flexion, while arching into Urdhva Dhanurasana (Upward Facing Bow Pose, or Wheel Pose) is extension. We walk or run with primary movements in this plane.

Transverse Plane: The transverse plane bisects the body into upper and lower halves. Movement in this plane is described as rotation. All spinal twists occur in the transverse plane, as do external and internal rotation of the limbs.

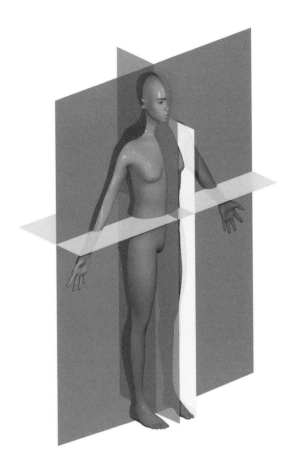

Figure 6.6: Planes of Motion

Terms of Movement

We describe movements in the planes of motion using the following specific terms. There are six general types of movement:

Abduction: Movements away from the midline of the body. *Example:* We abduct the arms to position them out level with the floor in preparation for Utthita Trikonasana (Extended Triangle Pose).

Adduction: Movements toward the midline of the body. *Example:* We adduct the arms when we cross the elbows in Garudasana (Eagle Pose).

Flexion: Bending movements that decrease the angle of a joint. *Examples:* Bending the elbow to bring the hand close to the shoulder, or bending the knee to bring the heel close to the hip. Also, folding forward, which decreases the angle of the spine.

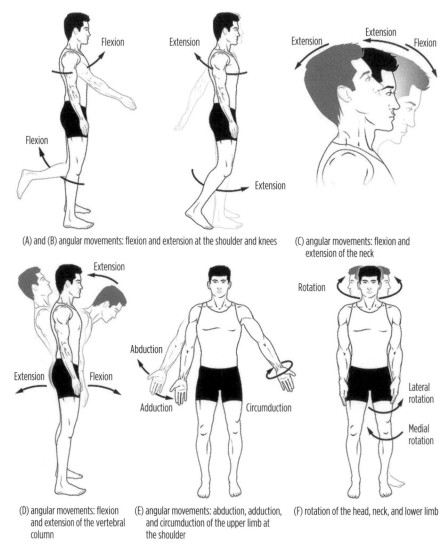

(A) and (B) angular movements: flexion and extension at the shoulder and knees

(C) angular movements: flexion and extension of the neck

(D) angular movements: flexion and extension of the vertebral column

(E) angular movements: abduction, adduction, and circumduction of the upper limb at the shoulder

(F) rotation of the head, neck, and lower limb

Figure 6.7: Types of Movement

Extension: Straightening movements that increase the angle of a joint. *Examples:* Straightening your legs or arms; also, arching your back in a backbend, which increases the angle of the spine.

External Rotation: Rotational movements in the limbs that turn them away from the midline. *Example:* Rotating the arms outward in a way that turns the palms forward and the thumbs back. This is also called lateral rotation.

Internal Rotation: Rotational movements in the limbs that turn them toward the midline. *Example:* Rotating the legs in a way that turns the feet to point toward the midline. This is also called medial rotation.

Circumduction: Circular movement in which the distal end of a limb moves in a circle while the proximal end is stable, thereby combining flexion, extension, abduction, and adduction. *Example:* The lower leg going around in circles from movement at the hip joint.

There are at least twenty-five other more specific terms of movement. Here we highlight the twelve most common terms of movement specific to certain parts of the body:

FEET/ANKLES

Dorsiflexion: Flexion of the ankle, drawing the foot toward the shin.

Plantar Flexion: Extension of the ankle, pointing the foot away from the shin. Yes, it seems odd to call this flexion, but remember: we are increasing the angle of the joint in the sagittal plane!

Inversion: Turning the sole of the foot inward as in Baddha Konasana (Bound Angle Pose).

Eversion: Turning the sole of the foot outward.

HANDS/FOREARMS

Supination: Externally rotating the forearm to turn the palm up (imagine you're holding bowls of soup in your palms).

Pronation: Internally rotating the forearm to turn the palm up (imagine spilling the bowls of soup).

SHOULDER GIRDLE

Elevation: Superior movement of the shoulders, as in shrugging the shoulders toward the ears.

Depression: Inferior movement of the shoulders, as in dropping them down from the shrugged position.

Protraction: Forward movement of the shoulders causing the shoulder blades to move away from the spine. Also called *abduction*.

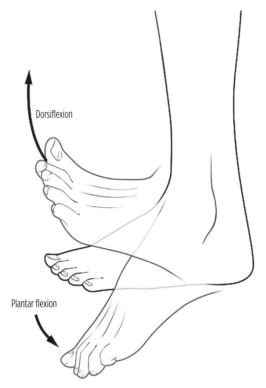

Figure 6.8: Dorsiflexion and Plantar Flexion

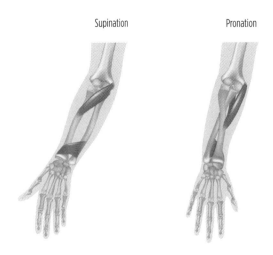

Figure 6.9: Supination and Pronation

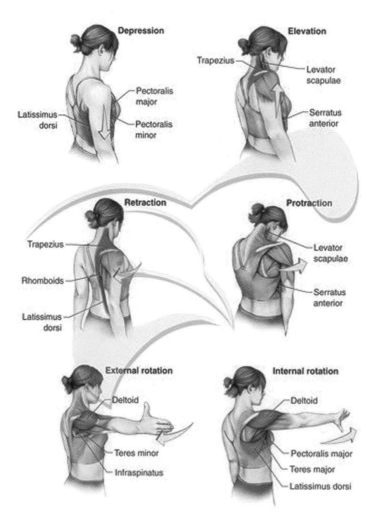

Figure 6.10: Shoulder Movements

Retraction: Backward movement of the shoulders causing the shoulder blades to draw toward the spine. Also called *adduction*.

SACROILIAC (SI) JOINT:

Nutation: Movement of the sacrum anteriorly and inferiorly, causing the coccyx to move posteriorly, thereby widening the lower opening of the pelvis. Generally occurs only during delivery or with hypermobility.

Counternutation: Movement of the sacrum posteriorly and superiorly, causing the coccyx to move anteriorly, thereby widening the superior opening of the pelvis. Generally occurs only during delivery or with hypermobility.

Common Bone and Joint Pathologies

Bone health across the span of life is cumulative: the healthier our bones when they are growing, the healthier they are when we are much further along the life path. Bone mass—a measure of bone size and strength—is largely determined by genetics, diet, and exercise, particularly when we are rapidly growing and up until around age 25, when we reach maximum bone density. Poor diet (particularly lack of adequate calcium intake), lack of weight-bearing exercise, smoking tobacco, and excessive alcohol consumption decrease bone mass, especially when we begin to naturally lose bone density after around age 40.

In a natural process called remodeling, the body continuously regenerates bone tissue. However, after around age 40 remodeling gradually diminishes, causing lower bone density and greater bone brittleness in a condition called osteoporosis. Osteoporosis is greater among women than men, particularly with the onset of menopause due to lower estrogen levels. In addition, diabetes, colitis, gout, and other conditions can cause arthropathy (joint disease). The leading joint disease—arthritis—is either a degenerative disease (osteoarthritis) or an autoimmune disease (rheumatoid arthritis). The following terms are associated with bone and joint disease:

Arthritis: There are numerous forms of arthritis, which involves inflammation of one or more joints. The most common, osteoarthritis, arises from wear and tear, leading to the breakdown of articular cartilage and potentially bone.

Bursitis: Repetitive movement and undue pressure on the joints can inflame the small bursa sacs containing synovial fluid, resulting in pain and tenderness in the affected areas, especially when moving. Bursitis is also caused by trauma, autoimmune disorders, and infection.

Bunion: Although there is disagreement over whether tight shoes or genetic factors best explain this deformity in the first metatarsal and the big toe (hallux), there is strong evidence that it is primarily due to too-tight shoes.[6] Force on the tendons and ligaments causes the deformation, leading to an inflamed bursa sac, pain, and a greater potential for developing arthritis in the joints of the toe.

Breaks, Strains, Fractures: Bones can break due to traumatic force or pathological weakening such as osteoporosis. Most are incomplete fractures in which there is a crack in the bone tissue, in contrast to complete fractures in which the bone fragments are entirely separated.

Ligamentous laxity and joint hypermobility: Whether caused by inheritable connective tissue disorders, injury, or repetitive stretching beyond one's safe range of motion, joint instability can lead to painful movement, subluxation (partial dislocation), or full dislocation.

Osteoporosis: A progressive bone disease in which bone mineral density is reduced, osteoporosis arises from multiple possible causes, mostly commonly a postmenopausal decrease in estrogen production. The bones are more frail and susceptible to fracture.

Kyphosis: Although this term refers to the normal curvature of the thoracic segment of the spine, it also refers to its pathological curvature (also called hyper-kyphosis). Its primary cause is poor posture (slouching). Scheuermann's kyphosis is idiopathic (of unknown or unclear cause) and cannot be corrected. Congenital kyphosis arises in the womb and can manifest later in childhood. See Chapter 23 for further exploration.

Scoliosis: This potentially crippling idiopathic deformation of the spine can worsen due to secondary factors such as spina bifida or cerebral palsy. It is not only of largely unknown cause, but its degree of progression is entirely unpredictable.

Spinal defects: Many spinal defects are interrelated, with one condition causing or exacerbating another. Spinal stenosis, in which the spinal canal narrows, can be caused by osteoarthritis, spondylolisthesis (intervertebral instability), fractures, tumors, and aging.

Cultivating a Healthy Skeletal System

A healthy skeletal system requires calcium-rich foods, vitamin D (which increases intestinal absorption of calcium, iron, magnesium, phosphate, and zinc), moderate weight-bearing exercise (excessive weight-bearing exercise causes premature loss of articular cartilage), and moderation in the consumption of alcohol. A general yoga practice that is appropriate for one's age and overall condition and that does not introduce repetitive stress to joints provides a balance between weight bearing and joint use that can maximize skeletal health throughout life.

In ayurveda, bones and cartilage are considered *asthi dhatu*, pervaded by air and space and thus the province of vata. Excessive vata is seen as causing most bone and joint problems.[7] Seasonal *snehana* therapy—loving the body internally and externally with herbs and substances that force negative substances from the body—is offered for many bone and joint pathologies, including fractures and arthritis. *Nadi Sveda* practice applies localized steam to areas affected by painful joints, sprains, and aches. Dietary recommendations are given for reducing vata. Although this practice promises to relieve bone and joint problems, there is no presentable evidence of the efficacy of these treatments actually doing so.

7

Muscles:
The Muscular System

The painter who is familiar with the nature of the sinews, muscles, and tendons will know very well, in giving movement to a limb, how many and which sinews cause it; and which muscle, by swelling, causes the contraction of that sinew; and which sinews, expanded into the thinnest cartilage, surround and support such muscle.
—LEONARDO DA VINCI

CONTRARY TO HALLOWEEN IMPRESSIONS, the skeleton does not stand or move on its own, the heart does not beat on its own, nor do vessels allow blood to flow on its own. Rather, each has movement and thus gains functionality in significant part because of the muscles, which have three distinctive types:

Skeletal Muscle: Voluntarily contracts and releases to stabilize and mobilize the skeleton and moves other structures such as the eyes. We further explore skeletal muscle in a moment.

Cardiac Muscle: This is heart tissue (it forms the heart—the myocardium), which is also found in the tissues of the aorta, pulmonary vein, and superior vena cava. Cardiac muscle involuntarily contracts under stimulation from the autonomic nervous system (ANS) to pump blood through the pulmonary and systemic circulatory systems. We further explore cardiac muscle in the section titled "The Cardiovascular System."

Smooth Muscle: Found in all of our various tubes, smooth muscle helps to shape and, with involuntary contraction stimulated by the ANS, to facilitate movement through vessels and hollow organs such as in the digestive and reproductive systems. The rhythmic contraction of smooth muscles in vessel walls creates the wavelike peristalsis that moves contents through the tubes. We further explore smooth muscle in the later sections on the digestive, reproductive, and lymphatic systems.

All three types of muscles are excitable (they respond to nerve stimulation), contractile (they have the potential to contract), and elastic (they have the potential to resume their noncontractile form). In addition to these capacities and functions, the muscular system adds overall form to the body and contributes to the maintenance of body temperature by helping to insulate the body from its external environment.

Here we focus on the skeletal muscle, reserving further discussion of cardiac and smooth muscle for later sections on the cardiovascular, digestive, and other systems.

The Skeletal Muscle

Skeletal muscle is contained in a protective sheath of connective tissue, the tendinous ends of which attach muscle to bone. Muscle functionality begins at the cellular level, with elongated muscle cells organized into threadlike muscle fibers with contractile properties. Muscle fiber consists of overlapping myofibrils that are made of proteins (from the Greek *myo*, meaning muscle), specifically actin and myosin filaments along with connecting titin filaments between them; these myofibrils are grouped into clusters called *sarcomeres* (from *sark*, flesh, and *meros*, unit) that run the length of the

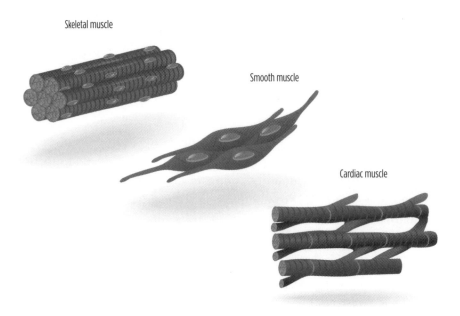

Figure 7.1: Types of Muscle

fiber. The striated appearance of skeletal (and cardiac) muscle fibers comes from the alternating layers of actin and myosin filaments. When stimulated by neurotransmitters, calcium ions in the muscle fibers trigger contraction, with the titin filaments facilitating the myosin filaments binding to actin filaments. Thus, the muscles fibers are turned fully on, causing contraction; when not on, they are off, giving us the all-or-none principle of muscle contraction.

Most skeletal muscle is bound to bone, cartilage, or ligaments through the cord-like tendons created by the convergence of connective tissue at the ends of muscles, with some attached directly to organs (such as the eyes and skin). With muscle contraction, the tendons pull on the bones. Imagine the muscle crossing over a joint from one bone to another (for example, a quadriceps group of muscles crossing from the thigh over the knee and attaching to the lower leg). Further imagine sitting on a table with your knees at the edge and your lower legs dangling down. With the quadriceps originating on the thigh (tendinous origin), crossing the knee, and inserting on the

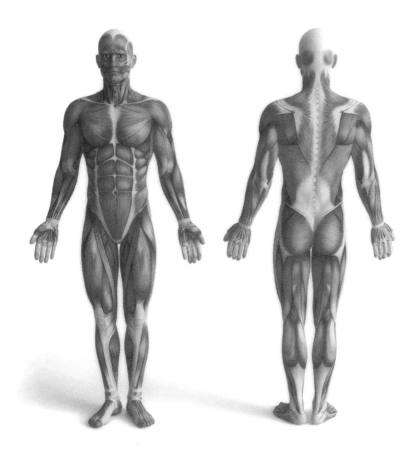

Figure 7.2: Skeletal Muscle Shapes

lower leg (tendinous insertion), when this muscle group contracts it causes the muscles to shorten, pulling the two tendinous ends toward each other. Put differently, the quadriceps are causing the lower leg to lift, thus extending the knee joint. Generally, muscles' origins are proximal and insertions are distal, with the direction of pull being toward the proximal origin and along the direction of the lines of the fibers. However, because the fibers are creating tension in both directions, movement will occur in either or both directions that the fibers run, depending on whether one or both bones are movable (as opposed to being anchored in a way that does not allow movement).

There are several different skeletal muscle shapes (often called muscle architecture), even though most have tendons and all have a fleshy belly. We define muscle length as the distance between its attachments. The macroscopic structural arrangement of muscle fibers inside the sheath of connective tissue gives each muscle its specific shape, and this shape largely determines the muscle's function. There are two basic shapes: parallel, in which the fibers run the length of the muscle and allow greater range of motion; and *pennate* (from the Latin *pinnatus*, "feathered"), in which the fibers run obliquely to their tendons and generate greater force. We can further classify these shapes as follows:

PARALLEL MUSCLE SHAPES

Fusiform: These cylindrically shaped muscles with a central belly and tapered tendinous ends create a direct line of pulling action between the attachments. *Examples:* The biceps and quadriceps.

Flat: Relatively thin, broad, and sheetlike, flat muscle has parallel fibers that spread out from a tendinous aponeurosis. *Examples:* The main muscles of the abdominal sheath—rectus abdominus, transverse abdominus, and the internal and external obliques.

Radiating: Also called fan-shaped muscles for their radiating shape, these muscles combine elements of flat and fusiform muscles, originating in an aponeurosis and attaching via a tendon to a single point. *Examples:* The trapezius and pectoralis major muscles are prime examples.

Sphincter: The circular sphincter muscles surround body openings, contracting to close them.

PENNATE MUSCLE SHAPES

Unipennate: The fibers are all on one side of the aponeurosis or tendon. *Example:* Biceps femoris.

Bipennate: The fibers are on both sides of the central tendon. *Example:* Rectus femoris.

Multipennate: Where the central tendon branches within a pennate muscle, with fibers on each side of each branch. *Example:* The deltoid muscle.

As discussed earlier, movement occurs when a muscle is stimulated. This stimulation causes the muscle to act in what is often called muscle contraction. The term *contraction* connotes shortening in length. However, muscle actions sometimes involve the muscle lengthening, even while creating tension. We can best clarify this language by emphasizing that muscle actions can cause, control, or prevent movement. They do so in three ways:

Isometric Contraction: Imagine lifting a baby from a crib and holding it in your hands with your forearms level with the floor. To stably hold your arms in position, there must be muscle action. It is the isometric contraction of your arm muscles that keeps your elbow joint bent and stabilized.

Concentric Contraction: How did you first lift the baby from the crib? Starting with your arms extended to reach down to take the baby into your hands, you next pulled your wrists toward your shoulders, what in weight lifting is called a half curl. This muscular action occurs primarily in your biceps muscles: their concentric contraction caused them to shorten, thus flexing your elbow joint to 90 degrees. Put differently, the force of the concentric contraction is sufficiently great to overcome gravity (or other resistance), thereby causing movement.

Eccentric Contraction: Now imagine easing the baby back down into the crib with steadily controlled movement. Starting with your forearms held level with the floor in isometric contraction, you slowly straighten your arms (extend your elbows). What keeps your arms from suddenly collapsing down and the baby falling into the crib? It is those same biceps muscles, but now their muscle action is eccentric: the muscle is lengthening while under gradually diminishing tension. Your biceps are thus still acting, working, even while stretching, lengthening, allowing controlled movement that resists gravity (or other resistance).

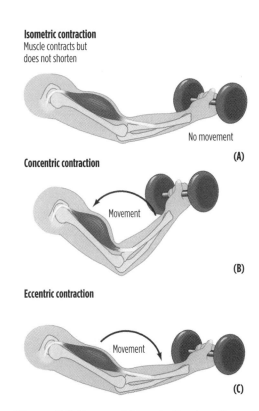

Isometric contraction
Muscle contracts but
does not shorten

No movement

(A)

Concentric contraction

Movement

(B)

Eccentric contraction

Movement

(C)

Figure 7.3: Types of Muscle Contraction and Movement

STRETCH REFLEX

Some movements involving voluntary muscle contraction happen automatically as a reflexive response to intended movements or external stimulation. Put dualistically, the body is producing unintended actions before you can think about it (without cortical direction). One such reflexive response, called *stretch reflex,* occurs when nerves react in response to overstretching or excessively fast stretching within the muscle. As the muscle is stretching, an automatic (and subconscious) protective nervous response is generated in reaction to the intended action, inhibiting or even stopping that action.

Looking more closely, sensory receptors called muscle spindles and Golgi tendons "read" the qualities of stretching in the muscle fibers (specifically the speed of the stretch) and send this sensory information to the spinal cord. This can cause motor neurons in the spinal cord to travel back to the muscle and "tell it"—with potentially greater force than the intended one—to contract in opposition to the stretching.

In folding forward into Uttanasana (Standing Forward Fold Pose), the hamstrings are engaged in eccentric contraction (lengthening as they work). Ideally, we move slowly and steadily in this hamstrings stretch, allowing the muscle fibers to lengthen free of strong stretch reflex, which in general is trying to keep the muscle in its natural resting length. When moving quickly, the force of stretch reflex can overwhelm the lengthening of the muscle, yet with the effort to keep moving plus the force of gravity, a muscle tear is increasingly likely.

Stretch reflexes limit the development of flexibility and must be circumvented through countervailing muscular actions to cultivate full flexibility (not to be confused with hypermobility, in which one exceeds safe range of motion [ROM]). When students or clients move very quickly in and out of asanas, they are likely to trigger stretch reflexes that not only limit flexibility but also increase the risk of straining muscles (and spraining ligaments). As we explore in some detail when discussing how to "play the edge," listening to the body's natural feedback through the breath, heartbeat, and nervous-system messages is the key to moving with ease and stability, all of which happens more easily and naturally when moving more slowly.

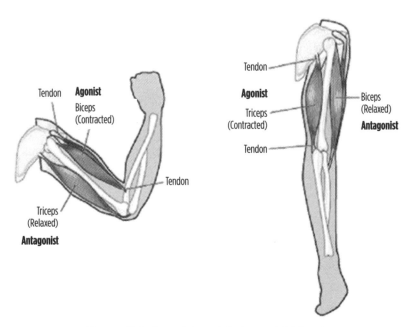

Figure 7.4: Agonist and Antagonist Muscles

When concentric or eccentric muscle action creates movement, it receives support and cooperation from other muscles, thus giving muscles different roles:

Prime Movers: Also called agonists, the prime movers are primarily responsible for creating the movement of the body in any given range of motion. In contracting, whether concentrically or eccentrically, the prime movers generate the force that moves the bones. For example, the hamstrings are the prime movers when flexing the knee joint to bring the heel back and up toward the hip.

Antagonists: All agonist muscles are matched with antagonist muscles that must relax for the agonists to generate the intended movement of the body. Referring to the previous example of knee flexion, for the hamstrings to succeed in flexing the knee the quadriceps must relax; were the quadriceps—which are knee extensors and those that oppose the knee flexors—to contract while hamstrings were attempting to flex the knee, the opposing force would either stop, inhibit, or overwhelm the force of the hamstrings.

Synergists: Sometimes called helpers or neutralizers, synergist muscles complement the prime movers to help ensure that the intended movement occurs by preventing undesired actions. For example, in flexing the elbow, the biceps are the prime movers, with help from the brachioradialis and brachialis.

Stabilizers: Also called fixators, stabilizers fix one part of a limb in place so that movement can occur in distal joints. For example, in strumming a guitar, wrist extensors and flexors cocontract in isometric contraction to stabilize the wrist joint (hold it in place) while the finger flexors and extensors work to strum the guitar strings.

The Musculoskeletal System

With our skeletal and muscular nomenclature and concepts in mind, we can now look at how their integrated actions give functionality (stability and movement) to our skeletal and muscular structures. We will work our way from the ground up.

The Feet and Ankles

With twenty-six bones that form twenty-five joints, twenty muscles, and a variety of tendons and ligaments, the feet are certainly complex.[1] This complexity is related to their role, which is to support the entire body with a dynamic foundation that allows us to stand, walk, run, and have stability and mobility in life. In yoga they are the principal foundation for all the standing poses and active in all inversions and arm balances, most backbends and forward bends, and many twists and hip openers. Meanwhile they are also subjected to almost constant stress, ironically one of the greatest stresses today coming from a simple tool originally designed to protect them: shoes. Giving close attention to our feet—getting them strong, flexible, balanced, aligned, rooted, and resilient—is a basic starting point for building or guiding practically any yoga practice, including seated meditation.

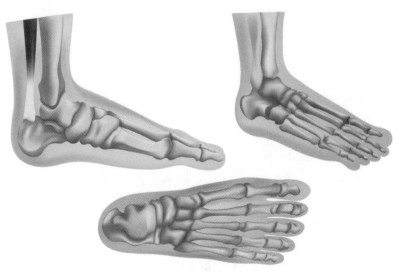

Figure 7.5: The Feet and Ankles

To support the weight of the body, the tarsal and metatarsal bones are constructed into a series of arches. The familiar medial arch is one of two longitudinal arches (the other is called the lateral arch). Due to its height and the large number of small joints between its component parts, the medial arch is relatively more elastic than the other arches, gaining additional support from the tibialis posterior and peroneus longus muscles from above. The lateral arch possesses a special locking mechanism, allowing much more limited movement. In addition to the longitudinal arches, there are a series of transverse arches. At the posterior part of the metatarsals and the anterior part of the tarsus these arches are complete, but in the middle of the tarsus they present the character of half domes, the concavities of which are directed inferiorly and medially, so that when the inner edges of the feet are placed together and the feet firmly rooted down, a complete tarsal dome is formed. When this action is combined with the awakening of the longitudinal arches, we create pada bandha, which is a key to stability in all standing asanas (and a key source for discovering and awakening mula bandha).

However, the feet do not stand alone, even in Tadasana, nor do they independently support movement. Activation of the feet begins in the legs as we run lines of energy from the top of our femur bones down through our feet. This creates a rebounding effect. Imagine the feeling of being heavier when riding up in an elevator, or lighter when riding down. The pressure of the elevator floor up against your feet not only makes you feel heavier, it has the effect of causing the muscles in your legs to engage more strongly. Similarly, when you intentionally root down from the tops of your thighbones into your feet, the muscles in your calves and thighs engage. This not only creates the upward pull on the arches of pada bandha (primarily from the stirruplike effect of activating the tibialis posterior and peroneus longus muscles) but creates expansion through the joints and a sense of being more firmly grounded yet resilient in your feet while longer and lighter up through your body.

It is helpful to divide the feet into the heel foot and the ankle foot. The heel foot derives from the lateral arch, which is connected to the fibula bone in the lower leg, a non-weight-bearing force distributor. Positioned in relation to the calcaneus and cuboid bones, and from there to the fourth and fifth metatarsals and phalanges, it creates more direct grounding and stability. The ankle foot—relating the tibia to the talus, navicular, cuneiforms, and the first three metatarsals and phalanges—is more resilient and a source of refined movement. Thus, in standing balance asanas such as Vrksasana (Tree Pose) or Virabhadrasana III (Warrior III Pose), you can guide more stable balance by asking students to bring more awareness to grounding down through the inner heel of their standing leg. At the same time, rooting through all four corners of each foot while cultivating pada bandha gives greater overall balance and stability amid a feeling of more resiliency.

To point or flex? In many asanas we either point or flex the foot, movements that in anatomy are described respectively as plantar flexion and dorsiflexion. Dorsiflexion creates greater stability in the ankle joint as the wider (anterior) part of the wedge-shaped talus is lodged in the space between the fibula and tibia. In plantar flexion the narrower part of the talus moves into this space, creating less stability but an easier sense of radiating energy out through the feet.

The Legs and Knee Joints

Connecting the femur to the tibia, the knees receive considerable stress from above and below, making their stabilizing muscles and especially ligaments among the most frequently strained in physical yoga practices. Athletes, runners, even committed sitting meditators discover that the stress created in the knees from their athletic or spiritual avocation can lead to debilitating injury, especially when they lack the beneficial effects of a balanced, appropriate practice of physical asanas. Even in a balanced yoga practice, the knee still must handle considerable forces, primarily from bearing weight but also due to twisting forces exerted from above and below. In more strenuous yoga practices, the knee has to handle very powerful physical forces. Primarily a hinge joint

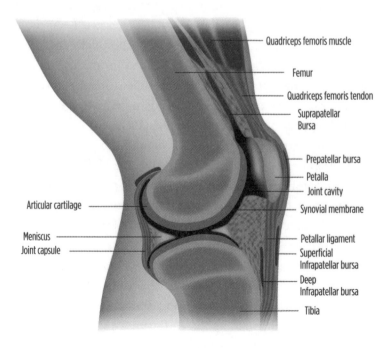

Figure 7.6: The Knees

capable of extension and flexion, with minor capacity to rotate when flexed to about ninety degrees, sudden or excessive movement in any of these motions can tear one of the supporting ligaments or cartilage. Understanding and honoring the knees is one of the keys to guiding a sustainable yoga practice. Let's take a closer look at the knee, which is two joints:

- The femorotibial joint, which links the femur and tibia
- The femoropatellar joint, where the patella is situated within the anterior thigh muscle and a groove that it slides through on the front of the femur.

The distal femur and proximal tibia are expanded into condyles that increase their weight-bearing capacity and offer larger points of attachment for supporting ligaments. The convex shape of the femoral condyles articulates with the concave tibial condyles. The joint is cushioned by articular cartilage that covers the ends of the tibia and femur as well as the underside of the patella. The medial meniscus and lateral meniscus are C-shaped intra-articular pads made of fibrocartilage that further cushion the joint, functioning as shock absorbers between the bones and preventing the bones from rubbing each other. Tears in the medial meniscus are common in yoga, whether originally injured during an asana or exacerbated in an asana such as Padmasana (Lotus Pose) or others where forced rotation at the hip joint can transfer stress into the knee when the foot is held in place by the floor or another part of the body. With little or no blood supply, they heal slowly—if at all. A set of ligaments, all of which are in the fully stretched position when the knee is extended (leg straight), help to stabilize the knee. When the knee is flexed, the ligaments are softened (shortened), allowing rotation in poses such as Padmasana.

The medial and lateral collateral ligaments (MCL and LCL) run along the sides of the knee and limit sideways motion. The MCL, extending vertically from the femur to the tibia, protects the medial side of the knee from being bent open by force applied to the outside of the knee, such as when a student presses down on the outside of the knee of the back leg in Parsva Dhanurasana (Side Bow Pose). The LCL protects the lateral side from an inside bending force, such as when a student inappropriately places the heel of the right foot against the inside of the left knee in Vrksasana. Muscles that run outside them support both of these ligaments.

Inside the knee joint are two cruciate ligaments. The anterior cruciate ligament, or ACL, connects the tibia to the femur at the center of the knee. Its function is to limit rotation and forward motion of the tibia away from the femur; without it the femur would slide forward off the knee. We will revisit this when looking at a variety of poses, especially lunges such as Warrior I or II, where the ACL is both a crucial source of stability and at considerable risk if the knee is not properly aligned. The posterior cruciate ligament, or PCL (located just behind the ACL), limits excessive hyperextension (backward motion) of the knee joint. Injury to the PCL is rare, especially in yoga, where there are no asanas that place great force on this ligament. The patella ligament is sometimes called the patellar tendon because there is no definite separation between the quadriceps tendon, which surrounds the patella, and the area connecting the patella to the tibia. This very strong ligament helps give the patella its mechanical leverage and functions as a cap for the condyles of the femurs.

The muscles acting on the knee from above—the abductors (primarily the glutei and tensor fascia latae, acting through their attachment to the iliotibial band), adductors (primarily the gracilis), the quadriceps (for extension), the hamstrings (for flexion), and the sartorius (a synergist in flexion and lateral rotation)—help the ligaments to stabilize the knee when contracting from their various origins on the front, back, and bottom of the pelvis. The gluteus and tensor fascia latae attach to the iliotibial band, which in turn attaches to the lateral tibial condyle below the knee, contributing to lateral stability. The medial side of the knee is given more balanced stability through the actions of the gracilis, sartorius, and the semitendinosus (one of the hamstrings) as they pull up and in from their attachments on the medial tibia just below the knee: the gracilis from the pubic ramus at the bottom of the pelvis, the sartorius (the longest muscle in the body) from its origin at the anterior superior iliac spine (ASIS), and the semitendinosus as it runs up the back of the leg to its origins in the ischial tuberosity (most commonly known as the sitting bones). These medial and lateral stabilizers also play a small part in the rotation of the tibia on the femur when the knee is flexed and the foot is drawn toward the hip in poses such as Vrksasana or Padmasana.

While lending stability to the knee, the quadriceps and hamstrings are the most powerful muscles involved in knee extension and flexion. The most powerful group of muscles in the body, the quadriceps (so named in Latin for its "four-headed" origins) has just one "foot" as the four parts combine to form the quadriceps tendon, which extends across the front of the knee to become the patellar tendon and inserts on the proximal edge of the patella, which then transfers their action via the patellar tendon to the tibia. Three of the four parts of the quadriceps—vastus medialis, vastus lateralis, and vastus intermedius—originate from the femoral shaft, while the rectus femoris arises from the top front of the pelvis, giving the rectus femoris a strong role in hip flexion as well as knee extension. This combined action is involved in Utthita Hasta Padangusthasana (Extended Hand-to-Big-Toe Pose). Their collective power in knee extension is increased through the fulcrum-like structure of the patella. Their concentric or isometric contraction extends or holds the knee in extension to stretch the hamstrings in a variety of standing and seated poses and contributes to lifting the body through eccentric contraction in backbends such as Setu Bandha Sarvangasana (Bridge Pose) and Urdhva Dhanurasana (Upward Facing Bow Pose).

The three-and-a-half hamstrings are the principle flexors of the knee. The semi-membranosus and the semitendinosus originate from the ischial tuberosity and run down to the medial side of the knee, giving medial support to the knee as well as assisting in medial rotation. The biceps femoris originates on the back of the ischial tuberosity and the back of the femoral shaft, merging along the way before crossing the lateral side of the knee—contributing to lateral stability—and inserting via a common tendon on the head of the fibula. The partial origin of the biceps femoris (its "short head") on the back of the femoral shaft also leads up to the attachment of the adductor magnus, giving the adductor magnus a "half hamstring" function that, when tight, adds further limitation to wide-angled forward bends such as Upavista Konasana (Wide-Angle Seated Forward Fold).

The Pelvis and Hip Joints

Mediating between the upper body and the legs, the pelvis is the hub of the body. Cradled within we find our deep abdominal organs and the resting place of the kundalini-shakti energy long ago revered by the ancient yogis. As a principal center of stability

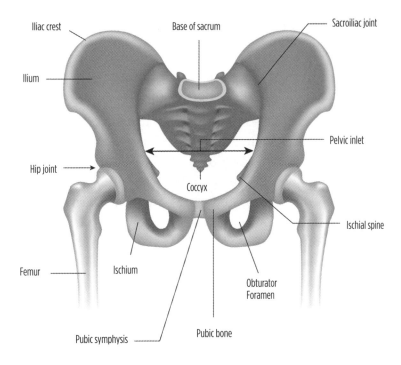

Figure 7.7: The Pelvis and Hip Joints

and ease, we both originate key movements and cushion the impact of those movements through the bones, muscles, ligaments, and energetic actions emanating from
within and around this vital structure. As a strong stabilizing structure, pelvic postural
imbalances, traumas, and injuries tend to manifest below in the knees or above in the
spine and upper body, although wear and tear in the hip itself can cause debilitating
pain that in some cases finds relief only through replacement of the joint. When the
pelvis is strong, balanced, and flexible, it lends these same qualities above and below.
With around thirty muscles giving support to hip movement and stability, there is
much here to work with in nearly every family of asanas.

At the lower front side of the pelvis is the acetabulum, the hip socket that receives
the ball of the femoral head in creating the hip joint, joining the thighbones to the
pelvis and supporting the weight of the body while allowing mobility through its ball-
and-socket structure. It is formed at the intersection of three bones that are fused into
one in infancy: the ilium, ischium, and pubis. The articular portions of the acetabulum
and the femoral head are covered with cartilage, allowing smooth movement of the
femoral head. The outer rim of the acetabulum has a strong fibrocartilaginous ring,
the labrum, which increases the depth of the socket and lends to greater stability in the
joint. This capsule is reinforced by four ligaments that wind around the head of the
femur, twisting and untwisting as we move the femur bone to create stability that also
limits the range of motion. In Virabhadrasana I (Warrior I) and Ashta Chandrasana
(Eight-Point Crescent Moon Pose) the tension created by these ligaments, especially
the iliofemoral ligament, limits the depth of the lunge and/or causes the pelvis to pitch
forward, creating lordosis as well as possibly excessively pressuring the intervertebral
discs of the lumbar spine. These same ligaments are also what keep the thighbone
from popping out of the hip socket in Virabhadrasana II (Warrior II) when the back
leg is fully extended and externally rotated. The length and girth of the femoral head
and neck vary by individual, giving further limitations to the allowable movement
of the femur that shows up in a variety of poses, especially when the femur is fully
abducted in poses such as Upavista Konasana. Women's acetabula are generally wider
apart than men's, another factor affecting range of motion and stability. The left and
right hips are joined at the pubic symphysis by a fibrocartilage disc and to the sacrum
by the sacroiliac (SI) joint.

The hips gain further stability in supporting the weight of the body plus precision
mobility through a complex set of muscles running in every direction. Six deep lateral
rotators with various origins inside the pelvis insert on different parts of the greater
trochanter of the femoral head, creating several refined movements of the femur: piriformis and quadratus femoris create lateral rotation when the sacrum is fixed and
the thigh is extended or cause adduction when the thigh is flexed (as in Vrksasana);
obturator internus and externus along with gemellus superior and inferior give more

refined lateral rotation movements depending on the position of the femur. The muscles you feel being stretched in Upavista Konasana and Baddha Konasana are primarily the five hip adductors: adductor magnus, the largest and strongest of the adductor group; adductor longus and adductor brevis, which extend from the medial pubis to the linea aspera; pectineus, running from the lateral pubis to a line connecting the lesser trochanter to the linea aspera; and gracilis, a long, thin muscle running from the medial pubis to the tibia just below the medial condyle. The strength of the adductors is crucial in a variety of poses, from arm balances such as Bakasana (Crane Pose) to Salamba Sirsasana (Supported Headstand Pose), where their ability to draw energy to the medial line of the body is essential.

The psoas, as Mabel Todd expresses in *The Thinking Body,* is the most important muscle in determining upright posture.[2] Arising from the vertebral bodies of T12 through L5, its fibers run downward through the anterior pelvis, where they join in a common tendon with the iliacus muscle, which arises from inside the ilium. The iliopsoas then reaches down to the lesser trochanter of the femoral head, creating the prime flexor of the hip joint—you feel it in Navasana (Boat Pose)—and one of the prime limiters in hip extension asanas such as backbends and lunges like Anjaneyasana (Low Lunge Pose). When the femur is fixed, as when sitting in Dandasana (Staff Pose), the psoas and iliacus create different movements (lumbar flexion and hip adduction plus anterior pelvic rotation, respectively). In creating lumbar flexion, the psoas acts on the SI joint relatively independently of the position of the hips. When short and tight, it causes potentially severe lumbar lordosis and compression of the intervertebral discs in the lower back. When weak it can contribute to a flat back. As we will see later, the iliopsoas also plays an important role in deep core stability as well as the integrity of breath and movement in the upper body, in part due to its shared connection at T12 with the crura of the diaphragm and the lower fibers of the trapezius.

The pyramid-shaped piriformis muscle originates on the anterior sacrum, passes under the sciatic notch (inflammation can cause painful pressure on the sciatic nerve) and inserts on the top of the greater trochanter. With the sacrum fixed, the piriformis laterally rotates the extended leg or abducts the flexed thigh, helping open the hips in poses such as Padmasana. If the femur is fixed, its contraction tilts the pelvis back, opposing the action of the psoas and creating more balanced stability and movement in the SI joint.

Earlier we looked at the role of the hamstrings and gluteus muscles in relationship to the knee; they also bear significantly on the pelvis, primarily as extensors. Contraction of the hamstrings brings the pelvis into a posterior tilt when the femurs are fixed or brings the legs into extension when the pelvis is fixed. Tight hamstrings limit forward bending by bringing the sitting bones (the ischial tuberosities, where the hamstrings originate) closer to the back of the knees in poses such as Uttanasana or Paschimottanasana (Seated Forward Bend Pose). Weak hamstrings contribute to lumbar lordosis when the hip flexors are tight.

The largest muscle in the body, gluteus maximus, is both a hip extensor and a lateral rotator, creating different movements depending on which of its fibers are activated. Its upper fibers are lateral rotators, helping open the hips out in poses such as Virabhadrasana II. Its lower fibers act as prime movers in hip extension, along with the hamstrings, assisting the movement into backbends such as Salabhasana (Locust Pose) or Urdhva Dhanurasana, where we want to rotate the femurs internally as a means of softening pressure on the SI joint. Typically, students will squeeze the entire gluteus maximus in backbends as they create hip extension, thereby creating the unintended effect of internally rotating the thighs—which, as a therapist, you will see plainly as the client's feet turn out in poses such as Setu Bandha Sarvangasana. With insertions on the iliotibial tract, gluteus maximus is an important stabilizer of the hip in standing poses. The lesser-known gluteus medius is one of the primary stabilizing muscles in one-legged standing poses such as Vrksasana and Ardha Chandrasana (Half Moon Pose). As an abductor it is also the prime mover in abduction of the hip into Ardha Chandrasana. Even lesser-known is gluteus minimus, a small muscle lying superficial to gluteus medius, which assists gluteus medius in abduction of the hip and assists in hip flexion and medial rotation.

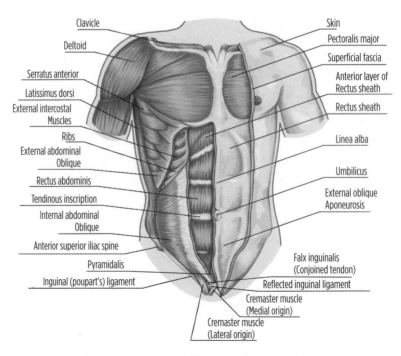

Figure 7.8: The Abdominal Core Muscles

The Core

We can usefully begin our exploration of the abdominal core by considering the belly button. The umbilicus is an important landmark on the abdomen in part because its position is relatively uniform among people, the motionless center of human gravity as represented in Leonardo da Vinci's *Vitruvian Man*. Perhaps even more important is the psychophysiology of this center of the belly, the portal of nutrition and development in the nine months of our embryonic life. Throughout life it is a potent well of emotion, and for many, a focus of obsessive attention and sculpting connected to feelings or projections of sexuality and power. It is also the home of the manipura chakra, the subtle energetic source of willfulness in the world.

Looking more deeply, we find the vital abdominal organs: liver, spleen, pancreas, stomach, large and small intestines, gallbladder, and appendix. Four abdominal muscle groups combine to completely cover these organs: rectus abdominus, transverse abdominus, internal oblique, and external oblique. Looking inferiorly into the bowl of the pelvis, we find the reproductive organs and a supporting structure of muscles and ligaments that are the physical source of mula bandha and uddiyana bandha, two of the essential energy locks first described hundreds of years ago in the earliest writings on Hatha yoga. Superiorly we have the diaphragm, the principal respiratory muscle. Long erector spinae muscles at the back of the torso lie parallel to the vertebral column, and deep to these muscles (i.e., underneath them) the multifidi lie in the gutter next to the spinous processes. Psoas, iliacus, piriformis, and quadratus lumborum also play vital roles in the body's core. When in balance this group of muscles supports standing with stability and ease, allows full and safe range of motion in the lumbar spine, supports the internal organs without compressing them, and allows the breath to flow strongly and freely.

Transverse abdominus (TA) is the deepest of the four main abdominal muscles. Its fascia wrap all the way around the waist to attach to the transverse processes of the lumbar vertebrae, while in front it is joined by a fascial sheet at the linea alba, thus giving its horizontal fibers a girdling effect as if a single muscle. It attaches below to the inguinal ligament, running from the iliac crest to the pubic tubercle. When you laugh until your belly aches, you are feeling your TA. It is also the muscular focus of kapalabhati pranayama, discussed in Chapter 21. When properly toned, this muscle keeps your organs in place while giving support to the lumbar spine. When habitually gripped, it compresses the organs and lends to abdominal hernias and digestive problems.

The internal and external oblique muscles (IO and EO, respectively) rotate the ribcage on the pelvis or the pelvis under the ribcage. The IOs are just outside the TA, with most fibers running anteriorly and superiorly from the lower ribs to the hips. When contracted together (right and left sides) the IOs flex the spine and compress the belly.

Contracting one side causes side bending such as Parivrtta Janu Sirsasana (Revolved Head-to-Knee Pose) and assists the opposite-side EO in rotation of the lower trunk to the same side as the contracted IO. The EOs run anteriorly and inferiorly from the outer surfaces of ribs 5–12, superficial and roughly perpendicular to the IOs, with fibers heading to the linea alba, inguinal ligament, or the pubic bone.

The most superficial abdominal muscle is the rectus abduminus (RA). Attached to the pubic symphysis and xiphoid process and located inside a sheath formed by the TA, IO, and EO, RA contracts to shorten the distance between these attachment points, pulling equally on both ends to flex the spine. When highly toned, its transverse grooves at three tendinous intersections create what is popularly called "six-pack abs" (it is a four-pack). Overemphasis on strengthening this muscle makes it hypertonic, overwhelming other muscles as it pulls the ribs closer to the pubic bone, pulling the ribs out of shape, restricting the breath, and lending to kyphosis and neck problems. As RA travels down to the pubic bone, it becomes less superficial—anatomically as well as functionally for the bandhas. A few inches below the belly button, the obliques and TA all pass in front of the RA, with the RA suddenly becoming the deepest abdominal muscle and one that plays an important role in uddiyana bandha. In looking at the anatomy and actions of uddiyana bandha, we must first return to the feet and the deep pelvis to explore the relationship between actions lower in the body and in the abdominal core.

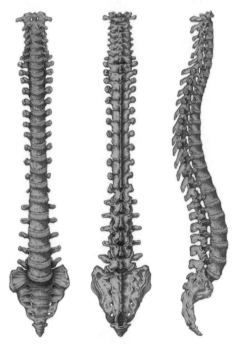

Figure 7.9: The Spine

The Spine

The spine is at the center of yoga. In the traditional yogic literature we find it as the sushumna channel, carrying life-force pranic energy up through the subtle body. Its relative stability, mobility, and overall functioning are among the primary sources motivating people to try yoga initially. More than any other part of the skeleton, the spine is directly involved in every asana. Weakness in support for the spinal column is a leading source of distraction in sitting meditation. With greater and more stable range of motion in the spine we experience more ease and sensory awakening throughout the entire body. "At its essence the spine is really a system of skeletal, neurological, electrical, vascular, and chemical input that when balanced and connected," Susi Aldous Hately says "creates magically fluid movement, much the same way a well-balanced and connected orchestra creates awe-inspiring music."[3] When unbalanced due to overdeveloped or weak muscles, repetitive stress, organic tension, or emotional gripping, we begin to see a variety of problems: lordosis, kyphosis, bulging or herniated discs, and other painful conditions that compromise the delicate balance, stability, and mobility of the spine.

A column of thirty-three vertebrae, the spine curves up from the coccyx to the base of the skull. Viewed laterally, the vertebral column presents four curves corresponding to different regions of the spine: sacrococcygeal, lumbar, thoracic, and cervical. The sacral/coccygeal curve consists of four separate coccygeal vertebrae and five fused sacral vertebrae, the latter forming the sacrum. Twenty-three intervertebral

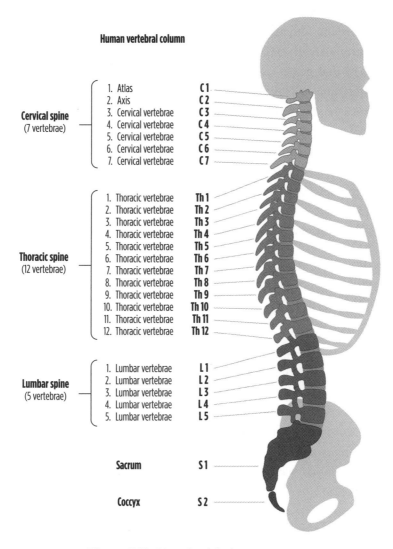

Human vertebral column

Cervical spine
(7 vertebrae)

1. Atlas — C 1
2. Axis — C 2
3. Cervical vertebrae — C 3
4. Cervical vertebrae — C 4
5. Cervical vertebrae — C 5
6. Cervical vertebrae — C 6
7. Cervical vertebrae — C 7

Thoracic spine
(12 vertebrae)

1. Thoracic vertebrae — Th 1
2. Thoracic vertebrae — Th 2
3. Thoracic vertebrae — Th 3
4. Thoracic vertebrae — Th 4
5. Thoracic vertebrae — Th 5
6. Thoracic vertebrae — Th 6
7. Thoracic vertebrae — Th 7
8. Thoracic vertebrae — Th 8
9. Thoracic vertebrae — Th 9
10. Thoracic vertebrae — Th 10
11. Thoracic vertebrae — Th 11
12. Thoracic vertebrae — Th 12

Lumbar spine
(5 vertebrae)

1. Lumbar vertebrae — L 1
2. Lumbar vertebrae — L 2
3. Lumbar vertebrae — L 3
4. Lumbar vertebrae — L 4
5. Lumbar vertebrae — L 5

Sacrum — S 1

Coccyx — S 2

Figure 7.10: Vertebral Segments

articulations allow it to bend and rotate in a variety of directions while its central column protects the delicate spinal cord that branches off into nerves sending and receiving information to and from most of the body. Viewed from the back, the spine looks like two pyramids, one short and inverted at the bottom (the coccyx and sacrum), the other tall and increasingly slender with each successively higher vertebra in the lumbar, thoracic, and cervical segments. This pyramid-like structure gives the spine its inherent structural stability.

The vertebrae in each segment are numbered from top to bottom: C1–C7 (cervical spine), T1–T12 (thoracic spine), L1–L5 (lumbar spine), and S1–S5 (sacral spine). The vertebrae in each segment of the spine have certain unique distinguishing features, starting at the bottom with the sacrococcygeal segment. Four vertebral remnants at the tail of the spine make up the coccyx, commonly referred to as the tailbone. Although most anatomy texts describe the bony segments as fused (and indeed sometimes they are ossified), several studies show that a normal coccyx has two or three movable parts that gently curve forward and slightly flex if we slump back in poses such as Dandasana or Navasana. It provides an attachment for nine muscles, including the gluteus maximus and the levator ani. The top of the coccyx articulates with the sacrum (from the Latin *sacer*, meaning "sacred"), a large inverted triangular set of five fused vertebrae wedged between the hip bones (the ilia) to complete the pelvic ring. The bodies of the first and second sacral vertebrae may not be fused. In most people the sacroiliac points are tightly bound and immobile, although some can rotate the sacrum a few degrees forward or back (nutation and counternutation, respectively). In women the sacrum is shorter, wider, and presents a slightly different curvature and tilt than in men.

The fifth lumbar vertebra rests on the slanted top of the sacrum, creating natural shear forces in the lower lumbar spine that are ideally balanced by muscles and ligaments in the lower back and abdominal areas. The lumbar vertebrae are the largest and strongest of the movable vertebrae, bearing more body weight than their vertebral siblings above as well as having the most flexibility, a dual role that makes this segment the most susceptible to injury and strain. The spinal cord comes to an end between L1 and L2, splitting off into nerve roots that exit between each of the lumbar vertebrae and gather together lower down to form the sciatic nerve. Compressed or herniated intervertebral discs in the lumbar spine, often caused by an excessive lordotic curve (remember that tight psoas muscle?), can affect these nerve roots and contribute to sciatica, which is experienced as pain radiating down the back of each leg into the feet.

The twelve thoracic vertebrae are unique in articulating with the twelve pairs of ribs. Increasing in width from T1 down to T12, they are distinguished by facets on the sides of their bodies for articulation with the heads of the ribs and by facets on the transverse processes of all but T11 and T12 for articulation with the tubercles of the ribs. The width of T1 closely resembles the width of C7 resting above, whereas T11 and T12 approximate the size and shape of the lumbar vertebrae.

The cervical vertebrae are the smallest true vertebrae and can be most readily distinguished from thoracic and lumbar vertebrae by a hole in each transverse process through which the vertebral artery passes. C1, called the atlas, rotates left and right on top of C2, called the axis, giving the cervical spine most of its rotational capacity. C3–C6 are similar to one another, all small and broader from side to side than front to back. C7, called vertebra prominens, is unique in its longer and more prominent spinous process.

Intervertebral discs cushion each vertebra, forming a joint that allows slight movement of the vertebrae while keeping them separated. The disc is formed by a ring called the annulus fibrosus, formed by layer upon layer of fibrocartilage, each layer running in a different direction. This ring surrounds the inner nucleus pulposus, a gel-like substance that absorbs impact in the spine. The intervertebral discs allow the spinal column to be flexible while absorbing shock from walking, running, and other physical activities. In deep forward bending (flexion) of the spine, the front of the disc compresses and pushes the nucleus back as the posterior side of the disc expands; just the opposite happens in extension (back bending), while in side-bending poses such as Parighasana (Gate Pose) the nucleus moves to the opposite side. Injury and aging can cause the expanding side of the disc to bulge and possibly herniate. This most commonly occurs in the posterior part of the disc, precisely where major spinal nerves extend out to different tissues and extremities. While the herniation tends to happen more commonly in forward-bending asanas, the associated pain is more likely felt when standing or in back bending.

Along with the malleable intervertebral discs, a complex and finely integrated system of ligaments and muscles brings further stability and mobility to the spine. Three ligaments extend the entire length of the vertebral column: the anterior and posterior longitudinal ligaments and the supraspinous ligament. In spinal flexion (think of folding forward) the posterior longitudinal ligaments absorb some of the pressure from the disc nucleus pressing back, although with excessive pressure, bulging occurs just to the outsides of the ligament (laterally). The anterior and posterior longitudinal ligaments limit extension and flexion, respectively. Other vertebral ligaments connect adjacent vertebrae. All create stability while limiting the degree of rotation, flexion, extension, and lateral flexion.

The two psoas and two posterior transversospinal muscles form four muscular bundles arranged around the lumbar spine that can contract together to create balanced lengthening in the lower back. Some have suggested that the upper and lower segments of the psoas lend to this balance because the lower fibers pull L5 and L4 anteriorly into lumbar hyperextension while the upper psoas fibers pull T12 and L1 toward the groin in lumbar flexion. But the psoas as a whole pulls the lower lumbar vertebrae forward, bringing the sacrum along in tilting the pelvis forward. Recalling that the psoas is a powerful hip flexor (bringing the knee toward the chest), we can appreciate how hypertension in this powerful muscle not only potentially compresses the lumbar discs but creates a major limitation in all back-bending asanas. Also note that when the psoas on one side contracts alone, this creates side bending or rotation of the spine. If it is relatively more tense on one side, then a variety of asymmetries arise that cause imbalance or strain in the SI joint and up through the spine, many of which we can easily observe when a student is standing in Tadasana or inverted in Salamba Sirsasana. A strong yet supple and balanced psoas is thus one of the most important sources of overall stability and mobility in the spine and the body. Asanas such as Anjaneyasana, Virabhadrasana I, and Supta Virasana (Reclining Hero Pose) stretch the psoas, while Navasana and Utthita Hasta Padangusthasana strengthen it.

A close neighbor of the psoas, quadratus lumborum originates from the posterior iliac crest and inserts on the transverse processes of L1–L5 and rib 12. With ipsilateral contraction (or hypertonicity on one side) it draws the pelvis and ribs on one side closer together; with bilateral contraction it creates spinal extension that is opposed by the psoas and abdominal muscles.

Several layers of deep muscles run up along the posterior spine, some connecting one transverse process to the next (intertransverse muscles), some connecting spinous processes (interspinales), and some connecting transverse processes to spinous processes (transversospinales). At the neck a set of muscles very similar to the transversospinales, the rectus capitis and oblique capitis, connect the spine to the lower rear part of the skull at the occiput. Depending on how these muscles are contracted, they can assist in extension, side bending, and rotation of the spine.

Superficial to the deep muscles of the spine are a set of erector spinae muscles and associated tendons that lie in the groove along the sides of the spinal column. In the lumbar region they arise from the thick, fleshy, tendinous mass of the lumbar aponeurosis, then split into three parallel columns of muscle rising along the spine. The primary action of these muscles is extension of the spine in poses such as Salabhasana and Pursvottanasana (Upward Plank Pose). In flexion these muscles control rather than produce movements; then they fall silent while being stretched in full forward-bending poses such as Paschimottanasana or Uttanasana. In twists and side bends, they are active on both sides in both producing and controlling movement. With each muscle crossing several segments of the spine, their contraction or relaxation has an effect in multiple vertebrae. They are most fully contracted and strengthened in prone backbends such as Salabhasana.

At the neck the erector spinae muscles are complemented by several other muscles that stabilize and mobilize the head on top of the spine like guy wires, including the splenius capitis, levator scapulae, longus colli, rectus capitis, scalenes, sternocleido-mastoids (SCMs), and the upper fibers of the trapezius. Here we find a fascinating world of nerves, muscles, and movements that for many yoga students is a common area of tension and strain. Typically overworked due to postural imbalances else-where in the body (and often excessively recruited in breathing), "pain in the neck" is very easily caused in some of the simplest asanas.

Three other muscles of the back—the latissimi dorsi, rhomboids, and trapezius—are discussed in detail later. For now we will summarize how they act on the back. The latissimi dorsi are the most expansive muscles in the body, covering almost the entire back and giving greater structural integrity to the trunk. The rhomboids draw the vertebrae toward the scapulae or release to allow easier movement into shoulder flexion backbends such as Urdhva Dhanurasana. The trapezius, with fibers running in three directions, can produce spinal extension as well as side bending.

The Shoulder Girdle

Much of human life and consciousness is predicated on our ability not just to erect elaborate structures or actions in our complex mind, but also on our ability to fashion those ideas into material reality in the world. In this creative expression we largely depend on the manipulative abilities of our arms and hands, the relatively free move-ment of which rests on the mobility of our shoulders. Although our shoulder joints are the most mobile joints in the human body, they must also be strong enough to allow us to lift, push, pull, twist, and move with or against force in multi-ple directions. Indeed, human consciousness itself and the very fabric of human thought is inextricably inter-twined with this uniquely human ability to engage creatively with the physical world in often fine and elaborate ways allowed by the shoulder, arms, and hands. The humble shoulders, where we carry much of our responsibility, or sometimes a chip (and where the Hindu god Shiva carries a resting cobra), deter-mine much about our posture and movement in the world, on and off the mat.

Anatomically, the shoulder is not a joint but a com-plex structure comprising three bones—the humerus (upper arm bone), the clavicle (collarbone), and the

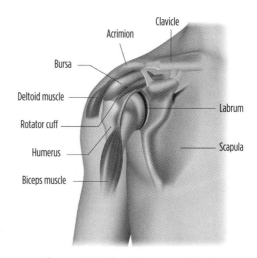

Figure 7.11: The Shoulder Girdle

scapula (shoulder blade)—tied together by muscles, tendons, and ligaments. The articulations among the three bones give us the three joints of the shoulder: glenohumeral,
acromioclavicular, and sternoclavicular. Working together they give the arms tremendous range of motion and stability, a balancing act that when off-kilter creates a variety of problems largely unique to this part of the body.

The glenohumeral joint is the primary joint of the shoulder, where the head of the
humerus rests in the glenoid fossa of the scapula, much like a golf ball on a tee. A ball-
and-socket joint that allows the arm to rotate circularly
or hinge out away from the body, the glenohumeral
joint is stabilized by four muscles that form a rotator
cuff around the humeral head to keep it secured to the
glenoid fossa: the supraspinatus, infraspinatus, teres
minor, and subscapularis, often referred to as SITS.
The tendons of these muscles connect to the capsule of
the glenohumeral joint, lending it further stability. Still,
the shallowness of the glenoid fossa makes this one of
the most commonly dislocated joints in the body, and
inappropriate hands-on adjustments in poses such as
Urdhva Dhanurasana have been known to cause this
joint to dislocate. The smooth movement of the upper
arm bone in the glenoid fossa depends on the balanced
strength, flexibility, and neurological functioning of
the rotator cuff muscles along with the soft tissue cap-

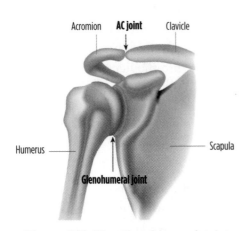

Figure 7.12: The Glenohumeral Joint

sule that encircles the joint and attaches to the scapula, humerus, and the head of the
biceps. Lined by a thin synovial membrane, the capsule is strengthened by the coracoclavicular ligament.

The acromioclavicular joint is at the top of the shoulder, located between the acromion process of the scapula and the distal end of the clavicle, and is stabilized by three
ligaments: the acromioclavicular ligament attaches the clavicle to the acromion of
the scapula; the coracoacromial ligament runs from the coracoid process to the acromion; and the coracoclavicular ligament runs from the scapula to the clavicle. The
movement of this gliding synovial joint allows the arm to rise above the head, helping
the movement of the scapula and giving the arm greater rotation for asanas such as
Urdhva Hastasana (Upward Arms Pose) and Adho Mukha Svanasana. At the medial
end of the clavicle is the sternoclavicular joint, where the convex shape of the manu-
brium interfaces with the rounded end of the clavicle. The scapula is a flat and roughly
triangular-shaped bone placed on the back of the rib cage, forming the posterior part
of the shoulder girdle. The relatively thicker lateral border of the scapula contains
the glenoid fossa, home to the upper arm bone's proximal end. The various physical

features of the scapula allow the attachment of seventeen muscles that give this bone its stability and the basic movements that allow greater range of motion of the arm.

Muscles that attach the humerus to other parts of the shoulder create movement of the upper arm bone. The infraspinatus muscle, assisted by the teres minor, externally rotates the arm, as when standing in Tadasana and turning the palms out or when wrapping the triceps side of the arm toward the ear in Utthita Parsvakonasana. The subscapularis adducts and rotates the arm medially, a rare movement in Hatha yoga (there is some internal rotation in Parsvottanasana [Intense Side Stretch Pose]). The supraspinatus abducts the arm, as when bringing the arms out and up into Virabha-drasana II. Again, these four muscles work collectively as the rotator cuff to stabilize the glenohumeral joint, keeping the humeral head in the glenoid cavity.

The Arms and Elbows

Two bones form the elbow joint: the distal humerus of the upper arm and the prox-imal ulna of the forearm. A second forearm bone, the radius, articulates proximally with the radial notch of the ulna and distally with the carpal bones of the wrist. The forearm can move in (1) flexion and extension (through hinge-like movement at the articulation between the humerus and ulna), and (2) pronation or supination, as when turning the palm alternately face up or face down while the humerus is fixed. The simple hinge joint of the elbow is made more complex by the articulation of the ulna and radius and the way these three bones share synovial cavities and ligaments. Like the knee joint (also a hinge joint), the elbow is very prone to hyperextension, a cause of misalignment and injury especially in weight-bearing arm support asanas.

Flexion and extension of the elbow joint arises from contraction of muscles from above: biceps, brachialis, and brachioradialis create flexion, while the triceps is the

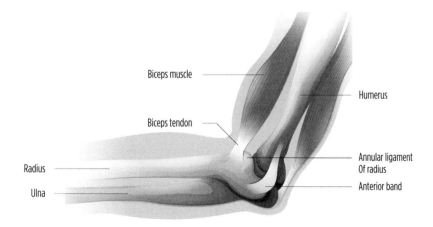

Figure 7.13: The Elbow Joint

primary extensor. In pronation and supination movements, the ulna and radius cross over each other to rotate the palm up and down. The pronator teres and pronator quadrates muscles are the primary pronators (assisted by brachioradialis from a supinated position) while the biceps and supinators create supination. The difficulty of pronation is evident when attempting to keep the palms fully rooted down in Pincha Mayurasana (Forearm Balance Pose), which is more challenging when the biceps muscles are tight.

The Hands and Wrists

Human evolution is largely due to our ability to hold and manipulate objects, an ability crucially afforded by our opposable thumb. Along with qualities of spirit, verbal cues, and demonstration of asanas, the hand is perhaps our most important teaching tool, enabling us to communicate with tactile precision, subtlety, and sensitivity. In asana practice, it provides one of the most important foundational anchors, included in all the arm balances, many backbends, even leveraged hip openers, twists, and forward bends. Given considerable mobility by the wrist joint, this precious tool is also one of the most vulnerable parts of the human body, and the wrist joint is one of the most commonly injured in asana practice.

The hand consists of five metacarpal and fourteen phalange bones linked by ligaments and surrounded by muscles, nerves, vessels, fascia, and skin. The wrist consists of eight small carpal bones, two of which articulate with the distal radius bone and four with the metatarsal, all essentially wrapped by transverse ligaments. The archlike structure of the wrist bones creates a central compartment containing flexor tendons, their sheaths, and fascia that support the positioning of the tendons. Movements of the wrist joint are seen in the hand: flexion draws the hand toward the inner forearm (which tends to elongate the fingers); extension draws the hand toward the top of the wrist (causing the fingers to tend to tighten, as in the tendency for the fingers and knuckles to rise from the floor in Adho Mukha Svanasana); abduction turns the thumb out when the palm is turned up; and adduction does the opposite. The thumb has considerable mobility in extension, flexion, abduction, and adduction.

The primary muscles acting on the wrist and hand originate along the forearm bones (radius and ulna),

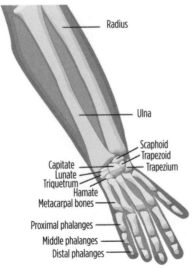

Radius

Ulna

Scaphoid
Trapezoid
Trapezium
Capitate
Lunate
Triquetrum
Hamate
Metacarpal bones

Proximal phalanges
Middle phalanges
Distal phalanges

Figure 7.14: The Wrist Joint

with long tendons inserting on the more distal bones of the wrist, metatarsals, and phalanges. Several small muscles intrinsic to the hand (four dorsal, three palmar) originate on the metatarsals or flexor tendons and insert on the phalanges, allowing flexion and extension of the palm and fingers. Several other small muscles cross over from the base of one finger to the first joint of the neighboring finger, allowing the fingers to abduct and adduct. Especially notable among these for our purposes are the thenar muscles, which move the thumb and its metacarpal; although we want to spread the fingers wide in cultivating hasta bandha in asanas such as Adho Mukha Svanasana and Adho Mukha Vrksasana (Downward Facing Tree Pose, or Handstand), abducting the thumb out as wide as possible easily strains the thenar ligaments and possibly the palmar branch of the median nerve.

Common Muscular Pathologies

There are several types of muscle pathology, including the following:

Muscle Cramp: Cramps are an expression of muscular tension that arises from myosin fibers not detaching from actin filaments in the otherwise normal relaxation of muscle fibers. This can occur due to inadequate stretching of muscles before exercising, hyperflexion of joints, dehydration, kidney disease, thyroid disease, or electrolyte imbalance.

Myositis: Whether caused by trauma (a common cause, or myositis ossificans) or more rarely idiopathic reasons (i.e., idiopathic inflammatory myopathies), here the muscles become weaker and inflamed. Autoimmune conditions may be involved in the idiopathic expressions.

Hypertonia: Although expressed as abnormally increased muscle tone, this is a central nervous system (CNS) condition in which damaged motor neurons increase the excitement of muscle spindles while decreasing synaptic inhibition. Put colloquially, one cannot relax certain muscles. Its extreme manifestation is rigidity.

Atrophy: This decrease in muscle mass most commonly arises from disuse of the muscles (as happens when the muscle is immobilized due to injury or illness) and less often from neurological impairment. It is often associated with cancer, AIDS, COPD, and other debilitating conditions that lead to inactivity.

Muscle Strain: Often called torn or pulled muscle, muscle strain is the tearing of muscle fiber due to overstretching. We explore several forms of muscle strain in Part IV.

Muscle Weakness: Whether true (a symptom of neuromuscular disease, which can be central or peripheral) or perceived (where one has a sense that greater exertion than usual is required, often as a result of muscle fatigue), muscle weakness compromises postural integrity, movement, and stability. It is related to chronic fatigue syndrome (CFS).

Cultivating a Healthy Muscular System

Much like the skeletal system, the muscular system health requires balanced use. Establishing a routine yoga asana practice that slowly warms the muscles, balances strength and flexibility of muscle tissue throughout the body, and reintegrates muscles after particularly strong use is a good way to develop or maintain this balance. In Chapter 20 we provide specific guidance on how to practice the asanas in this way, offering insights and tools that are appropriate for all ages and conditions. We also offer practices for several specific muscular ailments, such as strained hamstrings and unbalanced strength and flexibility in muscles that act directly on the major joints.

It is also important to properly nourish the muscles with oxygen, water, and food. Pranayama practices given in Chapter 21 can contribute to healthy respiration, which is a key to healthy cells that comprise muscle tissue. Drinking water to maintain hydration (being even slightly thirsty is a sign of inadequate hydration) contributes to muscle strength and endurance while it reduces the incidence of muscular cramping. Eating a well-balanced diet—healthy proteins supply the resources for muscle mass, carbohydrates from fruit supply immediate energy, vegetables and whole grains supply fuel, and healthy fats supply stored energy—is essential to optimum muscular function.

In ayurveda, muscle tissue is *mamsa dhatu*, which in its increased condition *(mamsa vruddhi)* causes muscle hypertrophy and flaccidity and in its decreased condition *(mamsa kshaya)* causes atrophy and fatigue. The muscular *srota* (channel), the impairment of which is caused by consumption of "heavy, greasy foods, excessive sleep, sleeping after meals, and a sedentary lifestyle," services the *mamsa dhatu*.[4] The health of the muscular *srota* might be supported with *samvahana* oil treatment, which may help to relieve "neuromuscular blocks" that arise from emotions getting "stuck" in muscles.[5] Meditation without expectation, being "motiveless," is seen as more fundamental to ultimately dissolving this tension in the *mamsa dhatu*.

8

The Nervous System

When we talk about understanding, surely it takes place only when the mind listens completely—the mind being your heart, your nerves, your ears—when you give your whole attention to it.
—JIDDU KRISHNAMURTI

THE SENSITIVITY TO TOUCH AND TEMPERATURE we discussed earlier in Chapter 5 when we were surveying the integumentary system depends on sensory nerves. The contraction of muscles and related skeletal mobility and stability depends on motor nerves. These nerves are part of the nervous system, which controls and integrates all of the systems in human beings. It is by far the most complex yet the smallest (in terms of weight) of all organ systems in the body. In its complexity, it provides immediate responses to changing environmental conditions (internal and external), receiving and sending electrochemical signals to affect the body's activities.

This rapid nervous communication occurs through specialized cells called neurons (also called nerve cells), which are the basic unit of the nervous system. These electrically excitable cells are composed of a cell body (*soma*, from the Greek word for body, not to be confused with the ritual Vedic drink of the same name found in the ancient *Rigveda*) and two processes—an axon and dendrite. Impulses arrive into the cell body through the dendrites that arise from the cell body, while the axon carries impulses away from the cell body. Most axons are coated by a myelin sheath that increases the speed of neural signals. As the electrical energy wave travels along the axon, it stimulates the release of chemical agents called neurotransmitters at nerve junctions called synapses. Although some neurons make direct connections through electrical synapses, most connections are made through chemical synapses by the neurotransmitters, which can either excite or inhibit another neuron. This occurs in a fraction of a millisecond, even if the effect on the stimulated neuron lasts longer. How much longer? The synaptic signal can lead to memory traces stored in engrams (which are theorized to be the neuronal basis of memory), giving indefinite awakening to the affected cells.

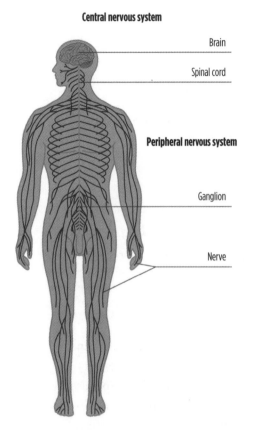

Central nervous system

Brain

Spinal cord

Peripheral nervous system

Ganglion

Nerve

Figure 8.1: The Nervous System

The nervous system can be described structurally as consisting of two parts that are an integrated unit: the central nervous system (CNS) and the peripheral nervous system (PNS).

The Central Nervous System

The CNS consists of the brain and spinal cord, which are the integrative, command, and control centers of the entire nervous system. It reacts to sensory input and issues motor commands. The brain receives and processes sensory information, stores memories, and creates thoughts; the spinal cord sends signals to and from the brain while also controlling reflex activities. Higher cognitive functions—thinking intelligence, memory, and emotions—are based in the brain, although, as we explore later with somatics, there seems to be intelligent function, memory, and emotion embodied through the human organism. Although we often follow ancient observers in casually describing the brain as gray matter, it and the spinal cord have both gray and white matter: nerve cells are the gray matter, whereas interconnecting fibers (myelinated axons) are the white matter. Membranous layers called meninges and cerebrospinal fluid surround the CNS, with the entire CNS contained within the bony structures of the skull and spine.

The Peripheral Nervous System

The PNS is fully connected and functionally integrated with the CNS, forming part of an unbroken whole of the overall nervous system. It consists of twelve pairs of cranial nerves (which exit through the cranial foramina) and thirty-one pairs of spinal nerves (which exit through intervertebral foramina). These nerves carry impulses to and from the CNS, providing communication lines that connect the CNS and the rest of the body. (The olfactory nerve [cranial nerve I] and the optic nerve [cranial nerve II] arise from the cerebrum, not the brainstem, and cranial nerve II is not considered part of the PNS.) The two directions in which the nerve impulses travel give us the division of the PNS into sensory nerves (also called afferent, meaning "carry into") and motor nerves (also called efferent, meaning "carry away"). Sensory nerves send information from the nerve receptors to the CNS, whereas motor nerves send information from the CNS to muscles and glands throughout the body.

In the sensory division of the PNS, afferent neurons convey nerve impulses from receptors (chemoreceptors, mechanoreceptors, photoreceptors, and thermoreceptors) in our sense organs to the CNS (specifically to the somatosensory cortex of the parietal lobe), giving us our commonly known experiences of smell, taste, touch, sight, and hearing. Neurologists debate whether there are other senses as well as about what constitutes a sense, with some positing the distinct qualities of nociception (perception of damaging stimuli), equilibrioception (sense of balance), and proprioception (sense of relative positioning and energetic action in movement).[1] We will revisit these questions when we discuss the kinesiology of movement as well as the experiences of pain and balance in Chapters 9 and 23, respectively.

In the motor division of the PNS, motor nerves send impulses from the CNS to muscles and glands in two ways: somatic motor nerves voluntarily convey impulses directly to skeletal muscles (free of synaptic junctions), and visceral motor nerves involuntarily convey impulses from the CNS to cardiac muscles, smooth muscles, and glands. These divisions give us the somatic nervous system (SoNS) and autonomic nervous system (ANS), respectively. We will return to the SoNS when we discuss neuromuscular actions in the kinesiology of movement in Chapter 9.

The ANS is often called the involuntary nervous system, which may trouble those yogis who claim they can consciously (voluntarily) control the entirety of their bodily activities (including heart rate, pupillary response, digestion, and reflex actions such as coughing and sneezing). To be sure, in the ANS, visceral afferent fibers are present along with the visceral efferent fibers that generate involuntary stimulation, allowing for perception of reflex and pain and conscious response. Regulated by the hypothalamus gland just above the brain stem, the ANS has two branches, the excitatory sympathetic nervous system and inhibitory parasympathetic nervous system, which in some exceptional circumstances such as sexual arousal and orgasm are simultaneously turned on.

The sympathetic nervous system—the concept of sympathy was first given medical expression in Galen's reference to how the CNS communicates with the viscera[2]—mobilizes our fight-or-flight responses through its extensive innervation of organs throughout the body. However, fight-or-flight can be misinterpreted to suggest that this system reacts only to extreme conditions. The sympathetic nervous system is constantly active, stimulating tissue metabolism and maintaining homeostasis. These pervasive functions are seen in multiple organs, from the dilation of pupils, bronchioles, and skeletal muscle to changes in heart rate, digestive peristalsis, and renin secretion in the kidneys. They are carried out through preganglionic neurons located between thoracic vertebra 1 and lumbar vertebra 2, ganglia located close to the spine, and in the adrenal medulla of each adrenal gland.

The parasympathetic nervous system (often abbreviated PN, and not to be confused with the peripheral nervous system [PN]) is sometimes called the "rest and digest" or "feed and breed" system.[3] This system distributes impulses only to the head, visceral cavities of the trunk, and to the clitoris and penis. PN neurons in the CNS enter and exit it through either the cranial or sacral parasympathetic outflow (cranial through cranial nerves III, VII, IX, and X, and sacral through the ventral roots of S2 through S4). Although the cranial outflow gives parasympathetic innervation to the head, its more dominant outflow through cranial nerve X— the vagus nerve—provides this innervation to the gastrointestinal tract from the esophagus to the large intestine.[4] In interfacing with the vagus nerve, parasympathetic innervation is delivered to all organs from the neck to the transverse colon (except the adrenal glands), thus affecting heart rate, digestion, sweating, and other organ functions. The PN's ganglionic neurons are found in or next to several organs, giving specific and local parasympathetic stimulation to the eyes, tear glands, heart, lungs, liver, kidneys, bladder, and erectile parts of the reproductive organs. Taken together, these functions of the PN generally allow us to relax, digest, and absorb energy.

Although we present these ANS divisions as though they are separate—indeed, the separate structures and functions just described are largely separate—there are many instance of duel innervation wherein most vital organs receive direction from both. The opposing effects of sympathetic and parasympathetic innervation are key elements in homeostasis, allowing our functional balance as complete human organisms. We will revisit vital organ innervation when we consider the organs themselves. We will also revisit the larger PNS when we discuss the neuromuscular basis of movement in Chapter 9.

Common Neurological Pathologies

There are several common neurological pathologies:

Neuropraxia: In this temporary disorder of the peripheral nervous system, there is a loss of both motor and sensory innervation due to impaired conduction. This disorder is most commonly caused by blunt force injury to skeletal nerve fibers and the consequent pressure on the nerves and neural lesions. Rest and physical therapy resolve most cases.

Axonotmesis: Like neuropraxia but typically involving a more severe contusion, axonotmesis damages the nerve's myelin sheath and can be mild to severe. Recovery depends mostly on space and time, with nerve regeneration occurring at a rate of about 1–3 millimeters per day.

Neurotmesis: Another form of peripheral nerve damage, neurotmesis is far more severe than neuropraxia and axonotmesis: complete healing, even with surgery, is rare. Most common in the upper limb and specifically with the ulnar nerve, it can be typically caused by overstretching or joint dislocation.

Stroke: Whether ischemic (lack of blood flow) or hemorrhagic (due to bleeding), stroke (technically called cerebrovascular accident or CVA) kills brain cells, can have serious long-term consequences determined by which areas of the brain are damaged, and may result in death. High blood pressure, tobacco smoking, obesity, and diabetes are common causes of stroke.

Brain Tumors: Cancerous or benign, the development of abnormal cells in the brain can cause headache (due to increased intracranial pressure), seizures, coma, and death. Tumors can manifest in the meninges, within the brain tissue itself, or in the spinal cord. Over half are gliomas that arise from the glial cells in the brain and can spread via cerebrospinal fluid through the brain and spinal cord.

Spinal Cord Injury (SCI): Trauma or disease can damage the spinal cord's motor, sensory, or autonomic functions. SCI is graded based on neurological responses and measurement of bilateral muscle strength in each dermatome. Incomplete injuries show varying degrees of recovery, whereas complete injuries show none.

Traumatic Brain Injury (TBI): Violence, car and motorcycle accidents, construction accidents, and sports-related injuries are the most common causes of TBI, which, depending on severity, can result in a variety of physical, cognitive, and emotional conditions or death. Mild TBI typically resolves in a few weeks, while more severe cases may not resolve.

Peripheral Neuropathy (PN): Systemic diseases such as diabetes, certain medications, traumatic injury, and some infections can cause PN, impairing sensation, movement, and organ function. It is classified based on the number and distribution of affected nerves as well as nerve type.

Metabolic Conditions: Metabolic neuropathy involves peripheral nerve disorders associated with metabolic-based systemic diseases such as diabetes, hypoglycemia, hepatic failure, and nutritional deficiencies. Here metabolic impairment causes demyelination (loss of the nerve sheath, which slows conduction) or axonal degeneration (the nerve cell body is destroyed, as with multiple sclerosis).

Inflammatory Conditions: Gastrointestinal tract and respiratory infections can lead to nerve dysfunction in a condition called Guillain-Barré syndrome, in which the immune system attacks nerve cells in the PNS, resulting in the quick onset of numbness, tingling, weakness, and pain that can be signs of the development of muscle paralysis. Although there is an 80 percent recovery rate, even with optimum care there is a 5 percent mortality rate.

Shingles: Caused by the same virus that causes chicken pox (varicella-zoster virus), shingles is often considered an integumentary system disorder due to its painful rash or a strip of blisters along the side of the torso. It can rest dormant near nerve tissue for many years and lead to postherpetic neuralgia, in which damaged nerve fibers send confused and exaggerated messages from the skin to the brain.

Cultivating a Healthy Neurological System

As with every system, diet, exercise, and rest are the essential keys to healthy functioning and longevity. Nerve tissue depends on a healthy intake of vitamins, minerals, monounsaturated fats, and polyunsaturated fats, with proper amounts of glucose being particularly important in healthy neurons. There is increasing evidence that select dietary factors are vital in brain plasticity and the healthy functioning of the central nervous system's synaptic plasticity.[5] Using one's brain in new and different ways on a daily basis also contributes to healthy neuroplasticity, with growing evidence in the emerging field of psychoneuroimmunology that active thinking can contribute to stronger immune system responses.[6] These insights are particularly important with greater age, with active brain use and physical exercise positively correlated with lower rates of diminished brain function and neurologically impaired proprioception and physical balance. We also find a growing body of evidence supporting the positive effects of meditation on brain function.[7]

Although the ancient pioneers of ayurveda did not understand the significance of the brain, modern Ayurvedic practitioners prescribe several methods for brain, spinal cord, and general neurological health. *Tarpaka*, one of *kapha's* waters, is said to flow in the brain as cerebrospinal fluid and to soothe the nervous system. Specific massage of the head, neck, and shoulders *(shirobhyanga)* in conjunction with *nasya* therapies, particularly *navana nasya*, is said to relieve headaches, earaches, and facial disorders, with even greater claims that this means of nasal insufflation creates "a healthy shock to the cranial system" that can ease "paralysis, neuralgia, cervical spondylitis, torticollis, and so on."[8] I recommend exploring more conventional treatments for such conditions under the guidance of a neurologist prior to considering these treatments for which there is no evidence of efficacy. Although the evidence is purely anecdotal, I can attest to the benefit of *shirobhyanga* and *navana nasya* in easing mild headaches and neck tension.

9

Kinesiology and the Biomechanics of Movement

The trouble with the fast lane is that all the movement is horizontal. And I like to go vertical sometimes.
—TOM ROBBINS

YOGA ASANAS ARE TYPICALLY DEPICTED in the yoga anatomy literature in the same static form that we find presentations of human anatomy more generally. We are given idealized perfect forms showing the precise position of the bones (and occasionally ligaments) in various asanas, with muscles added to show how the skeleton is held in that position. These portrayals help us understand the basic form of the asana and which muscles are doing what in support of it, sometimes including identification of the role played by each muscle. Many of the best of these published works on yoga anatomy are written by teachers with a primary background in Iyengar-style yoga, which emphasizes, in the words of B. K. S. Iyengar, the "perfect pose."

Moving into Stillness

The American yoga teacher Erich Schiffmann, whose early yoga roots initially grew during five years of study with Iyengar in India, gave his 1996 book, *Yoga,* the subtitle *The Spirit and Practice of Moving into Stillness.* In his foreword, he writes that yoga "will make you sensitive to the stillness, the presence, the hush, the peace of God. This deep inner stillness is at the core of your being."[1] But when Schiffmann discusses *how* we do asanas, he draws primarily from the teacher he "most notably" acknowledges—Joel Kramer, whose concept of "playing the edge" involves persistent inner listening and dynamic refinement. Although Schiffmann is true to his Iyengar roots and general yogic sensibilities in explaining stable and precisely aligned asanas, his subtitle is particularly suggestive in using *moving*, the verbal root of which, *move*, means to pass from one place or position to another: we are *moving into* stillness, not somehow always or already still. (The preposition "into" implies action, movement, going toward, a process, etc.)

This points to a profound limitation in the extant yoga anatomy literature: we see the final or idealized form of the asana, yet very rarely do we see how to get there. For example, we see Urdva Mukha Svanasana (Upward Facing Dog) and Adho Mukha Svanasana (Downward Facing Dog), along with the associated muscles primarily involved in holding them, but not how we move from one to the other. Because transitional movements are ignored, there is typically no discussion of the biomechanics or kinesiology of movement, including how the neuromuscular system functions to create movement and stability, thus the essential elements of what is happening are missed.[2]

Kinesiology considers human movement through the integrated application of anatomy, physiology, biomechanics, psychology, and neurology.[3] From the Greek term *kinesis*, meaning movement, a primary interest of kinesiologists is how the bodymind is an adaptive organism that changes physiologically (and psychologically) when exercised.[4] These changes, including many that involve neuroplasticity (brain adaptation), are found in many areas, including range of motion, muscular strength, cardiovascular endurance, neuromuscular control, emotional depression, immune system function, sleeping habits, and metabolic disease.[5] As such it potentially provides insight into asana and other yoga-based practices designed to accommodate the special conditions, needs, and unique intentions of many yoga students and yoga therapy clients. Although kinesiology can focus on any of several aspects of human movement, here we focus on the biomechanics of movement, including its neuromuscular dimension.[6]

The Nature of Human Movement

We are anything but static beings. We walk, stand, sit, run, dance, and move in many other ways. And as noted earlier, we move into asanas. In these transitions and once in an asana, no matter how much we aim for stillness, there is still movement: our heart beats, blood pumps through our vessels, our diaphragm and lungs expand and contract, and electrochemical messages move through our neurological system. Although many of these are purely involuntary movements, even when we aim for greater stillness we often find the most efficient and effective way through refining movements that allow us to more easily create and release the qualities of tension that give us stability and ease along the way. And as we are always "along the way" in a life or in specific practices such as yoga that never end, movement is at the heart of both life and the refinements we cultivate in yoga.[7] By doing so with Kramer's concept of playing the edge, we open more deeply, feel more consciously, and tend to experience deeper self-transformation.

Akin to Kramer's concept of playing the edge, biomechanics gives us the qualitative concepts of efficiency, effectiveness, and optimized movement. Efficient movement minimizes the required energy to create it. The more efficient we are in our activities, the longer we can sustain them. If we move appropriately, in keeping with how the body best works, we bring an effective quality to the movement, more likely fulfilling our intention in making the movement. Inefficient movement unnecessarily expends energy, leading to earlier fatigue or burnout, and making it less likely that we will be effective in our intention. When we are both efficient and effective, allowing greater sustainability in our actions—including practices we might wish to do on a regular basis for the rest of our lives—the more we benefit from them.

Yet in doing a practice in which one of our intentions might be personal transformation, we may not most fulfill our intention if our actions are always done with only minimal effort. On the other hand, maximizing our effort can cause fatigue. Yes, we want to have a sense of ease, but we also want to explore with sufficient intensity that we engender and embody intended changes. This requires endurance. Optimally effective movement usually optimizes efficiency, but optimally efficient movement might be biomechanically ineffective, even injurious. To explore this more clearly and deeply, we will return to a discussion of bones, joints, muscles, and nerves, this time looking through the prism of biomechanics.

Although we think of bone as being hard (it usually is in healthy adults) and unchanging, Wolff's law tells us that bone tissue remodels itself in response to how it is stimulated (i.e., how much or how little it is loaded with stress).[8] In this remodeling—called mechanotransduction—mechanical loading signals caused by physical stress to bones convert into biochemical signals that direct a cellular response in osteocytes (the most abundant cells in bone), leading to refined bone development that supports the stressing activity. This remodeling is continuous, even as bones increasingly ossify in normal human development, as we produce four types of stress on bone tissue:

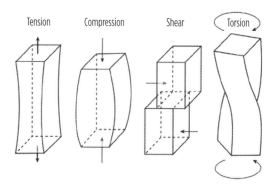

Figure 9.1: Tension, Compression, Shear, and Torsion

Tension: This is the primary load that occurs when muscles pull on bones. Recall our example of lifting a baby from a crib: the weight of the baby creates downward force on the hand while the force of the contracting biceps muscles pulls on the bones of the forearm. Also called tensile stress, tension occurs when these two forces pull in opposite directions.

Compression: The force of gravity causes whatever is above to press into whatever is below. The full weight of the body presses down into the feet, compressing the soles as we stand or walk. The weight of everything above lumbar vertebra 3 presses down on that vertebra, adding compression force to the intervertebral disc (and facets) just below it; each intervertebral disc is compressed by whatever is above it.

Shear: Here two objects slide over each other. Consider the knee joint, where the distal femur and proximal tibia join: if force is applied behind the tibia, it causes it to slide forward relative to the femur, creating shearing force in the joint.

Torsion: Torsional force occurs through twisting actions along a longitudinal axis such as the spine or a limb. We also create torsion with lateral loading, as when picking up a heavy object with one hand, causing lateral flexion in the spine. Further torsion is created in the combination of tension, compression, and shear in certain dynamic movements.

Each of these types of force pulls on bone in ways that stress it. The elasticity of bone is its ability to reform in response to this stress. During our growing years, as the bones are still ossifying, undue stress can disrupt normal bone development as well as the integrity of tendons, even creating a painful condition called Osgood-Schlatter disease in which the patellar ligament becomes inflamed where it attaches at the tibial tuberosity (most typically during adolescent growth spurts). Another common effect is stress fractures due to repetitive activities, especially in the more vulnerable joints such as the wrists, elbows, low back, and feet. Our bones continue to change even after they are completely ossified, with ongoing stress (or lack of stress) affecting bone density, mineralization, and strength. Hormones play a significant role in this, with reduced levels of estrogen in menopause being a prime factor in making women more vulnerable to osteoporosis.

In moving, we are firing muscles that pull on bones. In doing so we stress the articular connective tissues—primarily tendons and ligaments—that have varying degrees of elasticity (defined as the ability of a tissue to return to its original form). To stress does not mean to strain or sprain; those effects occur with excessive stress. When we stretch connective tissue beyond its normal elastic potential (or elastic limit) it will not return to its original form, causing a deformed condition called plasticity. Although there is evidence that we can increase elasticity through proper stretching—and playing the edge is a key part of how we do so with safe ranges of motion in yoga asana practices—with plasticity, we can also cause long-term joint instability. Here we return to the relationship between stability and mobility.

Joints gain the ability to safely absorb shock and support motion through the musculoskeletal tissues that surround them—primarily muscles, tendons, and ligaments. When these stabilizing structures are weak the joint is more prone to injury, including sprained ligaments, strained muscles, and articular dislocation.[9] When the stabilizing structures are strong, they make the joint more stable and thus less mobile. As noted earlier, it is possible to have both tremendous strength and mobility depending on the overall qualities of the joint and its supportive structures. How far we can move a joint—its range of motion—is defined by the total range through which the bones can move before being stopped by tight muscles, tight ligaments, or bone-on-bone contact. In exceeding safe range of motion we can cause injury.

We all move somewhat uniquely depending upon the unique characteristics of our bodies. Height, weight, stoutness, and relative proportions are all factors affecting both range of motion and ease of motion. Certain proportions make it difficult to accomplish certain movements in large part because the proportions confer varying degrees of biomechanical advantage. For example, the longer our arms are relative to the length of our torso, the more leverage we have in actions such as throwing (as in baseball) or pushing off with force to the ground (as in using poles when skiing). Sitting in Dandasana (Staff Pose), a student with very long arms in relation to her torso has greater mechanical advantage in pressing her hands down into the floor to elevate her sitting bones off the floor. Thus, all other factors held equal, this student will have greater ease in lifting from Dandasana and drawing her legs into Lolasana (Pendant Pose) and then extending her legs into Chataranga Dandasana (Four-Limbed Staff Pose) than a student with shorter arms in relation to his torso.

These and other normal differences in dimension are found across the landscape of humanity. Although they are significant, there are several other variables that can compensate for one's relative mechanical disadvantages. Efficiency of movement, one's motor ability in doing so, muscular strength, flexibility, and endurance all come to bear in the effectiveness and optimal use of energy when moving.

In our earlier discussion of muscles and joint movement we distinguished between agonist and antagonist muscles—agonists being the prime movers that cause motion, whereas antagonists are those muscles capable of creating the opposite motion. In contracting agonist muscles to create movement, the antagonists must relax, thereby allowing whatever range of motion one is capable of in a joint. Consciously engaging the agonist muscle naturally causes the antagonist to relax and lengthen in a process called reciprocal innervation in which there is reciprocal inhibition; activating the agonist inhibits the antagonist. Let's more closely explore this and related musculotendon and sensorimotor relationships.

Muscular tension (contraction) is the primary force that creates movement (and stable positioning) in the body. When we tense a muscle, it pulls on the tendon that is attached to a bone, causing that bone to move (if the pull has sufficient force and if the antagonist is relaxing, resulting in isotonic contraction) or not move (if with insufficient force or if the antagonist is firing, resulting in isometric contraction). These musculoskeletal actions are controlled by the neuromuscular system.

In our earlier discussion of the neurological system we distinguished between the CNS and the PNS, the latter consisting of nerve branches from the CNS that are arranged in pairs on each side of the body, with twelve pairs of cranial nerves and thirty-one pairs of spinal nerves. The spinal nerves radiate out from the spine in four sets of nerve plexuses (a branching network of intersecting nerves) that are grouped by function, as follows:

Cervical plexus: Its muscular nerves (distinct from its four cutaneous nerve branches) innervate several neck muscles (primarily the scalenes) as well as the hyoid muscles, diaphragm, and pericardium.

Brachial plexus: The brachial plexus has roots at C5–C8 and T1 that merge to form its upper, middle, and lower trunks, which then divide to form six divisions that combine into three cords that innervate the muscles of the arms and shoulder girdle (except for the trapezius, which receives innervation from cervical nerve XI).

Lumbar plexus: The first four lumbar nerves (with roots at L1–L4) and the subcostal nerve (rooted at T12, thus the last thoracic nerve) form a plexus that passes through the psoas muscles before branching into segments that innervate the transverse abdominus and internal obliques, parts of the genitals, and several muscles that act on the hip joints and anterior part of the thighs.

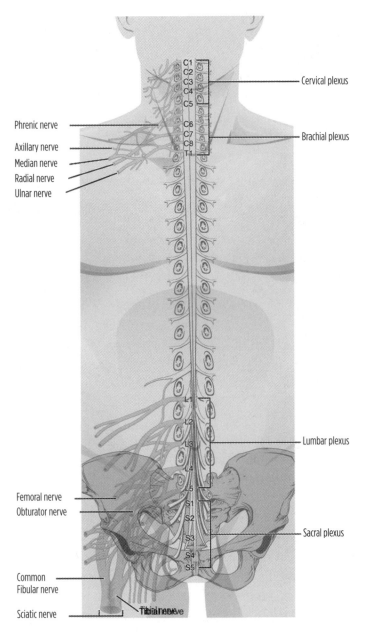

Figure 9.2: Nerve Plexuses

Sacral plexus: Lying on the back of the pelvis between the piriformis and anterior sacrum, the sacral plexus innervates the gluteus and tensor fascia muscles, posterior thigh muscles, most of the lower legs and feet, and the muscles of the pelvic floor. It is part of the lumbosacral plexus.

Although these nerve plexuses are primarily motor nerve conduits through which efferent messages flow to tell skeletal muscles to contract, we also find sensory nerves along their various pathways that send afferent messages to the CNS, which as we will soon see are important in refining our neuromuscular actions. As our neural pathways extend into the farthest reaches of the body, ending in a motor unit in a single muscle cell, that motor unit works with other motor units in that muscle to form a motor pool that innervates the entire muscle in keeping with the "all or none" law of innervation. Whether there is full innervation of all of the fibers in a given muscle depends on the condition of the muscle fibers and the quality of their neurological stimulation (if any).[10] This in turn affects the creation of muscular tension or force.

There are several types of muscle fiber that have differing effects on muscular tension. Their distinct characteristics can be distinguished by assaying their myosin activity under various conditions.[11] The two most pervasive muscle fiber types are slow twitch (ST) and fast twitch (FT), with various proportions of the two found in any given muscle. Slow twitch fibers (also called Type I) are smaller in size, contract slowly, have a low strength of contraction, and release energy slowly, making them relatively more efficient than FT fibers in using oxygen. This slower release of energy and more efficient work increases their endurance. The larger FT fibers contract quickly but release energy quickly, thus are more quickly fatiguing. Marathon runners perform best running with ST fibers while sprinters perform best with FT fibers. We cannot directly choose which fibers to fire; rather, we can change how we move to influence which fibers are recruited, which in turn affects their adaptation and further development. Thus, although the ST-FT ratio is genetically conditioned, with effort the gaseous exchange processes (metabolic capabilities) in both types of fibers can be refined.

Proprioception and Refined Movement

We can further refine our muscular tension (and relaxation) through steadier movements that affect the frequency and synchronization with which motor units fire. Where we intend to create a specific movement in the most efficient and effective way, we ideally initiate and sustain it with the synchronized contraction of nerve fibers. By learning to initiate and control movement with just the muscles we need, rather than unnecessarily recruiting other muscles or erratically engaging muscles, we can get the motor unit to concentrate firing in more optimal ways. Our ability to do this takes practice and is also affected by muscle warmth, which when generated through activity rather than an external source is significantly more effective in creating faster contraction and relaxation.[12]

How we move, including how fast we move, how far we move, how consciously we move, and the environmental conditions within which we move, are all part of the complex neuromuscular processes and sensorimotor mechanisms at play in yoga and movement in our larger lives. Fortunately, we have a set of natural sensory resources that provide guidance and control. As we have seen, we voluntarily move when neural stimulation (by efferent nerves) contracts skeletal muscles that pull on tendons that then pull on bones to mobilize (or stabilize) them in space. Meanwhile, our afferent (sensory) nerves are attuned to where we are in space (joint position sense) as well as how far, fast, and tensely our muscles are contracting. Sensory nerve receptors either connect synaptically to a motor nerve to stimulate a reflexive movement in reaction to what the sensory receptors are reading, or the sensory impulse continues to the brain, where, based upon conscious choice, new impulses are sent out through the PNS to provide more refined neuromuscular action. The sensory nerve receptors involved in this neuromuscular and sensorimotor refinement are called proprioceptors, which facilitate proprioception (from the Latin *proprius*, meaning "one's own"), a subconscious mechanism that helps us to control and refine posture and movement.[13]

Cutaneous receptors: There are several sensory receptors in the skin that sense qualities of touch, pressure, vibration, temperature, and pain: Meissner's corpuscles, Merkel's discs, Pacinian corpuscles, and Ruffini's end organ. These receptors contribute to one's ability to detect the position and movement of the body, particularly the limbs.[14]

Joint receptors: These specialized mechanoreceptors are in the capsular tissues of a joint and its surrounding ligaments, where they read relative speed and change of speed in the joint.

Golgi tendon organ: Located in the tendons, this musculotendinous receptor is sensitive to passive stretching in the tendons and active stretching of the related muscle tissue that is contracting to pull on the tendon. If there is a sense of excessive pull on the tendon, the Golgi tendon organ automatically inhibits contraction of the associated muscle (usually the antagonist). We will discuss the Golgi tendon organ further in relation

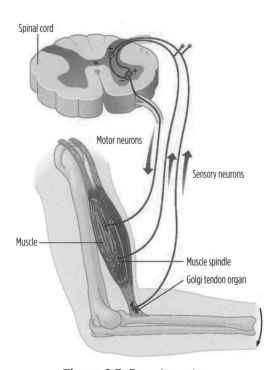

Spinal cord

Motor neurons

Sensory neurons

Muscle

Muscle spindle

Golgi tendon organ

Figure 9.3: Proprioceptors

to a healing and flexibility enhancement method called proprioceptive neuromuscular facilitation (PNF).

Muscle spindles: Also musculotendinous receptors, muscle spindles are located in the belly of muscles between and along muscle fibers, where they stretch along with the muscle. As muscle spindles detect changes in muscle length and speed, their sensory fibers communicate this to the CNS, which can change the rate of motor stimulation to the muscle to ensure one is moving safely. This is related to inhibitory stretch reflex.

Our proprioceptive faculties are constantly changing as we live our lives. When we are misusing part of our body, when we are injured, or when we are experiencing pain, we compromise the quality of our proprioceptive communication, creating an unclear or confused sense of our body in space and amid movement. Inflammation alone can be enough to disrupt normal proprioceptive awareness. Distorted proprioceptive awareness then leads to further misuse of our body and greater likelihood of further pain or injury, creating a cycle of dysfunctional use, dysfunctional proprioception, and greater dysfunctional use. Yet we can also consciously participate in the cultivation of our healthy proprioception, starting by using whatever qualities of self-awareness we presently have to position ourselves and move in the most conscious ways, free of pain and injuriously forceful action. In yoga asana practices, when we move with the breath, allow the barometer-like quality of the breath to guide us, move sufficiently slowly to respect every sensation we experience, and then use these sensory experiences to refine how we are doing whatever we are doing, we are already refining our proprioception.

It is common to think of forceful movement as contrary to yoga; if someone was trying to forcefully make their way into a certain asana, we might appeal to the yamas and counsel a different approach involving *aparigraha*, not grasping, and *ahimsa*, not hurting. Reconsidering this, it is important to appreciate that all human movement requires force. Indeed, one of the most important books in the history of yoga is titled *Hatha Yoga Pradipika*, a title that translates as *Light on Forceful Yoga*.[15] So the issue is not whether to use force, but the qualities of force and how we apply them in practice.

In physics, force is any action that tends to change the motion of an object, including beginning movement from a place of stillness. Any movement has distinct properties of force, including how much is applied (its magnitude), its direction (forward, backward, up, etc.), its point of application (what specific part of the body receives it), and its line of action (akin to Kramer's lines of energy, but always a straight line from the point of application to an indefinite point). Human movement occurs in a gravitational field (unless in outer space), with the earth exerting force on the body (and its segments) in proportion to the mass of the body. The effect is as though the gravitational pull were centered in the body, giving us our center of gravity, which we move around.

An external force against which there is resistance to gravity is required to move. In pressing from Chataranga Dandasana up to Phalakasana (Plank Pose), we press our hands against the floor, thereby generating a reactive force that gives practical expression to Sir Isaac Newton's third law of motion, the law of resultant force. This law states that, "When one body exerts a force on a second body, the second body simultaneously exerts a force in equal magnitude and opposite in direction on the first body." To further clarify this point, by "external force" we do not necessarily mean external to the body, but external to whatever segment is being asked to move (say, the arm, leg, or entire body). Thus, muscles pull externally on bones to move them, and we press externally against things to move the larger segment of our entire body.

Where external forces cause an increase in speed or change of direction, we call this propulsive force, whereas another external force that resists that motion is called resistive force. In moving any segment of our body, we create the greatest external force through the contraction of skeletal muscles that pull externally on tendinous attachments to bones. When we move our entire body, gravitational pull is greatest. Resistive forces, including oppositional muscular contractions, the resistance of connective tissue, friction, and the viscosity of fluids in muscles and joints, restrict these movements. The balance of propulsive and resistive forces contributes to stable movement within normal ranges of motion.

There are many other more specific concepts in biomechanics—including force and motion relationships, force and power, balance and equilibrium—that can inform how we look and approach yoga asanas and other physical practices. These will be explored when we look at conditions in which they most saliently apply. What we most wish to emphasize here is that in yoga asana practices, we must go beyond the static concepts of yoga anatomy and appreciate the significance of biomechanics and kinesiology, without which there is no functionality in functional anatomy.

10

Heart and Blood: The Cardiovascular System

It is only with the heart that one can see rightly;
what is essential is invisible to the eye.
—ANTOINE DE SAINT-EXUPERY

Heart and Soul

Although we find scientific insight into the cardiovascular system dating back as far as the early Egyptians, who saw the connection of the heart to the arteries and thought that air was circulated from the lungs and heart through the arteries, we find considerably more mystification than knowledge of this system in the long history of learning about the human body. In the *Rigveda*, the word for heart—*hridya*—is also used to mean mind or soul. The Chinese word *xin* is found in ancient writings to mean heart, intelligence, or soul. And Aristotle, with a sophisticated understanding of most of human anatomy, considered the heart, not the brain, the seat of reason. Even today, we say, "to know by heart" when we mean a strong and clear understanding of something.

Throughout the ages we see steady development in scientific understanding of the cardiovascular system and the larger circulatory system of which it is a part (along with the lymphatic system) presented in tandem with mystified conceptions that reflect humanity's grasp for meaning through powerful symbols. Although most of the mystified views have faded with further scientific knowledge, science does not explain everything, leaving plenty of space for persistent speculation and open-minded belief in the heart being something far greater than a pump. But pump it does.

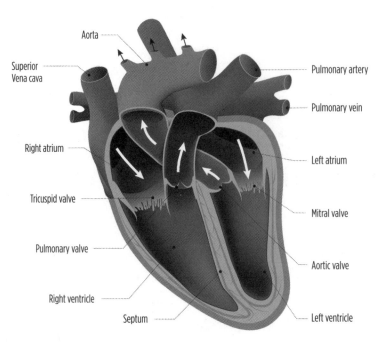

Figure 10.1: The Human Heart

The cardiovascular system, which consists of the heart, blood, and blood vessels, transports blood throughout the body in two distinct circulatory systems: the pulmonary circulatory system and the systemic circulatory system.[1] In pulmonary circulation the heart pumps deoxygenated blood through the lungs to oxygenate it, while in systemic circulation the heart pumps oxygenated blood to the body's tissues. Although blood never leaves the closed network of vessels that extend out from the heart, it absorbs and releases oxygen and other nutrients while absorbing carbon dioxide and other wastes as it constantly circulates through the lungs and tissues. We will look more closely at this circulation in the following pages.

The Heart and Circulation

The heart is at the heart of this system, beating around 100,000 times each day, 30 million times a year, about 2.5 billion times in a 70-year lifetime, to continuously pump about five liters of blood around and around. Fist-size and shaped like a cone, it rests directly behind the sternum in the pericardial cavity surrounded by a serous membrane called the pericardium. The pericardium along with pericardial fluid in the space between the pericardium and the heart provides a friction-reducing cushion for the heart. The heart is divided by septa into four chambers, with one atrium and one ventricle each for pulmonary and systemic circulation. Deoxygenated venous blood returns from the body through the superior and inferior vena cava to the right atrium, where it is pumped down through the tricuspid valve (also called the right atrioventricular valve) to the right ventricle. Once in the right ventricle, blood flows into the pulmonary trunk where it is pumped through pulmonary arteries to the lungs, where gaseous exchange reoxygenates the blood (see Chapter 12 on the respiratory system for what occurs in the lungs). This refreshed blood is drawn into the left atrium, and then pushed through the bicuspid valve (also called the mitral or left atrioventricular valve) into the left ventricle. The extremely thick wall of the left ventricle gives it the requisite power to pump the oxygenated blood up through the aorta and from there to every part of the body.

It might seem that the muscle tissue that forms the heart could directly absorb whatever nourishing blood it needs from all that is flowing through its chambers. Instead, the heart has a dedicated coronary circulatory system that starts with two coronary arteries that originate at the root of the aorta on the left side of the heart. These arteries transport oxygen-rich blood back to the heart through a maze of interconnected small arterial branches called anastomoses, ensuring relatively constant supply despite changes in blood pressure. Cardiac veins then carry the oxygen-depleted blood away from the cardiac capillaries, draining the blood into the coronary sinus from which it is pumped into the right atrium.

The heart is a very powerful pump, capable of pumping the entire blood supply (around five liters) in one minute in normal activity and five times that much during vigorous activity. Each heartbeat—which is one cardiac cycle—takes about one second. The heartbeat alternates between contraction (systole) and relaxation (diastole), with each chamber alternately contracting and relaxing in precise timing to properly pump or receive blood. While a property called autorhythmicity allows cardiac muscle cells to contract free of nerve stimulation, heart rate is fundamentally controlled by pacemaker cells in the sinoatrial node (or SA node, which is embedded in the wall of the right atrium next to the superior vena cava). These electrical impulses cause the steady rhythmic beat of the heart that we have when at rest.

Our heart rate increases or decreases from its resting rate as electrical impulses travel from the sinus node down through the atrial tissues to the atrioventricular node (or AV node, located between the atria and ventricles), which distributes the electrical impulses through the ventricles in a specific pattern that causes their tissues to contract and relax just so. The heart rate is increased or decreased based on the body's demand for oxygen, with impulses from the autonomic nervous system traveling to the SA node, AV node, and larger tissues of the heart to refine its pace of pulsation.

Although these are the gross mechanisms of heart rate, a variety of other players influence the rate and force of cardiac contractions in relation to activity. Heart rate and the force of contraction increases with a rise in body temperature, anticipation of an intense physical or emotional experience (activated through the limbic system), increased muscle firing (as detected by proprioceptors), introduction of stimulants such as caffeine, as well as changes in body chemistry related to nutrition. We find decreases due to the opposite kinds of activity, with relaxation, lower body temperature, reduced muscular activity, and various chemical changes (including less calcium or sodium, or more potassium). Thus, the combination of autorhythmicity, innervation, and body activity and chemistry create relatively precise regulation of heart rate in response to what the body needs.

With the heart pumping, blood flows to the body's tissues and back to the heart through a network of three types of blood vessels: arteries, capillaries, and veins.[2] In systemic circulation, arteries carry oxygenated blood away from the heart (except the pulmonary artery, which carries venous blood to the lungs), increasingly branching into smaller and smaller arteries, eventually so small that they become arterioles, the smallest arteries. Starting at the left ventricle and ending at the right atrium, oxygenated blood first flows through the ascending aorta into the aortic arch, which connects to the descending aorta. The ascending aorta feeds arteries that supply blood to the

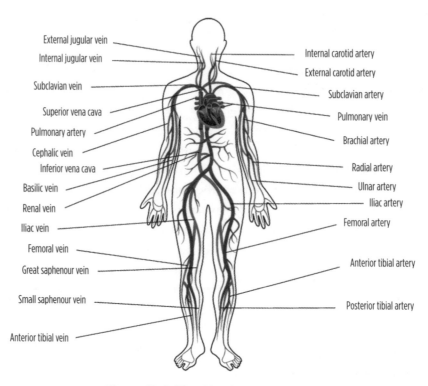

Figure 10.2: The Circulatory System

head, neck, shoulders, and arms, while the descending aorta supplies the rest of the body. Blood flows from these arteries into the arterioles and finally into capillaries, the smallest blood vessels in the body, which are interconnected to form capillary beds that permeate local tissues through diffusion to nourish them with oxygen.

For blood to so permeate our tissues, there must be adequate pressure to pump it all the way out into the capillary beds and bring it back through the venous system to the heart. Although blood pressure is generally measured as pressure against the arterial walls in systemic circulation, the pressure itself depends primarily upon cardiac output, the amount of blood present in the body (which directly affects cardiac output), and the resistance created mostly by arterial diameter and the viscosity of blood as it flows through the systemic system, the latter two of which decrease the farther from the heart the blood gets.[3] Each of these is in turn influenced by dietary salt intake (which increases blood volume), exercise (which increases heart rate and thus cardiac output), disease (the varying effects depending on the nature of the disease), stress (increases cardiac output), obesity (increases cardiac output and decreases arterial diameter), and other factors. Ultimately, the autonomic nervous system regulates these variables, allowing moment-to-moment changes in blood pressure to maintain homeostasis amid one's actual activities.

Systemic circulation continues with venous return—flow of blood back to the heart (not to be confused with "Mercury in retrograde").[4] The venous vessels are comprised of superficial veins, deep veins, and venous sinuses, the latter unique to dura matter (outermost covering) of the brain. The dual drainage provided through superficial and deep veins support the regulation of body temperature: when body temperature is too high, the deep veins push blood to the superficial veins to aid in cooling. (The superficial veins are visible through the skin and most accessible for obtaining blood samples or placing IVs, most commonly at the median cubital vein in the elbow crease.) Deep veins generally are paired with arteries (and nerves) of the same name (e.g., axillary vein, axillary artery, axillary nerve), with the veins and arteries contained in a common sheath. In fulfilling its function, the pumping action of the right atrium gains vital supplementary support from the musculovenous pump (rhythmic contraction and release of muscles in the arms and legs) and respiratory pump (placing pressure on the inferior vena cava). Blood flows through the veins to the superior vena cava (from the head, neck, chest, shoulders, and arms) and inferior vena cava (from organs and tissues located below the diaphragm) before reaching the right atrium.

A more specialized aspect of venous return is found in the hepatic portal system, which transports venous blood from the digestive organs—along with nutrients, wastes, and toxins—to the liver for storage, excretion, or to be metabolized for use. This is why some medications lose their potency when they are absorbed through the gastrointestinal tract rather than transdermally or sublingually. After passing through the liver's filtering capillaries, this venous blood gathers in the hepatic veins before flowing into the inferior vena cava en route to the right atrium.

As deoxygenated blood arrives back to the heart, pulmonary circulation transports it from the heart to the lungs to release carbon dioxide and pick up oxygen during respiration before reentering the heart. (We discuss this gaseous exchange in Chapter 12 on the respiratory system.) From the right atrium, the blood flows through the tricuspid valve down into the right ventricle, which in turn pumps it through the pulmonary valve and pulmonary arteries to the lungs. Once in the lungs the pulmonary arteries branch out into smaller and smaller arteries before reaching the lung's capillary networks, which surround the small air sacs (called alveoli) that are the sites of gas exchange. The oxygenated blood then flows through the pulmonary veins into the left atrium, from which it flows down through the bicuspid valve into the left ventricle. Thus, we have a complete and continuous cycle, from systemic circulation to pulmonary circulation to systemic circulation, mutatis mutandis, ad infinitum (or until the system fails or the larger human organism fades away).

Common Heart Pathologies

There are several common heart pathologies, including the following:

Atherosclerosis: Commonly known as hardening of the arteries, atherosclerosis is a disease in which plaque forms on arterial walls due to the accumulation of lipids. The lipids cause chronic inflammation and wall stiffening. This disease may remain asymptomatic for many years before manifesting as coronary occlusion, thromboembolism, and heart attack (cardiac infarction).

Cardiac Arrhythmia: Whether beating too fast (tachycardia) or too slow (bradycardia), cardiac arrhythmias are largely asymptomatic, quite common, yet potentially lethal. Although some arrhythmias arise from cardiac myopathy (usually in elderly people), it is essentially an electrical problem in which the nerve impulses that trigger heartbeats do not properly manifest in precise synchronicity from the sinus node to the atrioventricular node and then down into the ventricles.

Coronary Heart Disease: This most common form of cardiovascular disease includes stable and unstable angina as well as heart attack and sudden coronary death. Limited blood supply starves heart tissues of oxygen, causing heart tissue cells to die, inducing arrhythmia, and often leading to ventricular fibrillation and death. The most common causes are smoking, stress, obesity, and diabetes.

Hypertensive Heart Disease: This broad category of conditions that result from complications of high blood pressure can cause other conditions such as coronary heart disease, cardiac arrhythmias, and ventricular hypertrophy. Largely asymptomatic except for heart failure, it is often signaled by fatigue, shortness of breath, heart palpitations, and nausea.

Aortic Aneurysms: Largely asymptomatic until they enlarge and possibly cause pain, aortic aneurysms are most commonly found in the abdominal aorta (and secondarily in the thoracic aorta). They weaken the aortic wall, increasing the risk of rupture and potentially lethal bleeding. They are most commonly caused by abnormal elastin and collagen levels in the aortic wall, or may be caused by trauma or infection.

Cardiomyopathy: Literally "heart muscle disease," cardiomyopathy is the deterioration of the heart muscle's ability to contract. Although there are many types of cardiomyopathy, it typically refers to severe conditions that can lead to arrhythmia and sudden cardiac death.

Congenital Heart Disease: Primarily caused by genetic factors in association with environmental conditions, congenital heart disease takes many forms, most of which obstruct blood flow. There is also a wide range of severity, some requiring surgery and others not requiring any treatment. Maternal obesity may be a significant contributing factor.

Infective Endocarditis: This infection of the inner lining of the heart is caused by bacteria from elsewhere in the body spreading via the bloodstream and attaching to damaged areas of the heart, most commonly the valves. This causes inflammation of the affected cardiac tissue and inhibits immune system response. It is generally treated with antibiotics.

Peripheral Artery Disease: This common circulatory problem, a form of atherosclerosis, involves narrowed arteries due to plaque (fatty deposits) accumulating in the arteries. It can be a precursor to atherosclerosis. With limited blood flow to the extremities, there is greater potential for cramps, fatigue, impotence, and even nerve damage.

Cultivating a Healthy Heart

Loving and being loved—including by oneself—might be the key to a healthy heart, if only because it can lead to a variety of healthier behaviors. Mental and emotional stress are widely regarded as the prime sources of heart disease, in part because they are associated with poor sleep, high blood pressure, lack of healthy exercise, and other unhealthy behaviors. Engaging in pleasant, joyful, and fun activities every day, maintaining a healthy diet, and sleeping at least seven hours every night are thus important in cultivating a healthy heart.

Regular yoga asana, pranayama, and meditation practices can contribute to these healthy living practices. Yet yoga does very little for cardiovascular conditioning, a statement sure to raise the ire of many yoga purists who think that every health condition can be perfectly addressed with yoga alone. We often hear casual reference to the pioneering research of Dean Ornish on the benefit of yoga for patients with cardiovascular disease. It is important to note that Ornish's method included making significant changes in diet and lifestyle, with yoga postural practice a relatively small part of his approach.

11

Cleansing and Defending:
The Lymphatic System

*Like a welcome summer rain, humor may suddenly
cleanse and cool the earth, the air, and you.*
—LANGSTON HUGHES

ALTHOUGH FIRST BRIEFLY MENTIONED BY HIPPOCRATES in the fifth century BCE in his work *On Joints*, it was not until the third century BCE that Herophiles identified lymphatic vessels; Galen would soon after describe lymph nodes, but

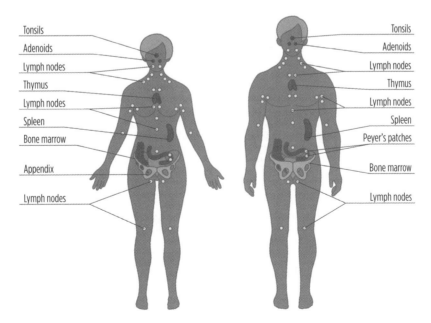

Figure 11.1: The Lymphatic System

it would be another 1,500 years until, during the Renaissance, we would get further insight into the lymphatic system.[1] Long confused with aspects of the cardiovascular system, the lymphatic system and cardiovascular system are close companions in the larger circulatory system of the human bodymind. Working closely with the cardiovascular system, the lymphatic system is an open circulatory system comprised of lymphatic vessels, a fluid called lymph (from the Latin *lympha*, water), and related organs made of lymphoid tissue (comprised of connective tissue and lymphocytes). This system fulfills two functions: 1) filtering and returning blood from the body's tissues to the bloodstream, and 2) defense of the body from infection and disease by snaring harmful organisms such as bacteria and viruses.

Moving Fluids

We have seen how the venous system removes carbon dioxide from tissues and organs and transports it to the lungs for release from the body. The lymph system complements this venous drainage and gaseous exchange system by returning interstitial fluid to the blood. Interstitial fluid (also called tissue fluid) surrounds and bathes the cells that comprise our various tissues, nourishing them with nutrients while providing a means of waste removal. Thus, interstitial fluid is found in extracellular spaces, giving it its name (from interstice, meaning an intervening space). The average person has around 10 liters of interstitial fluid that makes up about fifteen percent of body weight, which along with plasma—the major substance in blood—is the main component of our extracellular fluid.

The systolic force of the heart pushes the watery interstitial fluid out of vascular capillaries located throughout the entire body (except the central nervous system) and into tiny lymphatic capillaries where it flows into lymphatic vessels (where the interstitial fluid is now called lymph). Unlike the cardiovascular system's heart, the lymphatic system does not have a pump to push lymph through the vessels. Instead, skeletal muscular contractions that occur during normal movement squeeze the lymphatics, thereby pushing the lymph through the lymphatic vessels toward the venous system. Along the way the lymph empties into two ducts that collect lymph: the thoracic duct (which collects lymph from the left half of the head, neck, and chest as well as from the lower limbs, pelvis, and lower abdomen) and the right lymphatic duct (which collects lymph from the right half of the head, neck, and chest as well as the right side of the thorax superior to the diaphragm).

Lymphoid Tissues and Organs

There are two forms of lymphoid tissue: lymphoid nodules and organs. Lymphoid nodules are integrated into tissue linings (epithelia) throughout the digestive, respiratory, and urinary tracts, including in the five tonsils that help protect the openings to the digestive and respiratory tracts. If there are insufficient lymphocytes in a lymphoid nodule to destroy invading pathogens, infections such as tonsillitis and appendicitis develop. Lymphoid organs are not integrated into tissue linings but instead are separated from surrounding tissues by a fibrous capsule. There are three primary lymphoid organs:

Lymph Nodes: Lymph nodes are oval-shaped structures that vary in diameter from around 1–25 mm; there are over 500 lymph nodes (also called lymph glands) widely distributed throughout the body and linked by lymphatic vessels. They purify lymph on its way to the venous system by filtering out antigens and pathogens, including cancer cells.

Thymus: Composed of two lobes and located in the mediastinum (between the sternum and the heart). The thymus is the largest lymph organ and plays its greatest role as the site of T-cell maturation during neonatal and preadolescent development before it atrophies after puberty.

Spleen: Resting between the diaphragm, left kidney, and stomach in the left upper quadrant of the abdomen, the spleen filters out old red blood cells while holding a reserve of iron-rich recycled red blood cells and responding to antigens and pathogens in circulating blood. In the process of digesting red blood cells, the spleen produces bilirubin, which the liver uses to produce bile that is secreted by the gallbladder (and thus the liver plays a key role in the digestive system—and far beyond).

The lymphoid tissues produce lymphocytes, subtypes of white blood cells that are a vital component of the immune system.[2] The three major types of lymphocyte are T cells (T for thymus, these account for 75 percent of circulating lymphocytes), B cells (B for bone), and NK cells (NK for natural killer). This population of lymphocytes constantly circulates throughout the body. Both T cells and B cells identify harmful invaders and respond to eliminate them. The T cells attack cells that are infected by viruses, giving us cell-mediated immunity. B cells mature into plasma cells that secrete antibodies, giving us humoral immunity. NK cells continually monitor the body's tissues for infected cells and tumors, requiring no prior metabolic activation to carry out their function (thus the term "natural killers").

Natural Defense and Healing Systems

The human body offers other defenses that can successfully respond to pathogens well before they reach deeply inside of us and come into contact with the lymphatic system. First, we have a set of nonspecific innate defenses that can prevent the very entry of foreign substances into our bodies. Present at birth, our innate defenses include mechanical barriers such as the skin and other epithelial membranes, inflammation, phagocytes, fever, and interferon.

Anatomical barriers: The skin (with sweat, desquamation, and the presence of acids), gastrointestinal tract (with peristalsis, gastric acid, bile, flora, and digestive enzymes), respiratory airways and lungs (with surfactant), the nasopharynx (with mucus and saliva), and eyes (with tears) provide a set of physical, chemical, and biological barriers to pathogens crossing an epithelium (including the delicate epithelia that line the digestive, respiratory, urinary, and reproductive tracts).

Inflammation: Among the first responses of the immune system to attack, inflammation provides a localized tissue response to injury, irritation, or infection that also isolates the attacked area from neighboring healthy tissue. The immediate symptom of inflammation is localized swelling, redness, heat, and pain caused by increased flow of blood to the tissues. When tissue is attacked, a change in interstitial fluid sets in motion a chemical reaction in mast cells that causes dilation of blood vessels (and thus increased blood flow to the area) and related swelling, while also attracting phagocytes to engage in tissue repair.

Phagocytes: Phagocytes (from the Greek *phagein*, "to devour"), six billion of which are in a single liter of blood, remove pathogens by literally eating them. Present in circulating blood as microphages (small eaters) where they are on constant patrol for invading particles and pathogens, they leave the bloodstream to enter injured or infected tissues, wrapping their plasma membrane around the invading pathogen, killing and digesting it. They also manifest as organ-specific macrophages (large eaters, derived from white blood cells called monocytes) that move outside of the vascular system in pursuit of pathogens.

Fever: Defined as body temperature over 99° F (37.2° C), fever can be a useful defense mechanism by accelerating immune system responses, specifically increasing the mobility of leukocytes, enhancing phagocytosis, and increasing the distribution of T cells. However, there is considerable disagreement over the efficacy of higher body temperature in healing.

Interferon and Complements: These are proteins that play important roles in nonspecific defense, with interferon helping to produce antiviral compounds and stimulate NK cells, and complements enhancing phagocytosis and promoting inflammation.

In contrast to the nonspecific defenses, specific defense provides resistance to injuries and diseases caused by specific pathogens. Although some aspects of specific resistance are present at birth and thus unrelated to prior antigen exposure, it is precisely through such exposure that we develop acquired immunity. Also referred to as adaptive immunity, we acquire (adapt) immunity both actively (when antibodies are produced in response to antigens) and passively (when antibodies are transferred from another person). The adaptive immunity is highly specific to the offending pathogen, destroying the pathogens and their toxic friends while establishing long-lasting immunity. However, passive immunization is short term since the antibodies are gradually removed from circulation.

In specific response, the immune system first recognizes an antigen molecule that can be identified as "self" or "nonself" (foreign). The antigen might be a toxin from a bee sting or spoiled food, the protective protein coat of a virus, or a specific molecule in the membrane of pollen or other foreign cell. When the antigen is recognized and binds to a lymphocyte, it activates an immune response that varies depending on whether the lymphocyte is a T cell or a B cell. T cells directly attack the nonself cells in the process of cellular (or cell-mediated) immunity. When B cells are activated by an antigen response and subsequently divide, plasma cells are created and secrete millions of antibodies that circulate in plasma and lymph, binding to pathogens with the original antigen and neutralizing them. In both T-cell and B-cell immunity, memory cells are generated and make future responses to the pathogen more rapid and effective in a process called secondary response.

Common Lymphatic Pathologies

There are several common lymphatic pathologies, including the following:

Lymphoma: Cancer of the lymph system is called lymphoma, a group of white blood cell tumors that are known as "blood cancers," which represent about five percent of all cancers. Non-Hodgkin lymphomas can cause swollen lymph nodes in the neck, armpit, or groins, sudden weight loss, night sweats, chronic fatigue, and trouble breathing. There is a good prognosis with most non-Hodgkin lymphomas if detected and treated early.

Hodgkin's lymphoma: Also called Hodgkin's disease, this is a type of lymphoma in which a cancerous tumor develops in a lymph node. When symptomatic it causes pain in the area of the node (typically in the armpit or neck), itchy skin, night sweats, weight loss, and enlargement of the liver and/or spleen. Its development can weaken the body's immune system, especially as it potentially spreads into the liver, spleen, and bone marrow.

Lymphadenitis: This infection of the lymph nodes is a fairly common complication of certain bacterial infections such as streptococcus or staphylococcus; it also arises from immune system diseases. The most common symptom is swollen, tender, or hard lymph glands. It is generally treated with antibiotics and anti-inflammatories. With complications it can cause abscess formation, cellulitis, and sepsis (a bloodstream infection).

Lymphangitis: This is the inflammation of the lymphatic vessels and channels, most commonly caused by an acute streptococcal infection of the skin. A worsening condition indicates that the causal bacterial infection is increasing. The spread of streptococcal infection can be life threatening. Symptoms include chills, enlarged lymph nodes, fever, headache, loss of appetite, and muscle aches.

Lymphedema: When lymph builds up in the soft tissues rather than returning to the thoracic duct and then the bloodstream, it causes a type of swelling called lymphedema (also called lymphatic obstruction). (This condition is often confused with a different condition called edema, which arises from venous insufficiency.) It is primarily an inherited condition, although the secondary cause is injury to the lymphatic vessels, typically after lymph node dissection or radiation therapy. It is a disfiguring condition for which exercise, compression devices, skin care, and massage are key treatments.

Lymphocytosis: Lymphocytes comprise a significant portion of circulating white blood cells and are an important part of the immune system. Although lymphocytosis is not considered a pathology, lymphocytes temporarily rise in reaction to infection, thus providing a possible indication of a more serious condition such as blood cancer, chronic infection, or an autoimmune disorder. More specific causes include leukemia, mononucleosis, myeloma, tuberculosis, or vasculitis.

Cultivating a Healthy Lymphatic System

The body contains three times more lymph than blood but does not have a heart-like pump to move it. A healthy lymph system depends on regular movement, because movement is primarily responsible for pumping lymph through the body. This suggests the value of relatively dynamic yoga practices that are appropriate for one's age and overall condition. Doing so with healthy, spacious posture and expansive breathing causes lymph to move more easily through its dedicated ducts. A diet rich in anti-inflammatory substances—antioxidants—and healthy fats can help ensure that lymphatic vessels exiting the intestines are properly functioning. Since lymph is primarily composed of water, healthy hydration is vitally important. Drinking water containing antioxidants such as lemon juice may enhance the effectiveness of hydration in lymphatic health. Specific massage techniques can also assist lymphatic drainage. Some health conditions, including cancer, may contraindicate general massage techniques.

12

Breathing:
The Respiratory System

Breathe deeply, as though your life depends upon it.
—ANONYMOUS

Pneuma and the Exchange of Energy

While yogis in ancient India were pioneering pranayama as a somatic spiritual practice, the Greeks as early as the seventh century BCE were searching for knowledge about respiration, while Egyptian and Babylonian scientists were developing practical knowledge about the overall physiology of human beings.[1] The scientist-philosopher Anaximenes of Miletus (born circa 570 BCE) was close to the Indians and Chinese in

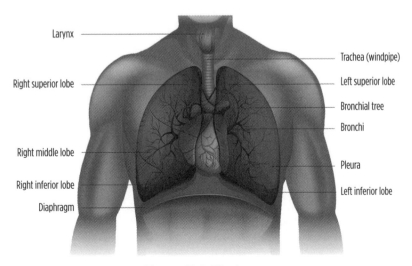

Figure 12.1: The Lungs

his belief that the essence of all things was air, or *pneuma* (literally, "breath"). He said, "As our soul, being air, sustains us, so pneuma and air pervade the whole world."[2] Yet alchemical and spiritual traditions giving sacred reverence to the breath often kept scientists at the threshold of discoveries about the nature of respiration. Only in the late eighteenth century CE would Antoine Lavoisier, the father of modern chemistry, develop the concept of oxidation that is at the scientific heart of breathing. With this discovery, Lavoisier and others laid the foundation for the detailed study of the natural respiratory exchange of oxygen and carbon dioxide that is essential to life.

In breathing we support a basic physiological reality: our cells need to keep generating adenosine triphosphate (ATP) to carry out their metabolic function (maintenance respiration), grow, and replicate.[3] This requires oxygen. Once oxidized, our cells need to flush out the resulting carbon dioxide. In the respiratory physiology, oxygen is delivered to cells via arterial blood from the lungs and heart, while carbon dioxide is returned to the heart and lungs as deoxygenated venous blood. Capillary membranes in the lungs, called alveoli, exchange these gases. This exchange, which we experience as breathing, happens about twelve to fifteen times per minute, or around twenty thousand times per day, with variations in rate depending on the health of the person's system, activity and emotional levels, and other factors.

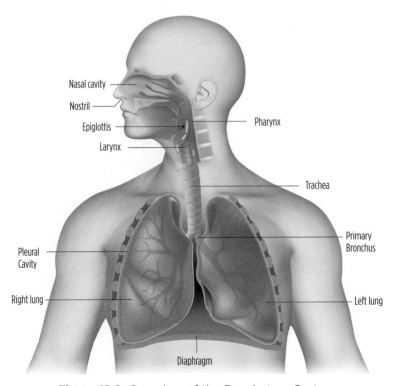

Figure 12.2: Overview of the Respiratory System

The mechanics of this exchange were long misunderstood as resulting from the pumping actions of the heart and lungs. Although the heart and lungs are essential in the respiratory process, they are in physiological service to the breath, not the physiological source of the breath. The mechanisms of breathing were first properly explained by Galen around 170 CE, and in much greater detail only in the sixteenth century by Leonardo da Vinci, who understood that when more space is made available in the lungs by the expansion of the thorax, the weight of the atmosphere forces air in through the trachea to fill the expanded space, a discovery that is directly relevant to how one practices pranayama.[4]

Modern science recognizes the same phases of breath highlighted by the ancient yogis: inhalation, exhalation, and the cessation of breathing, called apnea, which occurs naturally after each inhalation and exhalation. The volume, rate, sound, intensity, areas of relative physical movement or holding, and degree of passivity or activity can vary; the unique combination of these qualities gives us our experience of breathing. Each of these qualities can also be voluntarily affected, giving us the foundation for pranayama and other breathing practices.

The Organs of Respiration

Although we can sense and cultivate a feeling of the entire body breathing (or, depending on your perspective, being breathed), in scientific medicine the respiratory system consists of a specific set of interconnected organs: the nose (including the nasal cavity and sinuses), pharynx (throat), trachea (colloquially called the windpipe), bronchi and bronchioles (air passageways that branch into each lung), the lungs with their walls of alveoli (the gas exchange cells), and the diaphragm (which increases thoracic volume to cause inhalation). Let's look at these organs and their functions more closely.[5]

Air moves in and out of the lungs through a system of airway passages, starting with the nose or mouth. The nose is the more refined and refining organ for filtering air into the body and conditioning, purifying, and humidifying the air. This starts in the nostrils, where coarse hairs help filter out airborne particles. The nostrils open into a nasal cavity that is formed by facial bones, including the nasal septum that bifurcates the cavity into left and right chambers that consist of stacked turbinates (also called conchae). The shape of the turbinates slows the air movement and causes the air to swirl around in them, giving us a natural form of literal air conditioning. The air gains warmth and humidity while olfactory and other nerves in the turbinates allow more subtle sensitivity to the flow of breath, considerably more so than with air flowing through the mouth.[6] The nasal cavity is lined by a mucous membrane and flushed by mucus and tears that react to environmental conditions such as temperature change, allergens, and pathogens, further filtering the air that enters the body.

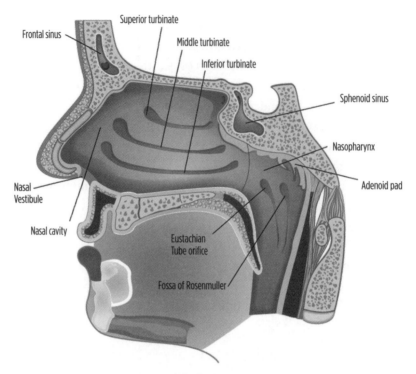

Figure 12.3: The Nose

Well conditioned or not—this depends on the condition of one's nose and nasal cavity—air flows from the nasal cavity into the upper region of the throat called the pharynx, a passageway shared with the digestive system. The pharynx has three portions, each of which has vital components. In the upper portion (the nasopharynx), which extends from the base of the skull to the upper surface of the soft palate, we find the pharyngeal tonsils and the entrances to the auditory (Eustachian) tube. The middle portion (the oropharynx) extends from the soft palate to the base of the tongue (at the level of the hyoid bone), with palatine tonsils in its lateral walls and an anterior opening to the mouth. Here we find the epiglottis, a flap of connective tissue that closes the glottis when we swallow food (thus preventing aspiration as air flow yields to food when we swallow). The lower portion (the laryngopharynx) extends down to where this common digestive and respiratory passageway divides into the larynx (for breathing) and esophagus (for digesting).

Commonly known as the voice box, the larynx receives air through the narrow opening of the glottis, where we cultivate the feeling of *ujjayi pranayama* in the throat, the same place we have sensation when coughing or gargling. The larynx contains the vocal folds (popularly known as vocal cords), which vibrate during exhalation to create sound and moderate the flow of air out of the body. The length and girth of the vocal folds determine the pitch of one's voice, with greater length and girth causing lower tones (with the tones further refined by the tongue, cheeks, and lips).

The trachea, its tubal walls supported by fifteen-to-twenty C-shaped rings of hyaline and cricoid cartilage, connects the larynx to the lungs. The posterior opening in the cartilage rings leaves a resilient membrane that allows the trachea to expand and contract under control by the autonomic nervous system (ANS) to accommodate the passage of food along the contiguous esophagus. The inferior trachea branches at the level of the sternum to become the left and right primary bronchi, which enter the lungs and further divide into secondary bronchi (also called the lobar bronchi) that supply air to the three lobes of the lungs. The branching continues as each secondary bronchus divides into ten tertiary bronchi, which in turn branch extensively to give complete form to the bronchial tree. As the bronchi branch they narrow and lose their cartilage, eventually becoming bronchioles, which divide into terminal bronchioles

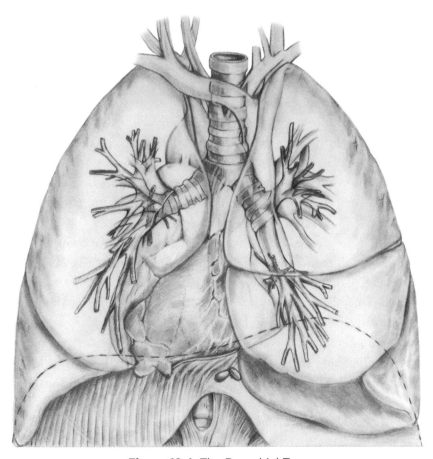

Figure 12.4: The Bronchial Tree

that branch out to become alveolar ducts. Impulses from the ANS cause the bronchi-oles to contract and relax, with the condition of one's neurological functioning and qualities of smooth muscles that form these tubes affecting their capacity for air flow.

Each lung has approximately 1,500 miles of airways and between 275 and 790 million alveoli, the cellular sacs where the exchange of oxygen and carbon dioxide occurs.[7] This is where the lungs receive deoxygenated blood from the pulmonary arteries. Each alveolus consists of a porous epithelial layer (much like the walls of cap-illaries) that is surrounded by a network of capillaries; they also contain elastic fibers that allow them to expand upon inhalation and compress upon exhalation (with their reinflation facilitated by a pulmonary surfactant that reduces surface tension). This very thin respiratory membrane (about one one-thousandths of a millimeter) allows the exchange of respiratory gases to occur very quickly and efficiently.

Each lung is enveloped in a two-layer pleural membrane that adheres to the ribs and diaphragm in separate pleural cavities located on either side of the heart, support-ing the lungs in place. Pleural fluid lubricates and reduces friction between the layers of pleural membrane, easing their movement as the lungs expand and contract. The air-filled passageways and alveoli make the lungs very light while the elastic fibers in the alveoli enable the lungs to tremendously expand, far beyond what is needed for basic oxygen requirements.

There are two types of breathing that involve different ways of moving the lungs: costal (sometimes called "rib breathing") and diaphragmatic (sometimes called "belly breathing"). In costal breathing, the rib cage opens with the inhalation and closes with the exhalation. In diaphragmatic breathing, the belly expands with inhalation and contracts with exhalation. Although neither type is "correct," they fit different cir-cumstances and can be combined to create variations that more or less support certain activities, movements, or energetic intentions. Diaphragmatic breathing is responsible for about seventy-five percent of our respiratory effort.

How fully and deeply we breathe is determined by how we breathe, which typi-cally is more habitual than conscious. In "normal" breathing there is relatively little volume, around five hundred milliliters (depending on physique, fitness, and health), while our respiratory capacity is four to seven times that much. The ability to breathe more deeply, steadily, and calmly—and to more consciously move energy throughout the body—can be developed through practices that make the skeletal and muscular components of breathing stronger and more limber (and the neurological impulses steadier). The movement of breathing itself maintains the suppleness and elasticity of the ribs, costal cartilage, and the muscles that support and mobilize the spine, although lifestyle, age, and genetics can diminish these qualities. The tendency is for the rib cage to expand either front-to-back or laterally, rather than mobilizing the ribs in both directions and thereby expanding breath capacity. Asana practice is an effective tool for developing the mobility of the rib cage in support of more expansive, calm, and balanced breathing.

The movements of the rib cage are blended with the positioning and movement of the pelvis, legs, and shoulders. The pelvis and rib cage are linked through the lumbar spine, where several respiratory muscles attach. Movement of the pelvis affects movement in the rib cage—and vice versa—along with movement of the organs contained in the pelvis and thorax. Movement of the legs into extension stretches the iliopsoas muscles from their insertions on the lesser trochanter of the femoral heads up through the pelvis and to their origin on the anterior transverse processes of the lumbar vertebrae and twelfth thoracic vertebra. This is the same place (T12) where the diaphragm attaches at its central tendon. The shoulder girdle, consisting of the sternum, clavicles, and scapulae, is involved in breathing via its bony articulations and muscular attachments with the rib cage. The arms and shoulders will enhance or constrain inhalations and exhalations depending on their positioning.

The diaphragm and muscles acting on the rib cage do the primary work of respiration. The diaphragm is responsible for about seventy-five percent of inhalation. It

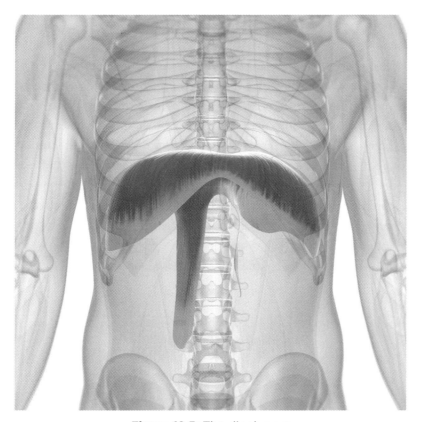

Figure 12.5: The diaphragm

is a double-dome-shaped muscular and fibrous wall located in the middle of the chest just below the lungs and heart, draping like a parachute over the stomach and liver.[8] Its base is formed at the back by asymmetrical vertebral fibers that attach to the third lumbar vertebra. It has a fibrous central tendon out of which muscular fibers rise to attach to the entire circumference of the rib cage, sternum, and deep surface of the lower eight ribs. The diaphragm flattens and draws down as it contracts, varying in shape depending on pressure from the ribs, lungs, and the muscles and organs in the abdomen. Like the heart, it works incessantly. As it contracts and lowers, displacing the soft contents of the abdomen, lung volume increases, reducing air pressure in the lungs and drawing in air from outside due to the relative change in internal and external air pressure. As the diaphragm relaxes, it moves up as the lung's natural elasticity pushes the air out, completing a cycle of breath.

Muscles acting on the rib cage, particularly the intercostal muscles between the ribs, assist the diaphragm. The external intercostal muscles contract to elevate the ribs. The pectoralis minor lifts the ribs forward, opening space in the upper chest and allowing breath more easily to fill the upper lungs. The sternocleidomastoid and scalene muscles also raise the upper rib cage, contributing to breathing into the upper regions of the lungs. Pectoralis major spreads the lower ribs and lifts the sternum, creating a more spacious inhalation that is lower in the lungs. Several muscles with attachments to the side and back ribs play additional roles: the serratus anterior helps maintain the posture of the rib cage (and assists with exhalation); the transverso-spinal muscles extend the spine and thereby help lift the rib cage; serratus posterior spreads the back ribs and eases breath into the back of the lungs. Intercostal muscles also assist complete exhalation by drawing the ribs closer together and compressing the lungs. Lung volume is further reduced by contracting the abdominal muscles: transversus abdominis girdles the waist; the obliques lower the ribs and compress the abdomen; and rectus abdominus further closes the anterior abdomen by drawing the pubis and sternum toward each other. Healthy pelvic floor muscles provide an adaptable foundation that withstands the expansive pressure from above while initiating the active lifting of core abdominal muscles with complete exhalations,[9] actions that are associated with mula bandha and uddiyana bandha.

Common Respiratory Pathologies

Bronchitis: An inflammation of the mucous membranes of the bronchi, bronchitis can be either acute or chronic. Acute bronchitis is associated with the common cold or flu (ninety percent of cases are viral) and generally resolves along with the virus. Chronic bronchitis, a form of chronic obstructive pulmonary disease

(COPD), typically caused by smoking tobacco, is a far more serious condition that involves a productive cough that lasts for several months in the absence of any other underlying disease.

Asthma: This long-term inflammatory lung disease inflames and narrows the airways, obstructing the flow of air and causing recurrent episodes of wheezing, chest tightness, shortness of breath, and coughing.

Emphysema: Smoking tobacco and inhaling other pollutants gradually damages the alveoli and inflames the lungs, leading to the breakdown of lung tissue and reduction of oxygen supply to cells throughout the body. This respiratory disease is a form of COPD, which often occurs with bronchitis. Although this disease is progressive, quitting smoking is the single most effective way to reduce the progression, relieve symptoms, and treat complications.

Pneumonia: This is a common inflammatory lung infection caused by a bacteria, virus, or fungi. About a half billion people are affected by pneumonia per year, resulting in about four million deaths. Its treatment depends on the source of infection, and most cases resolve within a few weeks. Without treatment and proper care, pneumonia can cause respiratory failure and other complications.

Tuberculosis: Dating to antiquity and in folklore associated with vampires, tuberculosis is an infectious and highly contagious mycobacterial disease that attacks the lungs, causing a chronic cough, fever, and potential infection of other organs. Recent hopes of completely eliminating tuberculosis through antibiotics have diminished as drug-resistant strains emerged in the 1980s.

Asbestosis: Although asbestos is a naturally occurring silicate mineral, inhalation of its microscopic fibers causes a chronic inflammatory condition and scarring around the alveolar ducts and walls. The scarring causes the walls to thicken, which compromises the gaseous exchange process, thereby reducing the supply of oxygen to the body and the removal of carbon dioxide. Although one can reduce symptoms such as shortness of breath and hypoxia, there is no cure.

Particulate Pollutants: Atmospheric particulate matter (also known as PM) is a complex mixture of acids, organic chemicals, metals, and dust particles that when inhaled causes potentially serious respiratory problems. Whereas larger particles are usually caught in the nose and throat, smaller particles can enter the lungs (causing lung cancer) and the circulatory system (causing cardiovascular disease, birth defects, and premature death).

Sarcoidosis: Most common among young adults, this disease involves the accumulation of inflammatory cells called granulomas in the lungs or its related lymph nodes due to respiratory infections, causing shortness of breath, fatigue, loss of appetite, loss of weight, coughing, chest tightness, and potentially hemorrhaging in the lungs. Although it may run its course and self-resolve, unresolved cases can affect the skin (causing lesions), nervous system (neurosarcoidosis), the endocrine system (by increasing prolactins), and the heart (affecting conduction). Left untreated, it can self-resolve or develop into pulmonary fibrosis.

Pleural Effusion: A fluid-filled pleural cavity surrounds the lungs. Accumulation of excess fluid inhibits full expansion of the lungs, causing chest pain, shortness of breath, coughing, fever, and rapid breathing. This is most commonly caused by congestive heart failure and is typically treated by intercostal drain.

Pulmonary Edema: This vascular disease is an abnormal accumulation of fluid in the air spaces of lung tissue most commonly caused by congestive heart failure, leaky heart valves, or sudden and severe hypertension. The fluid reduces normal air movement through the lungs, causing shortness of breath (especially when lying down), coughing up of blood, wheezing, and anxiety.

Pulmonary Embolism: A vascular disease, pulmonary embolism is a sudden blockage in a lung artery (usually from a deep vein thrombosis—a blood clot in the legs or pelvis). Symptoms include shortness of breath, rapid breathing, chest pain, and coughing up of blood. If untreated, mortality is around twenty-five percent; about fifteen percent of all sudden death cases are caused by this condition.

Pulmonary Hypertension: An irreversible vascular disease, pulmonary hypertension is high blood pressure in the pulmonary artery, vein, or capillaries (the lung vasculature), causing shortness of breath amid normal activity, fatigue, chest pain, and pain on the upper right side of the abdomen. While treatments can control these symptoms, there is no known cure.

Cultivating a Healthy Respiratory System

Respiratory health primarily depends upon what one breathes into his or her lungs. If one smokes tobacco, stopping is the primary behavior for improving respiratory health. It is also important to avoid exposure to common household and environmental pathogens and especially exposure to more severely toxic pathogens found in many workplaces in which dust particles and chemical solvents are present. Some dairy products may contribute to respiratory difficulties in some people, especially in children with asthma.[10] Cleanliness is important, including of the nasal passages, which can be effectively cleansed using a neti pot for saline nasal irrigation.

Even with a dedicated pranayama practice, one may often find their sinuses less than a cooperative participant in breathing. The nasal passages can be overwhelmed by the very impurities they are designed to filter out, including dirt, dust, and pollen, causing congestion, allergic reactions, colds, and other respiratory problems. If you are an avid surfer, you are already benefiting from an old folk medicine practice that in India is done ritually with the use of a neti pot: saline nasal irrigation. A neti pot makes daily nasal irrigation with a light and warm saline solution as easy as saying *namaste*.

To use a neti pot, follow these simple steps:

1. Purchase a neti pot and a supply of refined salt.

2. Place the recommended quantity of salt in the neti pot, fill the pot halfway with warm water, and stir.

3. Leaning over a sink, tilt your head to the side, place the nozzle into the nostril that is turned higher, and slowly tip the neti pot up to pour the saline solution into that nostril.

4. Continue pouring in the solution as it drains out the opposite nostril.

5. Switch sides and repeat steps 3 and 4.

Nasal irrigation with a neti pot is ideally done every morning as part of morning cleansing practices. The benefits are immediate, starting with the breath flowing more easily through the nostrils and sinuses.

Although a general yoga practice is beneficial for overall health, several specific yoga practices can enhance one's respiratory health. First, one can begin doing basic postural practices that support spacious, upright positioning of the spine that help ease breathing. Second, one can do a variety of yogic breathing exercises to develop or rehabilitate the neuromuscular mechanisms of respiration, as described in detail in Chapter 21. Third, one can do breath-as-mantra meditation practices as described in Chapter 22, including with mental visualizations that highlight a sense of comfort and ease in more spacious and energizing breathing.

13

Glands:
The Endocrine System

There is something bigger than fact: the underlying spirit,
all it stands for, the mood, the vastness, the wildness.
—EMILY CARR

FROM THE GREEK *ENDO*, "within," and *krinein*, "to distinguish," the endocrine system is all about distinguished specialization in supporting and guiding our adaptation to the constantly changing conditions of our bodymind. Although the ancient Greeks and other early medical pioneers were aware of endocrine glands (the Alexandrians were aware of the thymus gland in the third century BCE, Galen discussed the pineal and pituitary glands, and Acivenna discussed the symptoms of diabetes),[1] all they knew was rooted in the myths and mists of humoral conjecture until the mid-nineteenth century, when endocrine function was finally understood to be systemic. The chemistry and basic function of the individual hormones were identified and explained by the early twentieth century.

Unlike the immediate rapid-fire responses and effects of the nervous system, which turn off as quickly as they turn on, the endocrine system responds to stimuli more slowly but with far more lasting effects. Playing a vital role in growth, development, and homeostasis, this ductless system of vascular glands works closely with the nervous system to carry out its diverse array of functions, secreting hormones directly into the circulatory system for targeted transport to various organs.[2] In the late twentieth and early twenty-first centuries, researchers have developed a far deeper understanding of the interaction between the endocrine and nervous systems, leading to such insights as those described as psychoneuroimmunology that are highly relevant to the efficacy of yoga practices in developing a healing resonance.

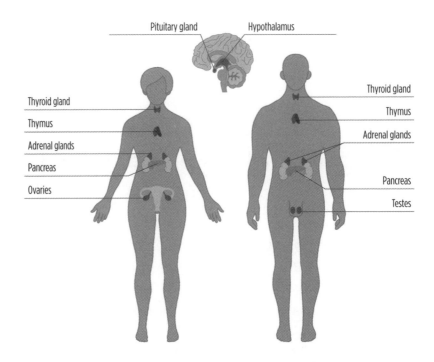

Figure 13.1: The Endocrine System

Hormones as Communicators

Like the nervous system, the endocrine system provides information signaling for communication between organs and tissues, helping to regulate such varied physiological and behavioral activities as digestion, metabolism, respiration, activation of the immune system, sleep, stress, sexual arousal, and mood. But unlike the nervous system, where signals occur only in preexisting nerve tracts, the endocrine system's hormonal signals can travel expansively throughout the circulatory system with relatively continuous yet varying effect depending upon the concentration of hormones (rather than being purely on/off).

Like the neurons of the nervous system, hormones are the endocrine system's agent of communication.[3] These chemical compounds are produced (biosynthesized) in specialized tissues in the endocrine glands and other specialized cells for secretion by the glands into the circulatory system. They are composed of either amino acids or lipids. Water-soluble amino acid–based hormones include the hormones of most of the endocrine organs (all except the adrenal and reproductive organs). There are two types of lipid-based hormones: steroid hormones secreted by the adrenal and reproductive organs; and prostaglandins, produced locally from fatty acids to coordinate local cellular tissue metabolism. Target cells in each hormone allow it to be recognized by associated cell membranes or intracellular receptors throughout the body, which enables a specific hormone to simultaneously affect different receptive tissues and organs throughout the body.

The rate of hormone biosynthesis and secretion varies based on negative feedback in which the endocrine system reacts to reduce or eliminate stimuli that present a challenge to homeostasis. We find direct endocrine response in the thyroid and parathyroid glands, which constantly read and respond (through the release of calcitonin and parathyroid hormone, respectively) to the body's calcium ion levels that are of vital importance to many physiological processes. But the activities of most endocrine glands are regulated by neurons in the hypothalamus, offering indirect responses to changes in the body's biochemistry.

The hypothalamus is an almond-size portion of the brain that links the nervous system to the endocrine system and regulates both systems in three ways:

Direct Control—Adrenal Medulae Release: The autonomic nervous system's direct sympathetic stimulation of endocrine cells in the adrenal medullae causes release of the neurotransmitters epinephrine (also called adrenaline) and norepinephrine (also called noradrenaline) by the adrenal glands into the bloodstream, where they increase heart rate, blood pressure, and set the body in its fight-or-flight mode.

Direct Antidiuretic Hormone (ADH) and Oxytocin Release: Here the hypothalamus functions as an endocrine gland by releasing 1) ADH, aka vasopressin, that increases the kidneys' water retention, and 2) oxytocin, which at the very least stimulates smooth muscle contractions in the uterus, mammary glands, and prostate gland. A rapidly growing body of research shows oxytocin's role in a vast range of other activities and behaviors, including social recognition, trust, orgasm, anxiety, maternal instinct, as well as maladaptive social traits like violence.

Indirect Control—Regulatory Hormone Release: Here the hypothalamus has a central neuroendocrine function, secreting two classes of regulatory hormones—releasing hormone (RH) and inhibiting hormone (IH)—that regulate secretion of endocrine cells in the anterior pituitary gland. RH controls the release of pituitary hormones while IH inhibits the release of pituitary hormones.

Endocrine Glands

The major glands of the endocrine system include the pineal gland, pituitary gland, thyroid gland, parathyroid gland, pancreas, ovaries, testes, hypothalamus, and the adrenal glands. Here we will look briefly at each, starting with what some refer to as the mysterious pineal gland, which is typically given little attention in the scientific physiology community.

THE ONCE MYSTERIOUS PINEAL GLAND AND PSEUDOSCIENCE

When we lack knowledge, we often make things up, what today might be called "alternative facts." Do bear in mind that it was not so long ago that we considered the Earth to be flat and did not know that germs exist; we bowed to the east every morning, praying for the sun to return, and we offered sacrifices to the gods or prayed to God in response to magico-religious explanations for common infections.

When Galen posited the presence of a "psychic pneuma" in the ventricles near the pineal gland, many others ran with this to proclaim the gland or the tissues near it as the localized site of consciousness, which Galen himself roundly rejected as unfounded speculation. To Descartes, who wrote extensively and with deep complexity about the pineal gland, it was the "seat of the soul" in a mechanical body otherwise devoid of cognitive or conscious capacity, whereas to Bataille it was the "pineal eye." With most early modern science considering the pineal gland to be vestigial, those who tended toward speculation in offering neat explanations for everything did as they were wont to do. Thus, for example, the consistently imaginative Madame Blavatsky imputed the pineal gland, unknown and thus unreported in original tantric texts, to tantra's ajna chakra, leading many modern-to-contemporary New Age imaginations to confidently posit it as the "third eye." Today a vast range of pseudoscientists attempt further validation of this notion by referencing the presence of hallucinogenic dimethyltryptamine (DMT) found in the pineal glands of rats, whereas others warn of what they describe as "calcification" of the pineal due to fluoride, vaccines, or "chemtrails" as a source of collective amnesia or confusion, the solution to which is typically an herb or supplement, or a detox diet.

Science is far from explaining everything. There will always be mysteries. We may eventually have a technology that reveals that the pineal gland does far more than it is known to do in seemingly miraculous ways: it translates the effects of light into a chemical that affects sleep. For now, we might well rest in that knowledge.

Pineal Gland

About the size of a grain of rice, this pine cone–shaped pineal gland is located in the roof of the diencephalon in the approximate center of the brain, directly back from what we colloquially call the third eye. Reacting to visual information about light and dark, it produces melatonin, which affects our sleep patterns in seasonal and circadian rhythms. There are wildly diverse pseudoscientific notions about its greater significance (as discussed above), ranging from its association with tantra's ajna chakra to Descartes's "seat of the soul" to Bataille's "pineal eye."

Pituitary Gland

Pea-size and located off the bottom of the hypothalamus at the base of the brain, the pituitary gland (also called the hypophysis) secretes eight different hormones involved in multiple physiological processes, including those that affect stress, growth, reproduction, blood pressure, the thyroid glands, and metabolism. Its anterior and posterior regions are functionally distinct structures. The anterior pituitary arises from the ectoderm, with its endocrine cells surrounded by two networks of capillaries that provide a direct path for hormones to flow from the hypothalamus through it and on into general circulation. Under the regulatory control of the hypothalamus's RH and IH (with GABA—gamma-aminobutyric acid—also involved in regulation), the anterior pituitary gland produces and secretes the following hormones (among others):

Corticotropes: Adrenocorticotropic hormone (ACTH) stimulates release of steroidal hormones by the adrenal cortex cells in the adrenal glands in response to biological stress.

Thyrotropes: Thyroid-stimulating hormone (TSH) stimulates the thyroid gland to trigger the release of the thyroid hormones thyroxine and triiodothyronine, which are involved in cellular metabolism throughout most of the body.

Somatropes: Growth hormone (GH, also called human growth hormone) is a peptide hormone that stimulates growth, cell reproduction, and cell regeneration. Age, sex, diet, stress, and other hormones affect its production and secretion, and its synthesized form is promoted in dietary supplements as a fountain of youth.

Prolactins: Prolactin (PRL) is primarily involved in the stimulation of the mammary glands for production of milk. It also plays an influential role in literally hundreds of other functions, ranging from postorgasmic sexual gratification to the formation of myelin coatings on axons in the central nervous system.

Gonadotropes: These endocrine cells produce the gonadotropins luteinizing hormone (LH) and follicle-stimulating hormone (FSH) that play vital roles in reproduction system regulation. LH induces ovulation and stimulates the release of estrogen and progesterone as part of a fertile woman's menstrual cycle, preparing the body for pregnancy. In men it regulates the production of testosterone. FSH also assists in production of testosterone in men, and further regulates female sex organs.

The posterior pituitary (also called the neurohypophysis) is more of an amalgamation of axons projecting downward from the hypothalamus than a glandular structure. These axons store and release the direct antidiuretic hormone (ADH) and oxytocin discussed earlier.

Thyroid Gland

Located in the neck just below the Adam's apple (which is thyroid cartilage, also known as the laryngeal prominence), the thyroid gland is a small butterfly-shaped gland that weighs less than one ounce yet controls the rate at which every cell, tissue, and organ functions. The pace of energy absorption, production of proteins upon which metabolic processes depend, and the sensitivity of the body to other hormones are all under the commanding control of the thyroid. Its secretions are regulated by thyroid-stimulating hormone (TSH) in the anterior pituitary, as discussed earlier, while TSH is in turn regulated by the hypothalamus.

The thyroid gland has scores of nodule-like follicles that release hormones into circulation, the most significant of which is thyroxine, which stimulates energy production in cells that causes increased cellular metabolism and oxygen consumption. It also produces calcitonin (CT), which helps to regulate calcium ion concentrations in the intestines (inhibiting calcium absorption), bones (inhibiting osteoclast activity and stimulating osteoblastic activity), and kidneys (inhibiting reabsorption of calcium so it can be released through urination).

Parathyroid Gland

The parathyroid glands, which resemble brown lentils in size and shape, generally consist of two pairs of tiny glands located on the posterior surfaces of the thyroid gland that share a similar arterial blood supply, venous drainage, and lymphatic drainage as the larger thyroid gland. They produce parathyroid hormone (PTH), which works in tandem with the thyroid gland to regulate calcium and homeostasis but with effects that oppose those of the thyroid. The PTH stimulates bone-dissolving cells (osteoclasts), increases calcium absorption in the intestines, and reduces urinary release of calcium.

Thymus

We discussed the thymus earlier as part of the immune system (see Chapter 11 on the lymphatic system and immunity). The thymus produces several hormones called thymosins, which support the development of lymphocytes. Again, this is the site of T-cell maturation during infancy through puberty, after which the thymus begins to atrophy, with only residual lymphocyte generation thereafter.

Pancreas

The pancreas is a dual-function gland with both endocrine and exocrine cells that lies in the abdomen between the stomach and small intestine, its head surrounded by the duodenum, its body behind the base of the stomach, and its tail extending to the spleen. About a million cells with endocrine function are clustered together to form islets of Langerhans (also called pancreatic islets) that are scattered among the exocrine-secreting cells.[4] The islet cells play an essential role in glucose metabolism and the regulation of blood sugar levels. There are four cell types in the islets, each of which produce and secrete different hormones:

Alpha cells: Secrete glucagon, which increases blood glucose levels.

Beta cells: Secrete insulin, which decreases blood glucose levels.

Delta cells: Secrete somatostatin, which regulates alpha and beta cells.

Gamma cells: Secrete pancreatic polypeptides, which self-regulate pancreatic secretions.

Adrenal Glands

The two triangle-shaped adrenal glands (the right adrenal gland is more pyramidal, the left more semilunar in shape) are nestled atop each kidney, surrounded by a capsule, and enclosed in the renal fascia that also encases the kidneys. Each has an outer adrenal cortex and inner adrenal medulla that produce different hormones—commonly called stress hormones—to help the body respond to stress.

Adrenal cortex: Produces glucocorticoids (the most important of which is cortisol) that accelerate glucose synthesis and glycogen formation, making more glucose—the brain's energy source—available for neurons. This steroid is an anti-inflammatory often used to control allergic rashes. The adrenal cortex also produces mineralocorticoids that target kidney cells, regulating sodium and potassium levels that in turn affect water retention, as well as sex hormones called androgens (also produced in the testes).

Adrenal medulla: Surrounded by the adrenal cortex, the adrenal medulla produces adrenaline and noradrenaline and releases it directly into the bloodstream, preparing the body for its fight-or-flight response to stressful environmental conditions.

Ovaries

Part of the female endocrine and reproductive systems (the latter discussed in detail in Chapter 16), the paired ovaries are located on either side of the uterus and produce eggs and hormones used in sexual reproduction. When stimulated by the hormone FSH, the eggs develop in a nest of follicles that produce estrogen, which along with FSH nurture the growth of the uterine lining in the period leading up to ovulation. These hormones determine secondary female sexual characteristics such as breast development and body mass. After ovulation the follicle cells produce progesterone, which prepares the uterus for pregnancy and, in conjunction with estrogen, promotes menstrual changes in the endometrium.

Testes

The testes, part of the male endocrine and reproductive systems (the latter discussed in detail in Chapter 16), produce androgens (male steroids), the most important of which is testosterone. This hormone causes the development of male sexual organs, stimulates production of sperm, and helps determine secondary sexual characteristics such as sex drive, hair distribution, and body mass.

Common Endocrine Pathologies

There are several common endocrine system pathologies, including the following:

Adrenal disorders: Adrenal gland disorders involve excessive or insufficient production of hormones, causing either hyperfunction or hypofunction. The various adrenal disorders arise from a variety of conditions, including genetic mutations, tumors, infections, pituitary problems, or in reaction to certain medicines. The consequent disorders are far ranging and include Addison's disease, hyperplasia, and Cushing's disease, with such symptoms as weakness, tiredness, dizziness when standing up, nausea, joint pain, and craving for salt.

Diabetes: If the pancreas fails to produce enough insulin (Type I diabetes) or the cells of the body do not properly respond to the insulin (Type II diabetes, cases of which account for ninety percent of all diabetes cases), blood sugar levels rise, which can damage the eyes, kidneys, and nerves. Over eight percent of the worldwide adult population has diabetes, which results in two to five million deaths annually. Treatment and prevention start with diet and exercise.

Thyroid disorders: Because the thyroid gland influences almost every metabolic process, its disorder can cause a variety of problems, ranging from goiter (a harmless swelling of the gland) to myxedema coma. If there is too much thyroid hormone (hyperthyroidism), every body function tends to speed up. With hypothyroidism, everything tends to slow down. The most serious disorder is thyroid cancer, which is three times more common in women than men. Unless the cancer is anaplastic, there is an excellent prognosis, especially if it is treated in Stage I or II (there is a ninety-eight to one hundred percent survival rate for papillary, follicular, and medullary forms).

Sex hormone disorders: Reduced activity of the gonads (hypogonadism) affects sex hormone biosynthesis and consequently sexual development and function. In men the effect is lower testosterone (which reduces muscle mass, energy, libido, erectile function, and mental acuity), whereas in women the effect is similar to experiences when moving into menopause (causing delayed onset of menarche and infertility). There are many other sex hormone disorders, including amenorrhea, hermaphroditism, and androgen insensitivity syndromes.

MEN Tumors: The endocrine glands can develop several distinct syndromes with associated tumors that are classified as multiple endocrine neoplasias (MEN). These rare conditions, which appear to have a largely genetic basis, can cause both benign and malignant tumors of the pituitary, thyroid, parathyroids, adrenals, pancreas, paraganglia, or nonendocrine organs.

Obesity: Although primarily a matter of diet, exercise, and genetics, endocrine disorders can contribute to obesity even as obesity causes some endocrine abnormalities.

Cultivating a Healthy Endocrine System

The key to maintaining or cultivating a healthy endocrine system is to maintain overall good health with food, sleep, and exercise. Aging has inevitable effects on our glands. The pituitary typically becomes smaller, we have lower production of growth hormone, and in women, the ovaries stop making estrogen and progesterone. Hormone imbalances can also arise from disease, physical, or mental stress, and environmental factors that introduce endocrine-disrupting chemicals (EDCs).

Eating healthy foods while minimizing the consumption of sugar, alcohol, and caffeine helps to maintain a healthy endocrine system. A balanced diet makes it easier to deal with stressful conditions, which in turn makes it easier to sleep. Doing a regular yoga practice and doing other simple exercises such as walking, cycling, or hiking also contribute to better digestion, less stress, better sleep, and generally better health. There is strong evidence supporting the efficacy of specific dietary practices, including the use of herbs and dietary supplements, to address specific glandular and hormonal problems.

14

Digestion:
The Digestive System

Let food be thy medicine and medicine thy food.
—HIPPOCRATES

How Much of You Is What You Eat?

The popular saying that "you are what you eat" has considerable truth, but there is a lot more to the story of how our tissues are our tissues. We start with what we inherit—the unique combination of traits given to us by our biological parents, which are immediately affected by the conditions within which they develop. This begins *in utero* (literally "in the womb") and is profoundly affected by our mother's internal and external environment, including how she nourishes herself with foods that affect her tissues. It continues throughout our lives as our own internal and external environments continuously affect our own tissues, perhaps most significantly through the foods with which we nourish ourselves and the interwoven systems that integrate those foods into every cell of our being.

Although our focus here is on what happens inside, it is important to acknowledge two external factors that can have an inestimably powerful effect on what does happen inside: the natural environment and the sociocultural environment, each of which influence what we eat and how we eat. Today most food is produced in an industrial model of cultivation and distribution involving extensive use of chemical fertilizers and pesticides, extensive processing (sometimes called "refining"), and packaging and shipping that can make the food we eat more a cause of toxicity than nutrition.[1] Our food consumption patterns and even how we eat—from our mental state to mastication and beyond—are influenced by pervasive cultural messages about physical appearance and attractiveness that cause many people to compromise their nutrition in exchange for the promise of something better. Meanwhile, as our bodies react to poor nutrition, we are inundated with advertisements for quick solution products for every conceivable digestive concern, from halitosis to overeating to gaseous indigestion to constipation, with more and more of such messages and products coming to us from "alternative health" sources. By better understanding what happens on the inside, we can better appreciate and navigate our available choices for how we relate to what comes to us from the outside.

The Digestive Tract

When one eats, food travels about nine meters (over thirty feet) from mouth to anus along a path called the digestive tract. The digestive tract (also called the alimentary canal) consists of the mouth, throat, and gastrointestinal (GI) tract; the GI tract is supported in its food processing activities by the liver, gallbladder, spleen, and pancreas. All along the way the food is broken down into smaller and smaller soluble products that can be absorbed into the bloodstream and assimilated into the rest of the body, with waste products eventually defecated via the rectum/anus. Yet before food ever arrives into the mouth, other systems are already affecting our digestive experience, starting with the hardwired visual and olfactory senses sending messages to the brain that can very much affect whether or how we will eat whatever is before us. Once we initiate our nutritional food processing in the mouth, we further churn and break down foods in the GI tract where chemicals reduce food to small molecules that can be readily absorbed by the digestive lining. Digestive system organs provide acids and enzymes to facilitate this processing, allowing more complete absorption of nutrients and elimination of waste. Let's look at this more closely.

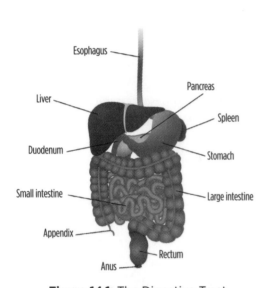

Esophagus

Liver

Pancreas

Spleen

Duodenum

Stomach

Small intestine

Large intestine

Appendix

Rectum

Anus

Figure 14.1: The Digestive Tract

The Mouth and Throat

Digestion begins the moment food enters the mouth, which is the first part of the alimentary canal. The mouth allows us to taste, chew, lubricate, and begin to chemically digest food. This oral cavity is formed by several structures: the mucus membrane–lined cheeks, which give way anteriorly to the lips (oral labia), gums, and teeth; the hard and soft palates, which form the roof of the mouth, separate the oral cavity from the nasal cavity above, and provide a sufficiently hard surface to bear the pressure of mastication; and the muscular tongue, which extends down into the pharynx and forms the floor of the mouth. The lingual tonsils, located at the base of the tongue, are lymphoid nodules with associated mucous glands that drain into pits called tonsillar crypts, helping to resist infection.

Once food is in the mouth, the chemoreceptors (the taste buds, the heart of the gustatory system) mainly on the upper surface of the tongue send information about the food via cranial nerves to the brain, which detects its qualities. If sensibly good or tolerable, we chew; if not, we might spit it out. Specific taste sensations—bitterness, saltiness, savoriness (or umami), sourness, and sweetness—trigger different responses. Bitterness can be a warning of poison, yet it can also trigger the release of calcium. Sourness—a sign of relatively high acidity—can be a sign of rotten food or a signal about acid balance. Saltiness interacts with sourness to control both acid balance and sodium balance. Sweetness promises energy. All the while, the nose thinks it knows; the olfactory receptors detect smells that combine with gustatory sensations to create the full experience of flavor.

When the choice has been made to chew, the tongue goes into greater action in moving food around in the mouth in coordinated movement with the teeth, gums, jaw, lips, and cheeks, stimulating secretion of saliva from three pairs of main salivary glands (plus close to a thousand minor salivary glands). The salivary glands produce about one quart of saliva daily, which despite being comprised mostly of water (99.4%), secrete sufficient supplies of digestive enzymes to initiate the chemical breakdown of food in the mouth. The largest salivary gland, the parotid, mainly secretes purely serous (not mucus) saliva containing the enzyme amylase, which plays a vital role in digesting carbohydrates. Other glands release amylase and other enzymes, including the digestive enzyme lipase (which breaks down fats). When not eating, the salivary glands continually release saliva into the mouth to help keep it free of harmful bacteria.

The Teeth

In chewing (masticating), the opposing surfaces of the teeth help to break down various food substances into sufficiently small particles to swallow. Beginning around age seven, our twenty primary teeth (deciduous teeth, popularly known as baby teeth) gradually give way to the emergence of thirty-two adult permanent teeth, all with roots embedded in the jaws and covered by gums. Each tooth has one of four specialized tooth structures that play different roles in the mechanical reduction of food to more digestible size. Eight bladelike incisors in the center front of the mouth have sharp edges useful in cutting. Four larger and stronger pointed cuspids (also called canines or eyeteeth) are effective in tearing, including through the tough connective tissues of animals and fibers of plants. The twenty remaining teeth are premolars (also called bicuspids) and molars with broad, flat surfaces and multiple ridges that effectively grind and mash food. So-called wisdom teeth—a full set of third molars—may erupt in adulthood (when one might be wiser), typically causing dysfunctional repositioning of other teeth; this problem is usually avoided by having the wisdom teeth pulled.

The roots of the teeth fit into sockets in the ridge-shaped alveolar bone that lines the upper (maxilla) and lower (mandible) jaws and are held in place by periodontal ligaments, specialized connective tissue that connects the alveolar bone to the soft, yet bone-like cementum layer covering the root of the tooth. The main substance of each tooth consists of dentin, a mineralized connective tissue located between the enamel or cementum and the pulp cavity that receives blood and nerves through a hole (root canal) at its base. A layer of enamel, which is the hardest and most highly mineralized substance manufactured in the body, covers the crown of the tooth.

After chewing, the masticated food—it's now called a *bolus* (from the Latin for "ball")—is swallowed, which sounds and typically is simple enough but nonetheless involves a complex set of neuromuscular activities, each controlled by a different neurological mechanism. The first of three phases occurs in the activities of the mouth and teeth just described, with the parasympathetic nervous system signaling the salivary glands to release saliva, the lingual nerve detecting the consistency of food on the tongue, the mylohyoid nerve stimulating movement of the tongue, the superior laryngeal nerve initiating the swallowing reflex, and a set of cranial nerves firing to begin the actual voluntary act of swallowing. Next, as the bolus moves downward into the pharynx (the throat), involuntary actions cause the nasopharynx and epiglottis to close and the hyoid to lift (thereby lifting the pharynx and larynx altogether), ensuring that the peristaltic actions in the throat push the bolus down into the esophagus. Entering the third phase, swallowing is now entirely under involuntary neuromuscular control, the pharynx and larynx elastically relax down from the hyoid, and peristalsis causes the further transit through the esophagus, an elastic muscular tube that contracts in waves and has valves (sphincters) at each end. Finally, the lower esophageal sphincter relaxes to let the bolus of food enter the stomach, and then the sphincter closes to prevent reflux (regurgitation).

The Stomach

After the mastication phase of digestion, the second phase of digestion occurs in the stomach (ultimately from the Greek *stoma*, "mouth"). This muscular and greatly distensible organic storage facility is capable of storing anything from a light snack to a full meal, enabling one to eat substantial meals and drink large quantities of water rather than needing to eat or drink only in small amounts. The stomach's expansion capacity arises from the composition of its walls, which consists of three layers of smooth muscle lined with mucosa. When relaxed, the walls fold into themselves, creating folds called *rugae* that disappear when the stomach expands. The outer structure of the stomach resembles a fetus or an expanded *J*, its large convex side called the greater curvature and the smaller concave surface called the lesser curvature. The outer surface of the stomach is draped with an apron-like structure called the greater omentum, a large peritoneal fold that extends below the greater curvature, over the small intestines, and as far down as the pelvis. The lower esophageal sphincter divides the stomach at its top from the esophagus, and the pyloric sphincter divides the stomach from the small intestines below; the closing of both sphincters contains the contents within the stomach.

The stomach greets each bolus of food with gastric juices, including proteases (such as pepsin, which breaks down proteins) and hydrochloric acid (which reacts to bacteria and facilitates the work of protein-digesting enzymes). The exact composition of the gastric juices is determined by the central nervous system (CNS) and glands found in the layers of the stomach. With the stomach churning in its peristaltic action and gastric juices swirling around, the agitated boluses are converted into a soupy mixture called chyme (pronounced "kime," which rhymes with "time"). The pyloric sphincter opens to allow the chyme to slowly move into the small intestine.

The Small Intestine

The small intestine might be a misnomer in that at 6 meters in length it is about four times longer than the large intestine, but the varied diameter of the small intestine (2.5–4 cm) is at most about half that of the large intestine (7 cm). Nor is the small intestine small in its digestive role, for it is here that most of the important digestive processes—specifically around eighty percent of the GI tract's absorption of nutrients and minerals—occur. It is composed of three regions, each with a distinct role in digestion:

Duodenum: The pyloric sphincter connects the stomach to the duodenum, which receives chyme from the stomach along with digestive enzyme secretions from the pancreas and bile from the liver via the gall bladder. These digestive juices break down proteins and emulsify fats.

Jejunum: Located in the midsection of the small intestine, this is the region where most digestion and nutrient absorption occurs. Its circular folds are covered with enterocytes and villi (which increase the surface absorption area) that allow only very small nutrient particles (all except for fats, which pass into the lymphatic system) to pass through to the liver in enterohepatic circulation.

Ileum: The longest section of the small intestine (about half its overall length), the ileum also contains villi and mainly absorbs vitamin B12 and bile. It gives way to the large intestine at the ileocecal valve, which controls the flow of chyme into the large intestine.

The Large Intestine

After digestion in the small intestine, whatever food remains moves into the large intestine (also called the colon) for around sixteen hours of final digestive activity, which begins at the ileum and ends at the anus. The slow movement allows maximum retention of water and other compounds. This last segment of the GI tract largely frames the small intestine and consists of three main parts: 1) the cecum, 2) the colon proper, and 3) the rectum. The general function of the large intestine is waste storage, water reclamation, and absorption of vitamin K (which the liver needs in synthesizing anticlotting substances), biotin (essential in glucose metabolism), and vitamin B5 (essential in the production of steroidal hormones and some neurotransmitters). Strong peristaltic actions from the transverse colon through the descending colon push any remaining fecal material into the rectum. Stretching the rectal walls triggers the defecation reflex and causes excretion of waste through the anus.

The Liver and Gallbladder in Digestion

The largest organ in the abdominal cavity, the liver is in the upper right quadrant of the abdomen directly under the diaphragm, with the intimately related gallbladder nestled into a recess in its right lobe. The liver has over two hundred functions that support almost every organ in the body, including its central role in synthesizing and secreting bile, regulating metabolism, and providing a blood storage reservoir. Its primary role in digestion is bile production.

Bile, which consists of mostly water (97%), salts, and cholesterol, helps to emulsify lipids and neutralize acids in chyme to aid in the digestion of fats. Bile passes through the liver's hepatic ducts and moves through the common hepatic duct to the gallbladder, a pear-shaped muscular organ that sits just beneath the right lobe of the liver and stores bile. While in storage, the bile becomes increasingly concentrated as water is absorbed, its salts potentially forming problematic gallstones. As fatty food enters the duodenum, it stimulates the release of the intestinal hormone cholecystokinin (CKK) into the circulating blood, which triggers the release of bile from the gallbladder, with greater amounts of bile release if the chyme contains a large quantity of fat.

The Pancreas

We previously summarized the endocrine functions of the pancreas, which is primarily an exocrine gland (only around one percent of its cells are endocrine cells, which produce insulin and glucagon). Located behind the stomach (between the duodenum and the spleen), it secretes pancreatic juices (digestive enzymes and buffers) that are transported to the duodenum to help break down carbohydrates, proteins, and lipids. Different pancreatic enzymes (lipases, carbohydrases, and proteinases) specifically break down lipids, sugars and starches, and proteins, respectively, as informed by hormones from the duodenum that are released in response to different compositions of chyme.

Common Digestive Pathologies

There are several common digestive pathologies, including the following:

Oral Disease: This broad category of digestive disorders includes dental and periodontal infections, mucosal disorders, oral and pharyngeal cancers, and developmental disorders, among others. Plaque-induced gingivitis is a common periodontal disease that leads to periodontitis, in which the gums deteriorate and expose the teeth to greater infection. Herpes simplex is the most common oral viral infection, causing recurrent blisters around the mouth and lips. Oral candidiasis is the most common oral fungal infection.

Esophageal Diseases: A wide variety of diseases and conditions, some derived from congenital conditions and others acquired later in life, affect the esophagus. The most common is gastroesophageal reflux disease (GERD, also known as acid reflux disease), in which the lower esophageal sphincter does not properly close. Dysphagia (difficulty swallowing due to mechanical causes or motility issues) and chest or back pain (sometimes associated with esophageal cancer) are also common.

Stomach Diseases: Diseases and conditions in which the stomach is inflamed due to infection are all called gastritis, which if chronic may indicate other diseases such as pyloric stenosis or gastric cancer. Gastric ulceration is a common condition that erodes the gastric mucosa, causing peptic ulcers. Common symptoms of a gastric disease are indigestion and vomiting.

Intestinal Disease: The many diseases of the small and large intestines can be caused by infection, autoimmune failure, or conditions in other organs. Common problems in the small intestine include intestinal obstruction, irritable bowel syndrome, peptic ulcers, celiac disease, Crohn's disease, and intestinal cancer. Inflammatory bowel disease is one of the most common problems in the large intestine. Appendicitis (caused by inflammation of the appendix), colitis (generalized inflammation of the large intestine), and hemorrhoids are other common conditions.

Liver Disease: Hepatic diseases are those affecting the liver. There are many kinds of liver diseases, including those involving inflammation caused by the hepatitis A, B, and C viruses. The yellowing of the skin, called jaundice, can be a sign of liver disease. Alcohol is the leading cause of liver disease and can lead to the chronic condition of cirrhosis, in which diseased liver tissue is replaced by scar tissue that may cause the liver to fail. The liver can also develop cancerous tumors.

Pancreatic Disease: There are several pancreatic diseases, including pancreatitis, in which the pancreas is inflamed when digestive enzymes begin digesting the pancreas itself (with rapid onset in acute forms, which are commonly associated with alcohol abuse). Inhibited insulin production by the pancreas leads to diabetes mellitus. There are also hereditary diseases such as cystic fibrosis in which cysts form in the pancreas, causing irreversible damage, inflammation, and premature death. Pancreatic tumors are among the most lethal of all cancers: the overall five-year survival rate is around five percent.

Gallbladder: The gallbladder normally stores bile and secretes it through the common bile duct to aid in digestion of fats. Gallstones, the formation of which is widely debated (with body chemistry, weight, and low-calorie diets all potentially involved), can block the ducts, causing painful inflammation. Many gallbladder problems are resolved by surgical removal of the organ.

Cultivating a Healthy Digestive System

When healthy, the digestive system functions to break down and absorb nutritious food into the body. We surveyed the basic ways this happens through ingestion, mechanical breakdown, chemical breakdown, absorption, and excretion. At the end of the day—indeed all day and night—the ultimate end of digestion is the maintenance of our tissues and fueling of the energy we require to live. We take in food that contains large organic molecules, many of which are insoluble and indigestible. If we can break down these molecules into digestible size and absorb them into our tissues, they will give us the ATP required in cellular metabolism; allow us to synthesize complex proteins, carbohydrates, and fats; and help ensure our healthy hydration. They will also give us a vital supply of what are often referred to as micronutrients: minerals, microminerals, trace minerals, vitamins, phytochemicals, antioxidants, and healthy intestinal flora.

Thus, a healthy digestive system begins with properly eating nutritious foods, which are organic whole foods, not foods that are heavily processed and refined, enriched, or fortified. First and foremost, since stress affects digestion—it can restrict blood flow to the GI tract, inhibit peristalsis, cause the esophagus to spasm, decrease the secretion of digestive enzymes, and contribute to ulcers and bowel dysfunction[2]— it is important to be relaxed while eating. This can be achieved by setting aside time for each meal, sitting, and signifying the sacred exchange of energy achieved in eating with a moment of silence, prayer, or other conscious act. Eating slowly, remaining relaxed, and being conscious that eating is one of the most important things in life all contribute to effective nutrition.

Second, proper eating involves thorough mastication, the lack of which can detract from effective digestive processes farther down through the digestive system.[3] Proper mastication is bilateral, thoroughly prepares food for swallowing, exposes food to saliva that starts the process of carbohydrate absorption, and increases overall nutrient absorption.

Third, we are inundated with diet fads—blood-type, detox, macrobiotic, Paleolithic, gluten-free, low-carbohydrate, high-carbohydrate, liquid, food-combining, raw, vegetarian, vegan, pescatarian—that tell us exactly how, what, when, and how much to eat. Although we appreciate the importance of special dietary intake with conditions such as celiac disease and lactose intolerance, a healthy diet is a nutritious one that contains abundant fresh fruits and vegetables, whole grains, legumes, nuts, seeds, lean meats, and fish.[4] Rather than developing stress over managing a precisely specified diet, it is more important to simply eat consciously, drink water, and enjoy what one is eating.

15

Letting Go:
The Urinary System

*Some of us think holding on makes us strong;
but sometimes it is letting go.*
—HERMAN HESSE

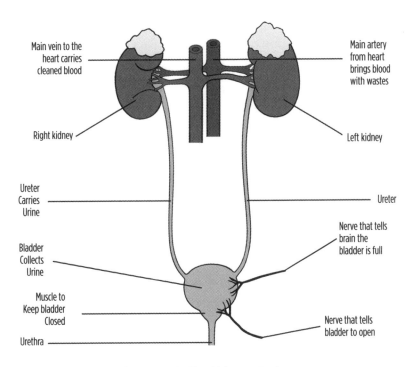

Figure 15.1: The Urinary System

Filtering

Although we do not ordinarily associate urine with blood, the primary role of the urinary system is to filter wastes that accumulate in the blood and discharge them via urination in a process that helps to maintain normal volume and composition of the blood. It accomplishes this by working in conjunction with the cardiovascular, respiratory, and digestive systems. The cardiovascular system both delivers nutrients to tissues and picks up wastes; carbon dioxide is eliminated via the respiratory system. The digestive system separates nutrients from waste, works with the liver to balance the concentration of nutrients in the blood, and directly excretes solid waste from the body. Any remaining water-soluble waste in the blood is filtered out by the kidneys in the process that creates urine, which is stored in the bladder for subsequent excretion. The urinary system also helps to regulate blood volume and pressure, electrolytes and metabolites, and blood pH.

The urinary system consists of two bean-shaped kidneys that produce urine, two ureters that transport urine to the bladder, a bladder for temporary urine storage, and a urethra for excreting urine form the body. The kidneys are located at the rear of the abdominal cavity on either side of the spine at about the level of the lower ribs with an adrenal gland nestled on top of each one. Each kidney and adrenal gland is held in place by the peritoneal lining and the renal fascia, which also help to cushion the kidneys from being jostled about. The kidney is divided into two main structures: an outer renal cortex and an inner renal medulla that has eight to eighteen cone-shaped renal pyramids (or lobes) where urine production occurs. The tip of each pyramid has small ducts that release urine into the minor calyses (which form a cup-shaped drain), which in turn empty into major calyces before flowing into the funnel-shaped renal pelvis that connects to the ureter.

The Kidneys

Each kidney has over a million urine-producing units called nephrons (from the Greek *nephros*, "kidney"), the key functional units that regulate water concentration and filter the blood. Each nephron has a renal tubule with a filter called the renal corpuscle. Blood arrives via efferent and afferent arterioles for filtration in the renal corpuscle, which yields a protein-free fluid called filtrate. The filtrate moves on through successive segments of the nephron for more elaborate filtering, becoming tubular fluid as it filters through the proximal convoluted tubule (where it reabsorbs nutrients such as glucose, acids, and ions), then into the loop of Henle where it flows into both an ascending limb (where ions are removed) and a descending limb that descends into the medulla (and moves water out via osmosis). The ascending limb gives way to the distal convoluted tubule, where ion transport regulated by the endocrine system occurs, before delivering the refined filtrate—urine—to the last segment of the nephron, the collecting duct. Multiple nephrons deliver urine to each collecting duct, and further absorption of water and/or secretion of sodium and other ions give the urine its ultimate composition. Urine leaves the kidneys through a pair of muscular ureters that begin at the renal pelvis of the kidneys and terminate in the urinary bladder. A layer of smooth involuntary muscles creates peristaltic waves through the ureters about twice per minute, pushing urine down into the bladder.

The Bladder

The hollow and highly distensible bladder collects and temporarily stores urine before contracting to push the accumulated urine into the urethra, which extends to the outside of the body. The male urethra carries both urine and sperm cells to the tip of the penis, while the far shorter female urethra carries only urine. The urge to urinate arises when the bladder is relatively full and there is sufficient pressure on the stretch receptors in its walls to trigger a reflex contraction that gives us the urge to urinate and stimulates involuntary contractions of the bladder. The contractions increase pressure in the bladder, which can be relieved by either relaxing the external sphincter (thus releasing urine) or not relaxing it, thus retaining the urine and causing the bladder reflex mechanism to reset and the bladder to further fill. As the bladder fills to capacity, eventually the external sphincter will relax, whether voluntarily or involuntarily.

With healthy urination, we release around 1,200 ml of water per day and about that same amount through sweat, feces, and exhalations. We gain water from the water content of food, directly from liquids, and from the destructive metabolic process of catabolism in which large molecules are broken down into smaller units. Around forty percent of body water is found in living cells (as the watery element of intracellular fluid, or ICF), with the rest found in extracellular fluid (ECF), which includes interstitial fluid, plasma, lymph, and other fluids. The ICF and ECF fluid pools contain very different fluid compositions: ICF contains mostly potassium, magnesium, and phosphate ions, whereas ECF contains mostly sodium, chloride, and bicarbonate. Changes in their respective concentrations affect pH balance and metabolic processes. Our sodium and potassium concentrations are particularly significant in determining our electrolyte balance (i.e., the balance of negative and positive ions), which in turn affects water balance (water in, water out) and cellular metabolism. Sodium concentrations in the ECF and potassium concentrations in the ICF reflect the balance between their absorption in the digestive tract and their release, primarily through the kidneys.

Common Urinary Pathologies

There are several common urinary pathologies, including the following:

Renal Failure: The kidneys are most commonly damaged by diabetes, hypertension, or inflammation of the kidney's filtration units (the glomeruli). Failure causes toxic wastes to accumulate in the body, raises blood pressure, and causes excess fluid retention. Other contributing factors include infection, heart disease, liver failure, blood clots, prostate cancer, colon cancer, and many others.

Kidney Stones: Also called renal calculi or nephroliths, kidney stones are solid pieces of materials that form in the kidneys from minerals in the urine stream. Ranging in size from a grain of sand to a small pearl, they typically pass out through the urine. If large enough to block the ureter, kidney stones can cause intense pain (called renal colic) that radiates into the groin and genitals. Different types of stones are classified based on their location and chemical composition, with calcium stones (very likely associated with high intakes of animal proteins) being the most common. Removal techniques range from painful patience in natural passing to surgical removal.

Urinary Tract Infections: Urinary tract infections (UTIs) can affect different parts of the urinary tract. In the lower tract they are commonly known as bladder infections, which occur far more commonly in women than men due to sexual anatomy: in women the urethra is much shorter and closer to the anus. Infection in the upper urinary tract (called pyelonephritis) is a kidney infection, which arises from bacteria spreading up through the urinary tract or traveling through the blood. The sexually transmitted disease chlamydia is a frequent source of this bacterial infection. Urinating immediately after intercourse, effective personal hygiene after urinating or defecating, and using alternatives to spermicides and diaphragms as means of birth control can help prevent the occurrence or recurrence of UTIs. The common alternative prescription of cranberry juice has proven in several studies to be effective only as placebo.

Urinary Incontinence: Involuntary urination arises from loss of bladder control. It is most common in women due to damage to the urethral sphincter during natural childbirth or other damage to the pelvic floor structures. Abdominal compression combined with bearing-down in the abdomen in athletic activities can cause what some call athletic incontinence. The most common cause in men is an enlarged prostate. Nerve damage that affects muscular control is another cause. Treatment varies widely depending on the specific cause of the condition, which is far ranging.

Prostatitis: An often painful condition that involves inflammation of the prostate and sometimes the area around it. There are four types of prostatitis: acute bacterial (least common, easiest to identify, and caused by bacterial infection), chronic bacterial (slower to develop and less intense), chronic pelvic pain (nonbacterial but idiopathic, with pain in the genitals), and asymptomatic inflammatory.

Cultivating a Healthy Urinary System

Effective hydration is the key to a healthy urinary system. The urinary system needs water to help flush out toxins and maintain healthy cellular metabolism. Carbonated water and water infused with caffeine, sugar, or alcohol all tax the urinary system and thus are not helpful in maintaining its healthy functioning. Drinking water throughout the day rather than waiting to feel thirsty, which is a sign of slight dehydration, is very important. How much water? The standard given by the American Dietetic Association is eight 8-ounce glasses per day, even though adults lose on average about a pint more than that per day. There is no danger in drinking more than ten glasses of water per day, although drinking a lot of water late at night can cause nocturia (frequent urination at night).

Salt is a significant factor in urinary health. Excessive salt intake causes unhealthy water retention (not circulation) and can contribute to the development of kidney stones. While salt (sodium) is essential for life in general and as an electrolyte and osmotic solute in mammals, in excess it also contributes to high blood pressure and hypertension (in both children and adults).

Urinary tract infections are often caused by a lack of basic personal hygiene. These infections are far more common among women than men because the urethra in women is much shorter, allowing bacteria to more easily travel into the urinary tract. It is thus important for both men and women to wash their external genitalia and groin area before having sex. Parents can also teach their daughters to wipe from front to back as doing the opposite can bring bacteria forward from the anus to the urethra.

So-called "pee-blocking," an exercise in which one halts the flow of urine once or several times before completely emptying the bladder, is an ill-informed method for trying to strengthen the urinary sphincter in women and to cultivate ejaculatory control in men. Pee-blocking disturbs the urinary system's neurological mechanism by prematurely signaling an empty bladder, which can lead to the inability to completely empty it even when trying to do so.

Although there is no scientific evidence for the effect of mula bandha and pelvic floor exercises on the condition of the lower pelvic organs (bladder, reproductive organs, and rectum), considerable anecdotal evidence points to the efficacy of these practices in heightened awareness of, and more subtle voluntary use of, muscles affecting these organs. Development and use of this musculature may have beneficial effects on circulation and the conscious, selective engagement and relaxation of specific muscles in the lower pelvis, including those that relate to the bladder and reproductive organs.[1]

16

Ultimate Human Creativity: The Reproductive System

Uncertainty is an uncomfortable position.
But certainty is an absurd one.
—VOLTAIRE

Sexual Reproduction

As with every aspect of our biological being, how we reproduce is now mostly a matter of scientific understanding rather than imaginative speculation guided by superstitious belief systems. In considering the anatomy and physiology of human reproduction, the ancient Greeks and Indians were equally confused yet wildly imaginative in offering their versions of human procreation. In ancient Hindu medicine and philosophy women are essentially a less developed human form than men (the great female hope is to be reincarnated as a man—as promised by male spiritual leaders). The ancient Greeks offered (and debated) at least two views: Aristotle's notion of sexual difference as minimal except for the size of organs, and Galen's notion of sexual commonality (he thought the uterus is an internal scrotum and the tip of the penis equivalent to the female pudendum). These ideas, along with many other myths and misconceptions, persisted well beyond the Renaissance. A clearer understanding only came with the advent of careful dissection combined with microscopic investigation.

Although human beings begin their development as sexually undifferentiated zygotes formed by the synthesis of male sperm cells and female egg cells, as fetuses we tend to differentiate into sexually dimorphic beings with primarily male or female sexual characteristics.[1] These differences are evident in our genes, chromosomes, gonads, hormones, anatomy, and, as contemporary neuroscience reveals, even in our psyche. While differences in sexual and related gender self-identity appear to be influenced by biological factors, our focus here is on the biology of reproduction, not the biology, psychology, or sociology of self-perception or self-identity (qualities that are explored elsewhere in this book).

In a curious irony, the human system, without which we cannot continue as a species, is precisely the one system we can biologically (individually) exist without. Take away the anatomical components of any of the systems we have surveyed thus far and life is not possible (no heart, no bones, no blood, no nerves, etc.), but take away the organs of reproduction and one can survive (even if with less joy and well-being). And although there are many philosophies of reincarnation that believe we live beyond this life, with sexual reproduction we directly extend our essence—or at least our genetic essence, the code that makes us much of who we are—into the future. Put differently, we develop as human beings from a process of fertilization in which male and female reproductive cells (*gametes*, from the Greek term meaning "wife") join to form a new organic human being with a cellular composition that is determined by the integrated gifts of genetic code given by our mating biological parents. If you have a lot of biological offspring, you have a high degree of biological reincarnation!

The reproductive system depends in its success upon fertilization through male and female sexual interaction, whether directly through sexual intercourse or indirectly through artificial insemination. This begins with meiosis, in which special stem cells in male and female gonads divide to become gametes. Our cells generally contain forty-six chromosomes, but in meiosis the cell division results in gametes containing twenty-three chromosomes. Successful fertilization combines the twenty-three-chromosome female and male gametes to produce a new single forty-six-chromosome cell—a zygote—that has the potential to develop into a fetus and a human being.

Although both male and female reproductive systems contain gonads that produce gametes and hormones, there is considerably greater difference than similarity in male and female sexual anatomy and physiology, starting in the gonads themselves. Both sexes have tubes that transport gametes, accessory glands that secrete fluids, and external genitals with functions in both reproduction and pleasure, but they have altogether different structures and functions.

The Male Reproductive System

Adult male gonads—two testes—secrete male sex hormones called androgens (primarily testosterone) along with around a half billion sperm cells every day (but fewer and fewer as one ages). The testes are contained within the temperature-sensitive scrotum where they are attached to a spermatic cord that is surrounded by the vas deferens, blood and

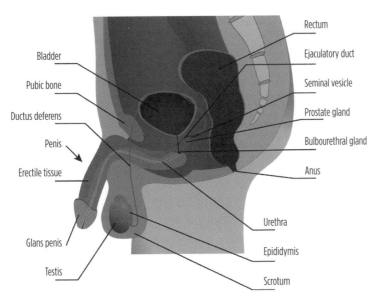

Figure 16.1: The Male Reproductive System

lymphatic vessels, and nerves. The location of sperm development in the temperature-sensitive scrotum is important because viable sperm require a lower than normal body temperature environment. Sperm cells (spermatozoa) are produced in around nine weeks through spermatogenesis, in which stem cells undergo meiosis. Although physically formed, the immature spermatozoa produced in the testes must undergo further development to become functionally mature and capable of locomotion.

The next stage in sperm development occurs in the epididymis (still within the scrotum's 1°C–8°C cooler environment), a 7-meter long tubule where the spermatozoa are bathed in organic nutrients for around two weeks, fully maturing before moving into the vas deferens, a long tube contained within the spermatic cord (sperm can be stored in the epididymis or vas deferens for several months). Secretions from seminal vesicles, the prostate gland, and the bulbourethral glands produce seminal fluid. The seminal vesicles produce around sixty percent of seminal fluid with secretions that are mostly fructose (with a quality of alkalinity that neutralizes acidic secretions from the prostate and vagina). The prostate gland, which surrounds the urethra as it leaves the bladder (and which when inflamed inhibits urination), produces around thirty percent of the volume of semen. The bulbourethral glands (also called Cowper's glands) secrete a thick, lubricating mucus that constitutes around five percent of semen. Where the vas deferens merges with the seminal duct to create the ejaculatory duct, seminal fluid and spermatozoa mix together to become semen, with the seminal fluid activating, nourishing, and buffering the spermatozoa. The very short (2cm) ejaculatory duct then empties into the urethra.

A series of muscular contractions in the penis, which is both a reproductive organ and part of the urinary system (and connected to a neurological system that registers pleasure and pain), ejaculates semen from the body. The three parts of the penis are the root (radix) that attaches the bulb of the penis to the body (and gains added support from the suspensory ligament); the body (corpus or shaft) that contains erectile tissue; and the epithelium, which consists of freely sliding shaft skin and foreskin (prepuce) covering the glans (the rounded end that surrounds the external urethral opening). (The foreskin is often removed in a surgical procedure called circumcision.) The body of the penis has three spongy columns of erectile tissue that consist of a network of blood vessels: two side-by-side corpora cavernosa on the dorsal side lying over the corpus spongiosum (which also contains the urethra). When sexually aroused, the autonomic (involuntary) nervous system stimulates vasodilation of the arteries supplying blood to these chambers, allowing them to fill with blood and causing the penis the lengthen, swell, and stiffen. Erection constricts the veins in the penis, which inhibits the outward flow of blood and maintains relatively constant erectile size. Erection allows sexual intercourse and other sexual activities but is not necessarily required for sexual activities besides intercourse.

The Female Reproductive System

Although the primary function of both the male and female reproductive systems is production of sex hormones and gametes, the female reproductive system has a second primary function: supporting a developing fetus and nourishing a newborn baby. This function is fulfilled with a distinct female reproductive anatomy. The main parts of the female reproductive system are the uterus, ovaries, vagina, and vulva. (Although breasts are related to the reproductive system—from sexual arousal to hormone generation to sustenance of a newborn baby—they are not technically part of that system.)

Adult female gonads—two ovaries—typically release one ovum (egg) per month. The ovaries are small, paired organs (about the size and shape of a large almond) located along the walls of the uterus and held in place by a fibrous cord called the ovarian ligament. Each end of the ovary has a distinct structure: at the tubal extremity we find the fallopian tube; at the uterine extremity we find the ovarian ligament. Ovum production occurs within ovarian follicles, which are the elemental foundation of female reproductive biology. At birth the ovaries contain hundreds of thousands of immature egg cells found in circular bundles called primordial follicles. Each follicle surrounds and supports a single oocyte (immature ovum). After puberty, rising levels of hormones periodically cause these cells to successively develop into primary, secondary, and tertiary follicle cells across about ten to fourteen days, with fewer and

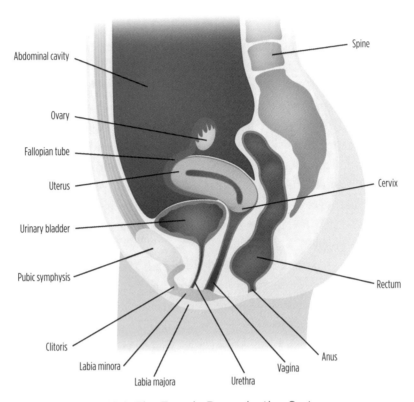

Abdominal cavity

Ovary

Fallopian tube

Uterus

Urinary bladder

Pubic symphysis

Clitoris

Labia minora

Labia majora

Urethra

Vagina

Anus

Rectum

Cervix

Spine

Figure 16.2: The Female Reproductive System

fewer taking each further step toward becoming a fully developed ovum. At around day fourteen of this cycle, one mature egg (rarely more) is released to the surface of an ovary, where tiny fimbriae (fingerlike projections) gently gather the ovum from the surface and slip it into the fallopian tube for transport via the movement of cilia on the inner linings of the tube to the uterus for potential fertilization by sperm. If left unfertilized, the ova disintegrate and are swept away during menstruation. If fertilized, the newly formed zygote undergoes rapid cell divisions before becoming implanted in the uterine lining for around nine months of gestation.

The uterus (from the Latin *uteri*, "womb") is a small, pear-shaped, hormone-sensitive, muscular reproductive organ located between the bladder and rectum. It is held in place by the bladder, rectum, and three suspensory ligaments (uterosacral, round, and cardinal). Its inferior dilating cervical end opens a short distance into the vagina while its rounded superior end opens into the fallopian tubes. The uterine walls consist of an inner endometrium lining and muscular myometrium capable of greatly stretching—so much that the uterus is the most expandable organ in the body. In the uterine cycle that begins with menstruation, the endometrial lining gradually deteriorates before breaking away and moving into the vagina, where peristalsis and intravaginal pressure—not one's relationship to gravity—cause the menses to flow out of the body.

The muscular tube of the vagina (from the Latin *vaginae*, literally "sheath" in what is surely a male concept), which extends from the cervix to its orifice at the vulva, plays a significant role in both sexual reproduction and pleasure. It receives the penis in sexual intercourse, which allows natural insemination. During labor it serves as the baby's pathway to independent life (another pathway being through the belly via cesarean section). It also serves as the passageway for eliminating menses. The vagina's elastic muscular walls have both circular and longitudinal fibers that can be voluntarily contracted. It is lined by mucus membrane and contains resident bacteria that metabolize to help maintain a slightly acidic pH environment, inhibiting the growth of pathogens. The vaginal opening is partially covered by the hymen, an elastic membrane that forms part of the vulva (external genitalia) and largely disappears after giving birth.

The fuller vulva consists of the mons pubis, labia majora, Bartholin glands, labia minora, and the clitoris. These structures protect the internal genital organs from infection, provide sexual pleasure, and allow sperm to enter the female reproductive system. The vagina initially opens into the vestibule, which is surrounded by the labia minora, small lips filled with a rich supply of arteries that when sexually aroused swell with blood to become more sensitive to touch. Here in the labia minora we also find the Bartholin glands, which secrete mucus to lubricate the vagina. The urethra opens into the vestibule near the vaginal orifice, and the clitoris—derived from the same embryonic elements as the penis—project into the vestibule. The clitoris is the female's most sexually sensitive tissue and the primary anatomical location of human female sexual pleasure as its internal erectile tissues fill with blood and thereby gain sensitivity and the potential for orgasm. The labia majora (literally, "large lips"), which are comparable to the male scrotum in containing sweat and sebaceous glands, produce lubricating secretions that reduce friction during sexual intercourse (with lubrication coming from the greater vestibular gland ducts that empty into the vestibule). The rounded mound of the mons pubis defines the outer region of the vulva. It is fatty tissue that covers the pubic bone and secretes pheromones that are involved in sexual attraction.

Fertilization and Human Development

Human development begins with the fusion of a sperm cell with an egg cell in the biological process of fertilization (also called conception). With over 200 million spermatozoa in the average ejaculate, it might seem that there are high odds of conception given that only one sperm cell is required to fertilize an ovum. Yet only around 10,000 sperm cells make it to the uterus and fewer than one hundred will reach the egg. Depending on the male's sperm count and the motility of sperm, the cells may never reach the egg. When first ejaculated, the sperm undergo capacitation (a bio-chemical event that increases motility and destabilizes the sperm head to allow for easier binding with the egg cell) in the vagina and uterus, where uterine secretions aid this change. Once sperm cells reach the egg they can relatively easily fuse with its plasma membrane; the challenge to fertilization that occurs here involves penetrating the relatively hard shell of the egg. But as a sperm cell approaches the glycoprotein layer surrounding the egg cell (the zona pellucida), the capacitated cell has an acro-some reaction that helps bind the sperm cell to the egg, after which a cortical reaction occurs to prevent fertilization by more than one sperm cell. Within around five days of fertilization, the new zygote undergoes rapid cell divisions in which it develops into a blastocyte, which forms into inner and outer cellular layers that later develop into an embryo.

During gestation, the human embryo develops within the same endometrial uter-ine lining that one otherwise sheds during menstruation. But viable implantation of the fertilized egg requires a favorable environment in the endometrial lining. The blas-tocyst itself releases a hormone called human chorionic gonadotropin (hCG). As the uterine gland cells within the endometrium break down, hCG helps to maintain a functional endometrial lining for the process of embryo formation. Once implanted, the inner cell tissues of the blastocyst divide into three layers—the ectoderm, meso-derm, and endoderm—which develop into specific tissues and organs in the complete new human organism. The outer layers of the blastocyst become the trophoblast, which develops into the placenta, connecting the developing fetus to the uterine wall and providing the nutrients, circulatory functions, and other nurturance that the fetus will receive from its mother throughout gestation.

Prenatal human development takes around nine months of gestation. In Chapter 25 we will survey various conditions of pregnancy by trimester and consider how one might have the healthiest pregnancy, delivery, and newborn child.

Common Reproductive Pathologies

Impotence: Also called erectile dysfunction (ED), impotence is a common male sexual dysfunction in which a man has difficulty getting or maintaining an erec-tion. Erection normally arises from sexual arousal as nerve signals travel from the brain to the penis. Cardiovascular disease, diabetes, neurological problems, exces-sive alcohol, drugs, and so-called performance anxiety are typical causes.

Dysmenorrhea: A painful period that interferes with daily activities is called dys-menorrhea, a condition that manifests as various types of pain in the lower abdo-men. The most common (70%) cause is endometriosis (note that most women with dysmenorrhea do not have endometriosis), while ovarian cysts, adenomyosis, and pelvic congestion are secondary causes.

Reproductive System Cancers: Several forms of cancer manifest in the reproductive system: cervical, ovarian, penile, prostate, testicular, and uterine. (Breast cancer is not technically a cancer of the reproductive system.)

Cultivating a Healthy Reproductive System

There are several practices one can do to cultivate a healthy reproductive system, with some differences for men and women. Both sexes can benefit from safe sex practices that prevent the sharing of sexually transmitted diseases. Both can benefit from the circulatory and neurological benefits of regular orgasms. Women can choose birth control wisely, be attuned to shifts in energy and emotion that might coincide with their menstrual cycle, and maintain a consistent yoga practice. Women can also prevent urinary tract infections and cervical cancer with healthy urinary hygiene, and men can contribute to this by cleaning themselves prior to having sexual intercourse. Women can prevent yeast infections with healthy hygiene, including wiping from front to back when using the toilet. Men can get prostate testing and also address erectile concerns with a doctor or other health adviser. Men can take care of their testicles by wearing loose-fitting underwear (or no underwear) and avoiding prolonged periods of time in hot baths. Specific reproductive health problems and related healing practices for men and women are discussed in Chapter 25.

Part III

Helping Others Heal with Yoga

THE PRACTICES OF YOGA THERAPY are ideally informed by a blending of ancient to modern experience-based wisdom with contemporary evidence-based insights into what heals and does no harm. Starting from this overarching premise, we can better navigate the vast and shifting seas of concepts, methods, and techniques across the world of yoga therapy. Here we look first to clarify the very concept of yoga therapy, differentiating it from yoga teaching and setting forth a coherent, inclusive, yet delimited scope of yoga therapy practice. When we are clearer in our identities as yoga therapists, we are better able to develop healthy relationships with clients, yoga teachers, and others in the healing arts and sciences. Chapter 17 attempts to offer such clarity.

Possessed of clearer self-identity and a specific scope of practice, we can then take the seat of the yoga therapist with a more wholesome foundation and motivation. The center of our practice is in the heart, in how we hold space with a client to foster healing resonance. This begins with the quality of our communication and overall interaction with clients, the topics that are discussed in detail in Chapter 18.

In Chapter 19 we dive into the nuances of assessing client conditions and developing practice plans for the delivery of therapeutic yoga services. The general assumption underlying this discussion is that informed assessment is an essential part of the therapeutic process, especially because it is the foundation for a plan of action. We are linking karma yoga with kriya yoga as we form and nurture relationships with individual clients. This process builds upon the healing resonance we first establish in client interactions and continues in the most comprehensive assessment of a client's intentions and conditions. This leads us to a practice plan, a living document open to modification in every breath shared along the healing path.

17

Integrity in Yoga Therapy: Teachers, Healers, and Therapists

*I have grown up as a card-carrying scientist, and
I know the power of science to answer many questions,
and for many questions I don't know of anything better
than scientific approaches to answer them.*
—DEAN ORNISH

IN RECENT YEARS, the International Association of Yoga Therapists (IAYT) has sought to clarify the nature of yoga therapy and to differentiate the work of the yoga therapist from that of the yoga teacher. Many yoga teachers who have for many years or decades provided what they call yoga therapy object to this distinction, maintaining that yoga is inherently therapeutic and any effort to differentiate yoga and therapy diminishes the true service of teaching yoga. There is also growing concern over some self-described yoga therapists who don lab coats, stethoscopes, goniometers, spirometers, and other medical tools, and walk the halls of clinics and medical institutions appearing to be medical professionals, which is said to cause confusion over roles and scopes of practice. In 2016, the U.S.-based Yoga Alliance, the leading registry of yoga schools and teachers, banned Registered Yoga Schools and Registered Yoga Teachers from using the term *yoga therapy* in any descriptive materials and communications in which Yoga Alliance is also identified. Here we try to unravel some of these issues in attempting to present a clearer definition of the work of yoga teachers whose work is specifically concerned with therapeutic yoga and healing.

In the fluid context of diverse ideas and extant and emerging practices, there is a growing consensus that the foundation of the yoga healer or therapist is first and foremost in having a personal yoga practice, and secondarily, yet vitally, in being a yoga teacher, whether one teaches one-on-one, group classes, or both. In becoming a yoga healer or therapist, one builds upon this foundation in practicing and teaching yoga to develop a deeper and more refined knowledge and set of skills for working in meaningful ways with diverse students and clients whose health needs indicate the value of more intensive and adaptive yoga practices in curing or healing. Although yoga therapy is not an established profession in terms of legal standards of training, competence, and licensing, IAYT has nonetheless promulgated a set of educational standards for training and certifying of yoga therapists. It has also established a certification committee charged with developing criteria, policies, and practices for granting IAYT certification as a yoga therapist, although IAYT itself presently does not have standing as an accrediting agency with any legally sanctioned accrediting body.

The self-healing effects of practicing yoga are an essential part of becoming either a yoga teacher or yoga therapist. In practicing yoga, we gradually learn about ourselves and develop a greater sense of wholeness and integration in our lives. We get to know our habits of bodymind and how to live in greater balance and harmony within ourselves and in our relationships. We develop skill in action as we explore the various techniques of asana, pranayama, and meditation, and we learn how to best apply the energies we are cultivating to our varied intentions in life on and off the yoga mat. We come to appreciate deeper qualities of self-awareness as we learn to listen inside for guidance, and we develop greater capacities for self-transformation by following our inner teacher in keeping with our conditions and related intentions.

In teaching yoga, one is both an educator and a guide, working with students to empower them as independent practitioners. The skills and insights we gain in our personal yoga practice are the essential starting point in sharing the practice with others. To do so in the most informed way, and thus gain basic competence in teaching, yoga students interested in the path of teaching first study and develop a deeper understanding of all they intend to teach.

If intending to teach asanas, ideally one first learns about their basic forms, alignment principles, energetic actions, risk issues, contraindications, modifications, adaptations, use of props, biomechanical and energetic relationship with other asanas, sequencing, and various means of teaching them to others. These teaching methods include specific qualities of demonstration, verbal instruction, and tactile guidance, all informed by a deepening understanding of yoga philosophy, learning theory, functional anatomy, biomechanics, and kinesiology. If teaching pranayama, one ideally learns about and practices extensively each technique before sharing it with others, teaching it based on personal experience and a growing knowledge of the anatomy and physiology of both the basic respiratory process, its modification in the various pranayama practices, and modifications in technique to accommodate special needs as well as contraindications. If teaching meditation, again, one is well practiced in a technique before sharing it with others and particularly attuned to the emotional and mental effects of a practice that can cause as much imbalance as it might relieve.

In all of this, the heart of the art and science of teaching is in the heart, in the compassionate, caring, and considerate qualities of interaction that most encourage students to feel safe and open to exploring and transforming more deeply inside. Yet, in addition to teaching from the heart, the teacher must also be informed by the best possible understanding of the students' objective conditions and how different yoga practices might affect them. Always a yoga student, always learning and growing, the yoga teacher comes to have new teachers in each one of his or her students.

In practicing as a yoga therapist, one draws upon these areas of knowledge and skill as a yoga teacher, including the ongoing personal practices that help in one's continual cultivation of the basic attributes of empathy, openness, and attentiveness. These are essential qualities in offering yoga as a distinctively healing practice, just as they are essential qualities in teaching yoga in general. When the teacher-student relationship moves into the realm of intentional healing, the yoga teacher steps onto the slippery slope toward interacting with the student in a more decidedly therapeutic manner. Here we come to blurry territory. If a yoga student comes to class complaining of low back pain, the teacher might suggest modifications to the asanas that result in reduction or elimination of the pain. This modification and benefit arises from the yoga teacher teaching yoga in an informed way, fulfilling his or her role in providing education about yoga methods and techniques, including specific modifications to support the student's special needs in the practice. Put differently, the yoga teacher is teaching yoga, not offering yoga therapy, a perspective widely shared among the IAYT leadership in helping to bring light and clarity to this distinction.[1]

Earlier in this book we explored the idea found in the most ancient to modern teachings on yoga—that yoga is a tool of self-transformation aimed at the root causes of suffering. This is perhaps most clearly expressed in the *Bhagavad-Gita*, the *Yoga Sutra of Patanjali* and the *Hatha Yoga Pradipika*. These texts offer us various therapeutic tools, ranging from moral and ethical practices to very specific methods of self-cleansing and strengthening that employ asana, pranayama, meditation, and other techniques. The yoga in these texts was traditionally taught one-on-one over many years by guru to disciple in such a way that the guru gained deep understanding of the conditions of the disciple; all conditions of imbalance were addressed as part of a closely guided practice. Going with this, many yoga teachers consider the heart of yoga to be *yogachikitsa*, "yoga therapy," seeing it as an inherent and essential aspect of yoga in general.[2] This perspective is clearly expressed by many yoga professionals (see every issue of *Yoga Therapy Today* and the *Journal of the International Association of Yoga Therapists* for scores of examples), making it less clear how to differentiate and distinguish the respective roles of the yoga teacher and yoga therapist.

Although this ambiguity may never be completely resolved, we can further clarify the distinction in practical terms by identifying the goals of healing with yoga. This clarification is important not only in giving clear guidelines and parameters to yoga teachers and students with respect to yoga therapy, but also to give those from outside the yoga community proper—physicians, nurses, psychiatrists, psychologists, physical therapists, respiratory therapists, acupuncturists, chiropractors, naturopaths, and others—clearer insight into the work of yoga teachers done in conjunction with complementary and integrative health practices. Since the U.S. Supreme Court ruling in *Dent v. West Virginia* (1889), it is also crucial to understand that states have the authority to define and regulate medical practice; practicing anything that is defined in statute as medicine without the required license is a felony. The state of Michigan offers a representative example of licensed medical practice, which it defines as "the diagnosis, treatment, prevention, cure, or relieving of a human disease, ailment, defect, complaint, or other physical or mental condition, by attendance, advice, device, diagnostic test, or other means, of offering, undertaking, attempting to do, or holding oneself out as able to do, any of these acts." Challenges to the *Dent* ruling on the basis of "medicine" being defined in allopathic terms have routinely failed, including in *Smith v. People*, regarding the laying on of hands, and more recently regarding acupuncture in *People v. Amber* (1973), iridology in *Stetina v. State* (1987), and homeopathy in *State v. Hinze* (1989).

As Cohen and Nelson point out regarding alternative medicine practitioners in general, there is a limited set of options for licensure in the context of *Dent*.[3] Licensed allied health professionals such as dentists, nurses, and radiological technicians, as well as licensed alternative medicine professionals, have "limited" licenses that define a narrow scope of practice. Dentists cannot legally set fractured bones, physical therapists cannot legally replace hearts, and acupuncturists cannot legally conduct brain surgery. If not licensed to practice a medical art as defined in law (whether under mandatory or title licensure), it is still possible in a few states to offer some services under certain exemptions to licensure. Short of licensure—and do note that as of 2017 yoga therapy is not a licensed profession in any U.S. state—a legal scope of practice for yoga therapy must be careful not to cross over into what is defined as medical practice.

Because many leaders and practitioners in yoga therapy circles wish to gain the requisite credibility and legitimacy for being accepted in the complementary and integrative health world, they are striving to establish yoga therapy as a recognized profession, starting with the clear statement of standards of training and competency. However, this very discussion—about defined practices and clear distinctions between yoga teachers, yoga therapists, and licensed health care providers—is disturbing to those who wish to exercise complete freedom to offer diagnosis and treatment based on their intuitive and/or other sense of appropriate service, of sharing the deeper practices of yoga. As Seitz points out, "efforts toward formalizing a profession are likely to cause apprehension and even conflict within the practitioner and school communities."[4]

Indeed, to the extent that yoga therapists wish to exchange referrals with licensed medical and mental health professionals and to most fully participate in integrative health practices, it will be important for them to move forward in defining standards of training and competence, gaining accreditation for yoga therapy schools, and moving toward some form of licensure. Even the first step of defining clear standards of education and competence is controversial within the yoga community, let alone the next steps of accrediting schools and providing regulatory oversight. If one's primary yoga mantra is freedom of practice in keeping with one's intuitive insights and understandings of yoga, it might be possible to carve out a somewhat more legitimate standing using softer methods of efficacy such as outcome-based therapy as discussed by Laurence.[5] Although this standard is unlikely to find acceptance among institutions engaged in complementary and integrative health, it may give solace to those who, as Forbes et al. put it, "elect to solidify their identity as 'renegade' practitioners or educators."[6]

In discussing training issues in yoga and mental health treatment, Forbes et al. offer an important distinction between psychotherapists who incorporate yoga into their work and yoga professionals who work with mental health issues.[7] They emphasize that the nonyoga professional who incorporates yoga into his or her work requires a level of training and experience in yoga at the 500-hour level plus additional training in yoga therapy. Meanwhile, to the extent that one accepts the traditional yoga concepts of *samskara, klesha,* and *avidya* as common conditions across all of humanity, all yoga therapists (and yoga teachers for that matter) are working with mental health issues—their own and those of their students or clients. Yet thorough understanding and practice of yoga philosophy and yoga psychology is not sufficient to prepare one for working with the ordinary range of mental health issues that are presented in psychotherapeutic relationships. Rather, if a yoga professional wishes to work with integrity in mental health treatment, he or she should complete the requisite clinical training and supervision required to do so competently and legally, thus being respectful of the legal line that defines a clinical psychologist in ways that are distinct and legal.

We can sensibly apply this as a general principle in the relationship between yoga and all health professions.

In going beyond teaching yoga as a holistic practice for cultivating health and well-being, we begin to approach the legally and ethically defined lines of professional scopes of practice. If we wish to cross the line from yoga teacher into any areas of legally defined professional health practice with integrity, we should satisfy the requirements for legitimately offering that practice. Put differently, if you wish to practice physical therapy, nursing, or cardiology as a yoga professional, first complete the required training to develop the related knowledge and skills, earn the related professional degree, obtain a license to work as a physical therapist, nurse, or cardiologist, and add training in yoga to learn how to complement your licensed professional health services with yoga techniques.

Given these important distinctions, how might yoga therapy be defined? The IAYT defines yoga therapy as "the process of empowering individuals to progress toward improved health and well-being through the application of the teachings and practices of yoga."[8] Considering this broad working definition in the context of complementary and integrative health, we can articulate a set of goals that can inform a yoga therapy scope of practice. Each of these goals is predicated upon supporting yoga practices that increase self-awareness and engage the client in lifelong self-care, including for specific conditions as diagnosed by a medical professional and/or the intentions of the student or client.

Many students primarily or exclusively choose alternative approaches to curing and healing, including comprehensive systems such as ayurveda, homeopathy, and naturopathy. As we discussed in Part I, ayurveda and yoga are closely associated; some assert they are inseparable. Given the intimacy of yoga and ayurveda, yoga therapists will encounter many clients who are patients of ayurveda practitioners. If a yoga therapist wishes to offer therapeutic services to a client who is receiving ayurveda care, he or she will need to be at least minimally conversant with ayurveda terminology and possess a basic foundation of knowledge about ayurveda principles and treatments, including their evidence-based efficacy, risks, and contraindications. We can apply this same principle to interaction with other alternative systems of care. In these interactions with conventional and alternative treatment providers, the yoga therapist ideally focuses on the basic goals of yoga therapy while working within a scope of practice that more clearly identifies and distinguishes the realm of yoga therapy.

Yoga Therapy as a Clearly Defined Practice

Nearly every country in the world uses health professional requisites such as licensure, certification, and proof of minimum training to define and control the quality of health workers practicing in their jurisdiction. Specific health professionals who wish to offer a particular type of health service are required to meet the jurisdiction's requisites as provided for by law. These requisites vary by country, and in many countries they vary by state, province, or other smaller jurisdiction with the authority to regulate health professions. In addition to required training and licensure, health professions are given more specific definition through scopes of practice that individuals with a license or other certification are legally permitted to perform.

The following example of Respiratory Care Practitioner can help shed light on the elements of a clear scope of practice. We choose this example in part because the breath is at the heart of all yoga practices, and much of our work addresses breathing patterns and practices. We also find some yoga therapists conduct respiratory assessments, which, depending on the nature of the assessment, can transgress into the Respiratory Care Practitioner's scope of practice. After prefacing language affirming the intent of the law regarding respiratory care ("… to protect the public from the unauthorized and unqualified practice of respiratory care …"), the field is clearly defined and delimited.

CALIFORNIA LICENSED RESPIRATORY CARE PRACTITIONER—SCOPE OF PRACTICE—BUSINESS AND PROFESSIONS CODE[9]

Respiratory care as a practice means a health care profession employed under the supervision of a medical director* in the therapy, management, rehabilitation, diagnostic evaluation, and care of patients with deficiencies and abnormalities which affect the pulmonary system and associated aspects of cardiopulmonary and other systems functions, and includes all of the following:

(a) Direct and indirect pulmonary care services that are safe, aseptic, preventive, and restorative to the patient.

(b) Direct and indirect respiratory care services, including but not limited to, the administration of pharmacological and diagnostic and therapeutic agents related to respiratory care procedures necessary to implement a treatment, disease prevention, pulmonary rehabilitative, or diagnostic regimen prescribed by a physician and surgeon.

(c) Observation and monitoring of signs and symptoms, general behavior, general physical response to respiratory care treatment, and diagnostic testing and

(1) Determination of whether such signs, symptoms, reactions, behavior, or general response exhibits abnormal characteristics;

(2) Implementation based on observed abnormalities of appropriate reporting or referral or respiratory care protocols, or changes in treatment regimen, pursuant to a prescription by a physician and surgeon or the initiation of emergency procedures.

(d) The diagnostic and therapeutic use of any of the following, in accordance with the prescription of a physician and surgeon: administration of medical gases, exclusive of general anesthesia; aerosols; humidification; environmental control systems and baromedical therapy; pharmacologic agents related to respiratory care procedures; mechanical or physiological ventilatory support; bronchopulmonary hygiene; cardiopulmonary resuscitation; maintenance of the natural airways; insertion without cutting tissues and maintenance of artificial airways; diagnostic and testing techniques required for implementation of respiratory care protocols; collection of specimens of blood; collection of specimens from the respiratory tract; analysis of blood gases and respiratory secretions.

(e) The transcription and implementation of the written and verbal orders of a physician and surgeon pertaining to the practice of respiratory care.

Nothing in this chapter shall be construed as authorizing a respiratory care practitioner to practice medicine, surgery, or any other forms of healing, except as authorized by this chapter.

---

* "Medical director" means a physician and surgeon who is a member of a health care facility's active medical staff and who is knowledgeable in respiratory care.

To the extent that one wishes to offer yoga in conjunction with the treatment practices of medical professionals and fellow alternative caregivers, the yoga professional must work within a similarly well-defined scope of practice that both informs and delimits his or her work. The alternative is to teach yoga and offer yoga therapy techniques in whatever ways one wishes, unconcerned about definitions and delimitations, which might be a beautiful way to go so long as one is open to foregoing the legitimacy that is generally required in complementary and integrative work.

As part of its effort to establish a yoga profession that bridges yoga and health care, the IAYT issued a set of baseline considerations "as a starting point for discussion" in establishing standards of yoga therapy, including its scope of practice, which it gives as follows:

Practices may include, but are not limited to, asana, pranayama, meditation, sound and chanting, personal ritual, and prayer. Teaching may also include, but is not limited to, directed study, discussion, and lifestyle counseling. Yoga therapy may address any of the dimensions of life. In the classical tradition, these are the *panca kosha* or the five sheaths of the human being. In contemporary terms, these may be approximated as the anatomical, physiological, emotional, intellectual, and spiritual dimensions.[10]

This is an exceptionally broad starting point, one that reflects the all-encompassing practices of yoga, and is meant to maximize inclusiveness across the nascent movement toward a yoga therapy profession. It behooves us to consider each of its elements:

- The preface "may include, but are not limited to," implies that yoga therapy could include any practice or treatment, which is overly broad in distinguishing yoga therapy from other methods.

- The specific reference to asana, pranayama, and meditation appropriately highlights the three most common areas of yoga practice and the three most studied in relation to curing and healing.

- The term *sound* is quite broad, and could include music, chanting, or listening to nature. *Chanting* refers to devotional practices that some consider the heart of yoga practice (in the various bhakti traditions), yet others find awkwardly esoteric, sometimes even in conflict with their spiritual values (some devout Christian yoga students consider chanting the names of Hindu deities sacrilegious). Although there is no evidence of efficacy for chanting in curing, it may have efficacy in fostering a sense of connection and wholeness.

- *Personal ritual,* which could include any imaginable activity, is far too broad to be a useful concept in defining a scope of practice, yet it is widely held as an essential element in developing safe, trusting, and open relationships with clients and offering techniques such as *bhavana* that may lend to healing resonance.

- *Panca kosha* is posited as "in the classical tradition," which, as we saw in Chapter 1, does not exist as such except in the minds of those who believe there is a singular classical tradition—which there is not. Rather, there are many yoga models that map the human being in keeping with a particular understanding of reality and yoga. Also, the panca kosha model does not so simply approximate the so-called dimensions of anatomical, physiological, emotional, intellectual, and spiritual. For example, one could translate the koshas as body, breath, mind, wisdom, and bliss. None of this is particularly helpful language if you are attempting to derive a clearly delimited scope of practice; rather, the practices are those techniques that have an effect on the so-called dimensions of being (which are not separate dimensions but what comprises the whole human being).

We can reframe these elements to offer greater clarity and specificity to the scope of practice for yoga therapy:

TOWARD A YOGA THERAPY SCOPE OF PRACTICE: A WORKING DEFINITION

- Asana, pranayama, and meditation are the primary techniques of yoga for the purposes of supporting curing and healing, while some yoga methods use sound, chanting, personal ritual, and prayer in support of healing with these techniques.

- Yoga applies these methods to help promote health and healing in ways that affect the physical, emotional, mental, and spiritual aspects of life.

- The specific application of yoga methods and techniques is informed by student assessments and preferences, and through open communication.

As a final note on this, it is important to reckon with similar issues regarding the legitimacy of the yoga teacher. For nearly twenty years, the very broad and minimalist standards set forth by Yoga Alliance have defined the legitimate yoga teacher: 200 hours of training and study. To obtain Yoga Alliance's legitimizing 200-hour Registered Yoga Teacher (RYT-200) badge, a Yoga Alliance Registered Yoga School (RYS) must certify the teacher. The RYS can be established by any RYT-200 yoga teacher with as little as two years of teaching experience. There is no oversight of yoga schools, allowing each of over 2,000 RYSs in the U.S. alone to certify that students have satisfied the 200-hour requirement while utilizing whatever specific curriculum and instructional methods that they wish. There is no requirement for any verification of learning or competence, let alone a certification exam that might demonstrate even the most basic competencies. As a consequence, there are tens of thousands of Yoga Alliance Registered Yoga Teachers and thousands of yoga teacher trainers who have no knowledge of even basic human anatomy or effective instructional techniques, this while they instruct their students in postural practices in which there is often significant risk of serious musculoskeletal or neurological injury.[11]

Although efforts have been made to make Yoga Alliance standards more robust, to implement an oversight system to ensure that yoga schools are teaching what they claim, and to have some form of standardized measure of yoga teacher competence, Yoga Alliance, a private organization with a self-perpetuating board of directors accountable only to itself, has opposed all such efforts. As a result, all is not so blissful in the yoga world, even amid the current yoga boom that has some 20 million Americans rolling out yoga mats and over 100,000 yoga teachers guiding them. Growing reports of student injuries raise serious questions about the standards of competence and accountability for teachers and trainers of teachers, especially as the diverse array of yoga teacher training schools in the U.S. churn out thousands of new teachers every year, and more and more yoga teachers offer classes in settings such as retirement homes, schools, and hospitals with populations at high risk of injury.

Anyone is presently entitled to teach yoga. In all but the very few states that require licenses, anyone can declare him or herself a yoga teacher, open a yoga studio, even train others to teach, without ever having done a single yoga posture or knowing anything about yoga. Although most yoga teachers have completed at least 200 hours of training, it is anyone's guess if even a trained and certified yoga teacher knows the difference between muscles and ligaments, types of joints, or the energetic and biomechanical relationships between various postures. With many yoga styles and teachers approaching yoga with a one-size-fits-all methodology, giving the same postures and instructional cues to everyone despite diversity in students' ages, conditions, and intentions, we have the makings of a yoga legitimacy crisis that begs the question: What should be the qualifications to teach yoga and to train those teachers?

With millions of people doing yoga and an increasing number of people getting injured in classes taught by teachers with little or no training, perhaps it is time to establish yoga teaching as a bona fide profession with specified core competencies, credentialing standards, and accountability measures that protect the public and give competent teachers the credibility they deserve. Along with this, the bar for the competence and accountability of yoga teacher training schools needs to be clearly defined and set to standards considered legitimate by the U.S. Department of Education, potentially qualifying yoga school students for the same financial aid, scholarships, and loans as other professional students.

To teach yoga well requires years of practice, study, training, and apprenticing. In the early years of yoga—think around 1,000 BCE—the practice was primarily about controlling the mind and coming into oneness with the divine. There was one yoga posture: sitting. There were also a variety of breathing techniques and myriad rituals intended ultimately to bring the yogi to a state of transcendence. After a few thousand years of development, yoga has evolved from being mostly ascetic and meditative practices related to transcendence to being mostly about living in a healthy and awakened way in the modern world. Until the twentieth century, there was nothing in the yoga world remotely comparable to the complex postural practices being done routinely today in thousands of yoga and fitness centers, schools, and offices. The 20 million Americans practicing yoga are mostly doing Up Dog, Down Dog, Tree Pose, and Wheel Pose, not living in an ashram, sitting in lotus position, and chanting the names of Hindu deities—although a sizeable minority of students in the West are immersed in the more esoteric practices considered by many to be at the heart of yoga.

The predominant forms of yoga today should inform the core competencies of today's yoga teachers. As with other professions, teaching yoga requires expert and specialized skills and knowledge, starting with an understanding of the human body in postural practices (the functional human anatomy, biomechanics, and kinesiology of movement and position). Other essential areas of basic teacher competence include how postures are sequenced, postural modifications and use of props to help ensure safe practices, ethics and techniques in giving hands-on guidance, practical understanding of yoga philosophy, how to guide pregnant students and others with special conditions or injuries, effective communication skills, methods of demonstration, and how to teach various breathing and meditation techniques.

Starting with evidence of best practices that inform the development of teacher training standards and curriculum, it is important to establish far more robust minimum standards of competence for teachers and training schools, a code of professional ethics, a professional certification exam, requirements for continuing education, and accountability for teachers, trainers, and any credentialing body. The national Yoga Alliance has done some work in some of these areas and could provide the leadership in moving from today's anemic standards to the stronger standards necessary for ensuring competent teachers and safe classes. Funded primarily by annual yoga teacher dues, Yoga Alliance could redefine itself as an accrediting entity and work with the National Commission on Certifying Agencies (NCCA) to establish a credentialing process for all yoga teachers in the United States, elevating teaching yoga to the professional status that competent teachers deserve and all yoga students should expect.

Establishing yoga teaching as a credible profession is a controversial idea in a yoga world that is as politically and philosophically diverse as the nation. Some oppose any standards or oversight that would disrupt what they consider an inviolable teacher-student relationship. Others say that yoga is too broad a discipline to define, let alone have consistent standards of competence for teaching. We can move beyond these ideological nonstarters by committing to a credentialing process that honors traditional approaches while embracing the realities of teaching yoga postural practices, pranayama techniques, and meditation in the twenty-first century. Although the politics and the issues are complex—much like the diverse practices of yoga and the more diverse conditions of those doing them—the vast growth and mainstreaming of yoga asks all who care to keep breathing deeply, to roll up their mats for a moment, and to commit to developing a viable yoga profession. Such a profession will go far in providing a partial foundation for the ongoing development of yoga therapy and yoga therapists.

18

Communicating and Interacting in Yoga Therapy

HUMAN BEINGS POSSESS INNATE POWERS of self-curing and self-healing. Even when our self-curing powers fail, our self-healing powers can make our lives better. To the extent that our self-healing powers are strong, they can support our self-curing powers and the power of curative treatments. Although there are many areas of illness and injury for which yoga offers curative treatment, the primary benefits of yoga are in cultivating a sense of overall well-being and a healing resonance. This therapeutic potential of yoga begins in one's personal yoga practice and in the relationship between the yoga therapist and his or her client. Working within the integrity of this relationship, we can better engage our clients and elicit their needs and intentions in curing or healing what ails them. With a deeper understanding of our clients' conditions, which we can help to illuminate and clarify through complementary yoga-related assessments (what we might also call *appreciations*), we can develop yoga therapy treatment plans with each unique client. Here we look closely at each of these steps in providing yoga therapy, starting with the healing relationship itself.

Guiding Principles in the Healing Relationship: Kriyas and Yamas

In teaching yoga either one-on-one or in a group class setting, we come into pedagogical (and hopefully inspirational) relationships with students. Teachers' varied instructional methods, personal styles of interacting with students, and qualities of energetic presence shape the nature of these relationships. Some yoga teachers teach yoga in a way that assumes the student must learn it all from the teacher, giving specific instructions that the student is expected to follow (directive method). Other teachers share their knowledge and insight with students while encouraging students to explore in ways that fully empower the student to learn from the experience and to adapt the practices in ways that make sense to them (nondirective method). Teachers who teach with a sense of kindness and compassion are found in both approaches. Teachers who teach without conveying much or any sense of kindness or compassion are also found in both approaches. As we cross the bridge from teaching yoga to yoga therapy, we follow Nichala Devi in highlighting the teacher-as-facilitator role and the qualities of kindness and compassion that help form the foundation of healthy relationships in which adaptive practices are fully explored in support of a client's goals and aspirations.[1] For some this creates a sense of healing energy—affirmative feelings and associations that foster trust and openness—that is an essential element in the healing process.

Yoga therapy is ultimately a form of self-healing that involves clarity about one's conditions, including conditions of emotional attachment and insecurity that can interfere with developing and maintaining a healthy relationship with one's students and clients. This highlights the importance of maintaining one's own personal yoga practice, especially in practices that instill emotional stability and mental clarity as awakening somatic beings. Patanjalian yoga points to two basic paths for this cultivation:[2] the purely contemplative path of mental refinement conducted in solitude, which is a form of *jnana yoga*, and the more practical path of action, or *kriya yoga*, which appreciates how the complexity of engaged social being presents a variety of difficulties and opportunities in seeking or opening to wholeness and offers a more accessible path. We will often look to the path of solitude for ways of deepening self-understanding and self-awareness, even as the main path is one of conscious actions directed toward germinating and growing from the seeds of that understanding and awareness.

There are three essential, interrelated, and underlying foundations for the yoga of action (which also appear as *niyamas*):

Tapas: First, we must care for ourselves in the physical dimension of our lives, purifying ourselves by eliminating all that stands in the way of our health and well-being. This involves *tapas*, the root word of which, *tap*, is a Sanskrit noun meaning warmth or heat. Thus, tapas implies the self-disciplined effort to work with what intensity (or "fire") one can muster and sustain to burn away whatever binds oneself to a constrained, confused, or overly complicated outlook and mode of being. Taken by some to the extremes of penance and bodily mortification,[3] here we tap tapas as a tool of special observance and sacred learning aimed at willfully relieving ourselves of unhealthy behavioral habits to more fully live with healthy behaviors and conditions. By staying in the fullness of our personal practices, including asana, pranayama, and meditation, and taking care in what we bring into our bodyminds (qualities of food, air, ideas, social experiences), we manifest a vital foundation of self-healing and a greater capacity for supporting our clients in theirs. With tapas, we steel the container of our journey.

Svadyaya: Second, the yoga of action invites us into deeper self-reflection or self-study, or *svadhyaya*, a term more rich in underlying meaning than typically conveyed by its ubiquitous interpretation as "self-study."[4] The root words here are *sva*, meaning "one's own," and *dhya*, meaning "thinking," which is the root word in *dhyana*, which is usually translated as "meditate." The suggestion in the combined root words is to reflect on one's own thinking. The direction or intention of this reflection is enriched by incorporating a sense of the closely related terms *svad*, meaning "to taste well, be sweet, or pleasant," *svadhita*, meaning "well-studied, repeated, solid, or firm," and *svadha*, meaning "self-position, inherent power, habitual state, one's own place, or home." In self-reflection and self-study, we thus open ourselves to more clearly seeing and understanding our habitual patterns of thought and behavior and to discovering the reality of where we are in every aspect of our lives. The sweet or pleasant quality suggests that these practices of getting to better know ourselves help us move toward deeper self-acceptance, feeling better about ourselves, and being more attuned to the inherent power of better caring for ourselves. In recognizing and appreciating the habits of our own bodymind, we increase our capacity for holding the space with our clients for them to do the same. With *svadyaya*, we become clearer.

Ishvara-Pranidhana: The yoga of action also invites us into *pranidhana*, from *prani*, "to attend to" or "advance," and *dhana*, with "fixing" or "exertion." Thus, *pranidhana* is about commitment or dedication in attending to or advancing with focus and exertion toward … what?[5] This is prefaced in the *Yoga Sutra* by the term *ishvara*, which most commentators, offering us various (often conflicting) theistic interpretations, interpret as "God." However, in his adherence to Samkhya philosophy, Patanjali never uses the term God, never refers to deities, but does refer to "ishvaras" in the plural. This suggests that the path he charts is not about devotion to God or dedication to an external source or force; rather, the source (of consciousness, *purusha*) is found within, with ample suggestion that it is found in the heart, the place of ultimate surrender into self-acceptance. This echoes the contemporaneous suggestion in the *Bhagavad-Gita* that an essential path of yoga is found in the heart (*bhakti yoga*), and that opening to love brings us to the third source of balanced foundation on the healing path of yoga. When we live more consciously through the wisdom of the heart, we open ourselves to being better able to create and hold space with clients as a *punya mandala*, a sacred circle in which one feels safe and supported in exploring and awakening to every aspect of one's being, free of personal judgment. With ishvara-pranidhana, we live more consciously in a life of abundant meaning.

This balanced foundation in the yoga of action gains more practical and specific expression through the *yamas*. The literal definition of *yama*, "to contain" or "to control," refers to the moral container of our actions, which brings our interrelated intrapersonal and interpersonal integrity into focus. We can fruitfully reflect on these moral and ethical principles as sources of deeper insight into our healing relationships, as follows:

Ahimsa: Literally "nonhurting," *ahimsa* is often interpreted as "nonviolence." It begins with respecting one's own bodymind and extending this respect to all other beings in the world. In yoga, this wisdom applies directly by creating a safe space to feel, learn, and heal. It suggests interacting with students with compassion and empathetic understanding, and offering qualities of guidance that do not cause physical or emotional harm. Because yoga teachers and yoga therapists work with a vast range of student and client vulnerabilities, there is a greater than usual risk of unintentionally and unknowingly causing harm. This underlines the importance of well-developed communication skills, working within a clear scope of practice, and offering only those treatments one well understands, including how they affect and are affected by other treatments a student or client is receiving.

Satya: *Satya* means "truth," the principle of being honest with oneself and others in every aspect of one's life. Being truthful begins with being true to oneself, to one's own values and sense of wholeness. When through self-awareness, self-observation, and self-reflection we discern tension between how we feel or what we think about something and what is being asked of us, we can fruitfully pause and reflect more deeply on the truths of the situation. Rather than suffering the confusion of cognitive dissonance—the emotional stress that arises amid contradictory beliefs or values or when confronted by new information that conflicts with one's understandings—yoga therapists can be open to recognizing both the insight and limitations of what they know.[6] On just the other side of what we know is what we do not know. Acknowledging our limited knowledge can help us to more easily appreciate and respect the knowledge of students and other caregivers. In these relationships, this involves both attentive listening that maximizes understanding and honest expression of the limits of one's knowledge. In living and working in our truth, we more naturally act with integrity in sharing all we know, including in finding ways to express what might be painful truths in the most honest and nonhurting ways.

Asteya: The essence of *asteya*, "not stealing," is freeing oneself from the desire to have something that one has not earned or paid for. Citing greed as one of the seven spiritual sins, Mahatma Gandhi emphasized that wealth without work is wrong. Some yoga teachers extend this to their yoga classes by encouraging students to "pay their dues" on the yoga mat before expecting the fruits of the practice or even the teacher's considered assistance. Creating ways for students to experience a sense of abundance in their practice while honoring what is not readily there for them is one way of expressing this principle in teaching, this while appreciating that there are even sweeter fruits further along the path. But there are some things for which there should be no price, starting with a sense of wholeness and well-being. We cannot take or steal wholeness (although we can disturb it). Rather, the potential for wholeness is natural and innate. But where one is cultivating wellness and wholeness amid illness or injury, there can be a strong tendency to take all one can from any and every source that holds the promise of feeling better. Thus, we need to be aware of the tendency of some students to take more than is being offered, including time, emotional energy, and whatever other resources one offers. We also need to monitor ourselves for any tendency to take from our students in any unnecessary ways, including their time, emotional energy, and financial resources. On the latter, there is inestimable value in reflecting on what you sell and why you sell it, especially if whatever is being sold is not helpful or has a less expensive yet suitable alternative—including your yoga services.

Brahmacharya: This *yama* is typically given loose and perfectly ambiguous interpretation as the "right use of energy." Although Iyengar points out that the literal definition of *bramacharya* means "a life of celibacy, religious study, and self-restraint," he goes on to write, "without experiencing human love and happiness it is not possible to know divine love."[7] The concept originates in the *Bhagavad-Gita*, which stresses that living in the truth of Brahma "a man's heart ... is never again moved by the things of the senses." The *Bhagavad-Gita* also goes on to say that, "The yogi should retire to a solitary place and live alone."[8] But here we are, alive in a social world and in our senses, including the sense of sexual desire and attraction. Even if one chooses renunciation, the power of desire can overwhelm one's values, as we see all too often among spiritual leaders who preach sexual abstinence while sexually exploiting those over whom they hold power or influence. The essence of this sutra is about honoring yourself and others in intimate relationships, including the inherent intimacy of teacher-student and therapist-client relationships, as we discussed earlier with yoga ethics.

Aparigraha: *Aparigraha* means "noncovetousness." This is often interpreted as not being greedy, or being free of desire. Stated affirmatively, it is about living with generosity of spirit and action, giving without expecting something in return. Applied to asana and pranayama, this principle can help us approach our practice with an attitude of patience in which steadiness and ease is more important than getting into a pose. It goes much further when applied to yoga therapy. The principle of aparigraha invites deepening self-acceptance on the path of curing and healing. As yoga teachers and therapists, we extend this value to our students and clients by relieving them of whatever expectations we might have that come outside the *punya mandala*—the sacred circle—of the relationship. We listen more attentively to better hear our students, meeting them in their intention—*sankalpa*—rather than attempting to impose ours on them. We also encourage and offer guidance and support to our students in their own deepening self-acceptance, and with it, a growing sense of *santosa*, contentment, amid the immediate realities of one's conditions.

The foundations of *kriya yoga* and *yama* inform the entire practice of yoga. It can be helpful to pause in one's work from time to time to reflect on how each of the elements is being expressed in our interactions with students. Just as in our personal yoga practice, there is no limit to how we can strengthen and refine these essential foundations in establishing and sustaining a healing relationship with students, the qualities of which are an integral part of the healing process itself.[9]

Principles and Skills for Interacting with Students and Clients

In practicing yoga, we interact with ourselves. In teaching yoga, we interact with others. The principles and skills that inform this interaction—with students, yoga teachers, health professionals, and others involved in a student's or client's well-being—are an essential foundation of yoga's therapeutic efficacy. This brings skillful, informed, heart-centered communication to the forefront of yoga therapy. Unfortunately, as Frymoyer and Frymoyer show, many physicians are relatively poor communicators;[10] yoga teachers and therapists are not always very good communicators either. This matters because the quality of teacher-student and therapist-client communication affects not only student and client satisfaction, it also affects student and client adherence to practices and improved outcomes.[11]

With improved communication skills, we can do a better job in every aspect of yoga therapy, which is predicated upon appreciating and respecting our clients as whole beings in a client-centered process of nurturance. Yoga therapists have invaluable contributions to offer—in addition to yoga practices themselves—in every aspect of client-centered care, including these:

Honoring Clients: Many clients are frustrated by a feeling of not being fully seen or heard by their caregivers, particularly physicians in conventional medical settings. In client-centered healing, yoga therapists can play a key role in respecting their clients as whole beings, including being attuned to their expressed values, preferences, and needs and reinforcing their right to be heard by others. This begins with how we query our clients about not only their condition but their life—their concerns, fears, dreams, relationships, priorities, and core values.

Integrating Care: Care can only be as integrated as allowed by the qualities of communication and information management found in any care setting. Yoga therapists can advocate for their clients' care by staying abreast of their clients' various services, including tests, consultations, and procedures offered by other caregivers.

Sharing Knowledge: We all want to know our condition (diagnosis), how to stay well, the likely course of various conditions (prognosis), and what we might do to make things better. Yoga therapists can educate their students about how to be well and offer a variety of practices to help their clients at least feel better, if not find better paths to healing what ails them.

Providing Comfort: Stress reduction and a variety of palliative yoga-based practices can support clients in reducing the suffering caused by pain as well as the pain itself, giving yoga therapists many tools for making clients more comfortable. This involves timely, individualized, and informed attention to the conditions of a client's suffering.

Offering Emotional Support: Fear and anxiety accompany most illnesses and injuries, with "fear of pain, disability or disfigurement, loneliness, financial impact, or the effect of illness on one's family" topping the list of causes.[12] The breathing and contemplative practices offered by yoga therapists can give clients added emotional support for more easily moving through the fear and anxiety of illness and injury, treatment and healing.

Involving Friends and Family: Social isolation is a major factor in suffering, while social connection, particularly with close friends and family, is a major factor in healing. Yoga therapists can work with students to invite the client's friends and family into their circle of care, even into their *punya mandala*, bringing the inestimably powerful resource of love more fully into the client's healing experiences.

Developing Healing Communication Skills

All of this is predicated upon refined communication skills. As we develop our communication skills, we are able to more skillfully engage with our clients, better understand their needs and conditions, and more naturally establish trusting rapport with them, thereby better empowering them to make the best choices they can in curing and healing. This begins with personal yoga practice, where cultivating the attributes of self-awareness, self-care, and self-acceptance allow us to be more fully present in our interactions with others. In later chapters we look closely at the techniques with which one might best engage in this cultivation in his or her yoga practice, the heart of which is self-study and the art of which revolves around reflective self-consciousness in asana, pranayama, and meditation practices.

We can also go beyond our yoga practice to further develop our communication skills; the IAYT Competencies Profile lists these first under its basic principles of the healing relationship, which include listening, presence, directive, and nondirective dialogue as general communications competencies, which we explore later.[13] In mental health professions, in which interaction with one's patient or client is an integral aspect of practice, considerable attention is given to these and other forms of both diagnostic and therapeutic communication. However, medical schools (and many alternative health training schools) have typically slighted the importance of physician-patient communication, focusing instead on objective measurement of conditions and physician-directed care, leading many patients to feel disconnected from their care and far from being recognized and treated as whole human beings. Today, all medical schools in the U.S. are required to teach students basic communication skills.[14] However, there is less focus on this during clinical rotations when medical students are most engaged with actual patients and even less once medical students begin to specialize (except in primary care), further highlighting the need to better focus on communication skills—a concern that extends to all the healing arts professions.

The American Academy on Communication in Health Care and other organizations are now providing concentrated communications skills trainings to health care professionals, who utilize role-playing, standardized scenarios such as breaking unfortunate news, and watching videos of interactions with patients. Going further, in 2001 the American Academy of Orthopaedic Surgeons (AAOS) initiated a communications skills development program in conjunction with the Bayer Institute for Health Care Communication that combines Bayer's "4Es" (engage, empathize, educate, enlist) with orthopedic videos and trains orthopedic surgeons as mentors to train others in their field in effective doctor-patient communications.[15] Here we adapt and expand upon this model, adding elicit, encourage, and ease to give us the 7Es of yoga therapy communications.

With practice, the 7Es of yoga therapy communications give richer character to our listening, presence, directive, and nondirective dialogue skills. With role-playing we can better develop skills in each of these seven aspects of communication with clients. In doing so, we want to emphasize that it is important to appreciate how your values, intention, and specific approach to yoga practices are embodied and expressed in how and what you do in communicating. Different yoga therapists offer different kinds of yoga, some well within a yoga scope of practice and others working at the edges of that scope as they offer practices that approximate those of other healing arts and sciences.

THE 7Es OF YOGA THERAPY COMMUNICATIONS

Engage: Establish a personal connection with your client through a warm, nonjudgment-oriented greeting to set the stage for further interaction with him or her; use eye contact and gentle speech that emphasizes your presence of mind and heart.

Empathize: Listen to your client in order to understand his or her values, concerns, thoughts, and feelings, and demonstrate your understanding and concern by affirming what you hear.

Educate: Provide what information you can to help your client learn more about their conditions and what they can do to feel better and more whole.

Enlist: In acknowledging that your client is—or should be—in control of his or her treatment plan, ensure that the client not only has the best understanding of his or her condition but is integrally involved in deciding on practices.

Elicit: To best involve your client in decision-making, proactively yet sensitively elicit his or her thoughts and feelings in discussing practice options.

Encourage: Give your clients affirmative support for their decisions and regularly check in to determine how they are feeling with the choices they are making and support either adherence to an existing practice plan or consideration of alternatives.

Ease: Reflect upon your own emotional reactions to issues raised by your client, then examine and learn to express your thoughts and feelings in ways that give highest priority to easing your client's condition, including their fear and anxiety.

As we discussed earlier, if you offer services outside the yoga scope of practice, it is important to be trained and licensed to do so and to follow the standards and guidelines given by those other health professions. For example, if you are a licensed clinical psychologist, you will have learned certain modes of intake interviewing that support working within the clinical psychology scope of practice. Now, expanding your offering to include yoga, you will ideally refine your intake interview techniques to integrate the 7Es. In this integrated approach, you might fruitfully consult sources such as Weintraub's *Yoga Skills for Therapists*, which offers specialized insight into how a yoga therapist can best communicate in his or her counseling practice.[16]

If you are not licensed to offer therapeutic services but you are working with clients receiving treatment services, it will be helpful to comprehend at least the basic indications and contraindications given by other health care providers so that you can communicate about them with your student and his or her other caregivers. This is part of the value of expanding one's knowledge to include deeper understanding of human organ systems and their interactions and common disorders, as we explored in Part II. But if you are not trained and licensed to work within a particular scope of work, for example, as a physician, physical therapist, or respiratory therapist, it is not for you to conduct the medical diagnostics offered by those professions, even as you might use some of the tools of medical diagnostics—such as pulse, heart rate, range of motion, and respiratory capacity—to assist a client in monitoring his or her conditions.[17] As a yoga therapist you will be fully prepared to do yoga diagnostics, not other diagnostics, unless of course you do those other diagnostics by profession. It is not for you to determine if your client has autism, COPD, or osteoporosis, but it is for you to have sufficient lay understanding of these conditions if it is within your intention to appropriately work with your students who have them.

Mindful Listening

We add the adjective "mindful" to this discussion to emphasize that effective communication is an active process in which one is consciously engaged in listening.[18] This starts by cultivating self-awareness and self-acceptance, which is an integral aspect of doing yoga. With greater self-awareness and self-acceptance, we are less likely to succumb to the leading barriers to active listening: internal or external distraction, insistence upon one's own opinions and beliefs, or simple misinterpretation. Our personal meditation practice can help us to recognize and overcome these barriers by allowing us to more clearly see our various tendencies toward certain qualities of judgment, expectation, and fear; our attachment to personal beliefs or notions of truth; and our propensity to over-interpret—and thus misinterpret—what someone else says or does.

Rather than listening only to words, in mindful listening, we strive to hear the complete message, which might be conveyed by body language as much or more than by words. With this quality of comprehension, we move closer to the shared understanding and retention of information that allows us to stay truly engaged with clients. Rather than passively receiving the words or other messages of a client, we more actively engage by being responsive. This can be as simple as saying "yes" or "uh-huh" in affirmative response to a client's statements, posing questions that convey empathy and elicit greater responses, and paraphrasing back to the client his or her words to confirm that one is hearing the client's intended message. Rather than arguing when in disagreement with what a client says, we find positive ways to affirm our client's immediate sense of things and confirm our understanding and appreciation of what they are saying, yet also gently offer our view, inviting our client to consider a different perspective.

Here it behooves us to recall the punya mandala and to consider inviting our clients into that safe space for feeling and sharing. Using the basic tools of yoga, starting with sitting comfortably, tuning in to the breath, and taking a moment to be more calm and self-aware, you can go far in helping students feel more comfortable and trusting in communicating with you. Weintraub offers specific techniques for this centering practice, focusing on moving closer to clear intention.[19]

In listening beyond words we can first tune in to body language, including posture, facial expression, eye contact, gestures, and qualities of speech such as pace, clarity, and tone of voice. Insecurity, defensiveness, and depression are often betrayed in crossed arms, downcast eyes, limited facial expression, and minimal arm and hand gesture. The extent to which one is present as well as qualities of mood are also found in sitting or standing posture, in which tendencies toward active presence versus dissociative states tend to find various patterns of postural expression. We can often detect relative happiness, sadness, anger, or depression through the combined ways that the eyes, eyebrows, and other facial movements express mood. Qualities of touch are very revealing, whether it is the firmness or softness of a handshake, or either an apparent need for strong and long hugging versus avoidance of all touch.[20]

To develop your mindful listening skills, it can be helpful to explore self-reflective journaling in which you consider how you listen and how you speak. Going further, role-playing is a very effective means of developing and refining mindful listening. Video-taping the role-plays allows you to easily observe, appreciate, and assess your skills.

Attentive Presence

The idea of "being present in the moment" is quite ancient; it is, to be sure, at least implied in ancient yogic approaches to meditation and the first *Yoga Sutra*, "to still the fluctuations of the mind." It is further elevated in Buddhist contemplative practices, including *vipassana* (recently recoined and further popularized as "insight meditation").[21] Krishnamurti wrote extensively about the power of being present to one's immediate experience, and Eckhart Tolle has further popularized the idea as a tool of spiritual practice in which one's awareness of being in the present moment helps draw him or her out of the confusion, worry, and anxiety that arise in preoccupation with the past or future.[22] Kramer and Alstad agree that "to be either preoccupied by the past or projecting into the future, both of which we do so much, is to remove your attention from the immediacy and ongoing movement of what's happening within or around you. This separation, which lives in thought, changes the experience by coming between you and the experience."[23]

In being as fully present in the moment as you can be, you will be better able to be fully attentive and present with a client. Again, we can usefully look to our personal yoga practice in cultivating this attribute. The earliest recognition of being present usually comes in recognizing its opposite: absence. In doing asana practice, especially asanas that one finds challenging, we gradually learn that paying attention allows us to more easily feel and navigate through whatever creates difficulty. If our gaze wanders, our mind wanders. If our thoughts drift to extraneous topics, we immediately inhibit our inner attunement, causing further difficulty. As we learn to tune in to the breath and sensations arising through the bodymind in reaction to our actions, we come to more subtle and nuanced awareness of tension, which suggests where to place our attention. In this way of being in the practice, distractions fade, boredom evaporates, and we gain more focused insight into what is happening.

When interviewing, teaching, and guiding clients, attentive presence—which is predicated upon and supports mindful listening—conveys genuine caring, one effect of which is greater trust and thus openness in sharing one's thoughts and feelings. It is the most essential quality of the punya mandala, as without it there is no circle. Our clients get a stronger sense of our attentive presence when we fully exercise mindful listening through awareness of our own body language, including being upright, facing our clients, and maintaining comfortable (not piercing) eye contact. Attentive presence might also involve simply being in the punya mandala, sharing in silence—whatever feelings seem to be in the air. With a deepening connection and openness through this practice, one can more easily be attentively present even amid less favorable conditions, such as when one is reacting to something that is intense. Just as one might most easily develop meditation skills sitting alone in a quiet space, it is amid the complexity and even chaos of life when these skills most serve us, allowing us to be more present regardless of what is happening inside and outside.

Directive Dialogue

This concept, which is rooted in psychiatry (and to some extent in personnel administration), describes a therapist-driven course of therapy.[24] Here it is assumed that clients come to yoga therapy for guidance on matters with which the yoga therapist is considered to have superior experience and training. This results in general deference to the therapist in determining practice methods and techniques. Much of conventional medicine is based on a directive relationship between the health care provider and patient.

In considering the underlying values of holistic health and treatment, particularly treating the whole person in ways that fully involve the client or patient in decision-making, directive dialogue can seem off-putting. But consider situations in which it is abundantly clear that a client has very low or skewed self-awareness. For example, you might have a client with severe disc degeneration who believes Power Yoga is his best hope for feeling well because his twin brother—with no disc issues—raves about how good it makes him feel. Or imagine a client entirely new to yoga, thus with very little sense of what doing yoga might be like. In either case your greater knowledge and experience with yoga gives you greater responsibility in directing the dialogue about how to approach the client's condition, including suggesting certain practices that you understand as being of likely benefit to the client.

Regardless of the extent to which a specific client's condition points to the value of relatively greater directive engagement, the other qualities of communication discussed above retain value. Mindful listening and attentive presence can be even more important so that there is a stronger connection with the client that results in his or her greater adherence to the informed suggestions you offer. By being explicit with your client that this is how you are working with him or her and emphasizing that one goal is his or her steady assumption of self-care through growing self-awareness, you are more likely to engage the client in ways that make that goal more attainable.

In doing directive dialogue, we give specific direction in every aspect of the relationship, including in doing an intake interview, setting goals, identifying methods, and guiding the student in specific practices. This can reach deeply into the interior experience of the client with such techniques as suggesting mental imagery in meditation. Depending on the client, this approach can reinforce feelings of inadequacy and self-judgment, thereby making it increasingly difficult for the client to develop the self-awareness and self-confidence that are cornerstones of holistic health. Precisely due to such potential adverse effects of directive guidance, it is important to steadfastly work toward less directive dialogue, gradually incorporating this objective as part of the practice goals and process.

Nondirective Dialogue

Here we return to Carl Rogers and the idea that the client has the greatest insight into his or her condition and how best to heal. Rather than directing a student or giving interpretation to everything, the yoga teacher assumes more of a facilitator role, working with the student to bring light and clarity to the conditions and options at hand through interaction that helps awaken the student's inherent intelligence and insight. Here again we fully tap into mindful listening and attentive presence, making the relationship itself a source of healing.

In Rogers' early work in nondirective psychotherapy, he coined the term "healthy person" to describe someone who is motivated to develop his or her potential as fully as possible, what Maslow defines as "self-actualization." Rogers identified five qualities of such a fully functioning person, each of which we relate to nondirective dialogue in communication and interaction:[25]

Openness to Experience: Through mindful listening and attentive presence in the punya mandala, we reflect back to the client the client's self-perception of feelings, conditions, and experiences.

Existential Living: Openness to experience opens us to living more in the present, which the therapist reinforces with the client by affirming the client's statements and actions that embody being in the moment rather than dwelling in the past or future.

Organismic Trusting: A key to healing resonance, we know what is good for us and what is bad for us. We can affirm this self-trust and the self-confidence it instills each time we recognize it in our client's words and actions.

Experiential Freedom: Being amid even the greatest difficulty, we still have the freedom to make choices in healing and thus the quality of our lives. We can point to the many options in ways that further empower clients to exercise this freedom within realistic circumstances.

Creativity: We are all creative beings whose bodyminds are inherently creative and capable of contributing to the world in positive ways. We can forget this when hurting; we can help forgetful clients remember this capacity through mindful listening that affirms the creative ways the student is presently expressing his or herself.

All of this assumes that one is doing his or her homework by staying in their personal yoga practice in ways that continuously cultivate the attitudinal qualities of *verstehen* (empathetic understanding), congruence, and unconditional positive regard for the student.

19

Assessing and Planning Healing Practices

It takes as much energy to wish as it does to plan.
—ELEANOR ROOSEVELT

Self- and Client-Assessments

Self- and client-assessment practices are ideally designed and implemented to elicit accurate and insightful information that is relevant to whatever practices one might suggest. Since yoga is a holistic practice that attempts to appreciate, engage, and support the needs of the whole person, yoga therapy assessments begin with a wide spectrum of queries into a client's general condition and lifestyle. If as part of a client's yoga practice there are certain areas of more specialized therapeutic focus or treatment, assessments should give greater attention to the related conditions and intentions of the client.

Many yoga teachers have training, expertise, and credentials that qualify them to work in other health professions. If you are a yoga teacher and a physician, psychotherapist, physical therapist, respiratory therapist, massage therapist, acupuncturist, chiropractor, or other licensed health profession treatment provider, you will have intake instruments and assessment protocols unique to your specialized field. You will appreciate the subtle aspects of your evaluations and having working knowledge of how to apply them and evaluate their effects. You may also have insight into how yoga practices might best complement whatever other treatments you prescribe, including how your patient's or client's conditions might contraindicate certain yoga practices. Where you lack knowledge of yoga practices, you can consult resources such as this book and scores of other published sources of information on the nature, requirements, and effects of yoga techniques, including a growing body of research into the relative efficacy and risks of those techniques for specific health conditions, as presented in Part IV.

Without the study and training that prepares licensed health professionals to work in their various areas of expertise, they would not be able to responsibly carry out the relevant assessments and offer the related treatments that are informed by them. This is the practical reality of most yoga therapists and clients. Thus, it makes little sense for yoga therapists in general to assess for conditions that we neither understand nor treat or are outside of yoga. Although it can be tempting to offer guidance and even treatments on any and all conditions, the principles of *ahimsa, satya,* and *aparigraha* remind us to stay with what we know and to refer our clients to others whose expertise is relevant to a client's condition when it is beyond our expertise.[1] Staying within our field we more assuredly stay in our integrity in working with all of our students, particularly those whose conditions might be extraordinarily complex.

Yoga-based assessment is predicated upon trying to understand and appreciate clients not merely as clients but as whole human beings whose life histories, lifestyles, values, dreams, and immediate conditions provide hints to appropriate yoga practices for any given individual client. We add "appreciation" to "assessment" to better emphasize this caring and holistic attitude and practice, thereby underlining how we seek to honor, respect, and support each client for who he or she is as a person. In doing so, we apply the principles and skills of communication and relationship discussed in the previous pages to what is more generally called "intake" and we refer to this as the initial client interview.

Interviewing and Assessing

There are three successive steps in doing client assessment: 1) gathering a personal history and intention; 2) assessing current conditions; and 3) developing a shared working assessment. Each is described here in detail.

Step One: Personal History and Intention

Eliciting a client's relevant history and core intentions is vitally important in gaining insight into his or her immediate conditions and in establishing a healing relationship, which potentially begins in the initial client interview. This is an ongoing process that extends from initial interaction or intake through the completion of healing practices. Most adverse conditions are developmental (developing over time) although some are incidental (due to a relatively discreet activity or event) yet no less within one's unique developmental experience. Background history is thus an essential part of understanding and appreciating a client.

Throughout this process, it is important to elicit, understand, and affirm a client's intentions, starting with his or her general intentions in life, and to revisit these intentions on an ongoing basis. Many if not most people come to questions of intention with all the ordinary doubts or uncertainties, starting with the question, "Who am I?" As Stephen Cope discusses, this brings us to discovering our *dharma*, our sense of life purpose that connects with our own character or genius and brings it forth in the world.[2] This realization is both an inherent part of being on the yoga path and one of the fruits found along that path as one comes to gradually clearer self-awareness. Eliciting at least an initial sense of this purpose will inform one's intention, which is discovered or set anew in deeper and deeper ways the more deeply one goes into yoga practices.

There are two basic methods for gathering a client's history and initial core intentions:

Traditional Interview: Utilizing directive dialogue and assessment instruments, we try to discover information that we consider important in offering appropriate practices, including baseline and boilerplate information. Questions are usually close-ended, allowing less elaboration and self-expression by the client; objective; and typically on a rating scale or dichotomous (yes/no) basis.

Ethnographic Interview: Using nondirective dialogue and assessment instruments, we engage with a client to elicit what the client considers important information to share. Here one uses open-ended questions that allow individualized and spontaneous responses from the client, mindful listening, attentive presence, and nondirective dialogue; avoids posing leading questions that create bias toward a certain response; and avoids asking "Why?" in keeping with nonjudgmental communication.

Combining these methods gives us both objective student indicators and subjective client understandings that can be refined with a variety of well-considered and tactful follow-up questions, starting with questions of clarification to help ensure that the client is feeling supported and being well understood. If we discern discrepancies or inconsistencies in the client's responses, it is important to seek further clarification without being confrontational. Paraphrasing a client's replies is one way to better establish accurate understanding and to convey to the client the feeling of being fully heard. Working at a more emotionally subtle level, we can offer a reflection of feeling, echoing the client's expressed emotions with as much intuitive awareness and sensitivity as we are able to. It is also helpful to look for connections among various responses, thereby tying various topics together and identifying themes that reflect the wholeness of the client.

Step Two (Part One): Issues in Assessing Current Conditions

Here we come to several significant difficulties that arise from the basic tension between an expansive concept of yoga, the actual skills and work of yoga therapists, and the importance of honoring the (often porous) boundaries of different health professions.

Given the holistic intent of yoga, it is tempting when considering a student's current conditions to assess everything and to conduct those assessments on one's own. The International Association of Yoga Therapists (IAYT) Educational Standards call for assessing "current conditions using tools relevant to the yoga therapist, including evaluation of the physical, energetic, mental, emotional, and spiritual dimensions of well-being"—categories some correlate with the *koshas* and that cover, well, just about everything in the known and unknown universe.[3] As noted earlier, the more ubiquitous rendition of *koshas* gives us the following dimensions or layers: physical *(annamaya)* the "food" sheath), energetic *(pranamaya* the "energy" sheath), mental *(manomaya)* the "thinking" sheath), intuitive *(vijnanamaya)* the "wisdom" sheath), and love or spirit *(anandamaya)* the "bliss" sheath).

Although the *kosha* model offers a useful heuristic device for mapping the yogic journey or describing in the most general ways the experience of moving from gross material experience to a sense of transcendence or bliss,[4] there are several problems in using it to categorize and assess human conditions in ways that translate into practical and specific treatments. To begin, the "physical" is never just so, unless without life. Living human beings are always and at once whole bodyminds. Dualistic thinking creates separations, starting with the separation into body and mind. The existence of the bodymind presupposes life, which in human beings involves the "energy" of breath. As stated in the *Chandogya Upanishad*, "no breath, no life." In our awareness as living bodyminds, we also have many qualities of consciousness, including those that arise from memory, reflection, and integrated sensation to give intuitive feelings/thoughts (the separation of feelings and thoughts is yet another expression of disembodied dualistic thinking, as though there are separate organs for this natural experience of awareness). The sense of spirit, love, or a power greater than oneself also arises in our organic consciousness as human beings, not somehow separate from the whole of our tissues, breathing, and cognition. It is very easy to lose our sense of this wholeness, especially when thinking about it (or not thinking about it while following someone else's thinking).

Given our wholeness, several issues arise in attempting to assess a client's conditions based on assumptions of dimensions, sheaths, and other concepts that are predicated upon separation or even interrelation (which assumes separate things in relationship to one another), which is reflected in the intake instruments found across much of the yoga therapy world. (This is not unlike how allopathic medicine has historically separated body and mind in assessment, diagnosis, prognosis, and treatment.) For example, a common yoga therapy intake instrument on "general satisfaction" asks clients to rate their "present state of distress or satisfaction" in "areas" (physical body, relationships, leisure/recreation, and total experience/happiness). On the physical body continuum, the opposing poles are: "I am experiencing intolerable levels of pain, discomfort, lack of energy or sexual functioning, sleep, or other physical problems" and "My physical body, sleep patterns, eating, drinking, and sexuality are at their highest level." Each of these statements implies an energized bodymind, not a separate physical body. Clearly, health and other human conditions cannot be reduced to such a separate mindless body or body somehow separated from the mind: "pain" requires a perceiving mind, which is a cognitive function of the brain in neurological communication with every part of the bodymind, even as it is experienced in part through the prism of memory and myriad elements of our general state of being (including sense of spirit). Nor is "lack of energy" or "sexual functioning" reducible to a physical body that is somehow separate from the whole of one's being, including one's emotional state. Thus, the instrument assumes and reinforces several dualisms or separations, which can distort or otherwise misrepresent the wholeness of a client's conditions.

A second and potentially more pernicious issue is found in standard evaluation forms used in yoga therapy client intake interviews that ask for pulse, blood pressure, radiologic and imaging findings, and information on surgeries and drug prescriptions, plus extensive measurements of range of motion, gravitational balance, respiratory function, and strength. Here we come to a rather different problem in assessment of conditions: qualification to do so, and qualification to interpret results and integrate them into a meaningful overall assessment one can then use to prescribe or recommend yoga therapies. If a yoga therapy clinic has a licensed medical doctor, nurse, radiological technician, physical therapist, and respiratory therapist on staff, or if a yoga therapist is working in a full-service health care setting to offer complementary services as a member of a collaborative or integrative health team, these assessments, done by qualified health professionals, could be very useful. But as we have it these assessments are well within other scopes of practice, not that of yoga therapy, leaving the yoga therapist who independently offers services to clients at a loss in doing such assessments, let alone knowledgably interpreting and applying them.

To make this point clearer, consider this hypothetical case that utilizes the intake assessments just described:

> You learn that your student is a fifty-seven-year-old woman, she had a pulse rate of 75 (when it was measured), blood pressure of 127/78 (when it was measured), had a lumpectomy eight months ago to address metastatic breast cancer, recently underwent radiation therapy, is currently taking an aromatase inhibitor to help keep the tumor from getting the hormone it needs to grow, and notes "advanced osteoporosis" under "warnings and contraindications" on the standard evaluation. Spirometry tests indicate FEV1 = 2.5% and PEF = 325 L/min (when they were measured). Range of motion tests have not been conducted, but since you recently learned how to use a goniometer in your yoga therapist training, you decide to give it a try in order to complete this part of the intake.

Ready to measure? Before you begin, here is *your* test:

1. You decide to begin at the top of the physical exam form, which calls for testing thoracolumbosacral spine range of motion, utilizing Uttanasana (Standing Forward Fold Pose) to test flexion by measuring the distance of the fingertips from the floor. You:

   a. Ask the client to bend her knees to better focus on flexing her spine and to more purely measure spinal flexion rather than hip flexion. (Do note that flexibility in the hamstrings, gastrocnemii, and glutei is a significant factor in how close one's fingers come to the floor.)

   b. Ask the client to first warm up and stretch her hamstrings for five minutes before holding Uttanasana for two minutes while flexing her spine.

   c. Ask the client to keep her legs fully extended to better isolate and measure her spinal flexion, asking her to hold Uttanasana for one minute.

   d. Do not ask the client to do this test because it is contraindicated by at least one of her conditions.

Let us assume that you chose the correct answer. This brings us to the next question:

2. Why is this test of lower spine flexion contraindicated for this client?

   a. Her blood pressure is too high to safely do the inversion.

   b. She has advanced osteoporosis.

   c. The inversion aspect of the asana is contraindicated by the aromatase prescription due to risk of thrombosis.

   d. Her FEV1 score contraindicates lowering her head beneath her heart.

Again, let us assume that you chose the correct answer because you learned in your 500-hour yoga teacher training or elsewhere that advanced osteoporosis contraindicates spinal flexion (due to risk of vertebral body fractures). What about the other conditions? Is there a high blood pressure issue? No. Is there a heightened risk of thrombosis with an aromatase drug? Slight. However, this is extremely unlikely in the absence of symptoms such as shortness of breath or feelings of being faint. Plus, her blood pressure is not an issue, and her FEV1 score is not a significant factor. But most yoga therapists are not trained within a scope of practice for these assessments and thus do not have this more specific and discerning knowledge.

We will explore one further permutation of this assessment puzzle—the question of testing range of motion and applying that information. Consider for a moment three different students (A, B, and C), all apparently free of any musculoskeletal issues, who have come to you for help with chronic depression. Since you are likely to recommend some aspect of asana practice, you once again decide to try your goniometer skills to assess ranges of motion in the major joints, this time free of concern about contraindications. To test hip abduction in relation to hip flexion, you ask the three clients to come into *Upavista Konasana* (Wide-Angle Seated Forward Fold). Student A abducts his legs to nearly 180 degrees and folds forward until his chest is on the floor without flexing his spine or allowing his femurs to internally rotate. Student B has her legs abducted to around 45 degrees and is barely able to sit upright, let alone rotate her pelvis forward. Student C's range of motion is in between that of Students A and B. The question is this:

3. These differences in range of motion are the result of which of the following?

    a. Muscular flexibility

    b. Relative retroversion of the acetabulae

    c. Relative length and girth of the femoral head and neck

    d. Relative length of the iliofemoral ligament

    e. A combination of all of the above

    f. B and D only

Here there is no correct answer because the question is framed to allow too many options (even choice E could be incorrect). The point is that any of these variables could be a factor in any of the three student cases, or not.

This raises another crucial question: What is the practical relevance of so precisely measuring or knowing range of motion in the absence of a far more detailed differential diagnosis that might explain the differences, thereby indicating or contraindicating certain asanas or approaches to asanas? We are not suggesting the irrelevance of any of these measures. Quite to the contrary, yoga therapists working with clients in asanas should do their best to understand and interpret these various conditions, and then only with sufficient knowledge of indications and contraindications give guidance on how a unique person might explore a particular asana. Although conducting and interpreting detailed range of motion analysis for diagnostic purposes is beyond the scope of practice of the yoga therapist, it is well within that scope to appropriately guide clients in asanas as informed by such analysis and interpretation that is provided by a licensed physical therapist or a physician. Furthermore, a yoga therapist can use range-of-motion measurements to monitor a client's progress. The remaining question for the yoga therapist addressing that knowledge and skill is this: Do you have the training and competence to relate a physical therapist's stated indications and contraindications regarding a specific client to asana practice for that client? Now ask the same question for assessments you might receive from a client's cardiologist, respiratory therapist, psychotherapist, and so on, and consider them in relation to pranayama, meditation, and other yoga practices.

Conducting, interpreting, and applying medical assessments requires certain areas of specialized knowledge without which one is likely to gaze with something like a blank stare at the assessment data and the client. It is not for the yoga therapists to conduct diagnostic medical tests, nor to interpret them except within his or her level of knowledge to do so while working within a yoga therapy scope of practice. To reiterate, we as yoga therapists should conduct only those assessments that are well within our scope of practice, that we are trained and permitted to do, and that we know how to interpret and apply. If we do not possess such knowledge and skills, and if we wish to work with such medical assessments, we should turn to those qualified to do them and collaborate with them to explore which yoga methods and treatments are likely to best support a student in curing or healing. Going further in our studies, we can learn how to work with assessments conducted by other caregivers yet still consider consulting with the source of the assessments to gain their insights into risks, contraindications, and indications.

There are three reasons one might reject this perspective. First, you might think yoga therapists should be free to assess, interpret, and treat without the skill, knowledge, or license to legally do so, perhaps believing that your legitimacy is conferred by a higher source than mere legal statute or relative consensus on professional health care ethics. With this belief, perhaps you consider the mainstream medical profession essentially corrupt and best avoided, instead charting a renegade path of unfettered service to all who wish to be healthy. Second, you might be confident of the medical assessment knowledge and skills you learned in your yoga therapist training and have no concern about crossing into other scopes of practice (for example, in using a spirometer to diagnose respiratory function, you are working as though a licensed respiratory therapist, and you are comfortable doing so despite the legal issues). Third, you might think all such assessments are flawed methods of allopathic analysis that have no place in yoga; that our work should proceed based on personal experience, intuition, and prayer; and that true yoga therapy is found in ayurveda, tantra, and other related approaches.

As a final preface to assessing current conditions, we wish to highlight what for some might be the proverbial elephant in the room: the idea of assessing *intuition,* the *spiritual dimension,* or "*spirit.*" Spiritual assessment is something of an oxymoron, even if it is at the core of some religions, perhaps most glaringly in Scientology. Would we be measuring one's biological proximity to God, as Mormons purport to do through extensive genealogical analysis, or to Brahma or another deity, as some Hindus attempt with respect to caste and reincarnation? Would we partner with neurologists to detect changes in alpha waves as a measure of a lucid, quiet, or balanced mind (and which is it)? Would we pose qualitative questions regarding quality of life and suggest that this provides a measure of one's experience in the so-called spiritual dimension? Do we follow the lead of some yoga schools and ask clients to rate their status with respect to each of the eight limbs of ashtanga yoga? (As an example, clients are asked to rate their progress toward *samadhi* or transcendence.) Can we even agree on the meaning of *spiritual,* let alone a protocol to assess it?

Asking about quality of life, self-concept, and connectivity with others might very well point toward the spiritual dimension of one's life—and this can be insightful—but we should be careful not to place this on a scale to weigh the gravity or levity of someone's unique sense of spirit, as though anyone could.

Step Two (Part Two): Assessing Current Conditions Within the Yoga Therapy Scope of Practice

Here we proceed on the assumption that most yoga therapists wish to honorably work within a clear yoga therapy scope of practice, to conduct only those diagnostic assessments for which they are legally and technically qualified, and to make use of other health professionals' assessments and interpretations in providing services to clients within a yoga therapy scope of practice. This is not to suggest that one does so free of any of the earlier concerns about the limitations of mainstream methods. Rather, the suggestion is to work within one's integrity as a yoga therapist while considering how best to work in the often complex, confused, and confusing real world of complementary and integrative health.

Exploring with this assumption, we can start by generally stating how yoga therapists might best assess a client's current conditions.

- First, refer to the background interviews (traditional and ethnographic) discussed in Step One to identify significant issues, particularly in relation to the client's reported conditions and intentions in first coming to you for help.

- Second, ask your client to provide assessments and professional health recommendations from other caregivers. If you do not understand those assessments or the related treatment recommendations, work with your client to seek clarification from the caregivers who conducted and interpreted them, particularly to discuss their relevance in the yoga practices you think might be beneficial to your client.

- Third, conduct further assessments within the yoga therapy scope of practice.

Conducting further assessments specifically within the yoga therapy scope of practice can help you and your client to more fully learn about your client's current conditions regarding doing asana, pranayama, and meditation practices. These assessments should be given in the light of all you have learned from the background interview and other assessments, especially in regard to honoring contraindications and doing no harm. As many yoga therapists utilize Ayurvedic philosophy and practices, Ayurvedic assessments are a further consideration. Although some take a different view, here we consider every yoga therapy approach to health an option to be considered and ultimately determined by the client, not the yoga therapist. Despite one's commitment to learning and openness to applying every known technique, not every technique is appropriate for every client. Thus, it makes little sense to assess common conditions while thinking of every possible treatment, but rather to focus on the client's immediate concerns and whatever he or she chooses to share in the initial interview. Should a relationship develop between you and a client, you can revisit conditions, assessments, and treatments in the new light that emerges through your shared experience with the client.

The assessments in Table 19.1 use mnemonic devices to remember each query.

Table 19.1: Basic Medical Intake Assessments

OPQRST	SOCRATES
Onset: What was the client doing when the presenting condition started? Does the client think the condition is due to that activity? Was the onset sudden, gradual, or related to a different ongoing chronic problem?	**Site**: Where do you feel this condition?
Provocation or Palliation: What movement, pressure, or other external factor makes the problem better or worse? What is the effect of rest on the problem?	**Onset**: When did it start? Was it sudden or gradual? Is it progressive or regressive?
Quality of the Client's Pain: Pose questions that elicit the client's description of the presenting symptoms. Ask whether it is sharp, dull, burning, throbbing, constant, or intermittent.	**Character**: What is it like? How does it feel?
Region and Radiation: Where are the symptoms most felt? Do they seem to radiate into other areas?	**Radiation**: Do you feel these symptoms moving into other areas?
Severity: What is the intensity of the condition on a scale of 1–10, with 1 being the least intense and 10 being the most intense? Offer an imaginative comparison: "Compared to your finger being smashed in a car door … "	**Associations**: What else do you feel when experiencing this symptom?
Time: How long have you experienced this condition? How has it changed over time? Do you recall prior instances of the same or a similar condition? If you are no longer experiencing it, how long has it been since the condition resolved?	**Time Course**: Do the symptoms seem to follow a pattern, such as being greater at a certain time?
	Exacerbating or Relieving Factors: What, if anything, exacerbates or relieves the symptoms?
	Severity: How intense is it?

PHYSICAL ASANA ASSESSMENT

One of the most important skills of the yoga teacher is the ability to look at, see, and understand what is happening with unique students in each of whichever asanas the teacher is teaching. This skill is predicated upon sufficient knowledge of functional anatomy and biomechanics to inform the understanding of healthy human positioning as well as deviation from that ideal. In studying basic anatomy, we observe anatomical illustrations and skeletons that are generally presented as perfectly symmetrical and balanced. In studying biomechanics, we go slightly deeper, learning safe ranges of motion for each joint while also discovering how naturally diverse structural conditions (primarily bone shape and ligament length) often limit or extend those ranges. We begin to better appreciate that human beings exhibit a vast array of beautiful deviations from the idealized skeletal models we see in anatomy textbooks. In learning to understand what is happening with students in doing asanas at this gross level of observation, we gain further insight based on the contrasts between idealized forms we have studied and the actual forms exhibited by a certain person.

We also begin to sense that we are unable to easily see everything that matters in doing asanas. As noted earlier, unlike postures, which are static and lifeless, asanas are alive with the invisible qualities of energy and awareness. Because the essential elements of asana include energy and awareness, which in part reflect the principles of *sthira* (steadiness) and *sukham* (ease), we are invited to try to appreciate the qualities of these elements in a student's asana experience. For instance, qualities of energy are revealed in breathing patterns, facial tension, and fatigue. Qualities of awareness are revealed in breathing patterns, gaze, and sustained attention to detail. Although difficult or even impossible to measure, these qualities are nonetheless notable and worthy of recording in asana assessment. They are also qualities that can be highlighted and explored in conversation with clients, starting with asking, "How do you feel?" This also makes the assessment experience an educational opportunity for each client by conveying knowledge about yoga and how certain yoga practices might make his or her life better.

There are several elements of asana practice that make it more accessible and sustainable and thereby more deeply transformational: ujjayi pranayama, modification to accommodate one's conditions and intentions, cultivation of steadiness and ease, perseverance and nonattachment, and each of the yamas and niyamas. These do not easily translate into measurable assessment questions but rather point to qualitative appreciation of a client's understanding of the principles of asana and how to realize them in practice.

There are three steps in considering a student's musculoskeletal condition in relation to asanas: 1) basic postural analysis, 2) basic strength and flexibility tests, and 3) basic balance tests. We look at these in turn.

OBSERVING CLIENTS IN ASANAS

Self-reporting is not a guarantee that you will get accurate or complete information on a client's condition; many people are reluctant to share personal information with relative strangers, are unaware of a condition, or are in denial about the significance of some conditions. Your ability to accurately see and better understand clients in asanas starts with learning to see bodies more generally, specifically learning to see and understand different bodies from various perspectives. This essential skill is best developed through anatomical and asana observation clinics in yoga workshops, including the basic methods of partner standing observation, asana laboratory observation, and practice teaching observation, the insights from which you will further develop in apprenticing with a mentor teacher and ideally for as long as you are teaching yoga. This observational skill development is best done in conjunction with learning the fundamentals of functional anatomy in the context of learning how to teach yoga.

It is important to note that deviations from idealized anatomical forms are both part of human diversity and potentially an indication of imbalance or a pathological condition. In appreciating any such deviation, there are innumerable possible causes. Rather than attempting to cover all such possibilities, in Part IV we will apply the observational insights to various specific conditions, what best explains them, and how best to work with them as a yoga therapist.

Step 1: Standing Observation

Using the Client Postural Observation Worksheet to record your observations, ask your client (if mobile) to take a few marching steps forward and then stop and stand in a normal position as if waiting in line. They will be in this position for a few minutes. Ask them not to try to change or correct their posture as you observe and take notes. Do not ask your client to stand in Tadasana (Mountain Pose) because this will influence how they stand (and here we want them to stand as they most naturally or habitually do). Ideally the client's clothes allow his or her posture to be easily observed from feet to head. Consider reviewing the chapters on the muscular and skeletal systems (Chapters 6 and 7), biomechanics (Chapter 9), and common musculoskeletal conditions (Chapter 23) to better inform your observation.

BEGIN YOUR OBSERVATION AT THE FEET AND MOVE UP, OBSERVING AND NOTING AS FOLLOWS:

Feet: Are the feet straight? One foot out, one foot in? Flat-footed or high-arched?

Achilles: Do they evenly align, or veer toward the midline or laterally?

Calves: Look and feel. Is there more tension in one calf than the other? Is there more tension on the outside or the inside of the calf?

Knees: Is the back of the knee hard or soft, flexed, extended, or hyperextended?

Hips: Place the palms flat on the hips facing downward with thumbs straight across the sacrum. Are the hips level?

Arms: Do they hang evenly at the side, or is one hand more in front than the other? Where are the palms facing? Is there a carrying angle at the elbow?

Shoulders: Are they even or level? Does one shoulder ride higher than the other?

Head: Is it centered between the shoulders? Does the head tilt or rotate to the side?

NEXT, STAND TO THE SIDE OF YOUR CLIENT AND OBSERVE THE FOLLOWING:

- What do you now notice about your client's feet? Are they noticeably different from this view?
- Does the knee line up over the ankle? Is it hyperextended?
- Do the kneecaps point forward? Do the knees collapse to the midline, are they straight, or do they bow to the side?
- Does the hip line up over the knee? Is the pelvis pitched either forward or back?
- Does the pelvis show anterior or posterior rotation?
- Does the shoulder (glenohumeral joint) line up over the hip? Are the shoulders either slumping forward or pulled back?
- Is the upper back hunched (kyphosis)? Is the chest collapsed?
- Does the earhole (external auditory meatus) line up over the shoulder? Is the head forward or behind the shoulders?
- Does the earhole line up over the ankle?

NOW STAND IN FRONT OF YOUR CLIENT AND OBSERVE THE FOLLOWING:

- Is one arm more anterior than the other?
- Where do the hands fall by the side?
- Do the forearms reveal a carrying angle?
- Are the shoulders still at the same level?
- Is the client's head level?

Step 2: Asana Observation

The yoga teacher–training asana laboratory is one of the most effective setups for learning to look at, see, and relate to clients in the asana practice. Preparation for this exercise includes prior reading about the asana under focus; study of its basic functional anatomy, alignment principles, and energetic actions; plus experience practicing the asana under different conditions (time of day, time of year, moods, qualities of well-being, and so on). The basic method is to look separately at each of three or four "model" students—usually coparticipants in a teacher-training program or continuing education workshop—whose varied expressions of the selected asana display the different challenges typically found in a class of students: tightness, weakness, hypermobility, instability, misalignment, and so on. After you have honed this skill as a yoga teacher, proceed as described in the following pages in working your clients. Here we use the example of *Parivrtta Trikonasana* (Revolved Triangle Pose) precisely because of its complexity and thus its many windows of observation. Use other asanas as appropriate for your client (applying the maxim of "do no harm"), and use a sufficient variety of asanas to "see" through the unique prisms of their forms.

- Encourage your client to honor his or her needs for safety and comfort, including the option to modify or come out of the asana whenever they wish.

- Ask your client to come into the asana based on their sense of how to do so. If they are new to yoga or appear to be about to do something potentially injurious, give guidance. Otherwise, refrain from giving any initial verbal cues so you can observe how your student naturally moves. If the asana has left and right sides, observe both sides.

- Take about a minute to observe the client in each asana, walking 360 degrees around him or her to achieve a more complete observation.

- Bring your observation first to whatever is most at risk in the asana. While asking yourself what is happening there, ask the client how he or she feels in that part of their body.

Now look more comprehensively at your client's entire expression of the asana:

Breath and General Vibe: How is he or she breathing? Does your student look comfortable? Anxious? Balanced? Steady?

Feet and Ankles: How are they aligned? Is the front foot turned out ninety degrees? Does it appear that the feet are rooting and awakening with pada bandha? Where does the weight appear to be—inner foot, outer foot, balanced? Are the toes softly rooting or clenching? What is happening with the arches?

Knees: Is the kneecap aligned toward the center of the front foot? Is the knee bent into flexion or hyperextension? Is the kneecap revealing activation of the quadriceps?

Pelvis: Is it level and even, pitched forward in anterior rotation, back in posterior rotation, or close to neutral? Does he or she appear to be drawing the sitting bone of the front leg back and down as if toward the heel of the back foot?

Spine: What is its position in the lumbar area as it extends from the pelvis? Is there an extreme lateral bend or twisting? Does there appear to be any compression in the spine? What curves do you see going up into the thoracic and cervical sections of the spine?

Rib Cage: Are the lower front ribs protruding out or softening in? Are the back ribs rounded? Are the upper side ribs protruding? What do these observations tell you about the spine?

Chest and Collarbones: Is the torso aligned straight out over the front leg, or is it leaning forward? Is the torso revolving open, lateral to the floor, or turned toward the floor? Is the chest expansive? Are the collarbones spreading away from each other?

Shoulders, Arms, Hands, and Fingers: Are the shoulder blades drawing down against the back ribs, or tending to draw up toward the ears? Is the lower shoulder rolled forward or drawn back and down? Are the arms reaching out away from each other perpendicular to the floor? Are they fully extended? Are the elbows straight, bent, or hyperextended? Are the palms fully open and the fingers fully extended?

Where is the client's energy being applied? Is it rooting down strongly from the tops of the client's thighbones through his or her feet? Is it extending long through the spine and out through the top of the head? Is it radiating out from the client's heart center through his or her fingertips?

Throughout this observation process, try to look at each client as the unique and beautiful person he or she is in the moment. Explore how you can share what you are seeing in a way that helps that client to see and more naturally experience his or her own bodymind, breath, and practice with a growing sense of wholeness.

BASIC STRENGTH, FLEXIBILITY, AND BALANCE TESTS

Muscle and range of motion testing are distinct and essential physical therapist skills. With muscle testing, physical therapists use specific manual procedures to assess relative strength and weakness, typically in relation to range of motion.[5]

Electromyography (EMG), which detects the electrical potential generated by muscle cells when activated (electrically or neurologically), provides more refined insight into medical abnormalities, activation levels, and muscle recruitment order in dynamic movement. Physical therapists use goniometry (from the Greek *gonia*, meaning angle, and *metron*, to measure) in measuring angles created at joints by the bones of the body and the total amount of movement available at a joint. Using a goniometer, the physical therapist identifies impairment, establishes a diagnosis, and offers a prognosis along with treatment goals and a plan of care. Superficially simple, the art and science of this musculoskeletal assessment quickly becomes more complex when considering the neurology of muscular activation and the arthrokinematics (various joint surface movements) and osteokinematics (gross movement of shafts of bones) of range of motion (ROM), especially in combination with each other (considering how strength affects ROM).

Here we consider very basic strength and ROM testing as a means of helping clients better understand their condition, thereby providing further insight into conditions that might benefit from yoga and/or referral to a licensed medical professional. Thus, well short of conducing medical diagnostics, the yoga focus is on appreciating a client's condition and offering what insight and support one might have as a yoga therapist.

Strength Testing

Strength is the force with which we make a movement or hold a position. In testing strength, we aim to test specific muscles even while muscles typically act in combination, which as Kendall and Kendall first recognized permits substitution of stronger muscles for weaker ones.[6] The ability to do so is predicated upon knowing muscle attachments, direction of muscle fibers and their line of pull, and the function of related muscles (antagonists and synergists). It also requires specific skill in proper positioning, stabilizing, and moving, and the ability to identify substitution patterns, contractile activity, and joint conditions. With this knowledge and the well-honed skill for conducting accurate tests, manual muscle testing proceeds on a graded basis. Here we will first further introduce manual muscle testing and grading, then suggest strength tests utilizing basic yoga asana transitions for specific assessments.

There are two basic types of muscle test: the break test and the active resistance test.

BREAK TEST (MOST COMMONLY USED)

1. Ask (or in cases of inability, assist) the client in comfortably maximizing any given range of motion. For example, fully extend the elbow in preparation for testing strength in elbow flexion.

2. Ask the client to hold that position.

3. Apply manual resistance to the distal extreme of the body part being tested (in the example of elbow flexion, press on the wrist), and ask the client to try to "break" the hold.

ACTIVE RESISTANCE TEST (OFTEN EQUIVOCAL RESULTS DUE TO TESTING SKILL):

1. As in the break test, ask (or in cases of inability, assist) the client in comfortably maximizing any given range of motion.

2. Apply resistance to the distal extreme of the body part being tested (if testing elbow flexion, press against the wrist).

3. Ask the client to move the body part (in this case, flex the elbow); gradually increase resistance until the client is unable to create further movement.

In conducting either type of test, we look to Harry Eaton Stewart for the basic principles of muscle testing.[7]

PRINCIPLES OF MUSCLE TESTING

- Determine just what muscles are involved by careful testing, and chart the degree of power in each muscle or group to be tested.

- Insist on such privacy and discipline as will gain the patient's cooperation and undivided attention.

- Use some method of preliminary warming up the muscles.

- Have the entire body part free from covering and supported to not cause strain [from gravity or antagonists].

Clearly, given the variable roles of the examiner and student, strength assessment is an inexact method shaped by objective and subjective factors in both roles.[8] Add in variations in client conditions, including affected age (consider the difference between a healthy child, an adult athlete, and an elderly person), and you come to further challenges in conducting practical tests. Your own sensitivity to differences in muscle contour and bulk, consistent use of proper positioning and stabilizing techniques, and ability to conduct tests under varying conditions (particularly client conditions but also the setting) can influence test results. The client's true effort, attitude, and understanding of how to participate in the testing—all affected by personal factors and the quality of therapist-client communication—are further sources of potential bias in test results. This points to the value of experience and the gradual development of discerning judgment to bring a greater modicum of insightful interpretation to these tests.

Results from manual muscle tests are graded on a scale with numerical scores ranging from zero to five and related qualitative statements, as shown in Table 19.2. Unlike EMG muscle-specific testing, manual testing involves groups of muscles involved in certain movements. Thus, the grading is for muscle groups involved in the observed motion, not individual muscles, and is based on the student's available ROM, not normal ROM.

TABLE 19.2: Grading Strength

GRADE	CONDITION	DESCRIPTION
5	Normal (100%)	Client can complete full ROM against gravity and maximum resistance.
4	Good (75%)	Client can complete full ROM against gravity and moderate resistance.
3	Fair (50%)	Client can complete full ROM against gravity but not against resistance.
2	Poor (25%)	Client cannot complete full ROM against gravity.
1	Trace Activity	Client cannot complete full ROM with gravity eliminated, but muscle palpation detects slight contraction.
0	No Activity	No contraction is detected.

Here is a set of widely accepted guidelines from Lamb to help make muscle testing and grading more meaningful (all of which can be further refined with plus [+] and minus [–] labels):[9]

Grade 5: You are unable to break the client's held position *and* the client is able to complete full ROM.

Grade 4: The muscle(s) can withstand considerable but less than "normal" resistance, the client is able to move through full ROM, and the client can tolerate strong resistance without breaking the test position.

Grade 3: The client can complete full ROM against gravity but not with other resistance.

Grade 2: The client cannot complete full ROM within the horizontal plane of motion.

Grade 1: You can see or feel muscular activity (for example, a tendon pops up), but the contraction does not create movement.

Grade 0: There is no indication of muscle activity.

Whereas muscle testing assesses the physical force with which we can make a movement or hold a position, flexibility testing assesses our ROM at a joint. Although they require distinct tests, strength and flexibility are interrelated: the strength required to move a body part varies in relation to flexibility in the parts of the body asked to move. For example, to the extent that the hamstrings are tight, more strength is required of the quadriceps in active extension of the knee (to overcome the resistance of the antagonist hamstrings). Thus, passive range of motion, in which the therapist assists the movement and thereby the client's muscles are more relaxed (less antagonistic), allows greater ROM. If pain occurs in either active or passive testing, it is a sign of stretching or tension in either contractile (muscles and tendons) or noncontractile (ligaments, joint capsules, bursa sacs, fascia, or skin) tissues. It is preferable to test passive range of motion to better identify limitations in the noncontractile tissues, which are typically evident well within normal range of motion, whereas limitations of contractile tissues are more evident at the end of passive ROM.

Except for rotations in the transverse plan (twisting the spine, and either internally or externally rotating the appendages), the starting position for ROM measurements is Tadasana (Mountain Pose) or a neutral (not anatomical) position. The measurements are made in reference to normal ROM. Although there are various notation systems, the most common (and suggested here) is the 0- to 180-degree system called the *neutral zero method.*[10] Hypomobility and hypermobility refer to decrease or increase in normal ROM, respectively. Hypomobility can result from the shortening or tightening of contractile or noncontractile tissues, inflammation, bone fractures, arthritis, and neurological issues. Hypermobility is typically caused by lax muscles, ligaments, or joint capsules and also by trauma and various hereditary disorders such as Ehlers-Danlos syndrome or Marfan syndrome. Age and gender also influence ROM, with older adults typically having less ROM than younger adults, and women typically having slightly greater ROM than men.[11]

In measuring passive ROM, we are testing potential muscle length in the antagonist muscle while also gathering insight into tension in related tissues. This measurement is made using a *goniometer*. It is not within the scope of this book to provide training in the use of a goniometer, competency with which requires specialized knowledge (joint structure and function, normal end-feels, testing positions, required stabilizations, bony landmarks, and instrument alignment) and specialized skills (how to correctly position and stabilize, how to move a body part, how to determine the end of ROM, how to align the goniometer with bony landmarks, and how to read and record the measurements). For readers with this knowledge and these skills, standard forms for recording measurements are easily found online (one can also use pictorial charts to record ROM measurements). In making these measurements, we consider the degrees of deviation from standard ROM.

Balance Testing

Balance becomes an increasing challenge with age. With a rapidly growing elderly age demographic, balance is of growing importance in yoga therapy.[12] Our ability to maintain balance might seem simple but it always involves a complex sensory, cognitive, musculoskeletal process.[13] Thus, one of the first tasks in assessing balance is to attempt to determine the extent to which imbalance arises from ability to correctly sense the environment (sensory), integrate this information in the central nervous system in a way that allows an appropriate motor command (cognitive), and then carry out the motor command (musculoskeletal). Medical issues such as diabetes, Parkinson's disease, and stroke; a history of head injuries, ear infections, or serious musculoskeletal injuries; and the effects of medications and presence of mind all affect balance.[14] This range of causes makes localized medical diagnosis difficult, especially as many balance disorders have multiple sources. Medical professionals utilize vestibulo-ocular reflex (VOR) tests such as electronystagmography (ENG) to test vestibular function (and provide insight into site of lesion) and computerized dynamic posturography (CDP) to test gaze and postural stability, providing insight into appropriate medical treatments.

We can assess balance in simpler ways utilizing static and dynamic balance tests that employ yoga postures and movements. Where these tests indicate great difficulty with balance, the client should be referred to a medical professional for further assessment. There are many types of both static and dynamic balance tests. Here we describe the most common:

STATIC BALANCE TEST

1. Tadasana (Mountain Pose) on a firm surface with *dristi* (gazing at a specific point)

2. Vrksasana (Tree Pose) on a firm surface with dristi

3. Tadasana (Mountain Pose) on a firm surface without dristi

4. Vrksasana (Tree Pose) on a firm surface without dristi

5. Tadasana (Mountain Pose) on a soft surface with dristi

6. Vrksasana (Tree Pose) on a soft surface with dristi

7. Tadasana (Mountain Pose) on a soft surface without dristi

8. Vrksasana (Tree Pose) on a soft surface without dristi

DYNAMIC BALANCE TEST

The first four items of this test are considered by Marchetti as equivalent to the full eight-item test given here.[15] On the eight-item test, see Shumway-Cook and Woollacott.[16]

1. **Gait on a level surface:** Client is asked to walk at a normal pace for twenty feet.

    a. Normal (3) = Walks twenty feet free of assistance with normal gait and balance.

    b. Mild Impairment (2) = Walks twenty feet using assistance with mild gait deviations.

    c. Moderate Impairment (1) = Walks twenty feet with abnormal gait and evidence of imbalance.

    d. Severe Impairment (0) = Unable to walk twenty feet free of assistance, gait deviation, or imbalance.

2. **Change in gait speed:** Client is asked to begin walking at a normal pace and then, on cue, to walk as fast as possible.

    a. Normal (3) = Able to change gait speed without loss of balance or gait deviation.

    b. Mild Impairment (2) = Able to change gait speed only with gait deviation or use of assistance.

    c. Moderate Impairment (1) = Able to make only minor changes in gait speed or make them only with significant gait deviation.

    d. Severe Impairment (0) = Cannot change speed or loses balance when attempting to do so.

3. **Gait with horizontal head turns:** Client is asked to walk at a normal pace and then, on cue, to alternately turn their head to the right, then to the left, then straight while still walking forward.

    a. Normal (3) = Able to turn head with no change in gait.

    b. Mild Impairment (2) = Able to turn head with only a slight change in gait.

    c. Moderate Impairment (1) = Head turn causes moderate change in gait but client staggers and recovers.

    d. Severe Impairment (0) = Head turn causes severe disruption of gait.

4. **Gait with vertical head turns:** Client is asked to walk at a normal pace and then, on cue, to alternately turn their head up, then down, then level while still walking forward.

    a. Normal (3) = Able to turn head with no change in gait.

    b. Mild Impairment (2) = Able to turn head with only a slight change in gait.

    c. Moderate Impairment (1) = Head turn causes moderate change in gait but client staggers and recovers.

    d. Severe Impairment (0) = Head turn causes severe disruption of gait.

5. **Gait and pivot turn:** Client is asked to walk at a normal pace and then, on cue, to quickly turn 180 degrees and then stop.

    a. Normal (3) = Easily turns within three seconds and stops quickly with no loss of balance.

    b. Mild Impairment (2) = Takes more than three seconds to turn and stop with no loss of balance.

    c. Moderate Impairment (1) = Turns slowly and requires several steps to turn and stop.

    d. Severe Impairment (0) = Cannot safely or independently turn and stop with balance.

6. **Step over obstacle:** Client is asked to walk at a normal pace and then to step over a standard-size yoga block.

    a. Normal (3) = Able to step over block without changing pace or losing balance.

    b. Mild Impairment (2) = Must slow down and adjust steps to clear block.

    c. Moderate Impairment (1) = Must stop before stepping over block.

    d. Severe Impairment (0) = Cannot step over block free of assistance.

7. **Step around obstacle:** Client is asked to walk at a normal pace and then to step around a standard-size yoga block.

    a. Normal (3) = Able to step around block without changing pace or losing balance.

    b. Mild Impairment (2) = Must slow down and adjust steps to clear block.

   c. Moderate Impairment (1) = Must stop before stepping around block.

   d. Severe Impairment (0) = Cannot step around block free of assistance.

8. **Stairs:** Client is asked to walk up stairs, turn around, and walk down stairs.

   a. Normal (3) = Able to alternate feet with hands free of railing.

   b. Mild Impairment (2) = Able to alternate feet only with use of railing.

   c. Moderate Impairment (1) = Unable to alternate feet and uses railing.

   d. Severe Impairment (0) = Cannot do task safely.

ASSESSING DOSHIC BALANCE

Although a full and accurate doshic assessment might be best conducted by an ayurvedic doctor, there are innumerable tests for self-assessing one's doshic constitution. To use this chart, chart the characteristics most consistent throughout your life or the life of your client (circle more than one answer if more than one applies). Add the number of selections under the vata, pitta, and kapha columns.

	VATA	PITTA	KAPHA
PHYSIQUE	Lean, tall or short, thin boned	Moderately developed	Large, broad, big boned
BODY WEIGHT	Low weight, prominent bones	Moderate weight	Overweight
CHIN	Thin, angular	Pointed, tapering	Rounded, double
CHEEKS	Wrinkled, sunken	Smooth, flat	Rounded, plump
EYES	Small, sunken, dry, dark, active, nervous	Sharp, bright, blue, green, yellow/red, sensitive	Big, beautiful, blue, calm
NOSE	Uneven shape, deviated septum	Long, pointed, red tip	Short, rounded
LIPS	Dry, cracked, thin	Red, inflamed	Smooth, pale, full
TEETH	Protruding, big, roomy, thin gums	Medium, soft, tender gums	Healthy, white, strong gums
SKIN	Thin, dry, cold, rough, itches	Oily, warm, flushed, moles, freckles	Thick, balmy, cool, pale, smooth, soft

	VATA	PITTA	KAPHA
HAIR	Dry, thin, curly, brittle	Straight, oily, blonde, red, light brown, balding, early gray	Thick, oily, wavy, luxuriant
NAILS	Dry, rough, brittle, break easily	Sharp, flexible, pink, lustrous	Thick, smooth polished
NECK	Thin, tall	Medium	Big, wide, folded
CHEST	Flat, sunken	Moderate	Expanded, round
FACE	Oval	Triangular	Round
BELLY	Thin, flat, sunken	Moderate	Big, pot-bellied
HIPS	Slender, thin	Moderate	Heavy, big
JOINTS	Cold, small, cracking	Moderate, loose	Large, lubricated
APPETITE	Varies, anxious when really hungry	Intense, angry when really hungry	Not very hungry, steady
DIGESTION	Irregular, gassy, bloated	Quick, burning	Prolonged, forms mucous
THIRST	Often feel dehydrated	Moderate	Rarely thirsty
BOWEL MOVEMENT	Constipation, can skip a day	Regular, loose or diarrhea	Routine, thick, sluggish
PHYSICAL ACTIONS	Very active, always on the go, walk and talk fast	Think before doing, thoughtful and precise	Steady and graceful
MENTAL ACTIVITY	Hyperactive, restless	Moderate, impatient	Dull, slow, calm
STAMINA	Tire easily, work in spurts	Medium	Good stamina
SWEAT	Rarely	Profusely	Sweat if I work hard
EMOTIONS	Anxiety, fear, worry	Anger, hate, irritable, jealousy	Calm, caring, greedy, attachment
DECISION-MAKING	Change mind often	Make decisions and stick to them	Prefer to follow others

	VATA	PITTA	KAPHA
INTELLECT	Quick but faulty response	Accurate response	Slow, exact
VOICE	Weak, horse	Strong, loud	Deep, good tone
MEMORY	Remember quickly, forget quickly	Distinct, selective	Slow yet sustained, detailed
DREAMS	Quick, active, many, fearful	Aggressive, competitive, sexual	Water, romantic
SLEEP	Toss and turn, sleeplessness	Light sleeper	Heavy, deep, prolonged
HEALTH PROBLEMS	Pain, constipation, anxiety, depression	Infections, fever, heartburn, inflammation	Allergies, congestion, weight gain, digestive problems
SPEECH	Rapid, clear	Sharp, penetrating	Slow, monotonous
WEATHER PREFERENCE	Love warm and humid, dislike cool and dry	Love cool and dry, dislike warm and humid	Love warm and dry, dislike cold and damp
TOTAL			

Breathing and Pranayama Assessment

We discussed prana and its manifestations in our discussion of yoga and ayurveda in Part I, and we surveyed the respiratory system in Chapter 12, noting both the importance of the breath in healthy living and the tendency for breathing to be compromised by one's condition. Anxiety and depression, injury and illness, calm presence of mind or agitated thinking are reflected in our breathing patterns. Thus, assessing a client's breathing can provide deeper insight into the qualities of their life that affect curing and healing. Such assessment also provides clues for prescribing specific pranayama practices to help a student to refine his or her breathing, including the physical and emotional conditions and effects of breathing.

In clinical respiratory assessment, respiratory therapists generally work closely with physicians to conduct tests that allow physicians to determine medical diagnoses. This involves cognitive skills in communicating with both a physician and a patient or client and the knowledge to identify the patient's problems, clarify those

problems, decide upon appropriate assessment tests, conducts those tests, interpret
results, formulate a treatment plan, and evaluate the effectiveness of treatment. This
process begins with gathering the patient's health history, including his or her cardiopulmonary health history, to identify factors that might affect his or her breathing
and general health. Lifestyle (especially smoking), occupation, and environment are
particularly important in understanding respiratory conditions. Depending on what
one learns based on patient history and complaints, certain specific assessments are
indicated. The specific assessments arise from determining more specific details about
cardiopulmonary symptoms, including coughing, sputum production, shortness of
breath, chest pain, dizziness and fainting, mental status, snoring, and gastrointestinal
reflex. More intensive assessments involve physical examination, neurologic assessment, clinical laboratory studies, interpretation of blood gases, pulmonary function
testing, chest x-rays, and electrocardiograms. More specialized assessments are given
to neonatal and pediatric patients as well as older adults.

These assessments identify several measures of respiratory health: total lung
capacity, tidal volume, residual volume, expiratory reserve value, inspiratory reserve
value, inspiratory capacity, vital capacity, forced expiratory volume, peak expiratory
flow, maximal voluntary ventilation, and more. These specific measures are well
outside the yoga therapy scope of practice but nonetheless important to understand
in lay terms as the insights generated through comprehensive respiratory assessment
can be fruitfully applied in all aspects of yoga, particularly in guiding pranayama
practices.

There are several ways we can meaningfully assess a client's breathing without
crossing into areas that require the knowledge, skill, and license of a respiratory therapist or physician. Basic yoga breathing assessments utilize many of the same techniques one might recommend to a client as part of a balanced (and energetically
balancing) pranayama practice. The difference is that rather than guiding the fullness
of pranayama, here one is using the pranayama technique to gather more insight into
a client's condition, a process that has the added benefit of an opportunity to further
converse with and educate a client about healthy breathing.

Although pulmonary function testing typically uses a spirometer to evaluate the
respiratory system and identify the presence or extent of impairment, yoga breathing
assessments can use a timer and client self-reporting to assess respiratory rate and
provide clues to tidal volume and other respiratory measures. The findings of these
assessments are superficial from the standpoint of full respiratory assessment (for
example, they will not distinguish obstructive from restrictive pulmonary disorders,
and they do not identify reserve, capacity, or volume). However, they provide helpful
insight into a student's basic breathing experience and may point to the importance of

referring one's client to a medical professional for full respiratory diagnostics. There are five basic breathing assessments:

1. **Inhalation/Exhalation (the foundation of *puraka/rechaka*):** Ask your client to inhale and exhale as slowly as possible without causing gasping or discomfort. Do each test three times and record the number of seconds of each phase of breath (inhalation and exhalation).

    Test 1: Sitting comfortably upright.

    Test 2: Lying supine.

    Test 3: After three Sun Salutations or after walking with moderate effort for 5 minutes.

    Test 4: After walking up a set of 10 stairs.

    Test 5: Maintain the continuous flow of the breath for two minutes while breathing as slowly as possible. Count the number of complete non-stop inhalations and exhalations.

2. **Retention of Inhalation (the foundation of *antara kumbhaka*):** Ask your client to draw in a full inhalation and hold the breath in for as long as comfortably possible. Do each test three times and record the number of seconds of retention and flow.

    Test 1: Retention only.

    Test 2: Following the longest retention of the inhalation, cue the client to exhale as slowly as possible and time the length of that exhalation on each of three tries.

3. **Retention of Exhalation (the foundation of *bahya kumbhaka*):** Ask your client to completely exhale and hold the breath out for as long as comfortably possible. Do each test three times and record the number of seconds of retention and flow.

    Test 1: Retention only.

    Test 2: Following the longest retention of the exhalation, cue the client to inhale as slowly as possible and time the length of that inhalation on each of three tries.

4. **Breath Interruption (similar to *viloma pranayama*):** Ask your client to breathe comfortably deep, then cue them to hold the breath when halfway in and again when halfway out for as long as comfortable. Note the tendency for the breath to rush out of the pause. Cue the client to hold only as long as the subsequent movement of breath is slow and steady. Explore adding up to three total

pauses, with the effort to hold the breath in each pause for 1–5 counts. Record the number of pauses and counts in each test.

Test 1: One pause for 1–5 counts.

Test 2: Two pauses for 1–5 counts.

Test 3: Three pauses for 1–5 counts.

5. **Restricted Flow (similar to *nadi shodhana pranayama*):** Ask your client to press one nostril completely closed and repeat the tests given above.

Test 1: Right nostril closed.

Test 2: Left nostril closed.

Follow each assessment with a subjective, qualitative interview to elicit your client's experience, focusing specifically on how they felt during and following each test. Note these reactions. The full test results and concluding interview will provide useful baseline references for evaluating the benefit of ongoing yoga practices and other treatments or lifestyle changes your client takes on. Follow-up tests using the same testing procedures and protocol will give each client a measure of change in their breathing.

Meditation Assessment

There is considerable evidence of the benefits of meditation, some presented in Chapter 22. There always has been and probably always will be considerable speculation about what is happening inside when we meditate. Now there is growing scientific insight into what happens in the brain during meditation. Thus, we can imagine a future with assessments that determine that the brain is in a meditative state and to perhaps even measure the qualities of that state. Any such assessment would require clear definitions of concepts, starting with what one means by *meditation* or *meditative state*. For some, meditation refers to concentration on a thought, feeling, or deity, fully absorbing one's awareness in that experience, even "becoming one" with the object of one's meditative muse. In this view, concentrated prayer is a form of meditation. For others, it is a way of relaxing into a quieter mental state, cultivating some form of spiritual energy, or opening one's awareness and behavior to a different way of thinking, feeling, and behaving. Clearly, the idea of assessing meditation is at least as awkward as trying to define it.

Assessment of the meditation experience—we again emphasize the quality of appreciation ideally contained within all yoga assessments—is best done through the client's personal reflections and complemented by interviews that attempt to identify and clarify what occurs in any given meditation session.[17] To measure or otherwise appreciate changes, begin with a preassessment of the client's thoughts and feelings regarding these considerations:

MEDITATION PREASSESSMENT

1. What is the client's perception of his or her anxiety level?

   Rate this on a scale of 1–5 (1 = low anxiety, 5 = high anxiety)

2. What is the client's perception of his or her depression level?

   Rate this on a scale of 1–5 (1 = mild depression, 5 = deep depression)

3. If the client has prior meditation experience, does he or she recall it as beneficial?

   Rate this on a scale of 1–5 (1 = not beneficial, 5 = highly beneficial)

4. Is the client motivated to try meditating?

   Rate this on a scale of 1–5 (1 = not very open, 5 = very open)

5. Does the client have spiritual or other beliefs that might affect his or her openness to trying meditation?

   If yes, describe.

6. Is the client taking mood-altering drugs?

   If yes, describe.

7. Does the client feel good about himself or herself?

   Rate this on a scale of 1–5 (1 = low self-esteem, 5 = high self-esteem)

8. Is the client experiencing physical pain?

   Rate this on a scale of 1–5 (1 = none, 5 = almost intolerable)

9. Does the client feel socially connected?

   Rate this on a scale of 1–5 (1 = socially isolated, 5 = socially connected)

10. Can the client comfortably sit or lie for 15 minutes or longer?

   Rate this on a scale of 1–5 (1 = low anxiety, 5 = high anxiety)

Based on this preassessment and other background information contained in your client notes, now discuss with your client specific goals and intentions in meditating. (In Chapter 22 we discuss how best to guide—or not guide—different meditation techniques.) Put differently, you are trying to elicit your client's desired outcomes so that both you and your client are clearer in what meditation options might best support the client. For example, if the client wishes to reduce anxiety and other stress responses, you are likely to recommend (prescribe) a guided relaxation practice designed to reduce unhealthy stress responses. These consciously chosen practices are then the focus of evaluations following each meditation session.

PERSONAL REFLECTIONS ON MEDITATION EXPERIENCE

Ask your client each of these questions, discuss them in turn, and make summary notes for future reference and comparison.

1. Describe what you generally experienced while meditating.

2. Was there any physical discomfort? If yes:

    a. Where?

    b. How intense?

    c. For how long?

    d. What was your physical reaction to the discomfort?

    e. What was your mental reaction to the discomfort?

3. Describe what would make you more comfortable while meditating.

4. How often did your mind drift into thinking about things that are happening in your life?

    Rate this on a scale of 1–5 (1 = constantly, 5 = never)

5. When you noticed your mind drifting, did you refocus on breathing?

    Rate this on a scale of 1–5 (1 = never, 5 = always)

6. Did you enjoy the meditation experience?

    Rate this on a scale of 1–5 (1 = never, 5 = always)

7. How did you experience my meditation guidance?

    Rate this on a scale of 1–5 (1 = distracting, 5 = focusing)

    Rate this on a scale of 1–5 (1 = not helpful, 5 = helpful)

Step Three: Developing a Shared Working Assessment

Upon completing the initial client intake and assessments, the next step is to integrate them into a more comprehensive and holistic working assessment of the client's conditions, limitations, and possibilities. In essence, the objective here is to more clearly identify the root of the client's difficulties, which will later help inform goals in exploring yoga therapy. By *working assessment* we mean to emphasize that it is both the initial and ongoing primary basis upon which you and your client will collaborate in discussing, deciding upon, and evaluating a yoga therapy practice plan. In addition to whatever assessments you have conducted, you will ideally have as many of the client's assessments from other caregivers as possible. Bringing this all together, write a narrative summary that succinctly describes the client and his or her significant presenting conditions and stated intentions.

Here is an example:

Jane Smith is a 43-year-old Asian female who is married with two teenage children. She is a family law attorney. She reports chronic low back pain, which began three years ago. She is 5 foot 5 inches tall and weighs 155 pounds. The pain is interfering with her work, sleep, and exercise. She has consulted with her primary care physician and was referred to physical therapy based on a diagnosis showing L3–L4 and L4–L5 disc degeneration. She describes a happy and healthy home environment but a highly demanding and stressful job in which she sits for long hours every day working on complex family law matters that are typically highly emotionally charged. She has a well-balanced diet. She practiced yoga in college and recalls its calming effects. She is hopeful of curing her low back problems and having less stress in her life. Her family is very supportive. She has loosely defined spiritual values that she describes as Buddhist but without any regular related practices. She is open to exploring asana, pranayama, and meditation practices but is concerned about becoming more stressed with the required time commitment.

Next, work with your client to review all assessments and to identify areas of greatest significance to them. Here again is an opportunity to educate your client about health conditions borne out in the assessments that yoga therapy might help. For example, in discussing your client's perception of his or her primary presenting conditions, you can assist in identifying relationships between lifestyle choices, related conditions, and yoga practices. In the preceding example, you might discover and highlight how the client's approach to her work (sitting for long hours doing emotionally and mentally demanding work) might be a significant factor in her physical posture and related intervertebral disc problems, and how a daily meditation practice might lend to more mindfulness in how she sits and breathes while she is working.

Proceed in this way with each significant issue identified in the assessments that might be relevant both to the client's presenting condition and the overall quality of his or her larger life.

In reviewing the client's detailed assessments (yours and others), give particularly careful consideration to the recommendations and prescriptions given by professional health care providers. For example, if your client's physical therapist has identified contraindicated activities and prescribed certain specific exercises, incorporate them into your working assessment. If you do not understand those recommendations or prescriptions, ask your client's permission to discuss them with their source. If you are in a collaborative health service setting with colleagues whose training and expertise gives greater insight into specific conditions, solicit their thoughts on the assessments to better identify tendencies or patterns that you and your client might not otherwise see.

Complete the initial working assessment with a clear list of conditions, intentions, and contraindications. Revisit this on a regular basis with your client to assess and appreciate changes, obstacles, and new opportunities for addressing the presenting conditions and cultivating better general health. With this comprehensive working assessment now fully developed, you can move forward in developing a yoga therapy practice treatment plan.

Creating a Therapeutic Yoga Practice Treatment Plan

Whatever one's condition, the general purpose of yoga is to support people in healthier and more conscious living. In better understanding one's actual conditions as revealed through the assessment process, self-reflection, and intuition, the next step is to develop clearer intention—even if provisional—about what one wants with respect to curing and healing, and in some cases, preparing for dying. The yoga practice treatment plan then matches client conditions and both immediate and larger life intentions to specific practices that address them.

How might we clarify intentions? This question is at the heart of the *Bhagavad-Gita* (where it is framed as *dharma*, one's purposeful path in life) and indeed of most spiritual and philosophical allegories and epics. It begins with an even more basic question: Who am I? We usually first come to this question with superficial notions tied to a limited sense of possibilities in life. But as Cope discusses in *This Great Work of Your Life*, there are deeper layers of our being that can be plumbed through self-reflection and self-examination to more richly reveal essential qualities we might otherwise keep hidden from ourselves.[18] When dealing with challenges to our health, these qualities can recede further from awareness as uncertainty and fear come to the fore. But therein are important clues to dharma and intention, for, as Merton put it, "what you fear is an indication of what you seek."[19] Cope takes this further, quoting from the Gospel of Thomas: "If you bring forth what is within you, it will save you; if you do not bring forth what is within you, it will destroy you."[20]

Earlier we looked at self-reflective assessments that can reveal these deeper aspects of who we are. In getting closer to intention, we ideally bring these insights forward into another set of reflections, now more decidedly focused on the present and moving forward in one's life. Pausing to ask just how fully one is living within the realities of his or her life and bringing forth all one might by digging into one's unique treasure as a human being points even more toward one's calling, one's dharma, and one's actions on his or her life path. This points to the value of engaging with your client to specifically elicit this *sankalpa*, this definite intention and will that is formed in the mind and heart. Guided heart-centered meditation, self-reflective journaling, and focused conversation are ways of helping a client discover and articulate his or her *sankalpa*.

In this way and just as with assessments, practice planning becomes a form of treatment as it provides an opportunity to reflect, learn, and explore how life can be made clearer and better. Developed collaboratively, yet no less client-driven, here again you can use the 7Es of communication to convey empathy, warmth, and respect, and to deepen the trusting relationship with your client in the spirit of evoking his or her clearest intention. With this clarity, however provisional it might be, what to do and how to do it become clearer as well.

The practice plan identifies priorities, sets short- and long-term goals, and gives specific strategies to match practices to the client's conditions and intentions. In working with a client to identify treatment priorities, we want our client to express his or her wishes, appreciating that the time, space, and other resources one has might be relatively limited. In identifying priorities, we recognize these limitations while making informed choices that give greater attention to certain conditions. This is the basis of setting short- and long-term goals, with the understanding that perhaps several short-term goals—think of them as the means—will become the long-term goal.

In getting closer to specific goals, it is helpful to work both forward from where one is now and backward from where one imagines being in terms of conditions. We look forward from the immediate moment, informed as it is by all we have done to bring light to our conditions. In moving forward we begin with a single step oriented toward an initial goal. We take further steps forward from there toward our intention. In some cases our intention might be something we can immediately realize, such as showing up for an appointment or going for a daily walk. But before slipping into immediate action, it is helpful to look from the other direction.

Our greater intentions might be grander or not so immediately realizable as to be part of short-term goals, which points to longer-term goals. Whatever one's ultimate goal might be, its realization occurs through the actions one takes starting in the present. Nonetheless, without a sense of where we might ultimately want to go, we are likely to get lost along the way. Thus, the map of one's practice plan should identify the longest-term goals and then pose questions that lead to what we call a *gap analysis*. Here is your condition and there is your farthest yet grandest intention; how do you connect the dots? By first identifying whatever chasm might exist between one's immediate condition and longest-term goals, one can subsequently identify the series of steps to get from here to there.

This is all about *parinamavada*—the constancy of change—and *vinyasa krama*—to place in a special way in support of gradual progression toward a goal. Although these two concepts are more commonly applied to planning and sequencing yoga classes, they can be more expansively applied to life, health, and healing.[21] Our most immediate short-term goal should be informed by our ultimate ideal, just as that goal is informed by our immediate condition. This ensures that we take conscious steps that lead us forward in keeping with our intention and in the direction of whatever our intention most celebrates.

We want to be careful to devise practice plans based on student conditions and intentions and not to assume that every client will benefit from the same approach. We state this primarily because there is a tendency among caregivers in offering treatments to first or only consider what they personally offer. Go to a neurologist, acupuncturist, or ayurvedic doctor for a migraine headache and each will most likely recommend treatments that they offer. Thus, the ayurvedic doctor typically begins with doshic constitution and aims to pacify aggravated doshas and purify and strengthen the entirety of one's being through *panchakarma* therapies.[22] Although these treatments might be beneficial to a particular client, there are other treatments that might be more beneficial, including those that keep with the client's values, sensibilities, and financial health.

With these general principles and strategic sensibilities in mind, we turn to the practice plan itself. You might use a different form or no form at all. Regardless, we recommend having a written expression of whatever course of treatment you and your client agree upon. Consider including the details in Table 19.3.

Table 19.3: Practice Planning Background

ITEM	CLIENT INFORMATION
Date	
Name, gender, date of birth, contact info, emergency contact info	
Medical provider information	

ITEM	CLIENT INFORMATION
Doctor's name and contact info	
Current health history	
Subjective presenting complaints	
Describe severity of symptoms (minimal to severe) and frequency (occasional, intermittent, frequent, constant)	
Mechanism of onset for primary complaint	
Date of onset	
Onset	
• Acute trauma	
• Worsening of prior condition	
• Repetitive motion	
• Gradual onset	
• Chronic	
• Other	
• Describe the details of the onset as specifically as possible:	
Date(s) of significant changes (better or worse)	
Vital Signs	
Height, weight, blood pressure, temperature	
Summary of Assessments	
Physical	
Breath/energy	
Mental/emotional	
Other assessments (x-ray, blood pressure, range of motion, respiratory)	
Possible contraindications for particular yoga therapy treatments (explain checked items)	

ITEM	CLIENT INFORMATION
• Arthritis	
• Circulatory or cardiovascular disorders	
• Infection	
• Neurological disorders	
• Osteoporosis	
• Pregnancy	
• Scoliosis	
Concurrent care	
Provider	
Type of care	
Dates	
Consensus on concerns, diagnoses, and goals	
Practice plan	
Dates (beginning and provisional ending dates of treatments)	
Recommended treatments	
• Asana	
• Seated	
• Lying	
• Standing	
• Pranayama	
• Ujjayi	
• Viloma	
• Kumbhakas	
• Nadi shodhana	
• Kapalabhati	
• Other	
• Specific pranayama	

ITEM	CLIENT INFORMATION
• Meditation	
• Food	
Number and frequency of recommended practice sessions	
Number and frequency of recommended visits	
Client home care	
Complicating factors	

The quality of your relationship with a client and the related quality of your assessments and discussions with your client regarding their conditions and intentions will largely determine the quality of the practice plan. In building upon your existing relationship, you must now discuss what to do to address your client's health concerns and find agreement on a certain course of treatments over a defined period of time—all of which will change to some degree as the practices and your healing relationship with your client develop further. Now you will fully tap into your knowledge of all aspects of yoga, complementary healing practices, and your understanding of your client's disorders and pathologies.

- On the general application of yoga and complementary healing practices, see the chapters in Part IV.

- On the specific application of yoga and complementary healing practices to specific conditions, see the chapters in Part V.

- On human physiological systems and their discontents, review the chapters in Part II.

The practice plan should identify specific incremental steps leading to a set of short-term goals that in turn lead toward more of the client's long-term goals. Each step should specify practices, including their order, duration, and repetition. They should reinforce the short-term goals in tangible ways (and, if possible, measurably). The exact way that you and your client craft the practice plan will ideally embody realistic goals, informative exchanges, and creative exploration.

When John Steinbeck adapted a stanza of Robert Burns's 1785 poem "To a Mouse, on Turning Her Up in Her Nest with the Plough" to entitle his book *Of Mice and Men*, he left off the passage's preface—"the best-laid schemes"—as well as the kicker, which in English is "often go awry."[23] We start as best we can, we plan as best we can, and we serve as best we can. In serving we listen, and in listening we come to better appreciate that which we thought might not be so, or not just so. People, conditions, and intentions change. Experience in action generates new insights. The plan, what we may have once considered so perfect, always remains open as a living document to visit and revisit even as it is being implemented.

Implementing a Therapeutic Yoga Practice Treatment Plan

The treatment plan is a reflection of your relationship with a client. It is the template indicating what actions your client might take to improve his or her health. It provides a common reference for discussing progress toward your student's health goals. Yet it is only as valuable as the consistency with which it is implemented: the client's commitment to exploring actions given in the practice plan, your fulfillment of your role in guiding those actions and providing ongoing connection with your student, and your evaluation of ongoing outcomes. As C. Everett Koop famously quipped when he was U.S. Surgeon General, "drugs don't work in patients who don't take them."[24] Without strong adherence to the practice plan, the plan has little value.

This leads us to the first and most important point in implementation, which is to stay as attuned as one can to a client's progress through ongoing communication and scheduled follow-up conversations and evaluations of efficacy and progress. From the beginning, regularly check in with your client to assess how they are feeling about the practices. The following questions can help frame this dialogue:

- How do you feel today?

- What is new or different in what you are experiencing?

- How do you feel while doing the _____ practice?

- What, if anything, seems difficult or confusing?

- What part of the _____ practice feels best to you? Why do you think that is?

- What new experiences are you having that perhaps pertain to your conditions and intentions?

- What, if anything, in these practices would you like to change?

Most yoga practice treatment plans include personally and directly guided one-on-one practices as well as home-based practices in which the student practices independently. It is particularly important to discuss home practices as most yoga students are less focused and self-disciplined in home practices versus group classes in the presence of peers and one's yoga teacher. Conveying ongoing moral support to your client will reinforce their commitment to consistently doing what is recommended in their plan.

In providing consistent attention and follow-up with your client, take progress notes to highlight any observations you and your client make about the challenges and benefits of each part of the practices. Use these notes as an addendum to the plan, regularly revisiting and refining goals and how best to get at them. Set specific dates for more comprehensive reviews of experience and progress, modifying the plan in accordance with giving the greatest benefits to your client.

More specific aspects of implementation take shape around the specific practices given in the plan. In the following chapters we will look closely at essential yoga practices and other healing practices, specific elements of which can be adapted to the uniquely indicated conditions and intentions of a client. As such elements are incorporated into the plan, each should have corresponding evaluation components that provide formative assessments of their relative support of the client's health.

Part IV

Yoga Therapy Practices

A SEEMINGLY ENDLESS ARRAY OF yoga practices are offered in the contemporary world. Most tap into one or more of the many streams of yoga flowing from the past, even if only in name or claim, whereas others are more an expression of largely modern innovation. Some claim to fully embrace and teach an unadulterated ancient tradition thought to have been passed down through an uninterrupted lineage. Some eschew references to ancient sources, emphasizing only those modern influences that seem consistent with the modern values or cultural sensibilities to which one subscribes. Although confusing to many observers and practitioners, the beauty of this diversity for yoga therapy rests in the vast range of options for appropriately individualizing healing practices.

The other side of this beauty is confusion in describing or defining yoga in a way that is acceptable to all who practice it. Some of us must always start with a certain Veda, Upanishad, Sutra, or Shastra, with various lineages, styles, and brands claiming that this one is the original, true, or best source. Such a claim is often accompanied by the denigration of other approaches as distorted, fake, or even harmful. Given our focus on yoga therapy for curing and healing various maladies, we care less about specific or grand historical claims—many of which will likely remain a matter of assertion and speculation—than the evidence-based health benefits of specific practices. We are willing to bear the criticism of selectivity in focusing on some practices over others if only to support this intention. However, due to the widespread teaching of many practices that may or may not be healthy, we widen our discussion to give attention to a broad set of practices commonly taught in today's yoga studios and schools.

Here we focus primarily on the integrally interrelated asana, pranayama, and meditation practices of traditional Hatha yoga and their contemporary expressions that are most relevant to the adaptive treatments offered in yoga therapy. Although they are interrelated, we devote separate chapters to each practice.

20

Asana Practices

There are very few human beings who receive the truth, complete and staggering, by instant illumination. Most of them acquire it fragment by fragment, on a small scale, by successive developments, cellularly, like a laborious mosaic.
—ANAIS NIN

THE CONTEMPORARY WORLD OF ASANA theory and practice is like a vast sea of swirling currents and tides, some carrying the ships of defined methods and others appearing and disappearing with frequent yet unpredictable waves that blend creativity with relative continuity. Postural practices are common to most, even if different approaches are mutually unrecognizable and for some practitioners the cause of raised eyebrows when described as yoga. Some devoted traditional students might not recognize asana on paddleboards or entwined aerial silks as yoga, just as those devoted to the relatively dynamic practices of flow styles of yoga might not recognize a practice involving chairs, blocks, and straps as yoga. Each of the myriad approaches are said by their proponents to offer some benefit in living a better, healthier life, with some going as far as to claim complete self-transformation that leads to a spiritual or material promised land. Within these broad claims are specific assertions about the basic purpose, path, and fruit of yoga, with adherents of some approaches asserting that the practice must be done in a precisely prescribed way, typically under the unquestioned direction of a guru or elevated teacher, particularly when there are claims of *yoga chikitsa*, yoga therapy.

A growing body of evidence shows the effectiveness of asana practices in treating many health conditions, pointing to the potent potential of adapted yoga postural practices in yoga therapy.[1] This potential has been most avowedly pursued as part of the historical development of asana practices created through the overarching twentieth century teachings of Tirumalai Krishnamacharya and his direct students, particularly

B. K. S. Iyengar, K. Pattabhi Jois, and—more than any—T. K. V. Desikachar.[2] The underlying theory of the practices in this lineage is that the life force energy of prana is stagnant, aggravated, or otherwise out of balance as a direct manifestation of living a confused or unconscious life. Well-being occurs only upon opening to conscious living and consciously cultivating the life force, typically in specifically prescribed ways. The primary purpose of asana practice is to condition the physical body in ways that allow prana to flow more fully and in balance within the subtle channels of one's being.

Following the teachings given in Swami Swatmarama's early fourteenth-century *Hatha Yoga Pradipika*, the leading Krishnamacharya teachers all emphasize the importance (even the primacy) of asana (and for some, its supposed mastery) in order for pranayama to be beneficial rather than harmful. Going further, Iyengar and Desikachar emphasize the importance of postural modification to address the unique conditions of each individual student, including through the elaborate use of yoga props they have largely designed. Iyengar's major contributions revolve around alignment that is somewhat informed by functional anatomy, modified forms, and supportive props. Desikachar has given us more completely individualized practices based on comprehensive assessment and appreciation of each unique student, which he says was also his father's approach, called "the viniyoga of Yoga."[3] Desikachar writes that, "The spirit of viniyoga is starting from where one finds oneself. As everybody is different and changes from time to time, there can be no common starting point, and ready-made answers are useless." Going further, he writes, "Yoga is a mystery" that should be "offered according to the aspiration, requirement, and culture of the individual" and "in stages."[4] In this chapter we expand on this sensibility in exploring the essential elements and techniques of asana practice, starting with a little theory of yoga as a transformation method.

The Heart of Practicing Yoga Asanas

Part of the sublime nature of yoga is that there are infinite possibilities for deepening and refining one's practice. In playing the edges of effort and ease, exploring balance between surrender and control, and opening to self-understanding and self-transformation, there is no end to how far one can go along the path of awakening to clearer awareness, more integrated well-being, and greater happiness. There are also seemingly infinite styles and approaches to yoga, even different ideas about what yoga is, offering a rich array of practices that any of the seven billion of us sharing this planet might at any given time find most in keeping with whatever brings us to explore this ancient ritual for living in the most healthy and awakened way. It's a fascinating, challenging, often mysterious path that ultimately reveals the deepest beauty inherent in each of us as we gradually come to discover the balances that most complement and support our diverse values and intentions in life.

In doing yoga, the best teacher one will ever have is alive and well inside. In every breath, every posture, and all the moments and transitions in between, the inner teacher is offering guidance. The tone, texture, and tempo of the breath blend with myriad sensations arising in the bodymind to suggest how and where one might best go with focused awareness and action.[5] There is no universally correct method or technique, no set of rules, no single goal, and no absolute authority beyond what comes to the practitioner through the heart and soul of simply being in it, listening inside, and opening to the possibilities of the amazing qualities of being fully, consciously alive. It's a personal practice, even if one comes to it and finds in it a more abiding sense of social connection or spiritual being.[6]

At the risk of stating the obvious, in practicing yoga we all start from where we are—this in contrast to where someone else might think we are or where we ourselves might mistakenly think we are. Many teachers have preconceived or ill-informed ideas about the abilities or interests of their students while many students over- or underestimate their present ability. How might we best navigate these realities? By cultivating a personal practice that reflects our own values, intentions, and conditions, even as these all may (and likely will) evolve.

The Bodymind, Somatics, and Personal Choices in Health and Healing

Matters of self-understanding, self-concept, and sense of meaning in life affect how we might adopt and sustain a healthy lifestyle, something to which yoga and somatics directly speaks. Here we come to squarely focus on questions of bodymind, self-consciousness, and embodied awareness that are at the heart of yoga as a healing modality. Whether one seeks the meaning or purpose of life from methods found in ancient texts, such as the *Bhagavad-Gita, Yoga Sutra of Patanjali,* or *Hatha Yoga Pradipika,* or looks to more modern or contemporary sources for guidance and inspiration, or awakens to or cultivates conscious awareness, a more awakened being and a better, healthier life are constants.

Standing on the edge of the mythical battlefield of the Mahabharata War, Prince Arjuna was frozen in inaction due to misunderstanding the nature of his being; in finding his path *(dharma)* he became clear in his awareness and thereby able to act consciously and forthrightly in his life. Patanjali similarly identifies the source of human suffering *(klesha)* that motivates yoga as ignorance of one's true nature *(avidya)* that is rooted in a confused bodymind, offering an eight-step approach to betterment that includes moral and practical observances, asana, pranayama, *pratyahara* (relieving the senses of their external distractions), and meditation as a defined path to blissful being *(samadhi)*. Eleven hundred years later—in the mid-fourteenth century CE— Swatmarama elaborated a specific regimen of self-purification techniques to be followed sequentially by asana (he describes fifteen, mostly sitting), pranayama, mudra, and bandha practices designed to enhance health, curtail mental confusion, and open to liberation *(moksha)*—all practices that currently find expression across the global yoga landscape.

Seemingly a world away, the Greek philosopher Plato pleaded for "an equal and healthy balance between [body and mind]" as his teacher Socrates, who said "no citizen has a right to be an amateur in the matter of physical training … what a disgrace it is for a man to grow old without ever seeing the beauty and strength of which his body is capable," trained in dance to refine his bodymind in keeping with the embodied philosophical practice of the time.[7] "Even in the act of thinking," Socrates affirmed, "which is supposed to require [the] least assistance from the body, everyone knows that serious mistakes happen through physical ill-health." Although imbued with a dualist perspective consonant with the dualism found in classical yoga that posits the material world as an illusion *(maya* in the Vedas and Upanishads, "ideal forms" in Plato's thinking), we no less find here the path to a clearer, freer, happier, better life through bodymind integration, clarification, and transformation practices.

Although most of the ensuing development of Western philosophy would deny the importance of the physical realm—certainly in Cartesian, Kantian, and Hegelian forms of dualism that guaranteed conceptual space for the authority of religious doctrine and social forces that typically denigrate the body, much as in renunciative forms of fundamentalist yoga—by the late nineteenth century, we begin to find recognition that embodied intelligence matters in understanding experience and improving one's life. The pragmatist philosopher and pioneering psychologist William James affirmed the body's pervasive influence on awareness and the bodily dimension of thought and emotion, even if in keeping with the Western dualist tradition that situated the ultimate source of consciousness outside the organic human being.[8] In his view, we do embody experience, and the meliorative project of pragmatic philosophy and psychology—to make life better—must address how emotion and thought are inextricably interwoven in our tissues and expressed in every aspect of bodily condition.

The American philosopher and educator John Dewey drew from James's thinking and went further in advocating the integration of the bodymind in experiential ways as "the most practical question we can ask of our civilization."[9] Offering a holistic perspective in a spiritual and philosophical universe dominated by dualist thinking and various forms of theological predeterminism in which an autonomous ego or supernatural force manifests everything, Dewey boldly charted a different path, asserting that we have real choices in our lives—even if the realities of our lives are powerfully conditioned by habits of being, which in traditional yoga philosophy are explained as samskaras inherited from past lives and embodied in the totality of our being. "Habits," Dewey writes, "are demands for certain kinds of activity …," the predisposition of which are "… an immensely more intimate and fundamental part of ourselves than are vague, general, conscious choices."[10] Put differently, Dewey builds upon and moves beyond James's idea that mental and emotional life are embodied by fully situating consciousness in the bodymind and its environmental context, including our social relationships, giving us the idea of reflective body consciousness that is open to constant evolution through deliberate effort.[11] He calls for "conscious practice" not in pursuit of an idealized notion of some primordial being or transcendence of this plane of existence, but in the reality of this being, right here and now. Dewey's daily practice, taught to him by Frederick M. Alexander (as in Alexander Technique fame), focused on recognizing and releasing habitual, unhealthy, self-limiting patterns in the bodymind. As a holistic practice that potentially takes one to the deepest experience of their bodymind, yoga can take this awakening to an altogether deeper level.

The evolution of one's awareness is an integral aspect of yoga as a transformative process, and in Hatha yoga—the big umbrella over all styles, brands, and lineages utilizing postural and movement techniques—this process is one of awakening and integrating on the path to a more holistic, congruent, and healthy experience in being alive. Put differently, doing yoga is a practice for awakening to our embodiment as organic humans that happens the moment one is present to the experience of breathing and being in this bodymind. For many this is and always will be a spiritual path that is about "being in" (a oneness perspective) or "connecting to" (a dualist perspective) a sense of the infinite or consciousness beyond the bodymind. For others—even if not specifically describing yoga—it's about fully awakening to the spirit and reality of being a human being, finding meaning, as Mark Johnson proposes, "within the flow of experience that cannot exist without a biological organism engaging its environment."[12] Rather than human thought and experience being essentially illusory or somehow "cut off from the world," Johnson points us toward an "embodied, experiential view of meaning" expressed through this "phenomenal body"—not the folk concept of the body that's reduced to biological functioning, but one in which the bodymind is whole.[13]

Relating this approach to yoga therapy, we are tapping into the concept of somatics. From the Greek *soma*, meaning "living, aware, bodily person," somatics assumes that we are in our essence whole beings rather than having the body/mind duality that is pervasive in Western philosophy and medicine as well as Eastern spiritual philosophies, metaphysics, and even ayurveda. Originally drawing on the pioneering work of William James and Wilhelm Reich, a rich array of practices aimed at bodymind integration has developed in the field of somatics, including the Feldenkrais method, Hanna Somatic Education, Ideokinesis, Body-Mind Centering, Postural Integration, Rolfing, and the Trager approach.[14] As noted earlier regarding Dewey's practice of the Alexander Technique, these and other somatic practice methods start from the assumption that emotional and mental experience is embodied rather than residing only in the gray matter of the brain and somehow separate from the body. Embodied emotional and mental complexes are seen in turn as causing or exacerbating physical dysfunction or pathology, blocking the full inner manifestation—what Reich referred to as Life Force, a concept of the breath like yoga's prana. Indeed, much of somatics is consonant with yoga as a process of healing and self-transformation, starting with the idea of psychic adhesions (yoga's samskaras) inhibiting or even blocking healthy life on the path to clear awareness (yoga's samadhi) and health.

In the view of somatics, self-transformation must address how to release accumulated tension and thereby bring embodied experience to consciousness in a way that allows integration of one's entire being. Somatics typically uses hands-on techniques, including deep tissue manipulation aimed at releasing deeply held tension. Much of this work uses physical stimulation or manipulation in specific areas of the body to highlight stressful responses in which the sympathetic nervous system—the fight or flight response—is activated. Using specific breathing techniques—some are similar to ujjayi, kapalabhati, and bastrika pranayamas—one then gradually brings more subtle awareness to the overall experience of being in those feelings in the bodymind and with it comes a deeper calm as the parasympathetic nervous system is activated.

Much of the somatics field is concerned with emotional trauma and related therapies. Although much of the contemporary yoga scene eschews such work in favor of yoga as glorified exercise, yoga originated and has always had as its principle focus fundamental self-transformation that involves movement into clearer awareness or spiritual being. In the *Yoga Sutra of Patanjali* this is stated as *citta vrtti nirodha*, or "to calm the fluctuations of the mind," which are seen as the sources of ignorance of the reality of one's true being and thus the proximate cause of existential suffering.[15] Although Patanjali's approach to yoga does not involve doing asana practice beyond sitting, he offers a yoga psychology that first describes the condition of the confused mind and then a set of actions—a yoga technology—one can undertake to cultivate a clear and healthy mind. As we've explored, several hundred years later Hatha yogis and Tantrikas elaborated various systems of postural practices, breathing techniques, kriyas, and mudras designed as a simpler path to the same goal, albeit along a path of fuller integration of breath and bodymind, and with it the blossoming of the clear consciousness promised by Patanjali's method.

Part of the beauty of yoga asana practice is that each different asana highlights tension and other sensation in the body. With more mindful practice, we also come to detect how the different asanas stimulate different emotional and mental reactions; a certain posture done in a particular way, time, or other circumstance tends to generate its own somewhat unique effects on one's mental experience. Each asana also tends to affect the breath in different ways, however subtle the differences may be. Staying with the breath as we feel it and consciously directing it in the body through mindful visualization in conjunction with physical sensation, we come to realize that we can breathe into the body in conscious ways, consciously directing the breath to places of tension or holding, and in this way come to experience how the breath transforms bodily sensation, emotional feeling, and mental awareness.[16]

Ancient writings on yoga explain this with the *kosha* model in which prana—the life force that we cultivate through the breath—is the mediating force unifying body and mind. Rather than starting from the assumption that the body and mind are somehow separate, here we approach the practice as one of awakening to the existing reality of our whole bodymind that we might not think or feel to be whole due to the conditions of the bodymind itself, including the pervasive ideologies, belief systems, and linguistic formulae that reinforce the feeling of duality as being true and natural.

This awakening is not an automatic process; it takes volition and action—it is the practice! When we breathe consciously into a part of the body as directed by the tension highlighted in an asana, we are creating the opportunity to consciously awaken awareness there. Doing this in each of 840,000 asanas—the number mentioned in the *Hatha Yoga Pradipika* as a way of saying there is infinite possibility—we gradually awaken awareness throughout the entirety of our being, awakening and expanding embodied (albeit relatively hidden, dazed, and confused) consciousness that is already there.

The specific ways a unique individual's embodied intelligence manifests in their experience initially may make it practically impossible for them to independently find a way in the various practices that yoga and other healing modalities offer that is safe, sustainable, and effective, often resulting in the reinforcement of lifestyle habits that are self-limiting rather than wholesome and transformational. Even just the part of the nervous system that gives us proprioceptive—"perceiving of self"—awareness is often inaccurate, including our kinesthetic awareness of movement and positioning in space. Self-awareness of deeper qualities of being can be even more elusive in large part due to the psychological condition and philosophical orientation of the person. Clearly informed and appropriately given guidance can thus help in developing and refining self-awareness as one learns to more consciously breathe and cultivate being present and mindful in the bodymind, thereby more consciously opening to the lifestyle choices that best support health, healing, and an abiding sense of wholeness.

The Essential Qualities of Asana Practice

Although there are potentially infinite qualities of asanas as they come to be experienced by the unique persons doing them, we can highlight some qualities that are essential in cultivating yoga practice in a way that makes it more accessible, sustainable, and deeply transformational.

Sthira Sukham Asanam

Among the most important elements of asana practice is the idea that it is a personal practice, not a comparative or a competitive practice, despite some people doing their best to make it so.[17] Exploring with this basic sensibility, the practice will be more safe, sustainable, and transformational. It's a sensibility—a basic yogic value—that reflects the sole comment on asana found in the *Yoga Sutra of Patanjali*: sthira sukham asanam—meaning steadiness, ease, and presence of mind (the latter, from the root word *as,* meaning "to be," or "to be present," which I interpret to mean to be here now, fully attuned to one's immediate experience).

It is helpful to relate to these as qualities we are always cultivating in the practice. Do note that Patanjali is not describing anything even closely approximating the sort of postural practices that began evolving several hundred years later and eventually became Hatha yoga, which has evolved more in the past seventy-five years than in the previous thousand. Nonetheless, we find the sensibilities of classical yoga brought forward in the earliest verified writing on Hatha practice, the mid-fourteenth-century *Hatha Yoga Pradipika*, where Swami Swatmarama tells the yogi to have "enthusiasm, perseverance, discrimination, unshakable faith, and courage" to "bring success to yoga" and "get steadiness of body and mind"; later, Swatmarama mentions "being free of fatigue in practicing asana," suggesting the balance of steadiness and ease earlier emphasized by Patanjali.[18]

Exploring this, let's say for a moment that we're starting a practice standing at the front of the mat (bearing in mind here that the same concepts, qualities, and sensibilities are ideally cultivated regardless of one's initial postural position—sitting, lying supine, and so on). This standing posture might be Tadasana (Mountain Pose). In it, we are opening to being as steady, at ease, and present as we can be and thereby more naturally open to a deepening sense of balance and equanimity that is well expressed with another Sanskrit term: *samasthihi* (literally, "equal standing"). For some clients, this simple position is somewhat challenging, especially if held for several minutes or if a student has a condition such as general postural misalignment, advanced pregnancy, multiple sclerosis, leg length discrepancy, or basic weakness. With practice, it's likely to become easier to find and sustain a sense of samasthihi in this position, especially with proper alignment and energetic actions. If all one did was continue to stand and move into deeper equanimity (or sit or lie supine), this might become more of a meditation practice. But here we are presently focusing on asana, the postural practices that are best explored with conscious breathing and presence of mind (the reciprocal effects of which are further essential aspects of asana practice) and contain the potential for various qualities of self-transformation and healing.

Tapas, Abhyasa, and Vairagya

As we come to the experience in an asana in which we no longer feel any significant effect or effort in being in it, we might simply stay there, being in it, or we might find ourselves opening to a variation of it or transitioning to an asana in which we find it takes some effort to find stability and ease to be just as stable, relaxed, and present. However, if we always practice asanas in a way that involves no effort—that is one path—we might be missing an opportunity to awaken deeper awareness. In going deeper, we open to potentially greater effects through the intensity and diversity of experience that practicing asanas offers. To do yoga most deeply and lastingly, one shows up with the self-discipline *(tapas)* it takes to practice to the best of our ability, breath by breath, asana by asana, practice by practice, day by day, exploring the edges of possibility and discovering what happens amid it all. With persevering practice—*abhyasa*—we do stay with it; fully committed to the practice, we proceed with deeper experience and reflection, opening to and learning from the intensity of the experience each breath of the way, all the while allowing the most abiding sense of santosa, contentment.

This involves staying close to the edges of possibility in what we're doing in our practice, an approach Joel Kramer, a pioneering innovator of contemporary yoga asana practice who significantly influenced the evolution of the practice in the 1960s and 1970s, beautifully and richly describes. As we begin moving into an asana, we come to a place where we feel something starting to happen, what Kramer calls "the primary edge" (I call it the "aha moment").[19] Going further, we come to another "edge" where the bodymind expresses pain, discomfort, or simply blocks further range of motion (I call it the "uh-uh moment"). In a persevering practice, we "play the edge" by staying beyond the "aha" but well enough within the "uh-uh" to have the space to slowly and patiently explore small refining intentional movements. Breath by breath, the edges tend to move—we open more space and create more sustainable ease, thus more easily moving awakening energy throughout the bodymind. If right up against the final edge of possibility or if moving too quickly, there is no space or time for this sense-based refinement and awakening; instead we're likely to cause injury, reinforce unhealthy habits, or simply burn out on the practice.

As much as fully showing up in the practice and playing the edges of possibility and refinement are essential in doing yoga, there's another essential quality of the practice, what Patanjali gives as *vairagya*—nonattachment. In the practice of nonattachment we open to being in the practice with a sense that anything is possible, with spontaneity yet still with self-disciplined effort, all the while identifying more with the deeper intention in our heart—perhaps health, contentment, happiness—than with the performance of a pose or attainment of some static or predetermined goal. Abhyasa and vairagya are thus integrally interrelated elements of a safe, sustainable, and transformational yoga practice that allow us to progress from one place to another with steadiness and ease. Together they give us one of the most basic yogic principles: *it's not about how far you go, but how you go.*

Exploring the asanas with a balanced attitude of vairagya and abhyasa helps ensure that we are at least somewhat liberated from attainment-related expectation. By embodying this attitude in every aspect of one's practice, we more naturally find our way to our inner teacher, utilizing the intensity of physical sensation and the barometer of the breath to guide this effort in our personal practice.

Ujjayi Pranayama

Exploring the asanas with a balanced attitude of vairagya and abhyasa helps ensure that our practice is sustainable. Indeed, an essential element of this balanced approach to sustainable and transformational yoga practice rests in the breath. Curiously, although the classical writings on Hatha yoga give primary emphasis to pranayama (from *pra*, "to bring forth," *an*, "to breathe," and a combination of *ayama*, "to expand," and *yama*, "to control"), pranayama practice—basic yogic breathing—is typically given little attention in many contemporary yoga classes.[20] As with asana practice, with pranayama it's important to develop the practice gradually and with steadiness and ease.[21] However, soft, gentle, subtle ujjayi—"uplifting"—pranayama can be safely practiced by all, including complete beginners, pregnant women, and those with blood-pressure issues, infirmities, and other pathological conditions. The breath itself nourishes our cells and our entire being. The light sound of ujjayi helps us keep our awareness in the breath in a way that makes it easier to cultivate the smooth, balanced, steady flow of every inhalation and exhalation, providing immediate feedback on our movement in, through, and out of the asanas. As such, it is a perfect barometer for sensing and cultivating energetic balance in doing asana practices. If the breath is strained, it's a sure sign that one has slipped away from steadiness and ease. Rather than trying to squeeze the breath into the asanas and the movements within and between them, ideally our practice finds expression in and through the integrity of the breath.

Alignment Principles

The functional anatomy and biomechanics of each asana give us its alignment principles, which tell us how best to position the body in each asana. When the alignment principles of any given asana are embodied in the practice, we find easier access to stability and ease while further ensuring the maximum benefits of the practice. When one misunderstands or ignores basic alignment principles, the benefits of the asana can largely be lost while its risks are increased. It is thus important to have a clear idea of where one is going before going into an asana. It is equally important to adapt basic alignment principles to one's unique conditions.

Adaptation of the asanas through modified form and the use of props is of utmost importance in utilizing yoga asana practices for healing. Unfortunately, such adaptation is disturbingly absent, ill-informed, or underutilized in many yoga classes, causing many students to 1) have greater difficulty in establishing basic alignment, 2) unnecessarily strain in the asanas, and 3) injure themselves. In Part V we give clear guidance on modifications, including the use of props. Also see my earlier work on guiding the practice for detailed information on alignment, modifications, use of props, and hands-on adjustments, including 857 photos and captions depicting various modified asana forms and use of props in 101 different asanas.[22]

Energetic Actions

As discussed earlier regarding the balance of stability and ease in the asanas, it is important first to establish the foundation of each asana. From the foundation that one creates through grounding actions and alignment, it is easier then to create other energetic actions that help to refine the integrity of the overall asana. The concept of energetic actions expands on Joel Kramer's idea of lines of energy. Energetic actions start with running lines of energy to enhance grounding and to help create opening, then from this foundation move into extension, flexion, rotation, lateral flexion, contraction, and expansion, all of which can be highlighted with specific guidance from a skilled teacher.

For example, in Bakasana (Crane Pose, often erroneously translated as "Crow Pose," which is Kakasana), the fingers are spread wide apart (the thumbs not so wide as to overstretch the ligaments and place undue pressure on the nerves in the thenar space between the index finger and the thumb), and there is ideally equal pressure across the entire span of each hand as well as out and down through the fingers and thumbs. Meanwhile, one wants to work from this foundation to more fully root the shoulder blades down against the back ribs, fully extend the elbows, squeeze the knees against the outer shoulders (enhanced by the energetic action of pada bandha in the feet as the heels and sides of the balls of the feet are pressed together), elevate the heels toward the buttocks, lightly engage the abdominal core, and thereby elevate the pelvis higher. In Utthita Parsvakonasana (Extended Side Angle Pose), we run a strong line of energy down the back leg and foot to root down while stretching from that rooted foot out through the arm that is stretched overhead. To this we add several energetic actions: pada bandha in the feet, isometric outward spiraling of the front foot to foster alignment of the front knee, thigh, and hip, extension of the back leg, rotation of the torso, external rotation of the upper arm, lengthening of the lower side of the torso, a line of energy from the lower shoulder into the hand and the floor, and expansion of the heart center, all of which can be given with subtle hands-on cues—and all of which lend to the stability, ease, sustainability, refinement, and deepening of the effects of this asana.

Transitioning

How we approach an asana shapes how we experience it and how we can refine it, which in turn influences the experience of coming out of the asana with stability and ease. In transition in, it is important first to establish the initial foundation with the proper alignment of whatever will be the source of grounding along with energetic actions that enhance this foundation and facilitate stable, safe, and comfortable transitional movement. Once in the asana, we apply the breath and energetic actions to refine and deepen our exploration and expression of it. We then apply specific energetic actions to more simply and easily transition out. For example, strongly rooting down through the legs and feet in preparation for Utthita Trikonasana (Extended Triangle Pose) awakens the leg muscles and creates the foundation from which to lengthen in the torso out over the front leg. Once there, the slight energetic action of spiraling the front foot outward (without it moving) helps press the hip of that leg under, toward the other hip, which in combination with pressing the back leg more strongly in extension makes this asana more of a hip opener. In preparing to come out of the asana, if one runs a strong line of energy from the hip to the heel of the back leg, this will make it easier on the lower back in bringing the torso back upright.

Vinyasa Krama

In bringing these elements of practice more alive in all of practice, the key is to explore in a way that allows us to move more stably, easily, and joyfully in the wise progression of our asana exploration. One aspect of this is in the sequence of actions. In designing specific asana practices tailored to a treatment plan, we ideally create an arc-like structure with specific asanas sequenced in a way that makes the most complex or challenging ones most accessible, safe, and sustainable—and thereby more deeply healing.[23] Along the practice path it's helpful to move from simple to more complex postures, generally warming the body while giving focused attention to areas where one will soon explore and go more deeply. Anticipatory asanas open and stabilize the muscles and joints most involved in the peak, helping to further awaken the deeper embodied intelligence one will tap into when exploring the deeper, more complex peak asanas.

This approach reflects the concept of vinyasa krama, from *vinyasa,* "to place in a special way," and *krama,* "stage," referring to the effective sequencing of actions. The essence of vinyasa krama is the wisdom of gradual progression, exploring and evolving consciously and methodically, moving steadily and simply from where one is to wherever one is going with the integrated qualities of abhyasa and vairagya. In bringing fuller integration to this practice, we do *pratikriyasana,* from *prati,* "opposite," and *kriya,* "action," methodically and creatively resolving whatever tension arises along the path leading to Savasana (Corpse Pose) and beyond with compensatory asanas. Breath by breath, we evolve in and through the practice.

When doing a yoga practice, we come to various asanas. In approaching them, we're already experiencing sensations. If we're doing yoga rather than merely exercising, then we're breathing consciously and using the breath to refine how we're exploring the asana. Breathing consciously, we're bringing more conscious awareness into the bodymind, ideally as suggested by the sensations that are arising in the moment, adapting our movement and positioning to be more stable, relaxed, and present. So there's a dance of the breath with the bodymind, each affecting the other, all of it increasingly experienced as part of the whole of our being. This is the basic practice of always and forever integrating and awakening that is at the heart of yoga asana practice. In it, we can play with different breathing techniques, positions, and visualizations, exploring their various effects, including the inner dialogue and reactions that are an increasingly clear reflective mirror of our deeper qualities of being. These qualities are essential when using asana practices for healing acute or chronic health conditions.

Adaptive Practices

Adaptive practices for healing are ideally informed by the assessments and larger communication processes discussed in Chapters 18 and 19. One can then proceed to offer three forms of support: (1) a safe setting in which clients can explore within their own bodyminds how to move and hold in ways that facilitate the natural healing process; (2) modifications of asanas and use of props in those asanas that help reduce further injury; and (3) asanas that enhance healing. A primary focus is on how to support clients with asana practices that are informed by an understanding of the client's condition and integrated with other care he or she is receiving. Focused on cultivating healing, wholeness, balance, and radiant well-being, your role as a yoga therapist working with clients is to help them create a healing resonance, doing only what feels good in the practice, consciously moving energy in the sensitive areas, going slowly enough to listen, feel, adapt, and enjoy the process. This very general attitude then allows us to provide the more specific asana practices for healing specific conditions in ways that maximize efficacy and minimize harm. The more specific practice suggestions are given in Part V.

21

Pranayama Practices

BREATHING CONSCIOUSLY IS ONE of the most important parts of Hatha yoga yet often the most elusive. The breath nourishes and guides the asana practice. It is the source of energetic awakening throughout the body. Through conscious breathing we open in the asana practice to learning more about ourselves, cultivating wholeness in body, mind, and spirit. Yet the breath often disappears from awareness amid everything else that is happening in the asana practice. Slipping from awareness, the breath usually fades. Students tend to lose focus, their attention drifting or leaping away from the here and now.[1] As the breath fades, students lose subtle awareness of how energy is flowing in their bodies, of the subtlety of sensation in the body, of the unification of bodymind, of refinement in the practice. Maintaining attention to the breath can be especially difficult for new students who are trying to move their bodies into new and often awkward positions while in an unfamiliar place and situation. Even as students progress in their asana practice, their breathing practice typically lags. As asanas become more challenging, limited breathing skills inhibit the deep source of stability and ease found through full and conscious breathing. It is thus essential for teachers to guide students in basic yogic breathing—*ujjayi pranayama*—and to introduce students to more refined breathing techniques found in the larger art of pranayama.

Pranayama is among the most mystified aspects of yoga. Different schools of yoga describe even its most basic form, ujjayi, in different and conflicting ways. Is it *prana-yama*, which most agree translates as "breath control" or "control of the life force"? Or is it *prana-ayama*, which suggests the near opposite: "breath liberation" or "expansion of the life force"?[2] Even when demystified by some teachings and teachers, including such authoritative sources as the *Hatha Yoga Pradipika* and B. K.

S. Iyengar, it gains intrigue when students are cautioned that "until the postures are perfected, do not attempt pranayama."[3]

This chapter unravels the discovery, development, practices, and teaching of pranayama. We will look briefly at the ancient teachings for insight into the original intentions and techniques of different pranayama practices. We will visit the modern science of respiration for further understanding of the anatomy and physiology of breathing. With this background, we will explore the art of teaching pranayama, starting with helping students rediscover their natural breath. Staying with our emphasis on Hatha yoga, we will explore teaching basic pranayama as part of contemporary asana practices and explore how to teach several more refined pranayama techniques that further balance energy in the bodymind and lead to a deeper sense of integration and overall well-being.

The Discovery and Development of Pranayama

Reflecting on the discovery process of ancient yogis, Dona Holleman reasons that pranayama was first developed by ancient yogis through close observation of the natural cycles of breath in the laboratory of their bodies.[4] When simply observing the breath, we first notice the body's rhythmic movement with each cycle of breath. As we tune in more closely, we discover that slower breathing is more relaxing, faster breathing more energizing. Holleman claims that this awareness led to *kapalabhatipranayama* ("skull-cleansing" pranayama), in which intense rhythmic breathing energizes the body, which led to another discovery: increased energy can be brought from the "long, snaky circles of the intestines that whorl around themselves, that promote heat" up through the spinal column to the "winding passages" of the brain where chemical (and perhaps alchemical) changes in the brain transform one's perception and sense of being.[5]

Exploring natural breathing more closely, we notice the natural pauses between the breaths that, when expanded—especially when empty of breath—lead to the sensation of pranic energy rising along the spine. Done consciously, this is the practice of *kumbhaka*, or breath retention. Yet sometimes the energy gets blocked rather than rising all the way up. The ancient yogis called these blockages *chakras*, or wheels of energy. *Nadi shodhana pranayama*, alternate nostril breathing, balances the flow of prana up through the *ida* and *pingalanadis* (energy channels) that rise along and cross the spine at each major chakra, which, when made conscious, allows the upward flow of prana.

Although the breath is the principal vehicle for cultivating prana, pranayama is more than a set of breathing practices: it is a tool for "expanding our usually small reservoir of prana by lengthening, directing, and regulating the movement of the breath and then limiting or restraining the increased pranic energy in the bodymind."[6]

This practice of tapping the breath as a tool for cultivating prana—and with it, self-awareness and self-transformation—is found as early as the ancient Vedas, particularly in the *Rigveda* from more than four thousand years ago. It is given its first detailed discussion in the *Prasna Upanishad*, where its all-pervasive and life-sustaining nature is likened to the sun. (See Chapter 3 for more on prana.) We first find the emphasis on breath in asana practice in the *Yoga Sutra* immediately following Patanjali's definition of *asana* as *sthira sukham asanam* in his use of the word *prayatna*, which is typically translated as "effort." Srivatsa Ramaswami points out that prayatna is of three types, one of which, *jivana prayatna*, refers to "efforts made by the individual to maintain life and, more especially, breathing."[7] As we breathe, so we feel, and in breathing more freely and fully, we feel more freely and fully. Although asanas in contemporary Hatha yoga are far more evolved and complex than in Patanjali's time, the point is to explore asanas with and through the steadiness and ease of the breath, continuously connecting the breath with the bodymind.

The *Yoga Sutra* tells us that mastering asana precedes breath control, which requires a still body and a calm mind. Many leading teachers abide by this advice. "Attain steadiness and stillness in asanas before introducing breathing techniques," says B. K. S. Iyengar.[8] "When pranayama and asanas are done together," he stresses, "see that the perfect posture is not disturbed. Until the postures are perfected, do not attempt pranayama." In this traditional perspective, asana practice develops the physical and mental basis for safely and fully experiencing the benefits of pranayama. Just as asanas should never be forced or imposed, pranayama is best practiced once asanas have removed "the symptoms that arise from obstacles in the personality"—suffering, depression, restlessness, and irregular breathing—that impede the flow of prana.[9] Only then, it is said, can the practice of pranayama regulate that flow of prana throughout the body.

The approach taken here departs from this traditional path. If clients practice sthira sukham asanam, there is no danger in exploring pranayama. The table at the end of this chapter offers suggestions on when to teach and whom to teach different pranayama techniques (details on each technique are given in the following pages).

Pranayama enhances respiratory function, improves the circulatory system, and thereby improves digestion and elimination. When the respiratory system is functioning at its best, the natural purification systems of the physical body function better as well. Combined with asana practice, pranayama allows us to move energy more easily and thoroughly through the body, especially as the lungs, muscles, and nerves of respiration are refined. Learning to breathe consciously and efficiently, clients can relax more deeply, loosening their grip over unnecessary tension in the body and organs of perception. With deeper relaxation and clearer awareness, clients find an easier path to concentration, equanimity, and serenity. In this way, pranayama can help all clients have a healthier life right now while giving them additional tools for deepening and refining their asana and meditation practices.

Cultivating Basic Breath Awareness

Breathing happens naturally, involuntarily, and unconsciously. This "natural breathing" varies considerably depending on the person's physical, emotional, mental, and spiritual condition. It is compromised by depression, anxiety, tight or weak respiratory muscles, distraction, lethargy, or flighty energy.[10] Under these conditions, the breath is typically shallow, inefficient, and over-relies on secondary respiratory muscles rather than the diaphragm. Instead of assuming clients share a common baseline quality of breath, it is better to guide pranayama practices starting with the natural conditions of each individual student and build from that initial foundation. This starts with guiding clients in developing basic breath awareness. "Learning to breathe well is not an additive process in which you learn specific techniques for improving the breath you already have," says Donna Farhi. "It is a process of deconstruction where you learn to identify the things you are already doing that restrict the natural emergence of the breath."[11] This observation process anticipates and develops insight into the possibilities of pranayama as well as deeper somatic awareness, helping to consciously connect breath, body, and mind.

One can explore this initial awakening of breath awareness by lying on the back, eyes closed, and tuning in to the natural flow of the breath. In this type of exercise, "we do nothing," suggests Richard Rosen, "but observe what is."[12] In this exploration, notice the subtle qualities of breath sensation through each phase of the breathing cycle, as follows:

> **Inhaling:** What does it feel like? What do you feel initiates the inhalation? What first happens in your body? How does the sensation of the breath change as it flows in? Where do you feel the breath? What parts of your body are moving? What is the succession of movement? Does the flow slow down, speed up, or seem to get stuck along the way? What does the breath sound like as it flows in? How fully do you inhale? What changes in sensation do you feel in your heart center, across your face, between your temples, as the breath draws in? What fluctuations do you sense in your mind?

> **Filled with breath:** What do you feel at the crest of each inhale? What is the length of the natural pause? What sensations do you feel in your body? What fluctuations do you sense in your mind?

> **Exhaling:** Where do you first feel the movement into exhalation? Does the breath tend to rush out? How does the pace of the exhale change as the breath continues

to flow out? What changes do you feel in your body and overall awareness as the breath leaves? How completely do you exhale? What fluctuations do you sense in your mind?

Empty of breath: What do you feel when empty of breath? How long do you tend to hold the breath out? Do you feel any gripping or holding? What is the quality of your awareness when empty of breath? What fluctuations do you sense in your mind?

Repeat this process sitting in an upright position, exploring the differences in sensation in this new relationship to gravity. Once past this initial awareness practice, gain deeper insight by making these observations in a variety of different positions, particularly amid the flow of an asana practice.

Refining the Flow of the Breath

With this baseline of breath awareness, you explore the development and refinement of your breathing more subtly, discovering how to cultivate sthira sukham asanam more easily while breathing in a variety of different ways. This starts by feeling the contraction and release of your respiratory muscles and the related movements in your body with two types of inhalation and exhalation—puraka and rechaka.[13]

Puraka—The Inhalation

A single inhalation is termed *puraka*, referring to "the intake of cosmic energy by the individual for his growth and progress."[14] Depending on what other actions one is doing—certain asanas, pranayamas, or sitting in meditation—the breath can be received in ways that support those actions. The following exercises are designed to help clients develop and refine their awareness and practice of puraka. In guiding these practices, encourage clients to be receptive to the breath rather than grasp for it. With practice, the breath is received delicately yet fully, steadily yet easily, causing as little disturbance as possible to the bodymind.

DIAPHRAGMATIC INHALATION

1. Lying on the back, flex the hips and knees as if preparing for Setu Bandha Sarvangasana, placing one palm on the belly, the other on the heart center. Feel how complete exhales cause the abdominal muscles to contract.

2. With the following inhalation, feel how the belly expands outward. Continue to focus on this movement, which is caused by the contraction and descent of the diaphragm.

3. Play with varying the extent of exhalation, feeling how this affects the subsequent movement of the belly. Try to allow the spine and ribs to remain relaxed and move only with the movement of breath caused by the diaphragm.

4. Play with starting, stopping, and varying the rate and volume of each breath, concentrating this effort in the diaphragm while feeling the effects elsewhere in the body. Continue this exploration with the palms farther down the belly.

5. Explore directing different volumes of diaphragmatic inhalations into different areas (one side and the other, front and back, lower and higher) in various body positions: lying on the back with the arms extended overhead, curled on the sides, lying on the belly.

6. Finally, explore diaphragmatic inhalations while keeping the abdomen from expanding, using the hands on the ribs to feel the gradual spreading and lifting of the ribs. Try to allow this movement to arise from deep in the thorax rather than at the more superficial level of the ribs. Explore this in different positions.

COSTAL INHALATION

1. Sitting comfortably tall in Vajrasana (Thunderbolt Pose, propped if necessary to establish pelvic neutrality and neutral spinal extension), place the palms high on the side ribs.

2. Exhale completely, feeling the side and back ribs draw together and downward.

3. With the inhalations, push the ribs into the hands while allowing the ribs to expand away from one another as the serratus anterior muscles contract, lifting and pulling the ribs back and out. Try to create the movement just in the ribs, keeping the shoulders and belly relaxed while feeling the full expansion of the rib cage and lungs.

4. Next, activate inhalations with the pectoralis major muscles on the top of the chest: pulling the shoulder blades down gently against the back ribs, place the fingertips of one hand in front of the shoulders and the other fingertips on the front ribs in line with the xiphoid process (just below the line of the breast).

5. Inhaling and exhaling, try to feel the contraction of the pectoralis major raising the sternum while spreading the lower and middle ribs apart.

6. Drawing awareness into the higher regions of the chest and lungs, place the fingertips just under the clavicle and try to feel the ribs.

7. Keeping the shoulder blades relaxed down against the back ribs, try to concentrate the inhalation as if breathing into the clavicles, activating the pectoralis minor muscles to open the heart center fully.

8. Try to alternate inhalations using the pectoralis minor and major muscles, feeling how the difference in their resulting movements opens distinct areas of the rib cage.

9. Now explore the highest breathing using the sternocleidomastoids (SCMs) and scalenes.

10. With your fingertips in and slightly above the hollow space between your collarbones, lean the head slightly back to feel the SCMs awaken. Create quick "sniffing" inhalations to feel the SCMs contracting. Explore doing this after taking in and holding a full inhale, lifting the sternum, and noticing how this allows you to draw in more breath.

11. Place the fingertips lightly onto the sides of your neck and feel into the texture of the scalenes muscles, which descend from the transverse process of upper cervical vertebrae down and outward to the first two ribs. These muscles assist high respiratory movements.

Rechaka—The Exhalation

The exhalation is termed *rechaka*, "the process by which the energy of the body gradually unites with that of the mind," says B. K. S. Iyengar.[15]

ABDOMINAL EXHALATION

1. Sitting in Vajrasana, slowly and completely exhale out the breath while maintaining the neutral positioning of the lower ribs, feeling the natural contraction of the upper belly just beneath the lower ribs. Notice the tendency of the spine to round forward into flexion.

2. Placing your palms on your belly, repeat this exercise while the spine is extended.

3. Now add mula bandha, lightly contracting and lifting the transverse perineal and deep pelvic muscles.

4. Explore connecting the energetic and muscular lift of mula bandha with the gradual contraction of the abdomen, increasingly awakening the transversus abdominis muscles.

5. Next, try to successively engage the abdominal muscles from below the navel up to the lower ribs as the breath is flowing out.

COSTAL EXHALATION

1. Placing one palm on your heart and one on your belly, slowly exhale while pulling your sternum back toward your spine and minimizing the abdominal

muscles' contraction. This practice brings awareness to the transversus thoracis muscle, which closes the rib cage in the front. Try to feel the slight flexion of the upper spine as the breath flows out.

2. With the palms on the side ribs, repeat this exercise, feeling how the side ribs lower as the obliques contract and the spine slightly flexes.

3. Place the fingertips on the xiphoid process and repeat this exercise, feeling the front ribs draw lower and in.

Use these basic inhalation and exhalation practices in your clients' yoga practices to help develop the balance and integrity of their breathing. Most clients initially find the inhalations and exhalations differing in pace, texture, sound, intensity, and duration. Later we will explore variations in the pace of inhalation and exhalation, including equal and unequal ratios between them (sama vritti and visama vritti). With practice, puraka and rechaka come into balance and form the foundation for all other pranayama practices, including ujjayi pranayama.

Ujjayi Pranayama—Basic Yogic Breathing

The basic breathing technique in Hatha yoga is ujjayi pranayama. Here we breathe through the nose with a very slight narrowing of the throat at the epiglottis (where you feel sensation when coughing or gargling). This increases the vibration of the larynx, creating a soft sound like wind breezing through the trees or the sound of the sea at the seashore. The effects of ujjayi are threefold: (1) the breath is warmed when breathing just through the nose, thus warming the lungs, which warms the blood, which warms the body and helps to awaken the body to natural movement in asanas; (2) the sound and sensation of ujjayi helps in maintaining awareness of the breath flowing with steadiness, ease, and balance; and (3) the rhythmic sound of ujjayi helps to calm the nerves and create a quieter internal practice.

Some teachings insist that the technique of ujjayi, like other aspects of the practice, is a "secret" that will (and should) reveal itself if the breath is left free in the asana practice.[16] Others directly guide clients in ujjayi as part of both asana and pranayama practices. Whether one approach is better than the other is a question that is best resolved in practice, which creates a seeming conundrum: How would a person know if it is beneficial to learn it unless they learn it? Although there does not seem to be any danger in doing ujjayi pranayama in asana practice, it can be taught and practiced in a way that overly restricts the breath, especially when it is taught through the application of jalandhara bandha (an essential part of many other pranayama techniques, but not of ujjayi). As with much of the practice, keeping it simple allows one to utilize an initial sensitizing technique while refining it through one's own practice. Here is a simple way to explore in discovering and cultivating ujjayi:

1. Sitting comfortably or standing in Tadasana, close your eyes, open your mouth, and breathe as if trying to fog up a mirror. This immediately creates the sound and sensation of ujjayi, bringing awareness to the epiglottis area.

2. Try to create the same sound and sensation while inhaling and exhaling. (The tendency is to do it only on the inhale.)

3. Close your mouth and breathe through your nose with the same sound and sensation.

4. Play with it, creating more or less constriction in your throat and noticing how that affects the flow of breath, its sound, and the overall sensation.

5. Finally, begin treating your ujjayi with a sense of delicacy, exploring how you can breathe more deeply and strongly—yet just as delicately and softly.

You can immediately apply ujjayi pranayama in your asana practice. Here are some tips on exploring the connection between ujjayi pranayama and asanas:

- Make the steady, rhythmic, balanced, strong yet soft flow of ujjayi just as important as anything else in your asana practice, cultivating it in a way that changes as little as possible from the beginning to the end of the asana session.

- Ujjayi can be deliberately varied, using more intensity to fuel more difficult movements, and more ease to generate a deeper sense of calm.

- Explore the deepening of your asana practice around the integrity of the breath rather than trying to force the breath in attempting asanas.

- Tune in to ujjayi as a barometer of the energetic effort and physical intensity of the practice, a source of immediate feedback that you can use in refining your practice.

Deepening and Refining Pranayama Practices

The following pranayama techniques are designed to further refine the awakening of subtle energy and awareness in connecting body, breath, and mind. Each of these techniques builds upon the natural breathing and disciplined puraka-rechaka practices discussed earlier. Explore these deeper methods only after finding stability and ease with puraka-rechaka and ujjayi. As with exploring other breathing practices, be more interested in relaxation than full performance of the breathing technique. Apply the concept of sthira sukham asanam as a tool for safely exploring pranayama.

Vritti Pranayama: Fluctuating Breath

The breath fluctuates in a variety of ways, including in the relative length or duration of inhalations, exhalations, and the pauses in between them. In vritti pranayama, the ratios of these durations are regulated. There are two practices: sama vritti (equal fluctuation) and visama vritti (unequal fluctuation). We will first look at practicing these with the inhale and exhale; later, as part of introducing kumbhaka practices, we will apply these qualities to retention.

SAMA VRITTI PRANAYAMA

1. Begin with natural breath observation. Simply observe the breath without changing it in any way, noticing how it feels flowing in, out, and in the pauses in between. Allow the breath to flow smoothly.

2. Begin counting the duration of your inhalations and exhalations, noting the difference.

3. Next, bring a uniform duration to the inhalations and exhalations, starting with a comfortable count.

4. Gradually, practice by practice, expand the length of the inhalations and exhalations while keeping them in balance.

5. Try to make steadiness and ease more interesting than longer or deeper breaths, breathing only as deeply as you can while staying relaxed and comfortable.

VISAMA VRITTI PRANAYAMA

1. Start practicing visama vritti pranayama with sama vritti. At the end of a natural and balanced exhalation try to lengthen the inhalation by a one-count over the exhalation, staying with this for several rounds of breath.

2. Try to watch and sense changes in the quality of the breath as well as subtle physical and mental reactions.

3. Gradually increase the uneven ratio by further lengthening the inhalations, eventually inhaling for twice as long as exhaling.

4. Stay with this for several minutes before returning to natural breathing and then reverse the ratios, gradually lengthening the exhalations over the inhalations.

Kumbhaka: Breath Retention

Kumbhaka is the practice of staying with and expanding the natural pause between inhalations and exhalations.[17] In holding the breath in these pauses, the bodymind becomes more still and clear. There are two forms: antara kumbhaka is retention of the inhalation; bahya kumbhaka is retention of the exhalation.[18] It is important to develop these practices slowly, gradually refining the neuromuscular intelligence of the diaphragm, intercostals, and other secondary respiratory muscles. This practice should not cause any strain in the body or mind. Take it easy in expanding the duration of retention. Explore as follows:

ANTARA KUMBHAKA

1. Sitting in a comfortable upright position, come into natural breathing with balanced puraka-rechaka (sama vritti pranayama).

2. Bring in ujjayi pranayama, the gradual deepening of the breath. The spine should be naturally erect and relaxed, the heart center spacious and soft, the brain as light and quiet as possible in that moment.

3. Using the basic breath awareness practices discussed earlier, focus your attention on the natural pause at the crest of the inhalations, noticing what happens in your bodymind and larger sense of being in that space.

4. Allow a feeling of seamless movement into and out of the pause, staying with this simple practice for several rounds of breath.

5. Explore antara kumbhaka, retaining the inhalations for a few seconds.

6. Hold the breath with as little effort as possible while tuning in to the shifting sensations in your body and mental awareness.

7. In transitioning into the exhalation, the tendency is for the breath to rush out; if that happens, try a shorter duration of retention.

8. After one antara kumbhaka, do several rounds of ujjayi pranayama, restoring the lungs to their natural condition. The rhythm of inhalation and exhalation should be smooth and steady before initiating further antara kumbhaka.

9. Next, gradually lengthen the duration of retention, but only so far as there is no strain, imbalance in inhalations and exhalations, or gripping or collapsing in the lungs.

10. Explore expanding the retention by one or two counts in each sitting, eventually holding the breath as long as you can with complete comfort.

11. When you can easily retain the breath for fifteen seconds, you can fully develop the antara kumbhaka practice by engaging mula bandha, uddiyana bandha, and jalandhara bandha, thereby containing the pranic energy.

BAHYA KUMBHAKA

1. Begin bahya kumbhaka after you are at ease doing antara kumbhaka.

2. Start with ujjayi, bringing attention to the natural pause when empty of breath. Do several rounds of ujjayi, refining awareness of the movement in and out of that pause.

3. With the first few retentions of the exhalation, hold for just one count and then do several rounds of seamless ujjayi before repeating.

4. Gradually expand the count, staying with simple retention. Try to keep your eyes, face, throat, and heart center soft and not to grip in your belly.

5. Unlike inhalations, exhalations naturally stimulate mula bandha and uddiyana bandha. Explore activating the bandhas along with bahya kumbhaka, starting with trying to sustain mula bandha while breathing and retaining the breath.

6. Begin uddiyana bandha when you can comfortably hold the breath out for three counts. When pulling the belly back toward the spine and up toward the diaphragm, you may feel a gripping in the chest, throat, and head. If this happens, back off.

7. To release bahya kumbhaka, it is important first to completely relax the belly and thereby allow the diaphragm to do its natural work; then consciously ease the breath in.

8. If the breath rushes in, it was held in bahya kumbhaka for too long.

9. Gradually develop this practice by lengthening the duration of retention and by adding antara kumbhaka in the same rounds of breath.

10. Applying vritti pranayama to kumbhaka practice, first do sama in each of the four phases of the breath cycle: cultivate an equal duration in puraka, rechaka, antara kumbhaka, and bahya kumbhaka, starting with a three-count and gradually lengthening.

11. Pay close attention to the transitions between each phase while maintaining mental focus, emotional calm, and physical ease. When you can comfortably sustain this practice for a few minutes with at least a five-count in each phase, gradually begin visama vritti, varying the duration of puraka, rechaka, antara kumbhaka, and bahya kumbhaka in a gradual manner.

12. Working with breath ratios, start by increasing antara kumbhaka to 2:1 over puraka and rechaka, allowing the natural pause when empty of breath. Then gradually increase this ratio, working up to 4:1. When at 3:1, begin gradually extending the duration of rechaka eventually to a ratio of 2:1 over puraka.

13. Add bahya kumbhaka, starting with a two-count retention and working up to the same duration as puraka.

14. Continuing this practice, eventually puraka and bahya kumbhaka are the same duration, antara kumbhaka is 4:1 over puraka, and rechaka is 2:1 over puraka.

15. The tendency in this practice is to gasp for air; extend durations only as much as the rhythm remains steady.

After you have refined your vritti pranayama and kumbhaka practices, begin blending these practices, as follows.

Viloma: Against the Grain

The term *viloma*, which in literal translation means "anti-hair," refers to going against the natural line or movement of the breath. In viloma pranayama, one repeatedly pauses during puraka and/or rechaka while changing as little as possible in the positioning and engagement of the diaphragm, rib cage, and lungs. With practice, one's awareness is steady throughout each cycle of breath, the nerves calm and quiet in support of both flow and pause. Begin by sitting up comfortably tall and do several rounds of ujjayi pranayama, focusing on the balance and ease in the breath, then explore as follows:

1. After a complete exhalation, inhale to half your capacity and hold the breath there for a few seconds before completing the inhalation.

2. Repeat several times before adding a second interruption to the inhalation, continuing in this way until you reach five pauses, and only so long as there is no strain or fatigue.

3. Follow this with several rounds of ujjayi pranayama before resting in Savasana.

4. Next, repeat this exercise with pauses in the exhalations only. With each interruption, bring slightly greater awareness and engagement to mula bandha and a light, gradual uddiyana bandha.

5. When the lungs are empty, let the diaphragm relax and the belly draw farther back and up before easing into the inhalation.

6. After resting in Savasana for a few minutes, do viloma pranayama on both the inhalation and exhalation.

7. Experienced clients whose basic viloma pranayama is free of strain can do the full practice of this technique in which kumbhaka is performed.

8. Start with antara kumbhaka following a viloma pranayama inhalation in which there are one or more interruptions, keeping the diaphragm soft during the pauses.

9. With the antara kumbhaka, retain the inhalation for two or three seconds before rechaka, gradually holding for longer with mula bandha and uddiyana bandha.

10. After gradually developing this practice for up to ten minutes in each sitting, do viloma pranayama exhalations as described earlier, followed by bahya kumbhaka, gradually increasing the viloma interruptions and the length of bahya kumbhaka.

11. For the full practice of viloma pranayama, explore viloma inhalations and exhalations along with antara and bahya kumbhaka, slowly lengthening the practice.

Kapalabhati: Cultivating Light

Kapalabhati (from *kapala*, "skull," and *bhati*, "luster") pranayama energizes the entire body by tremendously oxygenating the blood supply and creating a feeling of exhilaration.[19] In natural breathing, the inhalation is active; that is, it is activated by muscles, whereas the exhalation is passive, resulting from contraction of the elastic lungs. This is reversed in kapalabhati pranayama: the exhalations are made active and inhalations passive. The technique described here is from the *Hatha Yoga Pradipika* (II.35). The *Gheranda Samhita* offers other forms of kapalabhati that blend this technique with nadi shodhana pranayama (which is covered in a bit).

1. Start by doing several rounds of ujjayi pranayama, warming and awakening the lungs while activating mula bandha.

2. After completion of an ujjayi exhalation, the breath is drawn in halfway and then rapidly and repeatedly blasted out through the nose, with a slight pause when empty of breath. The sound is in the nostrils, not the throat.

3. The inhalation happens naturally.

4. In the early development of this practice, do twenty-five rapid exhalations, then fill your lungs and perform antara kumbhaka for a few counts before releasing the breath and relaxing.

5. After this and each successive round, draw your attention to the sensations you feel in your head, perhaps sensing the calming and clearing effects of this practice.

6. Gradually increase to several minutes of sustained kapalabhati followed by kumbhakas.

7. Complete the kapalabhati practice with Savasana or move into the asana practice.

8. Explore kapalabhati sitting still, sitting while taking one to two minutes to reach the arms outward and up overhead, in Shishula Phalakasana (Dolphin Plank Pose) or in Ardha Navasana (Half Boat Pose).

Bhastrika: The Fiery Bellows Breath

Bhastrika ("bellows") pranayama is similar to kapalabhati, though more intense in fanning the flames of inner fire. Introduce clients to this technique only after they are comfortable in the kapalabhati practice. Here both the inhalations and exhalations are done through the nostrils vigorously and in rapid succession. Unlike kapalabhati, there is no pause after the exhalation.

1. Start sitting and doing ujjayi pranayama.

2. Initiate bhastrika by quickly blasting out the breath after a half inhalation.

3. Make the following inhalation just as strong and quick as the exhalation, followed by a strong and quick exhalation, completing one round of bhastrika. The sound should come from the nose, not the throat.

4. Do five to ten rounds, ending with an exhalation and several rounds of ujjayi pranayama, then repeat three or more times.

5. Gradually increase the number of cycles in each round and the number of rounds in each sitting, eventually sustaining bhastrika for five to ten minutes.

6. Rest in Savasana.

Sitali: Cooling Breath

The purpose of *sitali* ("cooling") pranayama is to cool and calm the physical body and mind. It can be done at any time, including during asana practice and after fiery pranayamas such as kapalabhati. Here the tongue is extended slightly out of the mouth and its sides curled up to form a channel. (The ability to create this channel is genetic; some people can do it, others can't. If you can't curl your tongue, visualize the curling and continue with the practice.) Explore as follows:

1. Sitting comfortably, close the eyes and relax.

2. Extend the tongue and curl its sides to create a channel for moisture.

3. Slowly and deeply draw in the breath across the tongue, sensing the breath becoming moist and cool as it passes across the tongue.

4. Then close the mouth and slowly exhale through the nose.

5. Repeat this ten times, then relax.

6. Gradually build up the sitali practice for up to fifteen minutes.

7. Over time explore variations that include antara kumbhaka (with mula bandha and jalandhara bandha) and viloma pranayama.

Anuloma and Pratiloma: Delicate Regulation of Breath

Anu, meaning "along with," and *prati*, meaning "against," give us pranayama practices in which one uses the fingers to delicately prolong the exhalations (in anuloma) and inhalations (in pratiloma). Done in stages, these practices help to cultivate stronger breath control amid deepening ease. Explore as follows:

1. Sit comfortably and do several rounds of ujjayi pranayama.

2. Beginning with anuloma pranayama, exhale completely and then slowly and deeply inhale through the nose.

3. At the crest of the inhalation, use the fingers to partially close the nostrils, being attentive to applying pressure evenly on each side of the nose.

4. Slowly and completely exhale, feeling the natural pause when empty of breath.

5. Release the fingers and take a deep inhalation, then reapply the fingers for a controlled exhalation. Make the exhalation about twice as long as the inhalation.

6. Continue for five to twenty minutes, then rest in Savasana.

7. For pratiloma pranayama, practice as described for anuloma, but switch to using the fingers and slowing the breath with the inhalations instead of the exhalations.

8. Experienced clients able to remain calm with basic anuloma pranayama and pratiloma pranayama can explore variations that include antara kumbhaka (with mula bandha and jalandhara bandha), bahya kumbhaka (with mula bandha, uddiyana bandha, and jalandhara bandha), viloma pranayama, and nadi shodhana (covered later).

Suryabheda: Stimulating Vitality

Suryabheda (from *surya*, "sun," and *bheda*, "to pierce") pranayama is said to pierce the pingalanadi and activate pranic energy. The pingalanadi receives prana through the right nostril. In suryabheda pranayama, the fingers are applied to the nostrils to regulate the breath:

1. Sit comfortably and do several rounds of ujjayi pranayama.

2. Draw the fingers to the nostrils as described in the following "Nadi Shodhana" section, blocking the left nostril.

3. Inhale slowly and deeply through the right nostril, close both nostrils, and perform antara kumbhaka for a few seconds with mula bandha and jalandhara bandha.

4. Release jalandhara bandha, open the left nostril, and exhale slowly and completely.

5. This completes one cycle of suryabheda pranayama. Repeat for up to thirty minutes, followed by Savasana.

6. Explore the permutations of viloma pranayama, as discussed earlier, with suryabheda.

Chandrabheda: Calming Energy

In chandrabheda (from *chandra*, "moon," and *bheda*, "to pierce") pranayama, energy is directed in through the left nostril to the ida nadi, calming the body and mind. The practice is precisely the opposite of suryabheda pranayama. There is nothing written about chandrabheda pranayama in the traditional Hatha yoga literature, but it is described in the *Yoga Chudamani Upanishad*.[20] Explore this practice with the same techniques applied in suryabheda, reversing sides and applying antara kumbhaka.

Nadi Shodhana: Alternate Nostril Breathing

The *Hatha Yoga Pradipika* and other classical yoga texts describe nadi shodhana pranayama without giving it this name. This practice is said to activate and balance the ida and pingalanadis and harmonize the hemispheres of the brain. In its basic form, nadi shodhana combines puraka as performed in pratiloma and rechaka as in anuloma. More advanced variations add kumbhakas and bandhas.[21] This highly contemplative practice is, as B. K. S. Iyengar puts it, "one of delicate adjustments. The brain and the fingers must learn to act together in channeling the in and out breaths while in constant communication with each other."[22] It is, he continues, "the most difficult, complex, and refined of all pranayamas. It is the ultimate in sensitive self-observation and control. When refined to its subtlest level it takes one to the innermost self." Explore this technique as follows:[23]

1. Sit comfortably and practice ujjayi pranayama for a few minutes.

2. Place the fingertips on one side of the nose, the thumb on the other side, just below the slight notch about halfway down the side of the nose. Try to place the fingers with even pressure on the left and right sides of the nose, maintaining steady contact while keeping the nostrils fully open.

3. While continuing ujjayi pranayama, play with slightly varying the pressure of the fingers, becoming more sensitive to the effects of the fine finger adjustments.

TECHNIQUE 1: BASIC NADI SHODHANA (WITH SURYABHEDA AND CHANDRABHEDA PRANAYAMA)

1. After a complete exhalation, close the left nostril and slowly inhale through the right.

2. At the crest of the inhalation, close the right nostril and slowly exhale through the left.

3. Empty of breath, fully inhale through the left, close the left, and exhale through the right.

4. Continue with this initial form of alternate nostril breathing for up to five minutes, cultivating the smooth and steady flow of the breath while remaining relaxed and calm.

TECHNIQUE 2: NADI SHODHANA WITH VILOMA PRANAYAMA

1. Begin as described for Technique 1 and do two or three rounds of basic nadi shodhana.

2. After a complete exhalation through the right nostril, inhale through the right to the halfway point of the inhalation, firmly close both nostrils and hold for a few seconds, then slowly complete the inhalation through the right nostril.

3. Whenever cued to hold the breath, use the fingers to close both nostrils.

4. Exhaling through the left nostril, stop halfway, hold the breath for a few seconds, then complete the exhalation through the left nostril.

5. Inhaling through the left nostril, hold at the halfway point for a few seconds, then complete the inhalation through the left nostril.

6. Exhaling through the right nostril, stop halfway, hold the breath for a few seconds, then complete the exhalation through the right nostril.

7. This completes one round. Explore deepening this practice by adding pauses and lengthening their duration, eventually pausing five times on each side for ten seconds each.

8. Make the steady, comfortable flow of the breath more important than the number or duration of pauses.

TECHNIQUE 3: NADI SHODHANA WITH KUMBHAKAS

1. Begin as described for Technique 1 and do two or three rounds of basic nadi shodhana.

2. Start with antara kumbhaka. After a complete exhalation through the right nostril, slowly inhale through the right nostril and hold the breath in for a

few seconds, closing both nostrils and engaging mula bandha and jalandhara bandha.

3. Maintaining mula bandha, release jalandhara bandha and slowly ease the breath out through the left nostril.

4. Ease the breath in through the left nostril and hold the breath in for a few seconds, closing both nostrils and engaging mula bandha and jalandhara bandha.

5. Maintaining mula bandha, release jalandhara bandha and slowly ease the breath out through the right nostril. Continue for several cycles.

6. Add bahya kumbhaka. Continuing as just described, at the end of the exhalation hold the breath out and engage uddiyana bandha, as described in introducing bahya kumbhaka.

7. Completely release uddiyana bandha before easing in the breath. Continue for several cycles, exploring longer retention with both antara and bahya (up to thirty seconds with antara and fifteen seconds with bahya).

TECHNIQUE 4: NADI SHODHANA WITH VILOMAS AND KUMBHAKAS

1. Start with the practice described in Technique 1, adding viloma pauses.

2. Start with one pause for a few seconds, then add more pauses, each held for a few seconds. When comfortable with three pauses held for three seconds each on both the inhalations and exhalations, add antara and bahya kumbhakas for a few seconds.

3. Gradually lengthen the pauses and retentions, working up to five pauses of five seconds each, antara kumbhaka of thirty seconds, and bahya kumbhaka of fifteen seconds.

TECHNIQUE 5: NADI SHODHANA WITH KAPALABHATI PRANAYAMA

1. This innovative pranayama technique should be practiced only when comfortable with the previous nadi shodhana practices. The effect is far more intense than the other techniques. Practice only as strongly as you can remain calm and quiet inside.

2. Do five rounds of nadi shodhana as described in Technique 1. After a complete exhalation, inhale halfway through the right nostril, keep the left nostril closed, and engage mula bandha.

3. Repeatedly and quickly blast the breath out through the right nostril for up to one minute (eventually several minutes), as described for kapalabhati pranayama.

4. Inhale deeply through the right nostril and hold the breath, antara kumbhaka, for as long as can be comfortably maintained, then slowly exhale through the left nostril. Inhale through the left and exhale through the right.

5. Do several rounds of soft ujjayi pranayama and switch sides.

6. Rest in Savasana.

Consciously Cultivating Energy

The heart of yoga practice is the conscious awakening and movement of energy that creates a feeling of being fully alive and aware of the wholeness of one's being in the world. Although asana practice is an essential part of this awakening, conscious pranayama most distinguishes yoga from physical exercise. If all you do in practicing yoga is breathe consciously and feel yourself more subtly and holistically through the breath as you explore in the universe of your bodymind and spirit, you will be healthier. Blending pranayama practices with asana practices and meditation will take you even further along the path of living joyfully and consciously.

Table 21.1: When and to Whom to Teach Pranayama

PRANAYAMA TECHNIQUE	WHEN	WHO
Natural Breathing	Excellent way to initiate all practices.	All clients.
Ujjayi	Teach at the beginning of every practice.	All clients.
Sama Vritti	Teach in conjunction with natural breathing and ujjayi.	All clients.
Visama Vritti	Teach in conjunction with natural breathing and ujjayi.	All clients.
Antara Kumbhaka	Teach in conjunction with ujjayi as a means of expanding and refining breath capacity.	Clients at ease with ujjayi and experienced with bandhas; *not* for clients who are experiencing eye or ear complaints, or for those with high blood pressure.
Bahya Kumbhaka	After developing ease with antara kumbhaka.	Clients at ease with ujjayi and experienced with bandhas; *not* for clients who are pregnant, experiencing eye or ear complaints, or for those with high blood pressure.

PRANAYAMA TECHNIQUE	WHEN	WHO
Viloma	Teach in conjunction with ujjayi as a means of expanding and refining breath capacity.	All clients, especially when experiencing fatigue or anxiety.
Kapalabhati	Teach at the beginning of practice to stimulate energy, awaken the breath, and more quickly warm the body; teach during asana sequences, especially as part of core awakening. If taught during asanas, teach with students who are either seated, ideally in Hero Pose (Virasana) or in Dolphin Plank Pose (Shishula Phalakasana).	Not for clients who are pregnant, experiencing eye or ear complaints, or for those with high blood pressure.
Bhastrika	Teach in a pranayama class or as a final energizing practice immediately before Savasana.	Not for clients who are pregnant, experiencing eye or ear complaints, or for those with high blood pressure.
Sitali	Whenever you sense clients can benefit from cooling.	All clients.
Anuloma	Pranayama classes.	Clients familiar and comfortable with ujjayi.
Pratiloma	Pranayama classes.	Clients familiar and comfortable with ujjayi.
Surya Bheda	Teach in conjunction with ujjayi.	All clients.
Chandra Bheda	Traditionally practiced on alternate days from suryabheda.	All clients.
Nadi Shodhana 1	Beginning of practice.	Experienced clients.
Nadi Shodhana 2	When comfortable, steady, and at ease with Technique 1.	Experienced clients.
Nadi Shodhana 3	When comfortable, steady, and at ease with Technique 2.	Clients at ease with ujjayi and experienced with bandhas; *not* for clients who are pregnant, experiencing eye or ear complaints, or for those with high blood pressure.
Nadi Shodhana 4	When comfortable, steady, and at ease with Technique 3.	Same as above.
Nadi Shodhana 5	When comfortable, steady, and at ease with Technique 4.	Same as above.

22

Meditation Practice

AS PART OF THE BEAUTY of yoga, meditation is the seed that can always immediately blossom into the thousand-petal lotus flower of happiness, wellness, and fullness as an awakened human being. It is both the ultimate form of yoga practice and an integral part of the entire path of discovering, loving, healing, and transforming the totality of one's being, and in this respect, it provides an essential means of healing. All the various paths of practice lead to meditation becoming a deeper yet easier method of feeling whole within one's self and connected as part of the whole of the universe. In meditating, we open the windows of the mind to clearer consciousness. To the extent that we refine the temple of the physical body through consistent asana practice, it gives us more unwavering support in allowing the windows to open smoothly. Similarly, consistent pranayama practices awaken subtle energy in a way that creates a stronger inner invitation to the currents of clear awareness, leading to a lighter and more balanced sense of being. Yet to meditate, we do not have to wait for some requisite level of asana or pranayama practice; rather, we can meditate without ever having done a single asana.

Many people say they can't meditate because their minds won't stop chattering. Frustrated, they often give up exploring meditation. This mindset expresses the common misunderstanding that meditating means having no thoughts. Although moving into inner stillness is one of the many fruits of meditation practice, it is not the goal of the practice itself. In fact, there doesn't have to be a goal. Much like the asana practice, when we go into meditation with a specific goal in mind, such as a perfectly quiet mind, it is frustrating because even the most practiced meditators have only rare moments of complete inner quiet and stillness. If, just like the asana practice, we practice meditation as a process of self-exploration, self-discovery, and self-transformation, we can experience the joy of it the first moment we try.

My first meditation teacher, Alan Watts, whose mid-1970s radio broadcasts offered mind-blowing kernels of insight into Eastern spiritual philosophy and practices, offered simple analogies to drive home the point that meditation is a process. "When we dance," he said, "the journey itself is the point. When we play music, the playing itself is the point, and the same is true of meditation. Meditation is the discovery that the point of life is always arrived at in the immediate moment." He thought that meditation should be enjoyable, not a chore. "It is an appreciation of the present, a kind of 'grooving' with the eternal now, and it brings us into a state of peace where we can understand that the point of life, the place where it is at, is simply here and now."[1] This take on meditation reflects a Buddhist influence; since thoughts will always come and go, much like clouds floating by overhead, they are something to play with. Interested without being attached, the playful practice of watching is the practice.

The Buddhist nun Pema Chödrön comments that by meditating we come to four realizations: (1) thoughts have no birthplace, (2) they are unceasing, (3) they appear but are not solid, which, since there's nothing to react to, together lead to (4) awareness of "complete openness."[2] But what about the *Yoga Sutra*, which defines yoga practice as *chitta vritti nirodha*, "to still the fluctuations of the mind"? The problem is that we do react to our thoughts, despite knowing they are just thoughts, and it is in these reactions that we find ourselves distracted, suffering, confused, unhappy, or hurting. The ancient yogis identified this problem as *klesha*, a deep form of confused perception. Traditional yoga philosophy, much like Buddhism, holds out the hope that through its practices, from asana and mantra to pranayama and puja, we can come to a place of samadhi, a blissful state free of thoughts where we realize our true self.[3]

Although the various strands of yoga philosophy offer different maps to attaining samadhi, most offer a path through pratyahara, dharana, and dhyana. Here we will consider these as useful tools for helping clients cultivate clearer self-awareness, self-understanding, and self-acceptance, which, taken together, tend to yield a steadier, easier, and ultimately healthier and more meaningful life. But rather than looking on all this as leading to certain promised outcomes, it is more fruitful to explore these tools as sources for guiding clients into deeper insight right here and now.[4] After looking at this classical yoga meditation process, we will explore how to infuse asana sessions with other practical meditation techniques, offering a variety of ways to help your clients discover the full joy of meditation as a healing practice.

Patanjali's Isolation Path: Pratyahara, Dharana, Dhyana

Earlier we explored Patanjali's eight-limbed path of yoga, which begins with essentially material practices: yamas to guide us in our social relations, niyamas for our intrapersonal life, asana and pranayama as tools of awakening that prepare us for a deeper journey into the self. Yet with these practices we are still scratching the surface, still working with *bahiranga*, the external life of the senses. Moving into the mystical realm of samadhi first requires relieving our senses of their external distractions, developing a single-pointed mental concentration, and then a meditative state. This is the path from bahiranga to *antaranga*, or internal meditative practice. In this traditional yogic view, before stepping into meditation and blissful supraconsciousness, we must first cross a bridge departing the material realm of sense awareness. Patanjali describes this practice as *pratyahara*, detaching at will from the senses. We are led to this bridge by following the path of yama, niyama, asana, and pranayama. Nothing is forced as we abide in the self-revealing truth of our being along this path. With asana we finally come to the physical and mental health that allows us to work easily and steadily with the breath; as we refine the breath and cultivate the life-force energy of prana, then "all that veils clarity of perception is swept away… and thought becomes fit for concentration." But before we can completely concentrate, we must tame the mind's attachment to the awakening of our senses. As Patanjali notes, "Withdrawal of the senses occurs when the sensory organs, independent of their objects, conform to the nature of the mind."[5] In other words, we can bring our mind into its own inner space, freed from external stimulation. Only then can we can completely concentrate.

It is helpful to offer clients a backdrop to pratyahara. Wherever we are, there are always sounds, sights, aromas, and other vibrations entering our senses—or, put differently, to which our senses are attaching. When you're sitting in class, it is likely that sounds are reaching you from outside and from others in the room. If there is any light, then there are visual impressions coming about through the eyes. The heart is felt beating in the chest, clothing or a draft is felt on the skin, and perhaps there is a sense of more subtle energy pulsating through one's entire being. There are all these vibrations, what Alan Watts termed "so many happenings."[6] With pratyahara, the idea is to just let them all be there. Sounds and other vibrations will come and go. Meanwhile, there are the happenings of the mind, habitually taking all these vibrations and reacting to them with more thoughts. The thoughts are also reacting to other thoughts. The mind is typically chattering away, reactively and imaginatively adding more vibrations. Without focusing on the breath or anything else, just following the breath as another source of vibration, you will notice that when empty of breath there is a natural quieting, an opening to the bridge from the world of the senses to the world of the true self. Staying in that awareness, without thinking about it, you are on the other side, the inside, in pratyahara, even as vibrations intrude.

So how do we guide students to stay inside without thinking about it and reintroducing intrusions? This is the practice of *dharana*, single-pointed focus of concentration. By intently focusing the mind on one thing, there's no space for anything else. It doesn't matter what you focus on. Commenting on Patanjali's advice that we "concentrate wherever the mind finds satisfaction," Sally Kempton suggests that we can recognize satisfaction when the experience is one of natural joy, peace, and relaxation. "If you have to work too hard at it," she writes, "that may be a sign that it is the wrong practice for you."[7] In concentrating, a person is aware that he or she is concentrating, aware of being in the practice of single-pointed awareness, conscious of being a meditator who is meditating.

In traditional dharana practice, the focus is a mantra, "a tool for the mind,"[8] but it could be the breath or, as we'll explore shortly, even an activity such as gardening or surfing in which our attention is wholly connected with what we're doing. For many years, I found my mind quite satisfied—in a state of natural joy, peace, and relaxation—when fully concentrating on carefully placing my foot on a tiny lip of granite on the face of a cliff hundreds of feet off the ground, my life literally in the balance. In this intense circumstance, I was definitely in the moment. What about complete concentration in less intense circumstances? Around this period I also had the privilege of sharing time with a group of visiting Tibetan Buddhist monks I was working with in the juvenile facilities of the County of Los Angeles. When we were together one weekend I suggested hiking to a tranquil meditation spot on top of a mountain overlooking the Pacific Ocean. They openly laughed at this idea, gently admonishing me that one could just as easily meditate while washing the dishes.[9] Although I appreciated their experience and wisdom, it also occurred to me that I hadn't grown up meditating in Dharamsala, India, and wasn't at their level of easy concentration. I was still with the yogis of old who had discovered that when we repeat a word or phrase over and over, it not only occupies our mental space, but opens an inner rhythm of quieting awareness. In some meditation traditions, the mantra is said to contain "the throb of shakti," the "original pulsation of divine energy that creates the universe and remains embedded within every particle of it."[10] Whether or not that is what is happening with mantra practice, one thing is clear: focusing the mind on a single thing, whether it's repetition of a word or phrase or following the breath or some other recurrent energy, the effect is a steadier mind in which thought slows down.

At the heart of Patanjali's approach to meditation is the idea that a steadier mind is a clearer mind. Clarity arises when "the senses are perfectly mastered" through pratyahara and dharana, bringing us further along the path to the pure meditative state of dhyana, "a current of unified thought."[11] In this state of consciousness, the truth of one's being as an expression of pure love is made manifest, as "perfect concentration on the heart reveals the contents of the mind."[12] Mantra now disappears as the person's awareness is completely at one with the divine (spirit, nature, the universe, the Self). "When purity of the peaceful mind is identical with that of the spiritual entity," Patanjali relates, "that is liberation."[13] Free of external stimulation, present in the moment, there is only the truth of one's being as love and light. There is a sense of directly knowing the essence of whatever one is meditating on, of being part of the whole of existence.

Where does this effort lead? *Samadhi*. The various origins of the term are insightful: *sam* ("together"), *a* ("toward"), and *dha* ("to get"); *sama* ("equal") and *dhi* ("intellect"). In either case, *samadhi* means moving into a sense of wholeness and balanced awareness. Pure bliss. The eight-limbed path of Patanjali's raja yoga is the classical formulation of moving into this state of blissful being. There are many other schools of yogic thought with different approaches to samadhi, ranging from laya samadhi's trance dance into joy to the vaishnava bhakti yogis' pathway through purely devotional love of God.[14] But as exemplified by the Tibetan Buddhists visiting Los Angeles several years ago, it's entirely possible to find that state of bliss doing practically anything. What Patanjali and others have bequeathed to us are some practical tools that we are free to adapt and apply in our lives here and now in ways that make blissful being that much more abundant and accessible.

Taking One Seat

When Patanjali summarized the received wisdom of earlier yoga traditions in the *Yoga Sutra*, he was succinct on asana: sthira sukham asanam. In earlier chapters we have focused on steadiness and ease. *Asanam*, "to take one seat," is a foundation for *chitta vritti nirodha*, "to still the fluctuations of the mind." Regular asana practice creates a foundation for the physical steadiness and ease we want when sitting in meditation. Similarly, refining the breath and cultivating life-force energy through pranayama yields more naturally awakened awareness in meditation. Through these practices we can sit more comfortably tall with the spine in its natural form, the heart center spacious, and the breath flowing effortlessly; pratyahara comes more naturally, it is easier to stay with dharana, and dhyana appears more frequently and stays longer.

In helping clients set up for seated meditation, ask them to choose a comfortable sitting position. The most important quality in sitting is comfort; over time, alignment of the spine will lead to greater comfort in sitting for longer periods. With practice, most clients will eventually be able to sit on top of their sitting bones with a neutral pelvis that allows their spine to be more easily held naturally erect. For some clients, this requires a chair, high cushion, or wall for back support. Over time and with practice (along with a supportive lifestyle and favorable genetics), students may find they are able to sit comfortably in Padmasana (Lotus Pose), the ultimate asana for sitting (although few Westerners, including those with lifelong meditation practices, can sit in this position for extended periods, perhaps because of having grown up sitting in

chairs, and as a consequence, they can injure their hips when sitting in Padmasana).
Guide clients into sitting with whatever props it takes to establish and maintain a
neutral pelvis; then ask them to consciously root down into their sitting bones, feeling
how that grounding action leads to a taller spine, more open heart center, more natural flow of breath, and a sense of their head floating on top of their spine. Exploring
this stable and eventually more sustainable position, ask clients to feel their spine and
the crown of their head extending taller as they feel more grounded through their
sitting bones, from there allowing the shoulder blades to release down their back
and their chin to release slightly down. The palms can rest together in the lap or in a
mudra on the knees.[15]

Six Guided Meditation Techniques

All the basic meditation techniques involve focusing the mind on a single thing. Here
we look at six different guided meditations using various objects of attention. Each
approach tends to evoke different qualities of meditative awareness. Play around with
how these feel in your own meditation practice before exploring them with clients.
Explore doing each technique at different times of the day, in different moods, before
and after practicing asanas, and after experimenting with some of the pranayama
techniques described in Chapter 21. As with the asana practice, there is no one correct
or best path, only infinite paths that you and your clients will find different and that
change in resonance across the course of your lives.

ONE: BREATH AS MANTRA[16]

1. Sit comfortably tall, drawing your attention to the breath.

2. Allow the breath to flow softly and quietly, simply watching it without trying
   to change it in any way.

3. Feel and visualize the breath flowing in through your nostrils, down through
   your throat, and into your lungs, receiving the breath as a pure form of beauty
   or a gift from the universe of the divine.

4. As easily and naturally as the breath flows into your body, let it flow back out
   just as effortlessly, a sense of giving back the gift we all share.

5. Allow your mind to become completely absorbed in the flow of the breath,
   noticing how and where it arises and what it feels like along the way.

6. When your mind wanders away from the breath, gently bring it back to the
   steadiness, the rhythmic flow of your inhales and exhales.

7. Staying fully absorbed in the breath and allowing it to continue flowing freely, notice the natural pauses between each inhale and exhale.

8. Notice the natural quieting and stilling of the mind that happens when you are empty of breath, allowing that sense of quiet to ride along with the following inhale.

9. At the crest of your inhale, feel a sense of the rising quiet expand into a feeling of openness and spaciousness in your mind, and just as simply let the breath flow out.

10. Stay with it, continuously coming back to the feeling of your thoughts as though enveloped in the breath, at one with the breath as it flows in and out of your body.

TWO: ACOUSTICAL MANTRA

1. Choose a mantra that works for you. If this is your first mantra meditation, consider using the words inhale-exhale or so-hum: *so* meaning "that," *hum* meaning "I am." Although you can use any word, keep it simple and consider using words that you want to embed more deeply in your consciousness, such as calm, clear, peace, or love. If you feel a deeper resonance using ancient Sanskrit words, try *aum* or *shanti* ("peace").

2. Do the breath-focused meditation for a few minutes, letting your awareness settle into the natural flow of the breath.

3. After completing an exhale, with your inhale, slowly say the word *inhale* (or *so*) while absorbing your awareness in the word, not the breath.

4. As easily as the breath draws in, allow it to flow out while saying the word *exhale* (or *hum*).

5. As with the breath meditation, notice and allow the natural stillness that happens in the pauses between the breaths. Then just as the breath moves, begin repeating the mantra.

6. As with all meditation techniques, your mind will wander—it will think. This is what it is good at and likes to do! Without thinking about the thoughts or judging yourself for thinking (or for judging), come right back to the mantra.

7. Rather than jumping from one mantra to another, stay with one for at least ten sessions to see what happens. One of the benefits of repetition is that the words themselves become less and less significant, the sound of the mantra in your mind gradually becoming like a neutral vibration, the "grooving" awareness described by Alan Watts.[17]

THREE: COUNTING[18]

1. Do the breath-focused meditation for a few minutes, letting your awareness settle into the natural flow of the breath.

2. With an inhale, say *one hundred* to yourself as the breath draws in, then say *ninety-nine* to yourself as it flows out.

3. With the next cycle of breath say *ninety-eight* with your inhale and *ninety-seven* with your exhale, continuing in this way until exhaling on *fifty-one*.

4. As other words and thoughts intrude, just come back to breathing and counting down.

5. Now inhale and exhale saying a single number to yourself, starting with stretching *fifty* across one complete cycle of inhale-exhale, continuing in this way until exhaling on *twenty-one*.

6. After exhaling on *twenty-one*, stop counting and simply follow the breath. As words and thoughts arise, just watch and come back to the breath.

7. Continue sitting and watching for longer than it would have taken to count down to zero, noticing how the mind slows and quiets along the way.

FOUR: CHAKRAS

1. Do the breath-focused meditation for a few minutes, letting your awareness settle into the natural flow of the breath.

2. More consciously grounding down through the sitting bones, bring more awareness to the floor of the pelvis, feeling with each breath a deepening sense of stability and rootedness. Watching the breath, with each exhale say to yourself *lam*, visualizing the vibrations of that silent sound stirring the upward release of energy, drawing in the energy of the earth. Repeat the mantra five times, bringing consciousness to the muladhara chakra.

3. Staying with the breath, bring your awareness up into the center of your pelvis, opening your imagination to the deep reservoir of creativity resting in the svadhisthana chakra. With each of five exhales, say the word *vam* to yourself while visualizing that silent sound stimulating your creative juices. Feel the richness of that creativity deepen with each sound of vam.

4. Drawing your awareness to the center of your belly, sense the latent determination resting in the manipura chakra. With each of five exhales, say the word *ram* to yourself, visualizing the vibrations of that silent sound sparking the fire of willful consciousness that opens you to easier laughter and joy.

5. Breathing as though you are doing it through your spiritual heart center, tap into feeling the love that you are in your essence. Connected with the breath, with each of five exhales, say the word *ham* to yourself, visualizing the vibrations of that silent sound opening your heart to the light and wisdom pulsating there along with each beat of your heart, each breath a sense of the love that you are radiating from your anahata chakra all through and around you.

6. With your awareness resting in the light of love and innate wisdom, draw your awareness to your throat, imagining your every word arising from the love and wisdom in your heart. Following the breath, with each of five exhales, say the word *vam* to yourself, visualizing the vibrations of that silent sound emanating from the vishuddha chakra creating a peaceful resonance with all the other sounds in the universe.

7. Feeling energy drawing up from the base of your spine, through your heart, and to your third eye, imagine light drawing into your third eye, opening your inner visual landscape to the purity of light. With each of five exhales, say the word *kesham* to yourself, visualizing the vibrations of that silent sound opening your ajna chakra to clearer awareness of yourself and your connection with the universe.

8. Now let your awareness rest more gently in the breath, feeling a sense of blissful being as energy rises effortlessly from the base of your pelvis out through the crown of your head. Visualize a feeling of the crown of your head opening like a thousand-petal lotus flower, the sahasrara chakra expanding the light of your being. Stay with it, with a sense of being whole and complete in this moment of blissful being.

FIVE: LIGHT

1. Either following the chakra meditation or breath meditation, draw your palms together at your heart in a prayer position, anjali mudra, the reverence seal.

2. Bring your awareness to the sense of energy rising from the base of your spine and out through the crown of your head. Imagine this energy like warm white light beaming out toward the sky.

3. With your awareness resting in the effortless breath and keeping your palms together, with an inhale raise your palms up past your face and slowly overhead through that beam of light, grounding down while reaching toward the sky, spaciousness all through you.

4. As you exhale, slowly extend your arms out and down, a sense of drawing that light out and around you as you bring the backs of your hands to rest softly on

your knees, feeling a sense of being warmly enveloped as though in a cocoon of nourishing light.

5. Staying with the breath, spread your fingers and palms wide open, a sense of radiating energetically from your heart center out through your fingertips and the crown of your head.

6. Bringing the tips of your thumbs and index fingers together into jnana mudra, let your thumbs symbolize all that you consider divine or beautiful in the universe, your index fingers all that is divine or beautiful in yourself, the touching of your thumbs and fingertips representing that yoking, the union, the whole of these qualities.

7. Breathing and following the natural flow of the breath, allow the three extended fingers on each hand to represent your release of the illusions in your life that keep you from feeling more whole, happy, and complete—the ego, fear, anger, and greed giving way to contentment and clarity of being.

8. Staying in the light of this awareness, keep following the breath, breath by effortless breath creating a sense of deepening self-awareness and self-acceptance in this perfect moment.

SIX: MALA

1. Holding a string of mala beads (108 beads) across the middle finger of your left hand, palms resting in your lap or on your knees, do the breath meditation for a few minutes.

2. Placing your thumb against the *semuru* (head bead), as the breath draws in, circle your thumb around the next bead.

3. As the breath flows out, use your thumb to move the mala to the next bead, circling it with your thumb as the breath flows in, rotating the mala to the next bead as the breath flows out.

4. Continue in this fashion until completing one mala, eventually going around 108 times.

5. In using your thumb to move the beads, become completely absorbed in doing just that, opening your awareness to each gentle push from your thumb drawing the energy of the divine, or the essence of nature, deeper into your consciousness.

When to Meditate

One can meditate at any time and place. When teaching classes, we can offer brief or extended periods of seated meditation at the beginning or end of class. Amid the flow of the class, you can always bring the students to samasthihi or to sitting for a few moments of self-reflective meditation. Going beyond asana classes, you may want to offer classes devoted entirely to meditation or a combination of pranayama and meditation. When you give clients more meditation tools for healing, they can also explore the time and settings they find the most conducive to deeper meditation. Most people find the most natural inner peace and quiet in the early morning hours, before the day fills their mind with new thoughts. Others find the asana-pranayama practice lends to the most favorable inner conditions for meditation. Here we will look at one approach to bringing meditation into the asana-pranayama practice itself.

Meditating amid the Body and Breath

In guiding meditation, we want to help clients explore at a place of safe, tolerable intensity in their physical, mental, and emotional experience because pure consciousness is especially close to us in moments of intensity, moments that might seem the opposite of peace. The entire yogic paradigm is based on the idea that there is something vast, loving, and spacious in the heart of reality; the practice is to live from that vast spacious source, going to the very core of ourselves to reveal the totality of our experience and dissolve it to its essence. Anything in our experience can provide a doorway to this quality of consciousness; developing the fortitude to hold steady with this intensity can bring us to a place of synchronicity, so we are not "doing" yoga but just being in that state of grace, in that awareness that it is all just happening.[19] This is where tantric awareness utilizing micropractices can gain practical traction, and where tantra brings deeper meditative awareness to the flow of asanas.

A good example of this: standing asana sequences. In most classes, we usually do standing asanas after warming up the entire body with Sun Salutations *(Surya Namaskara)* or other dynamic movements. The standing asanas continue to heat the body while opening and strengthening the hips and legs. But if you teach an inappropriately long, sustained sequence of standing poses requiring strength mostly from one leg, then muscle fatigue will eventually set in, compromising neuromuscular functioning and leading to the wrong muscles being recruited to do the required work. If you are coaching your students to "go for it" or to "push harder to find your true self," strain or even serious injury is probably not an "if" but a "when."

Surely our own thoughts can misguide us in various ways, leading us either to push too hard or to shy away from challenges, usually reflecting to some degree the behavioral patterns in our larger lives. One of the purposes of doing yoga is to cultivate a clearer mind and more balanced life. This clarity arises in the practice of yoga asana with the interplay of bodymind and breath, especially as we "play the edge" of the intensity of the experience with increasingly subtle awareness of what we are feeling. Ignore the feeling and there you are, back in the world of aerobics, or maybe yogarobics.

There is a far deeper level in guiding a yoga practice as one of conscious awakening to spirit, bliss, or inner peace. The key is in:

- Working with what we are feeling in the totality of our experience.

- Exploring, going with that feeling to a place of tolerable intensity.

- Opening oneself through refined breath, nuanced movement, and a sense of settling into stillness to experience a greater sense of spaciousness around that intensity.

- Tapping more deeply into the source(s) of our feeling/experience.

- Moving along with our shifting edge as our bodymind and breath invite us into a sense of expanded awareness, openness, inner strength, and harmony.

In applying this approach to the experiences in an asana practice, we can embrace the fullness of energy in a way that makes the asana practice itself a form of meditation. When fully absorbed in the flowing connection of breath and bodymind, we come to experience the present moment in a nonthinking state of awareness so direct that it leads to spontaneity and gives way to a joy that is no longer dependent on external circumstances of freedom or attainment. This is the essence of tantra as expressed in Hatha yoga. Creating the inner space to really feel takes us to the core of our being by including everything in our experience—the feeling of our feet grounding into the earth, the rhythmic pulsation of the breath and heart, the vibration of energy in our legs and through the spine, the emotions and thoughts swirling all through and around us—bringing us ever closer to a sense of essence. This practice fruitfully and ultimately extends well off the mat. In the simplest of experiences—tasting an apple, riding a bicycle, weeding the garden, standing in Tadasana, flowing from Up Dog to Down Dog—it is the same: to be conscious, to give yourself the space to breathe completely, to feel completely, to move with intuitive spontaneity in each moment of freedom and find there more bliss for an expanding moment amid a deepening sense of healing resonance and well-being.

Part V

Healing Common Conditions

AFTER ALL THE HISTORY AND philosophy, theory and methodology, practices and techniques, we come to the realities of human conditions. Here we apply yoga therapy's primary tools of asana, pranayama, and meditation to healing what might ail us. The application of these tools is ideally informed by all we have covered thus far. As we look at a wide array of musculoskeletal, mental health, and reproductive issues, constant mantras must be to do no harm, to be truthful in what we share, and to give with loving-kindness. Honoring these values will take us furthest in supporting our clients in healing.

23

Healing Musculoskeletal Conditions

THE MOST AILMENTS WE FIND in yoga are musculoskeletal. Many occur while doing yoga asanas, although many others are caused by activity (or inactivity) separate from yoga. Here we address the most common conditions.

Feet, Ankle, and Lower Leg Issues

Plantar Fasciitis

We begin with our roots, the bottom of the feet, where we most feel and establish our physical sense of grounding to the Earth. The foot is a highly complex biomechanical structure that consists of twenty-six bones and surrounding tissues that when healthy transfer our weight to the ground with balance, stability, and ease. The fleshy bottom of the foot consists of muscles and ligaments, including a flat weblike band of tissue that extends from the heel bone (at the calcaneal tuberosity) to the toes (at the distal heads of the metatarsal bones). The truer term for this tough ligamentous structure is *plantar aponeurosis,* which, by virtue of surrounding and connecting to bones (as connective tissue) and to the dermis of the skin, is also considered fascia. The springlike tension arising from the connection of its pliable-yet-strong collagen fibers between the heel and toes contributes significantly to longitudinal arch strength when the foot bears weight while also making one's gait more energy efficient.

THE PAINFUL EXPERIENCE

The painful pathological condition of plantar fasciitis is due to the structural breakdown of the collagen aponeurosis tissues—microtears and scarring, not inflammation as was thought until recently,[1] even though it causes inflammation. The pain typically occurs in one foot (not both), and worsens after rest (it is often most acutely and severely felt after rest, especially when taking the first few steps in the morning). If the pain persists at night, it is a possible sign of arthritis, nerve impingement, a stress fracture, or tarsal tunnel syndrome, and thus might not be a symptom of plantar fasciitis. With plantar fasciitis, point tenderness primarily tends to occur nearest the front of the heel where the aponeurosis attaches to the heel bone (calcaneous) as well as along the center of the bone. Pain tends to increase when drawing the toes toward the shin in dorsiflexion. It is also common with plantar fasciitis to find an abnormal bone spur at precisely the point where the aponeurosis attaches to the heel, where a protective bursa sac will typically develop and cause further pain.

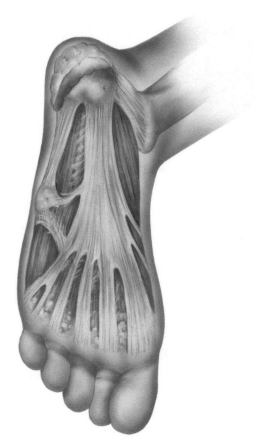

Figure 23.1: The Plantar Aponeurosis

THE KNOWN CAUSES

We often find contrasting or even conflicting assertions for the cause of this tissue breakdown and the consequent inflammation and pain, ranging from overuse to under use. There is a growing body of evidence that there are indeed many causes,[2] including excessive pressure in high-impact activities such as running, but also from obesity, heel spurs, long periods of standing, weak ankles (and interrelated collapsed medial arches), and age-related deterioration. It is also associated with tight calf muscles and tightness in the Achilles tendons, hypertonic feet, high arches or flat feet, and leg length discrepancy.

HOW IT HEALS

Although most cases of plantar fasciitis self-resolve with time and simple treatment (rest, ice, heat, weight reduction, and calf stretching and strengthening), if left unattended it can become a chronic and highly debilitating condition. Compensatory actions (modified walking or running gait) can then transfer up the body into ankle, knee, hip, and sacroiliac and lumbar spinal segment joints, causing imbalance, strain, and pain in those joints along with more general physical discomfort and thus diminished physical freedom.

The common conventional protocol for healing plantar fasciitis calls for gentle stretching, rest, and gentle use, as rest alone can result in further tightening of the affected tissues. When highly inflamed and chronic, most recommendations are for rest. The common prescription of ice for musculoskeletal injuries is now debated, with some medical researchers and healers claiming it reduces the body's natural inflammatory response and thus inhibits or delays healing. Medical doctors often prescribe nonsteroidal anti-inflammatory drugs (NSAIDs), which can effectively reduce inflammation and pain but may also detract from healing the underlying condition causing the inflammation and pain.

HEALING WITH ASANA PRACTICES

The primary focus of asana is on stretching and strengthening the calves (gastrocnemius and soleus muscles) and their tendon (the Achilles), along with small lower leg muscles whose actions or attachments affect the plantar aponeurosis. In the asanas suggested here, progress sequentially in the order in which they are presented.

DANDASANA (STAFF POSE) RESISTED ANKLE MOBILIZATIONS In setting up for the basic form of Dandasana, place a folded blanket, block, or other firm bolster under the sitting bones if unable to comfortably and stably sit fully upright with pelvis neutrality, fully extended legs, and the spine in its natural form. Explore alternately moving from plantar flexion to dorsiflexion (pointing and flexing the feet), backing away from even the slightest sharp pain in the bottom of the heel of the affected foot when creating the dorsiflexion movement. Do three sets of fifteen repetitions three to five times per day, gradually increasing range of motion, sets, and repetitions only to the extent that there is no increase in inflammation or pain within two hours of each stretching practice.

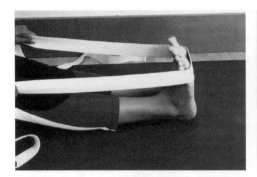
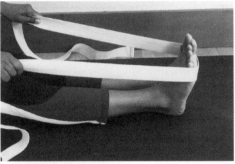
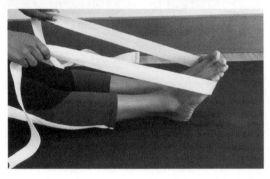

EKA PADA UTTHITA BIDALASANA (ONE-LEG EXTENDED CAT POSE)
Begin on all fours in Bidalasana (Cat Pose). Fully extend the leg of the affected foot, curl the toes under, and alternately press and release pressure back through

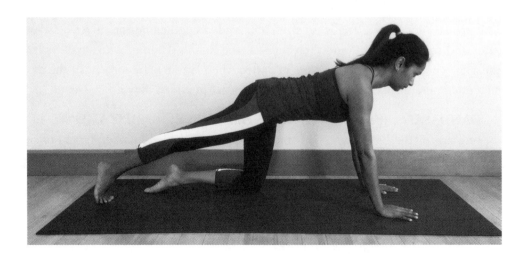

the heel. Do three sets of fifteen repetitions three to five times per day, gradually increasing pressure, sets, and repetitions only to the extent that there is no increase in inflammation or pain within two hours of each stretching practice.

PARSVOTTANASANA (INTENSE SIDE STRETCH POSE) When the stretching actions described for Adho Mukha Svanasana can be done with no increase in inflammation or pain, progress to a modified expression of Parsvottanasana. Stand facing a wall in the basic stance of Parsvottanasana, establishing the affected foot as the back foot while placing the front foot approximately one meter from the wall. Place the hands on the wall to support the upper body. With the back heel lifted, begin to gradually stretch it back and down toward the floor, alternately lifting it and gently stretching it farther back and down. Start with thirty seconds of this movement and gradually progress to two minutes, exploring this increase in sustained activity only so long as there is no increase in inflammation or pain within two hours of each stretching practice.

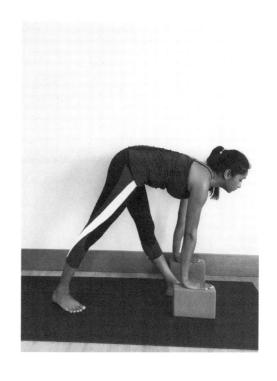

ASHTA CHANDRASANA (EIGHT-POINT CRESCENT MOON POSE) When the stretching actions described for Parsvottanasana can be done with no increase in inflammation or pain, progress to a modified expression of Ashta Chandrasana. Starting in Tadasana, step the affected foot back approximately the length of one's leg, initially keeping the front leg straight (fully extended) and the back knee slightly bent. Place the hands on the hips and use them to establish and maintain the neutral position of the pelvis (neither anteriorly nor posteriorly rotating it). Moving with the breath, on each exhalation bend the front knee (only so far as it does not travel past the heel) while gradually pressing back through the heel of the extended back leg. Back out of the lunge on the inhalations; then lunge more deeply on the exhalations. Focus on sensations in the calf, Achilles, heel,

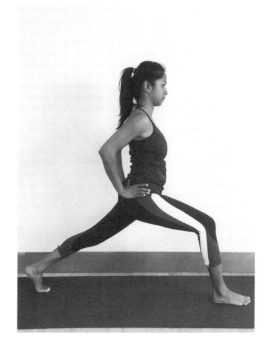

and plantar aponeurosis of the leg and foot, stretching only so far as there is no sharp pain. Explore doing three sets of fifteen repetitions three times per day, gradually increasing how far the heel is stretched toward the floor, sets, and repetitions only to the extent that there is no increase in inflammation or pain within two hours of each stretching practice.

TADASANA (MOUNTAIN POSE) When the preceding asana explorations can be done free of pain and any resulting inflammation, explore heel raises and stretches from the basic form of Tadasana. Fold a yoga mat to create a platform that is approximately the thickness of one's toes and the length of about one-third of one's foot. (As an alternative, use a similarly elevated door threshold.) Stand with the balls of the feet on this platform, placing most weight on the nonaffected foot. Gradually explore bringing equal weight to both feet with the heels at the same level as the platform. If comfortable, slowly and steadily lift and lower the heels, thereby alternately engaging and stretching the calf muscles, intrinsic foot muscles, and the plantar aponeurosis. Explore doing three sets of fifteen repetitions three times per day, gradually increasing how far the heel is stretched toward the floor, sets, and repetitions only to the extent that there is no increase in inflammation or pain within two hours of each stretching practice.

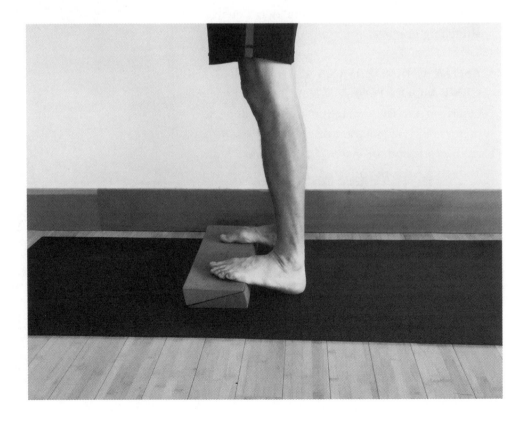

VIRASANA (HERO POSE)   Explore sitting in Virasana to help relieve tension that may arise in the bottoms of the feet or fronts of the calves in doing any of the modified asana actions suggested for plantar fasciitis. If the basic form of Virasana causes discomfort in the tops of the feet or fronts of the ankles or lower legs, sit on a stack of blankets with the ankles at the blanket edge, thereby reducing the forced plantar flexion that Virasana creates. If there is pressure in the knees or it is diffi-cult to sit with the pelvis neutral, place a block (or blocks) under the sitting bones.

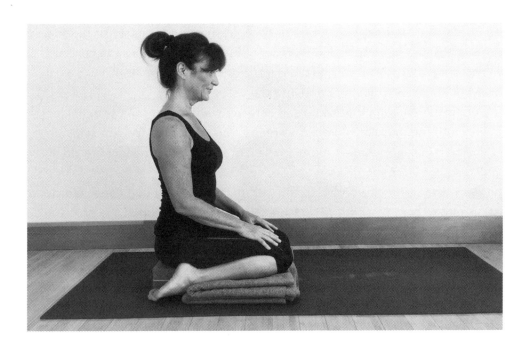

SELF-MASSAGE AND MANUAL MANIPULATION (WITH A BOW TO REFLEXOLOGY)

Reflect for a moment on the pressure your feet endure every day of your life. Without falling into a philosophical dualism or overly fetishizing the feet, con-sider the feet as giving you a lot of love—and how you might best reciprocate that loving energy. How do you care for your feet? How do you listen to, honor, and respect your feet—the part of you that most connects you with the Earth, gives you physical grounding, and allows you to traverse the world? When did you last give yourself a foot massage? Interested in deeper healing (and heeling)?

Rub your feet. Start lightly, gently pressing your fingertips into the center of the bottom of your affected foot. Wherever you feel intensity, press around it, and only very gradually move into it. If it feels good, play with increasing the pressure. Move gradually from the center toward the heel and toes. Being very sensitive and pain-free, play with manual manipulation of your foot, using your hands to alternately flex and extend the toes and to squeeze, twist, and otherwise move your foot in any and every way that feels good. Try to stay within around 75 percent of what you sense to be your maximum ranges of motion, even it feels good to go farther, and then get a sense of how it feels the next day before you go farther. If you want to press more deeply into the flesh, make a fist and use your knuckles to gently grind into the tissues.

Now go further, sharing this loving self-care with your other foot, your ankles, and deeply into the muscles of your lower legs. You are caring for yourself, nurturing yourself, making yourself more whole. Let it feel good as you are doing something so good for your life.

There's a wonderful alternative to this self-massage: have someone else do it! Just be sure to communicate very clearly about the sensation of the pressure and ask for more or less intensity if that's what you feel your bodymind inviting. Relax into healing.

Collapsed and Hypertonic Arches

Going more deeply into the feet, we can appreciate that with twenty-six bones that form twenty-five joints, plus twenty muscles and a variety of tendons and ligaments, the feet are highly complex structures. This complexity is related to their role, which is to support the entire body with a dynamic foundation that allows us to stand, walk, run, and have stability and mobility in life. In yoga, the feet are the principal foundation for all the standing poses and are active in all inversions and arm balances, most backbends and forward bends, and many twists and hip openers. They are also subjected to almost constant stress in transferring our weight to the Earth.

The tarsal and metatarsal bones are structured into a series of arches that support the weight of the body. The familiar medial arch is one of two longitudinal arches (the other is called the lateral arch). Due to its height and the large number of small joints between its component parts, the medial arch is relatively more elastic than the other arches, gaining important support from the tibialis posterior and peroneus longus muscles from above. The lateral arch possesses a special locking mechanism, allowing for much more limited movement.

Normal foot

Flat foot

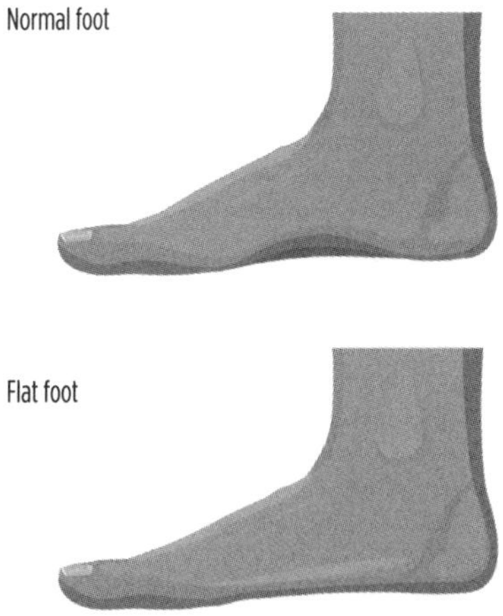

Figure 23.2: Collapsed and Hypertonic Arches

In addition to the longitudinal arches, there are a series of transverse arches. At the posterior part of the metatarsals and the anterior part of the tarsus these arches are complete, but in the middle of the tarsus they present with more of the character of half domes, the concavities of which are directed inferiorly and medially, so that when the inner edges of the feet are placed together and the feet are firmly rooted down, a complete tarsal dome is formed. When this action is combined with the awakening of the longitudinal arches, we create pada bandha, which is a key to stability in standing poses (and a source of cultivating mula bandha from below).

However, the feet do not stand alone, even in Tadasana (Mountain Pose), nor do they independently support movement. Activation of the feet begins in the legs as we run lines of energy from the top of our femur bones down through our feet. This creates a "rebounding effect." When you intentionally root down from the tops of your thighbones into your feet, the muscles in your calves and thighs engage. This not only creates the upward pull on the arches of pada bandha (primarily from the stirruplike effect of activating the tibialis posterior and peroneus longus muscles) but creates expansion through the joints and a sense of being more firmly grounded yet resilient in your feet while longer and lighter up through your body. Our primary focus here in on the medial longitudinal arch.

The basic integrity of the arch arises primarily from the shape of its interlocking bones (talus, calcaneus, navicular, cuneiforms, and three of the five proximal metatarsals) and secondarily from several plantar ligaments and the plantar aponeurosis. These structures all sustain significant stress in daily life but are given important support from the actions of muscles from above, specifically the tibialis (anterior and posterior) and the peroneus longus.[3] Several intrinsic foot muscles (such as the lumbricales, adductor halluces, and flexor digit minimus) add important arch support.

THE PAINFUL EXPERIENCE

Both collapsed and hypertonic arches lead to achy feet, especially in the arches. With weak arches there are also typically more wobbly ankles, which increases fatigue in the muscles of the lower leg and ankle that must overwork to compensate for the instability of the arches.

THE KNOWN CAUSES

When the plantar ligaments are lax and/or the muscles that support the medial arches are weak, the feet tend to pronate (eversion), often causing pain in the feet and ankles when standing or walking for long periods of time. Weak arches also result in wobbly ankle joints, which makes it more difficult to balance on one foot.

When the plantar ligaments are tight and the muscles intrinsic to or related to the feet are tight, the feet tend to be rigid and thus less capable of the resilient transfer of weight to the Earth. This rigidity also compromises both smooth gait and stability in standing, especially in standing balance asanas.

HOW IT HEALS

There are different strategies for collapsed versus hypertonic arches. Weak arches invite strengthening of the interrelated soft tissue support structures of the feet and ankles (muscles and tendons), while hypertonic feet invite manual mobilization and massage of the feet to introduce more softness, flexibility, and resilience.

Conventional medicine prescribes immediate reduction of symptoms such as inflammation through rest, ice, and NSAIDs. Physical therapy is often recommended along with orthotic devices and braces. Some even recommend injection of corticosteroids to reduce inflammation. There is also increasing focus on obesity and diabetes as high-risk factors in fallen arches, with related dietary interventions. Aside from physical therapy, these interventions are primarily to reduce symptoms, not to address the root cause of the problem. With some extreme conditions involving tarsal coalition (abnormal fusing of foot bones during early childhood), bone spurs, or tendon transfer, surgery is often recommended.

HEALING WITH ASANA PRACTICES

For weak or collapsed arches, the primary focus of asana is on strengthening the muscles and tendons that pull up on the bones of the medial arch. The secondary (and important) focus is on the intrinsic foot muscles.

PADA BANDHA PRACTICE Pada bandha is an active practice that stimulates the awakening of the muscles that create and sustain the arches. To do pada bandha:

1. Stand, placing the feet parallel to each other.

2. Create a feeling of more strongly grounding yourself from the tops of the thighs down through the legs and feet as if you are trying to root into the earth.

3. Maintaining this activation of the legs and the rooting action, lift the toes as high as possible, thereby more strongly and specifically rooting the inner portion of the first metatarsals (inner edge of the balls of the feet). This will further

stimulate the awakening of the tibialis posterior and peroneus longus muscles, which are the key muscles that create a stirruplike effect on the ankles and stabilize the medial arch.

4. By doing these actions in all standing asanas (and when waiting in line at the grocery store), one can condition the tibialis posterior and peroneus longus muscles to be more awake and thus create and sustain the medial arch.

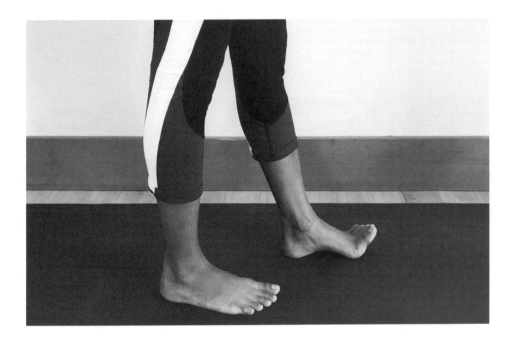

TADASANA (MOUNTAIN POSE) HEEL LIFTS
Standing in Tadasana, do the pada bandha practice just described. While maintaining the rooting of the inner edges of the balls of the feet and the lifting of the inner arches and ankles, very slowly and slightly lift the heels off the floor, and then slowly release the heels down. Lift only as high as possible without wobbling or otherwise creating uneven lifting of the inner and outer ankles. Repeat up to fifteen times, gradually lifting higher. Try to pause the lifting and lowering action two or three times and hold at each stage of elevation for a few breaths while consciously maintaining pada bandha actions and the stable positioning of the ankles.

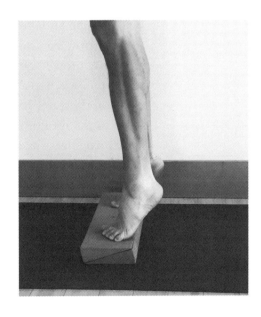

DANDASANA (STAFF POSE) RESISTED ANKLE MOBILIZATIONS   Sitting in Dandasana, place a strap around the feet; clasp each end of the strap while sitting upright with straight arms. Place the strap very specifically in such a way that it is immediately below the small toe and extends straight across the ball of the foot. Explore alternately moving from plantar flexion to dorsiflexion (pointing and flexing the feet) while maintaining moderate tension in the strap, thereby making the movements with resistance. Do three sets of fifteen repetitions three to five times per day. After doing the three sets, massage deeply into the feet and ankles for a few minutes.

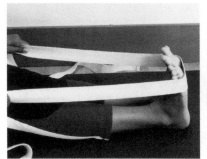 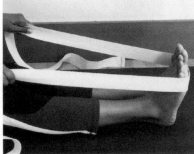 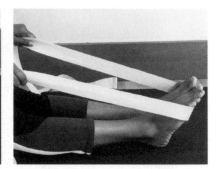

Achilles Tendon Pathologies

Achilles is the central heroic character in Homer's *Iliad* and the greatest of all warriors in the Trojan War; he is so named from the combination of the Greek words *akhos*, "grief," and *laos*, "a people." The hero is both an embodiment of the grief of a people, and through his heroic actions, the cause of grief to others in their defeat at the point of his arrow. Ironically, the connection with the term "heel" arises from Achilles himself being brought down by Paris's arrow to his heel. This is the source of the common turn of phrase, "my Achilles' heel," which is a literal misnomer in that there is no such physical thing (we have heels and we have an Achilles tendon that attaches to them), even as the turn of phrase clearly speaks to a personal sense of self-limitation that relative tightness manifesting through the real tendon symbolizes. This helps explain why the German surgeon Lorenz Heister (1683–1758), appreciating the vulnerability of this tendon, coined *tendo Achillis* from Latin root terms, referencing the most vulnerable spot on the Greek hero.[4] It is also called the calcaneal tendon.

Although the Achilles is the strongest and thickest tendon in the body, it is also the most commonly injured. It is vulnerable in yoga and other activities in which one intensely stretches it, as in Adho Mukha Svanasana (Downward Facing Dog Pose), or in springing actions through the feet and legs, especially in running but also as when jumping forward from Adho Mukha Svanasana. This vulnerability can manifest in several different ways, including inflammation and pain when aggravated, and in worse scenarios, partial or full ruptures. Such injuries can be at the boney insertion at the calcaneous (most common among those with nonathletic and sedentary lifestyles) or in the body of the tendon (especially among athletes who frequently or quickly spring from their feet).

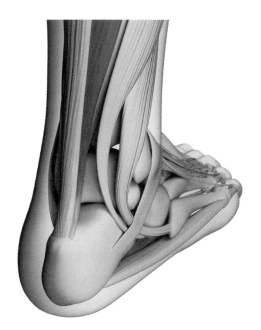

These conditions of injury have more specific medical definitions that provide clearer description than the common (and misleading) term *tendonitis*:

Tendonosis: Chronic degeneration of the tendon at a cellular level without inflammation (and possibly with little or no pain). If there is pain throughout full range of motion, it is most likely tendonosis.

Paratenonitis: An acute Achilles injury due to overuse in which the tendon sheath (the paratenon) is inflamed. If the painful area does not move in creating full range of motion, it is most likely paratenoitis.

Tendon rupture: Whether a partial or full tear, an Achilles rupture involves tears to the tendon tissues that may require surgical repair.

THE PAINFUL EXPERIENCE

Depending on the severity of injury, Achilles tendon pathologies can create symptoms ranging from mild tenderness to debilitating pain.[5] Rather than being purely painful experiences, Achilles injuries are often felt as a dull ache or stiffness anywhere along the tendon, from its boney insertion on the back of the heel up to the lower part of the calf muscle. Pain most typically arises when rising from rest, diminishes with mild use, but then increases with more active use. There can be intense pain (or somewhat more tenderness) when squeezing the sides of the tendon.

THE KNOWN CAUSES

The etiology and pathogenesis of different Achilles injuries vary from the unknown (especially with the chronic pain experienced in noninflammatory tendonosis) to the very specific in action-related inflammation, tears, and ruptures. Although overuse and repetitive strain are the leading suspects in Achilles injuries generally, weak arches, wearing high heels, and general tightness in the calf muscles (gastrocnemius and soleus) are also found to cause Achilles ailments.

Misuse is another important factor. A variety of neuromuscular and structural conditions affect the precisely coordinated movements of the foot, ankle, and lower leg in normal gait as well as in running. Where there is inhibition in the forces that otherwise create balanced movement, including from weak arches and lack of flexibility in the calves, there is a tendency to overly pronate, thereby causing the Achilles to work harder (this amid asymmetrical forces due to the excessive pronation).

Once the degenerative process of tendonosis begins, there is increasing risk of rupture (there is also increased risk of tears in the calf muscles), even as ruptures can occur in a healthy Achilles due to sudden eccentric stretching, as when a runner springs off the blocks in a sprinting race.

HOW IT HEALS

Slowly. Depending on the severity of the injury, healing can take a year or longer. All Achilles tendon pathologies invite patience as they are all slow to heal. If the proximate cause is overuse or misuse, rest is most indicated. If the strain is due to sedentary lifestyle and underuse, then very gradual introduction of use, combined with light stretching, is most indicated. If there is a full rupture, most medical professionals recommend immediate surgery, although there are some cases of self-healing free of surgery.

With acute Achilles tendonosis, most podiatrists and physical therapists recommend rest combined with orthotics to help stabilize the arch and ankle. If rest and orthotics are not successful treatments, many mainstream medical professionals still typically recommend the use of NSAIDs, this despite evidence from the past twenty years of research that the issue is usually not one of inflammation but rather degeneration (which NSAIDs can exacerbate).[6]

Where the condition arises from the physiological condition of paratenonitis, in which the tendon sheath (the paratenon) has poor blood supply, the tendon sheath is inflamed. Ice and mild compression are typically recommended to reduce pain and inflammation, after which some recommend various methods of blood flow stimulation therapy, although there is little medical research to support its efficacy.

HEALING WITH ASANA PRACTICES

The primary focus of asana is on gently stretching the calves (gastrocnemius and soleus muscles) and the bottoms of the feet. In the asanas suggested here, progress sequentially in the order in which the asanas are presented. In exploring, try to fully commit to *ahimsa*, nonhurting, and *aparigraha*, noncovetousness, by going very slowly and patiently, letting go of any expectation of rapid healing.

DANDASANA (STAFF POSE) In setting up for the basic form of Dandasana, place a folded blanket, block, or other firm bolster under the sitting bones if unable to comfortably and stably sit fully upright with pelvis neutrality, fully extended legs, and the spine in its natural form. Explore alternately moving from plantar flexion to dorsiflexion (pointing and flexing the feet), backing away from even the slightest sharp pain in the heel or bottom of the affected foot when creating the dorsiflexion movement. Do three sets of fifteen repetitions three to five times per day, gradually increasing range of motion, sets, and repetitions only to the extent that there is no increase in inflammation or pain within two hours of each stretching practice. After doing the three sets, massage deeply into the calf muscles for two to five minutes, helping to stimulate blood flow while breaking down adhesions. When able to comfortably hold Dandasana with the ankles in full dorsiflexion for one minute, you are ready to proceed to the next asana.

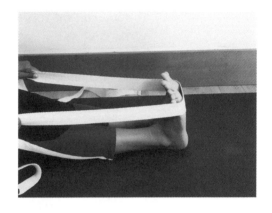

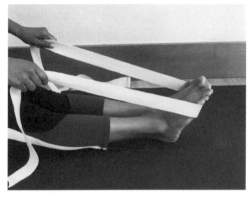

EKA PADA UTTHITA BIDALASANA (ONE-LEG EXTENDED CAT POSE)
Begin on all fours in Bidalasana (Cat Pose). Fully extend the leg of the affected

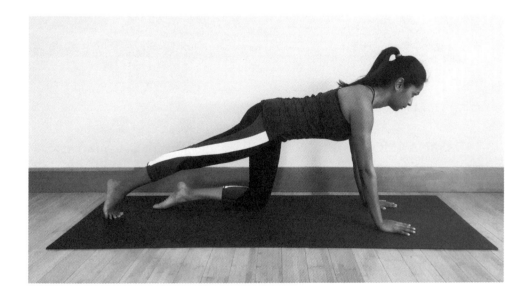

foot, curl the toes under, and alternately press and release pressure back through the heel. Do three sets of fifteen repetitions three to five times per day, gradually increasing pressure, sets, and repetitions only to the extent that there is no increase in inflammation or pain within two hours of each stretching practice.

ADHO MUKHA SVANASANA (DOWNWARD FACING DOG POSE) When the stretching actions described for Eka Pada Utthita Bidalasana can be done with no increase in inflammation or pain, progress to a modified expression of Adho Mukha Svanasana. Coming into the basic form of Adho Mukha Svanasana, bend both knees and begin to slowly bicycle the legs, very gradually drawing the heels closer to the floor. Do three sets of fifteen bicycling repetitions three to five times per day, gradually increasing how far the heels are stretched toward the floor, sets, and repetitions only to the extent that there is no increase in inflammation or pain within two hours of each stretching practice.

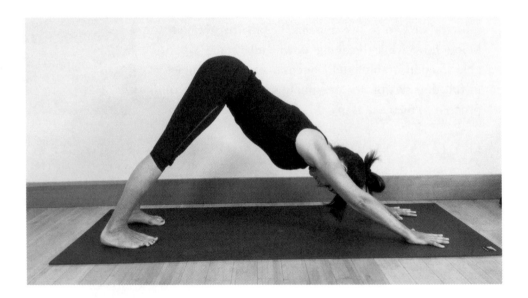

TADASANA (MOUNTAIN POSE) When the preceding asana explorations can be done free of pain and any resulting inflammation, explore heel raises and stretches from the basic form of Tadasana. Fold a yoga mat to create a platform that is approximately the thickness of one's toes and the length of about one-third of one's foot. (As an alternative, use a similarly elevated door threshold.) Stand with the balls of the feet on this platform, placing most weight on the nonaffected foot. Gradually explore bringing equal weight to both feet with the heels at the

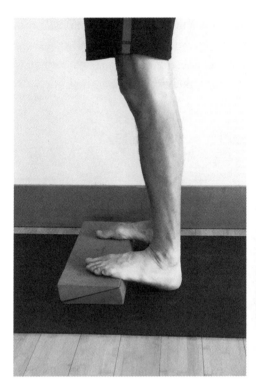
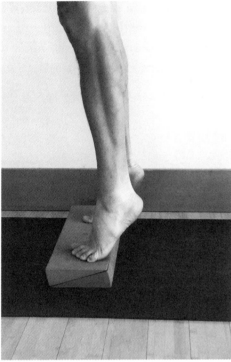

same level as the platform. If comfortable, slowly and steadily lift and lower the heels, thereby alternately engaging and stretching the calf muscles, intrinsic foot muscles, and the plantar aponeurosis. Explore doing three sets of fifteen repetitions three times per day, gradually increasing how far the heel is stretched toward the floor, sets, and repetitions only to the extent that there is no increase in inflammation or pain within two hours of each stretching practice.

Sprained Ankles

The ankle is the most commonly sprained joint in the human body. "Ankle"'s Proto-Germanic root, *ang*, "to bend" (also related to "angle"), perhaps understates this tendency. Rather than one type of sprain, the complexity of the joint gives us multiple types of potential sprains, with some so mild as to cause only a slight and very temporary limp and others so severe as to require surgery, months of rehabilitation, and uncertain healing outcomes. As the following text explains in greater detail, what we commonly understand as the ankle joint is several interconnected joints that collectively allow for complex functions, not merely the plantar flexion and dorsiflexion of the main hinged synovial joint. There are numerous ligaments connecting the bones of the ankle with one another and with the bones of the larger foot and the lower leg.

A sprain to any of them is considered a sprained ankle, although as we will see in a moment there are three main types of ankle sprain. Ankle sprains are among the most common injuries that students bring to yoga classes, and many yoga asanas place large amounts of stress on the joint and thus very likely exacerbate the injury.

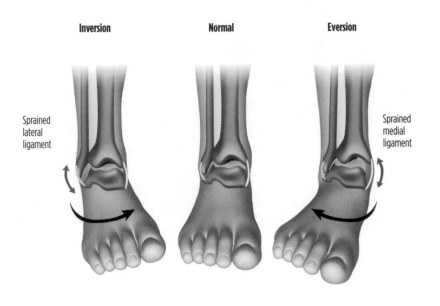

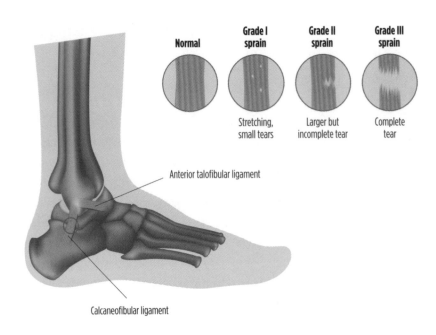

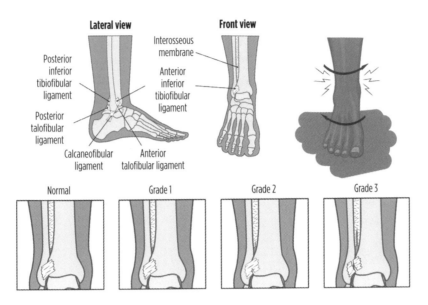

The basic ankle joint—specifically the talocrural joint—consists of three bones: the distal tibia, distal fibula, and talus. But in practical terms the ankle is an extraordinarily complex joint composed of seven bones. When medical school students learn anatomy, they often use the mnemonic device "The Children Need Milk" for TCNMILC, to help recall talus, calcaneus, navicular, medial cuneiform, intermediate cuneiform, lateral cuneiform, and cuboid. Although only the talus is part of the talocrural joint's up-and-down movement, when combined with the subtalar and transverse tarsal joints the ankle is capable of movement in multiple directions. Among the multiple directions, inversion (supination) and eversion (pronation) are most related to ankle sprains.

The three most common types of ankle sprain are:

Inversion Sprains: These occur when the lateral complex of ankle ligaments are overstretched, particularly the anterior talofibular ligament (ATFL). This type of sprain is common in sports with explosive lateral movements such as tennis and basketball, but it also occurs in simple accidents such as slipping off the side of a curb. ATFL damage is greatest when the ankle is in some degree of plantar flexion, whereas when the ankle has an inversion sprain while in dorsiflexion, the injury is more likely to the calcaneofibular ligament. Inversion sprains are by far (85%) the most common.

Eversion Sprains: These occur when the strong and thick medial complex of ankle ligaments—collectively called the deltoid ligaments of the ankle—are overstretched. The ankle's bony structure, specifically the position of the distal fibula, greatly reduces the potential for overstretching the deltoid ligaments (eversion accounts for only 5% of ankle sprains), and when there is a sprain it is typically accompanied by a fracture to the distal fibula.

High Ankle Sprains: These occur when the ligaments that hold the distal tibia and fibula together at the syndemosis of the ankle are overstretched. These two bones are connected along their entire length by the interosseous membrane and most significantly held together at the ankle by three ligaments: the interosseous tibiofibular, anterior-inferior tibiofibular (AITF), and posteroinferior tibiofibular (PITF). Although these only make up 10 percent of ankle sprains, a significant tear in these ligaments typically requires surgery and a year or more of physical therapy to restore healthy function.

THE PAINFUL EXPERIENCE

Ankle sprains are graded 1–3 depending on the severity of the ligament tears, which largely determines the intensity of the resulting pain. The body's natural inflammatory response sends white blood cells to the area, which causes swelling and thus increased pressure on nerves in the injured area. This causes throbbing pain that increases with added pressure when attempting to stand or walk. Swelling also reduces mobility in the joint and can cause a dull fatigued sensation up through the leg.

THE KNOWN CAUSES

The ankle is sprained due to excessively strong or sudden twisting and rolling of the foot in relation to the lower leg. Well over half of all ankle sprains occur when playing sports or moving on an uneven surface. The relative likelihood of a sprain is intrinsically increased when the ankle area has weak muscles and tendons, weak or lax ligaments, and/or poor proprioception. Extrinsic or external factors such as shoe structure (especially high heels), obesity, and ground surface are also significant. Functional instability in the joint and loss of proprioception are prime suspects in recurrent sprains.

HOW IT HEALS

The grade of a sprain from mild to severe (1–3) largely determines how it will heal, including how long it will take to heal. Many mild sprains allow immediate weight bearing with minimal pain and might even be "walked off." The RICE method (rest, ice, compression, elevation) is still recommended by most podiatrists and physical therapists. Whereas RICE reduces pain, its reduction of natural inflammation may cause a longer period of healing. Rest is the primary source of healing with inversion and eversion sprains, whereas high ankle sprains usually require surgery and long-term immobilization prior to undertaking physical therapy. With any severe sprain, a medical professional should conduct an examination to determine the type and severity of injury, utilizing active and passive movement tests, resistance movements, functional tests (pain allowing), palpation, and possibly x-ray to identify possible fractures.

The first phase of healing involves decreasing swelling and pain while protecting the joint from further injury. Considerable research shows that minimal back-and-forth plantar flexion and dorsiflexion with very mild resistance promotes healing so long as the movement is pain-free and does not cause further swelling. With reduced pain and inflammation, one can go further with this manual mobilization of the joint, giving it gradually increasing resistance. When this can be done pain-free and without further swelling, then one can do very gentle manual movements into inversion and eversion, using pain as a guide for less movement. The next phase of manual mobilization is to move the joint in all of its ranges of motion, but only so far as it is pain-free.

Lateral and medial sprains heal in much the same way except that medial sprains typically require twice as long to heal. In exploring modified yoga asanas, note that there are none with active eversion, although a wobbly ankle can stress the medial ligaments even in simple asanas.

HEALING WITH ASANA PRACTICES

TADASANA (TREE POSE), DANDASANA (STAFF POSE), AND VRKSASANA (TREE POSE)   As pain-free range of motion is gradually restored, one can begin restoring greater flexibility and strength to the foot, ankle, and lower leg utilizing

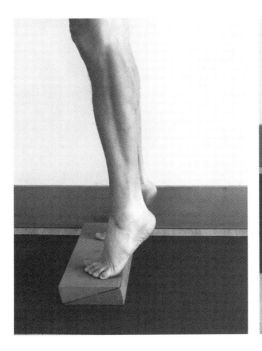
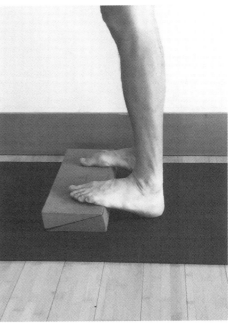

modified asana exercises. Start by standing in Tadasana and alternately lifting and lowering the toes as done in pada bandha exercises. Next, use a strap around the balls of the feet while sitting in Dandasana and make very slow movements with strap resistance through the fullest range of plantar flexion and dorsiflexion. When this is comfortable and there is no pain or resumption of swelling, do heel raises in Tadasana, gradually raising the heel higher and lower (by standing on a door threshold). Doing each of these exercises very slowly, and doing the standing exercises with the eyes closed, will also contribute to restoring proprioceptive function. When fully free of all pain in the joint, progress to doing Vrksasana and other standing balancing asanas to further restore healthy proprioception, exploring these very gradually with the support of a wall or using the other foot to give added support.

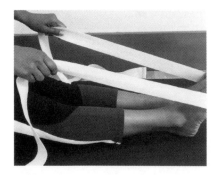

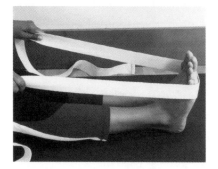

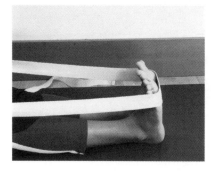

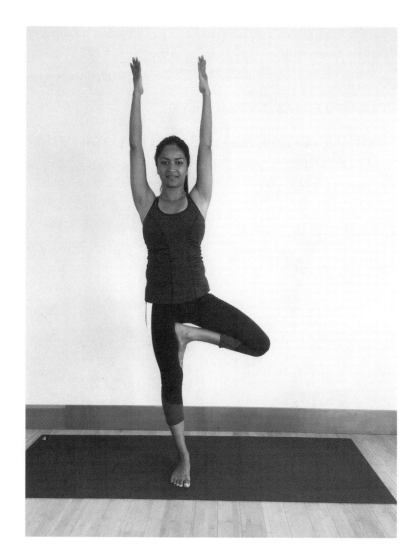

UTTHITA TRIKONASANA (TRIANGLE POSE) AND UTTHITA PARSVA-KONASANA (EXTENDED SIDE ANGLE POSE)   These two asanas involve different degrees of ankle inversion and thus are contraindicated if there is sharp pain in the ankle joint. The inversion angle is significantly less in Utthita Trikonasana and can be further reduced by placing a wedge under the back foot as shown here. The same wedge prop can be used under the back foot in Utthita Parsvakonasana and under the injured foot in Prasarita Padottanasana, significantly reducing or even eliminating inversion.

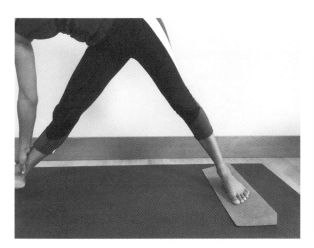
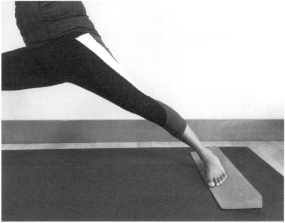

VIRASANA (HERO POSE) AND BALASANA (CHILD'S POSE)   Although increasing plantar flexion is important, the forceful plantar flexion caused in Balasana and Virasana can be injurious. Placement of a blanket under the shin and ankle in these asanas supports limited plantar flexion while allowing safe movement in that direction.

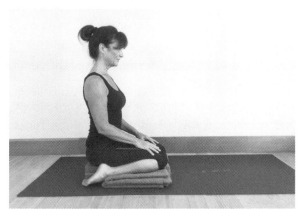
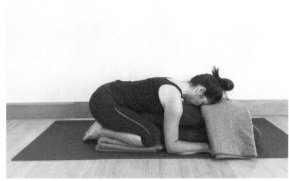

ADHO MUKHA SVANASANA (DOWNWARD FACING DOG POSE)   Adho Mukha Svanasana effectively stretches the calf muscles (gastrocnemius and soleus) as well as the Achilles tendon. Doing this with pada bandha to help stabilize the ankle while alternately lifting and lowering the heels will help with both stretching and strengthening the affected muscles and tendons without doing so forcefully and thus stressing the ligaments.

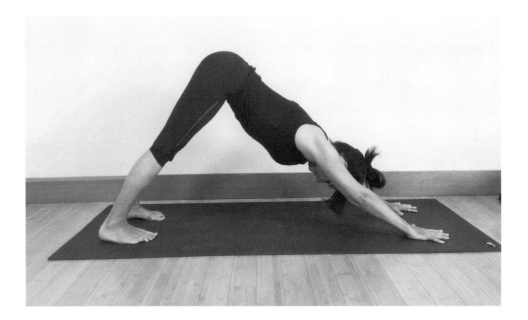

Shin Splints

Shin splint is a classic misnomer in that there is no splint involved in this condition. The term is even more problematic because it is often used to refer to very different conditions affecting both bone and soft tissues in the lower leg.[7] Here we will focus on the two most familiar and common soft tissue conditions generally referred to as shin splints: medial tibial stress syndrome (MTSS) and anterior tibialis strain (the latter term, "strain," is disappearing in favor of more specific identification of the condition as either stress fracture or compartment syndrome).

MTSS and anterior tibialis strain refer to painful conditions around the front and medial side of the distal two-thirds of the tibia. Knowledgeable physical therapists and osteopaths will conduct differential diagnosis to identify the specific injury, which in the general case of shin splints is important due to the overlapping symptoms of shin splints, stress fractures, nerve entrapment, and other conditions.[8] An MTSS diagnosis will identify damaged connections of the connective tissue (Sharpey's fibers) between the medial soleus fascia through the periosteum of the tibia. An anterior tibialis strain diagnosis will identify small tears in the tibialis anterior and in the periosteum covering the body of the tibia, what is increasingly categorized as anterior compartment syndrome (in which muscle swelling within a closed compartment increases pressure in that compartment, which results in pain).

THE PAINFUL EXPERIENCE

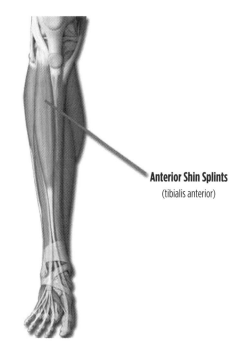

Anterior Shin Splints
(tibialis anterior)

Although shin splint pain is usually described as a dull ache, throbbing, or tenderness along the front to medial side of the shin, when highly acute, the pain can be sharp and persistent when walking or running. The pain may come and go even without healing the underlying condition, often leading to prematurely resuming regular activity that can cause deeper injury. For some, the painful experience is nagging yet sufficiently tolerable to allow continued regular activity, this too possibly worsening the condition.

THE KNOWN CAUSES

Shin splints are a classic repetitive stress injury most common among runners involved in excessive training. The condition is also common with a sudden increase in the intense use of the lower leg, as occurs when hiking long distances or running after a relatively sedentary period.[9] In either case the lower leg is being overloaded in ways that are exacerbated by poor biomechanics, specifically due to dysfunction of the tibialis posterior, tibialis anterior, and soleus muscles caused by changes in tibial pressure. Imbalance in the strength and flexibility between the anterior and posterior calf muscles—especially tight posterior muscles, including the gastrocnemius, soleus, and plantar flexors—are also significant factors.

One is more susceptible to shin splints if the medial foot arches are either weak or hypertonic, or if one runs or otherwise exercises the lower leg on hard surfaces, runs on tip toes, overpronates, or wears improper or worn out shoes. Physician and physical therapists can conduct closer evaluation of possible biomechanical abnormalities in the lower leg as well as knee abnormalities, leg length discrepancy, and hyperpronation of the subtalar joint, along with a more general evaluation of leg, pelvis, and spine mechanics and function.[10]

HOW IT HEALS

The first step in healing acute shin splints is to immediately reduce impactful use of the lower leg. This means resting the injured leg—that is, stop running. Physical therapy techniques such as whirlpool baths, electrical stimulation, unweighted ambulation, and ultrasound may help despite little evidence of their efficacy over other treatment options. There is significant evidence supporting the benefit of daily exercises to stretch and strengthen the calf muscles (especially with eccentric strengthening exercises) as well as strengthening the tibialis anterior muscles and those that help to stabilize the ankle joint.[11] A general program for correcting poor biomechanics in the pelvis, hips, and legs that addresses related musculoskeletal dysfunctions will further help reduce the occurrence or recurrence of shin splints.

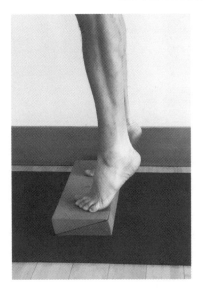

HEALING WITH ASANA PRACTICES

Many weight-bearing asanas that involve active engagement of lower leg muscles may be contraindicated with acute shin splints. So long as there is pain and inflammation, one should minimize active use of the lower leg. When pain and swelling have subsided, one can begin to explore strengthening and stretching the affected tissues.

TADASANA (MOUNTAIN POSE) HEEL LIFTS   Strengthening exercises should focus on the eccentric contraction of the calf muscles, starting in Tadasana with the balls of the feel elevated onto a block, wedge, or door threshold. Slowly raise and very slowly lower the heels through the full range of plantar flexion and dorsiflexion, doing three sets of fifteen repetitions twice daily for several weeks.

BALASANA (CHILD'S POSE) AND VIRASANA (HERO POSE)   The forceful plantar flexion caused in Balasana and Virasana can effectively stretch the anterior calf muscles. Placement of a blanket under the shin and ankle in these asanas supports limited plantar flexion while allowing safe movement in that direction.

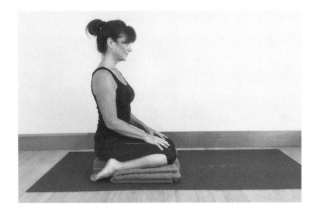

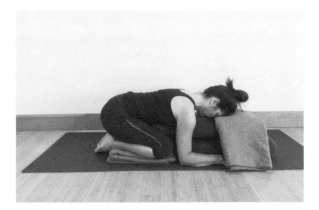

ADHO MUKHA SVANASANA (DOWNWARD FACING DOG POSE)   Adho Mukha Svanasana effectively stretches the calf muscles (gastrocnemius and soleus) as well as the Achilles tendon. Doing this with pada bandha to help stabilize the ankle while alternately lifting and lowering the heels will help with both stretching and strengthening the calf muscles.

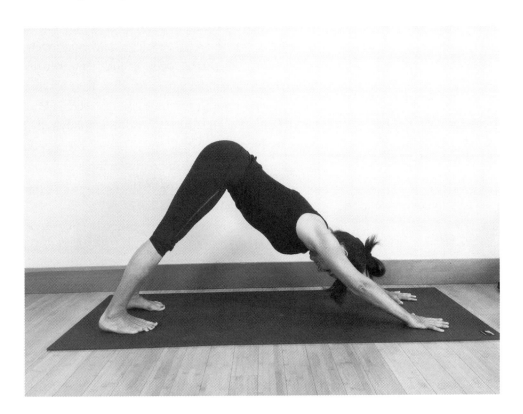

Knee Issues

The knees are perhaps the most complex joints in the human body and the ones that receive the greatest stress in yoga asanas and life. It is for this reason that we give them greater attention before discussing specific ailments and how to heal them in yoga.

The relative complexity of the knee joint is reflected in its varied classification as 1) a ginglymus joint (because it functions like a hinge, allowing extension and flexion), 2) a trochoginglymus joint (because it gains slight rotational capacity when flexed, which is important to note in teaching asanas such as Padmasana [Lotus Pose]), and 3) a double condyloid joint given its bicondylar structure. These three aspects of the knee joint proper gain greater complexity with the gliding patella, which gives us the patellofemoral joint (classified as an arthrodial joint).

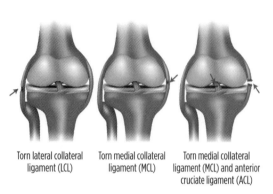

Torn lateral collateral ligament (LCL)

Torn medial collateral ligament (MCL)

Torn medial collateral ligament (MCL) and anterior cruciate ligament (ACL)

Figure 23.3: Knee Tears

Connecting the femur to the tibia, the knee receives considerable stress from above and below. This makes the knee's stabilizing muscles and especially ligaments among the most frequently strained in physical yoga practices. Athletes, runners, even committed sitting meditators discover that the stress created in the knees from their athletic or spiritual avocation can lead to a mildly nagging or debilitating injury, especially when they lack the beneficial effects of a balanced, appropriate practice of physical asanas. Even in a balanced yoga practice, the knee still handles considerable forces, primarily from bearing weight but also due to twisting forces exerted from above and below, especially in seated hip openers. In more strenuous yoga practices, the knee handles very powerful physical forces.

Primarily a hinge joint capable of extension and flexion, with minor capacity to rotate when flexed to about ninety degrees, sudden or excessive movement in any of these motions can tear one of the supporting ligaments or cartilage. Understanding and honoring the knees is one of the keys to guiding a sustainable yoga practice. Let's take a closer look.

The distal femur and proximal tibia are expanded into condyles that increase their weight-bearing capacity and offer larger points of attachment for supporting ligaments. The convex shape of the femoral condyles articulates with the concave tibial condyles. The joint is cushioned by articular cartilage called menisci (from the Greek *meniskos*, "crescent," for their crescent moon shape) that cover the ends of the tibia and femur as well as the underside of the patella. The C-shaped medial meniscus and lateral meniscus are intra-articular pads made of fibrocartilage that further cushion the joint. Thicker on their outside borders with a taper to a thin inner edge, they would easily slip about were they not held in place by small ligamentous fibers (the medial meniscus is larger than the lateral and has a more open form). Although both contain blood vessels during early infancy, with weight bearing their vascularity diminishes, leaving their center portion nourished only by synovial fluid. They function as shock absorbers between the bones and prevent the bones from rubbing each other. Tears in the medial meniscus are not uncommon in yoga, whether originally injured during an asana or exacerbated in an asana where forced rotation at the hip joint can transfer stress into the knee when the foot is held in place by the floor or another part of the body. With little or no blood supply, they heal slowly—if at all.

The medial and lateral collateral ligaments (MCL and LCL) run along the sides of the knee and limit sideways motion. The MCL, extending vertically from the femur to the tibia, protects the medial side of the knee from being bent open (valgus deviation) by force applied to the outside of the knee, such as when a student presses down on the outside of the knee of the back leg in Parsva Virabhadrasana (Side Warrior Pose, sometimes called Reverse Warrior). It also receives potentially injurious pulling forces in a wide array of asanas, extremely so in seated asanas such as Padmasana (Lotus Pose), Baddha Konasana (Bound Angle Pose), and Gomukhasana (Cow Face Pose). The LCL protects the lateral side from an inside bending force (varus deviation), such as when a student misplaces the heel of the right foot against the inside of the left knee in Vrksasana (rather than well above or below the knee). Muscles that run outside the MCL support these ligaments, although strain to those muscles can make the ligaments more vulnerable (and in the case of the MCL, excessive pulling on it can damage the medial meniscus with which it is partially interwoven).

Inside the knee joint are two cruciate ligaments. The anterior cruciate ligament, or ACL, connects the tibia to the femur at the center of the knee. Its function is to limit rotation and forward motion of the tibia away from the femur; without it the femur would slide backward off the knee. The ACL is both a crucial source of stability and at considerable risk if the knee is not properly aligned or supported muscularly in asanas such as Virabhadrasana II (Warrior II Pose) or when transitioning in or out of asanas such as Ardha Chandrasana (Half Moon Pose). The posterior cruciate ligament, or PCL, is located just behind the ACL and limits excessive hyperextension (backward motion) of the knee joint. Injury to the PCL is rare, especially in yoga, as no asanas place great force on this ligament. The patella ligament is sometimes called the patellar tendon because there is no definite separation between the quadriceps tendon, which surrounds the patella, and the area connecting the patella to the tibia. This very strong ligament helps give the patella its mechanical leverage and functions as a cap for the condyles of the femurs.

The muscles acting on the knee from above—the abductors (primarily the glutei and tensor fascia lata, acting through their attachment to the iliotibial band), adductors (primarily the gracilis), the quadriceps (for extension), the hamstrings (for flexion), and the sartorius (a synergist in flexion and lateral rotation)—help the ligaments stabilize the knee when contracting from their various origins on the front, back, and bottom of the pelvis. The gluteus and tensor fascia lata attach to the iliotibial band, which in turn attaches to the lateral tibial condyle below the knee, contributing to lateral stability. The medial side of the knee is given more balanced stability through the actions of the gracilis, sartorius, and the semitendinosus (one of the hamstrings) as they pull up and in from their attachments on the medial tibia just below the knee: the gracilis from the pubic ramus at the bottom of the pelvis, the sartorius (the longest muscle in the body) from its origin at the anterior superior iliac spine (ASIS), and the semitendinosus as it runs up the back of the leg to its origins in the ischial tuberosity (most commonly known as the sitting bones). These medial and lateral stabilizers also play a small part in the rotation of the tibia on the femur when the knee is flexed and the foot is drawn toward the hip in poses such as Sukhasana (Simple Seated Pose) or Padmasana (Lotus Pose).

While lending tremendous stability to the knee, the quadriceps femoris and hamstrings are the most powerful muscles involved in knee extension and flexion. The most powerful muscle in the body, the quadriceps—so named in Latin for its four-headed origins—has just one foot as the four parts combine to form the quadriceps tendon, which extends across the front of the knee to become the patellar tendon and inserts on the proximal edge of the patella, which then transfers their action via the patellar tendon to the tibia. Three of the four—vastus medialis, vastus lateralis, and vastus intermedius—originate from the femoral shaft, while the rectus femoris arises from the top front of the pelvis, giving the rectus femoris a strong role in hip flexion as well as knee extension. This combined action is involved in Utthita Hasta Padangusthasana (Extended Hand-to-Big-Toe Pose). Their collective power in knee extension is increased through the fulcrum-like structure of the patella. Their concentric or isometric contraction extends or holds the knee in extension to stretch the hamstrings in a variety of standing and seated poses and contributes to lifting the body through eccentric contraction in backbends such as Setu Bandha Sarvangasana (Bridge Pose) and Urdhva Dhanurasana (Upward Facing Bow Pose, also called Wheel Pose).

The three-and-a-half hamstrings are the principle flexors of the knee. The semimembranosus and the semitendinosus originate from the ischial tuberosity and run down to the medial side of the knee, giving medial support to the knee as well as assisting in medial rotation. The biceps femoris originates on the back of the ischial tuberosity and the back of the femoral shaft, merging along the way before crossing the lateral side of the knee—contributing to lateral stability—and inserting via a common tendon on the head of the fibula. The partial origin of the biceps femoris (its "short head") on the back of the femoral shaft also leads up to the attachment of the adductor magnus, giving the adductor magnus a "half hamstring" function that, when tight, adds further limitation to wide-angled forward bends such as Upavista Konasana (Wide-Angle Seated Forward Fold).

With these insights, we will now look at knee injuries and how to heal them, focusing on three of the most common conditions that appear among students in yoga classes: ACL tears and repairs; MCL tears and repairs, where we also consider issues with the medial meniscus; and knee replacements.

Anterior Cruciate Ligament (ACL) Sprains and Tears

ACL sprains and tears are among the most common ligament injuries and often occur in ways that also damage the MCL and the shock-absorbing medial meniscus. Focusing on the ACL, we have a ligament that is most stressed in high impact sports such as skiing, soccer, and basketball. There are three grades of ACL sprain:

Grade I ACL Sprain: The fibers of the ligament are overstretched to the point of mild damage but not torn, causing very little swelling and tenderness without making the knee feel unstable.

Grade II ACL Sprain: The fibers of the ligament are partially torn, causing tenderness, moderate swelling, and a sense of weakness and instability in the joint.

Grade III ACL Sprain: The fibers of the ligament are completely ruptured, tearing the ligament into two parts and causing tenderness, swelling, and a definite feel of instability and loss of control in the joint.

Although the tear may occur at the femur or tibia, most tears occur in the middle of the ligament. There is often a popping or cracking sound as the ligament tears, an initial feeling of instability that may diminish with extensive swelling, immediate pain, and inability to fully extend the joint.

THE PAINFUL EXPERIENCE

The intensity of pain varies depending on the grade of the sprain, although most tears immediately cause an intense searing or burning sensation. Severe pain indicates a strong likelihood of a Grade II or III sprain. Weight bearing will add pain, as will the greater swelling likely to occur within several hours of sustaining the injury. (Immediate swelling indicates a more serious sprain and could be a sign of bleeding inside the joint.)

THE KNOWN CAUSES

The most frequent causes of ACL injury are forced hyperextension of the knee, quick stopping, sudden change in direction of movement, and landing from a jump. The likelihood of an ACL tear is increased due to weak quadriceps and hamstrings muscles. In yoga, the ACL can be sprained in asanas such as Virabhadrasana II when the knee travels beyond the heel and splays medially, especially when quickly extending the knee joint from this lunged position.

There is recent discussion among orthopedic researchers, physical therapists, and sports injury physicians regarding the greater frequency of ACL tears among women than men. Most of this research points to a greater angle between the pelvis (specifically the ASIS) and the patella ligament, narrower intercondylar space, and lesser activation of the hamstrings during athletic cutting movements.

HOW IT HEALS

The healing of the ACL depends primarily on the grade of the sprain. Grade I sprains typically heal on their own when provided with adequate rest followed by strengthening the muscles that surround the knee. Grade I sprains are often supported with a knee brace. It is very different with Grade II and III sprains, and thus important to have a correct diagnosis, which may require an MRI of the knee.

While Grade II and III tears will not fully heal without surgery, nonathletes and those with less active lifestyles can use general knee strengthening exercises to maintain a quiet lifestyle free of pain.

With partial or full ruptures, a fibrin blood clot may form between the two torn ends of the ligament and provide a scaffold for rejoining the two ends. However, the synovial fluid that surrounds the ACL is likely to wash away the blood clot that is required for the release of growth factors that attract immune cells, which signal fibroblasts to start the remodeling of functional scar tissue. Given this, Grade II and III sprains usually require surgical repair if one wishes to resume active (particularly athletic) movement.

In all healing strategies, the initial focus is on restoring full range of motion in the knee joint. This should never be forced, which is precisely what occurs in asanas such as Balasana (Child's Pose) and others involving forced flexion of the joint. As range of motion is restored one should gradually rebuild the strength of all muscles that are related to the knee joint, giving primary attention to the hamstrings and quadriceps.

HEALING WITH ASANA PRACTICES

In exploring these practices, give soft tissue treatment (gentle mobilization and massage) to the patella, patella tendon, incision areas, and the back of the knee to help reduce fibrosis and increase range of motion. As the healing practices progress to strength building in the hamstrings, quadriceps and gastrocnemii, massage those tissues too. Throughout these practices, explore pada bandha exercises and any of the general healthy knee practices that are not contraindicated for one's specific condition.

Restoring Knee Flexion

To help restore knee flexion, proceed in three steps, going from one to the next over whatever time is required to do so without pain or the resumption of swelling.

DHANURASANA (BOW POSE)   First, begin lying prone with a yoga strap or belt positioned around the feet and draped up across the shoulders. Clasping the strap and maintaining taut tension in it, slowly bend the knees as for Dhanurasana, using the strap to gently explore gradually greater flexion in the knees. Do not forcefully flex the knee to the point of pain. Rather, use the strap to flex to the point of light resistance inside the knee, then back off slightly, pull slightly, and continue with these alternating movements for one to two minutes.

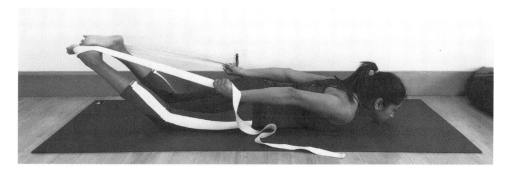

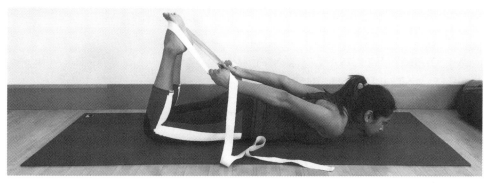

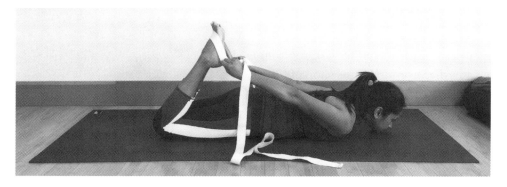

MODIFIED APANASANA (KNEES-TO-CHEST POSE)   Second, lie supine with the knees positioned above the hips and bent only enough so there is no pressure on the healing knee. Gently pull the knees toward the chest while allowing the heels to drop toward the hips as in Apanasana, going only so far that there is no pain in the knee. Then alternately release slightly away from and back into this range of motion in the knees ten to fifteen times before holding in the more flexed position for up to two minutes.

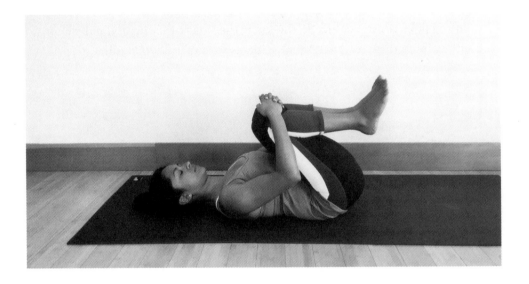

MODIFIED USTRASANA (CAMEL POSE) AND BALASANA (CHILD'S POSE)   Third, begin by kneeling as is done for preparing for Ustrasana (Camel Pose) but with a folded blanket (approximately two inches thick) placed behind the knees. Explore very gradually moving toward Balasana (Child's Pose). As always, use pain as a friend and back away from any sharp or intense sensation in the healing knee.

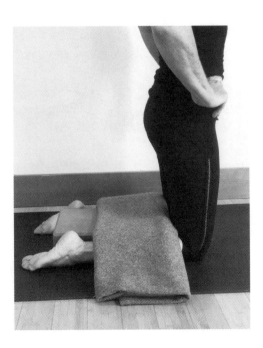

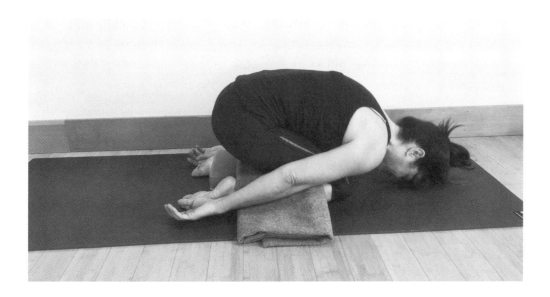

Restoring Knee Extension

Before beginning the process of restoring knee extension, *if there is a hamstring graft*, make sure to wait two weeks before working with the hamstrings. Otherwise, lie prone as described above in the first step for restoring knee flexion and place a strap around the foot of the leg with the healing knee. Very slowly flex and extend the knee joint, using the strap for passive resistance at the foot. Extend only so far as there is no intense pain while breathing deeply to tolerate mild intensity.

DANDASANA (STAFF POSE) Explore sitting in Dandasana with a bolster placed sufficiently high under the sitting bones and thighs to ensure that the healing knee is not forced beyond its presently safe physiological range of motion.

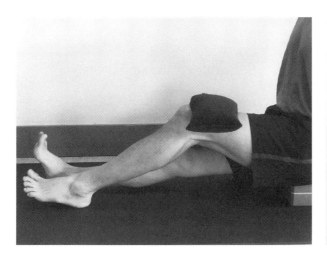

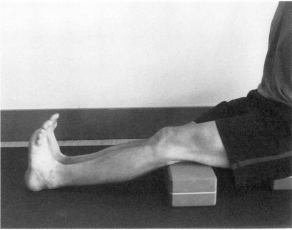

Place a sandbag just above the patella and explore gradually extending the knee. If free of pain, lower or remove the bolster and place a rolled blanket or foam roller under the knee to prevent full extension while gradually pressing the knee joint into greater extension.

Restoring Muscular Strength

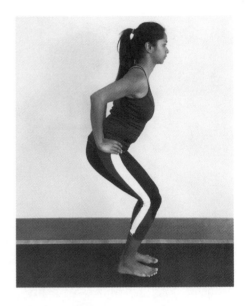

To help restore muscular strength, the first step is to do non-weight-bearing resistance exercises (that is, bearing less weight on the crutches and more weight on both feet while still using crutches).

TADASANA (MOUNTAIN POSE) TO UTKATASANA (AWKWARD POSE, OFTEN CALLED CHAIR POSE) When weight bearing is comfortably tolerable, begin slowly and steadily moving between Tadasana and Utkatasana until lightly fatigued yet pain-free.

ANJANEYASANA (LOW LUNGE POSE) AND ASHTA CHANDRASANA (EIGHT POINT CRESCENT MOON POSE) Explore Anjaneyasana and, if comfortable with it, Ashta Chandrasana (also called Crescent Pose and High Lunge Pose) to build greater strength in the quadriceps.

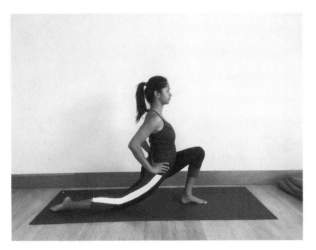
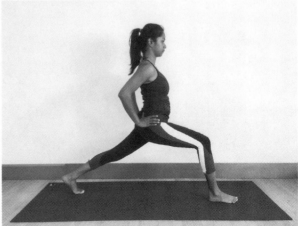

MALASANA (GARLAND POSE) SQUATTING MOVEMENTS As range of motion is restored and there is greater ease in the dynamic Tadasana to Utkatasana practice, explore moving slowly from Tadasana toward Malasana (also called Yogic Squat), going only so far as there is no sharp sensation in the knee. Gradually progress to full Malasana and slowly back to Tadasana.

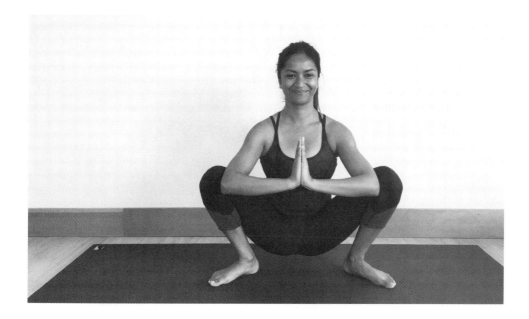

VIRABHADRASANA II (WARRIOR II POSE) AND UTTHITA PARSVAKONA-SANA (EXTENDED SIDE ANGLE POSE) Develop greater strength in the quadriceps by holding Virabhadrasana II and Utthita Parsvakonasana as long as comfortably possible. In doing so, be certain to align the knee with the center of

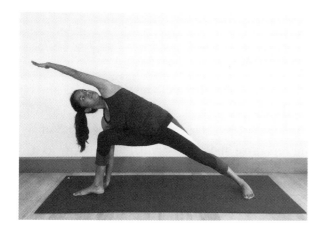

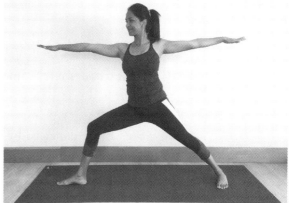

the foot and do not let the knee travel forward beyond the back of the heel. Move slowly and with added pressure to the heel of the front foot when pressing out of these high-lunge asanas.

TADASANA (MOUNTAIN POSE) TO UTTANASANA (STANDING FORWARD FOLD POSE), SALABHASANA (LOCUST POSE), AND SETU BANDHA SARVANGHASANA (BRIDGE POSE)   There are not many ways to strengthen the hamstrings with yoga asanas. One way is moving very slowly from Urdhva Hastasana to Uttanasana, thereby eccentrically contracting the hamstrings through most of their range of motion. Lying prone and extending the hip concentrically contracts the hamstrings as in Salabhasana, and pressing up off the floor into Setu Bandha Sarvanghasana also concentrically contracts them, with these two movements working the hamstrings at different degrees of hip extension.

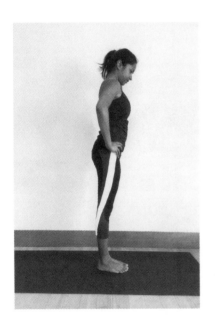 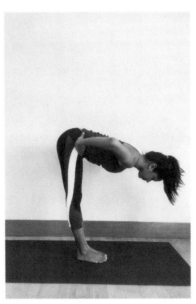 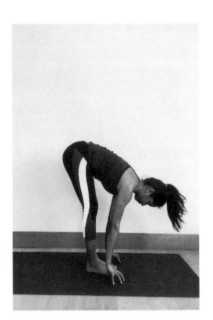

Medial Collateral Ligament (MCL) Tears

MCL sprains and tears are among the most common ligament injuries in yoga and typically occur in ways that also damage the shock-absorbing medial meniscus. The MCL is a ligament that is most stressed in intense sports such as football, skiing, and surfing, but it can also be damaged by strong repetitive abductive–adductive movements as in the breaststroke kick when swimming. There are three grades of MCL sprain:

Grade I MCL Sprain: The fibers of the ligament are overstretched to the point of mild damage but not more than 10 percent are torn, causing very little swelling and tenderness and without making the knee feel unstable. Pain increases with pressure to the outside of the knee.

Grade II MCL Sprain: The fibers of the ligament are partially torn, causing moderate medial tenderness, moderate swelling, and slight instability in the joint. Some physical therapists use 2– and 2+ to indicate injuries closer to Grade I or II, respectively.

Grade III MCL Sprain: The fibers of the ligament are completely ruptured, tearing the ligament into two parts and causing severe medial tenderness, swelling, limited range of motion, and instability in the joint in resisting valgus forces.

MCL injuries are often confused with other injuries, primarily meniscal tears, ACL tears (with which they sometimes occur), bone fractures, and patellar subluxation. An orthopedic physician or physical therapist can conduct differential diagnosis to correctly diagnose the injury. Failure to correctly diagnose the differentiated injuries (especially with combined injuries) can lead to incorrect treatment and chronic problems in the joint.

THE PAINFUL EXPERIENCE

The intensity of pain varies from mild to severe depending on the grade of the sprain, although most tears immediately cause an intense searing or burning sensation (very soon after hearing a popping or cracking sound). Severe pain indicates a strong likelihood of a Grade II+ or III sprain. Weight bearing will add pain and a feeling of the knee collapsing, as will the greater swelling likely to occur within several hours of sustaining the injury.

THE KNOWN CAUSES

MCL tears are caused by excessive force that pulls the medial femur and medial tibia away from each other. This most commonly occurs in general sports activities due to blunt force to the lateral side of the knee. The carving motion created in skiing, snowboarding, and surfing can also cause MCL tears. It occurs most commonly in yoga when attempting to mobilize the hip while the knee is bent into deep flexion, especially when attempting to add twisting movement into the knee joint as is required in all Lotus-like positions of the leg.

HOW IT HEALS

The healing of the MCL depends primarily on the grade of the sprain. Grade I sprains typically heal on their own within two to ten weeks when provided with adequate rest followed by strengthening the muscles that surround the knee. Most orthopedic physicians and physical therapists recommend the RICE method during the first two days after the injury occurs. Once swelling has subsided, isometric, isotonic, and resistance activities will strengthen the supportive musculature on the medial side of the joint, thereby adding support to the vulnerable MCL.

As with ACL tears, it is very different with Grade II and III MCL tears, and thus important to have a correct diagnosis, which may require an MRI of the knee. The paramount concern is protecting the torn ends of the ligament from further damage by avoiding stress to the medial side of the joint for about one month. If the injury is coincident with an ACL tear that requires surgery, the general protocol is to treat the MCL for about six weeks post injury and only then begin ACL repair.

With nonsurgical treatment of Grade II and III tears, the first two weeks of healing focus on reducing swelling by applying ice for fifteen to twenty minutes every one to two hours for the first two days, then three to four times per day until swelling subsides. It is important to avoid weight bearing during this phase of healing (full yet cautious weight bearing with a hinged brace can resume when normal gait is restored). Gentle stretching can be done to gradually restore pain-free full extension and flexion. Static strengthening can be done to strengthen muscles around the hips, in the quadriceps, and in the hamstrings so long as it is pain-free. If there is normal gait and no pain or swelling, then after about six weeks one can do more intense strengthening exercises, gradually including those that introduce rotational force inside the knee joint.

Although most Grade III ruptures can heal with nonoperative treatment, in cases of complete rupture in the presence of other injuries (entrapment of the end of the ligament, bone fracture) surgical repair is often required if one wishes to resume active (particularly athletic) movement or asanas that involve rotational forces in the knee joint. The postsurgical treatment protocol follows the protocols given above for Grade 2 tears.

In all healing strategies, the initial focus is on restoring full range of motion in the knee joint. This should never be forced, which is precisely what occurs in asanas such as Balasana (Child's Pose) and others involving forced flexion and partial rotation of the joint. As range of motion is restored one should gradually rebuild the strength of all muscles that are related to the knee joint, giving primary attention to the hamstrings and quadriceps.

HEALING WITH ASANA PRACTICES

In exploring these practices, give soft tissue treatment (gentle mobilization and massage) to the patella, patella tendon, incision areas, and the back of the knee to help reduce fibrosis and increase range of motion. As the healing practices progress to strength building in the hamstrings and quadriceps, massage those tissues too. Throughout these practices, explore pada bandha exercises and any of the general healthy knee practices that are not contraindicated for one's specific condition.

Restoring Knee Flexion

To help restore knee flexion, proceed in three steps, going from one to the next over whatever time is required to do so without pain or the resumption of swelling.

DHANURASANA (BOW POSE) First, begin lying prone with a yoga strap or belt positioned around the feet and draped up across the shoulders. Clasping the strap and maintaining taut tension in it, slowly bend the knees as for Dhanurasana, using the strap to gently explore gradually greater flexion in the knees. Do not forcefully flex the knee to the point of pain. Rather, use the strap to flex to the point of light resistance inside the knee, then back off slightly, pull slightly, and continue with these alternating movements for one to two minutes.

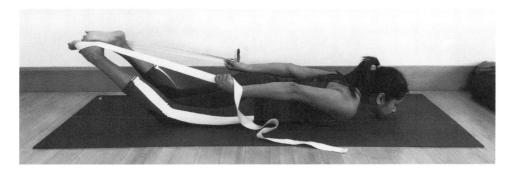

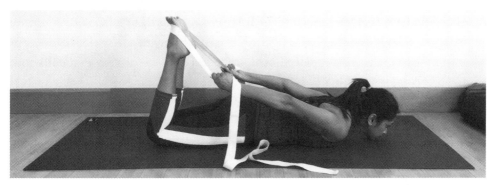

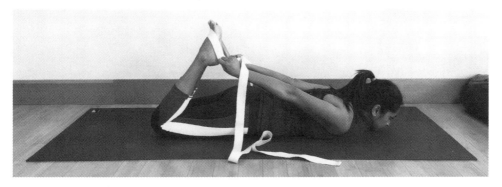

MODIFIED APANASANA (KNEES-TO-CHEST POSE)   Second, lie supine with the knees positioned above the hips and bent only enough that there is no pressure on the healing knee. Gently pull the knees toward the chest while allowing the heels to drop toward the hips as in Apanasana, going only so far that there is no pain in the knee. Then alternately release slightly away from and back into this range of motion in the knees ten to fifteen times before holding in the more flexed position for up to two minutes.

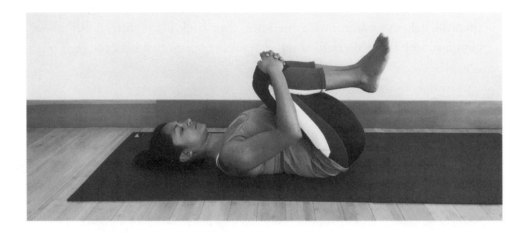

USTRASANA (CAMEL POSE) TO BALASANA (CHILD'S POSE)   Third, begin by kneeling as is done in preparing for Ustrasana but with a folded blanket (approximately two inches thick) placed behind the knees. Explore very gradually moving toward Balasana (Child's Pose). As always, use pain as a friend and back away from any sharp or intense sensation in the healing knee.

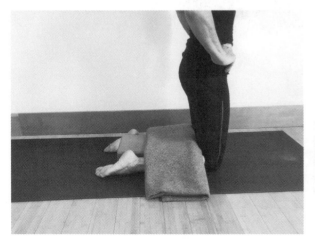

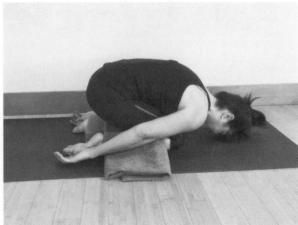

Restoring Knee Extension

Before beginning the process of restoring knee extension, if there is a hamstring graft, make sure to wait two weeks before working with the hamstrings. Otherwise, lie prone as described in the first step for restoring knee flexion and place a strap around the foot of the leg with the healing knee (the other foot can be placed on the floor next to the hip in a comfortable position). Very slowly flex and extend the knee joint, using the strap for passive resistance at the foot. Extend only so far as there is no intense pain while breathing deeply to tolerate mild intensity.

DANDASANA (STAFF POSE) Explore sitting in Dandasana with a bolster placed sufficiently high under the sitting bones and thighs to ensure that the healing knee is not forced beyond its presently safe physiological range of motion capacity. Place a sandbag just above the patella and explore gradually extending the knee. If free of pain, lower or remove the bolster and place a rolled blanket or foam roller under the knee to prevent full extension while gradually pressing the knee joint into greater extension.

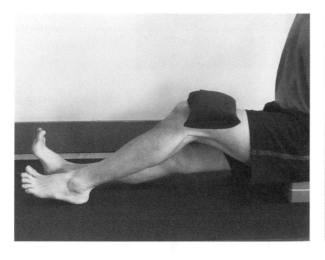 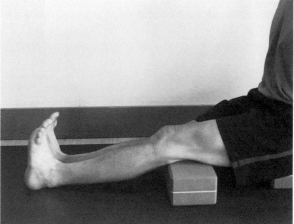

Restoring Muscular Strength

To help restore muscular strength, the first step is to do non-weight-bearing resistance exercises (that is, bearing less weight on the crutches and more weight on both feet while still using crutches).

TADASANA (MOUNTAIN POSE) AND UTKATASANA (AWKWARD POSE)
When weight bearing is comfortably tolerable, begin slowly and steadily moving between Tadasana and Utkatasana until lightly fatigued yet pain-free.

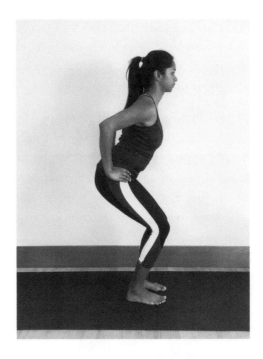

ANJENEYASANA (LOW LUNGE POSE) AND ASHTA CHANDRASANA (EIGHT POINT CRESCENT MOON POSE)   Explore Anjeneyasana and, if comfortable with it, Ashta Chandrasana to build greater strength in the quadriceps.

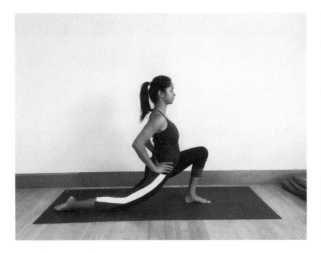
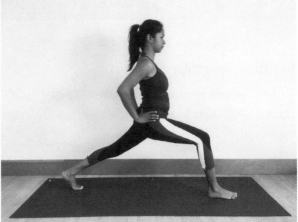

MALASANA AND BACK As range of motion is restored and there is greater ease in the dynamic Tadasana to Utkatasana practice, explore moving slowly from Tadasana toward Malasana, going only so far as there is no sharp sensation in the knee. Gradually progress to full Malasana and slowly back to Tadasana.

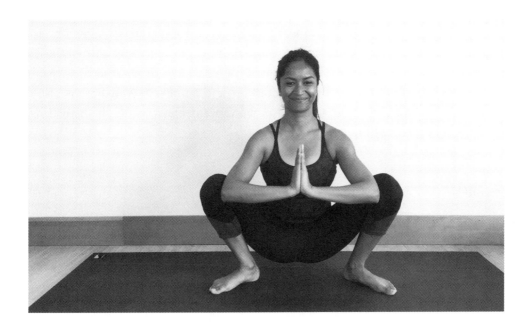

VIRABHADRASANA I (WARRIOR II POSE) AND UTTHITA PARSVAKONA-SANA (EXTENDED SIDE ANGLE POSE) Develop greater strength in the quadriceps by holding Virabhadrasana I and Utthita Parsvakonasana as long as comfortably possible. In doing so, be certain to align the knee with the center of the foot and do not let the knee travel forward beyond the back of the heel. Move

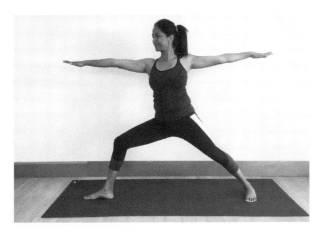

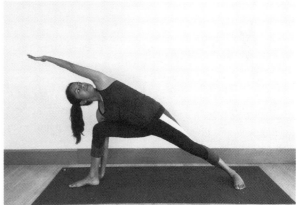

slowly and with added pressure to the heel of the front foot when pressing out of these high-lunge asanas.

TADASANA (MOUNTAIN POSE) TO UTTANASANA, SALABHASANA (LOCUST POSE), AND SETU BANDHA SARVANGHASANA (BRIDGE POSE)

There are not many ways to strengthen the hamstrings with yoga asanas. One way is to move very slowly from Urdhva Hastasana to Uttanasana, thereby eccentrically contracting the hamstrings through most of their range of motion. Lying prone and extending the hip concentrically contracts the hamstrings as in Salabhasana, and pressing up off the floor into Setu Bandha Sarvanghasana also concentrically contracts them, with these two movements working the hamstrings at different degrees of hip extension.

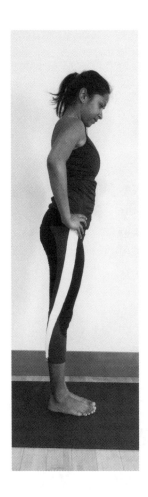
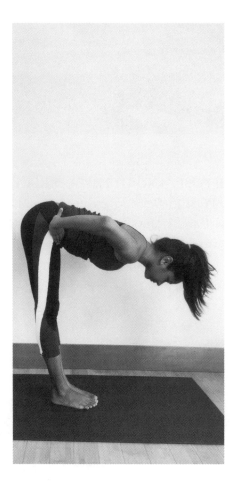
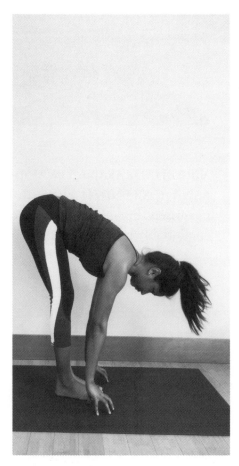

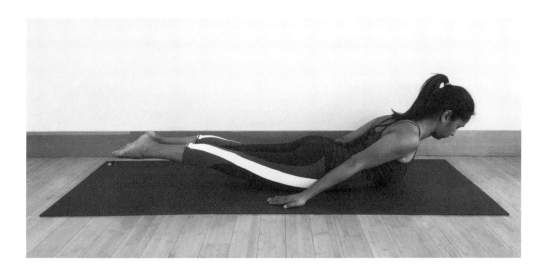

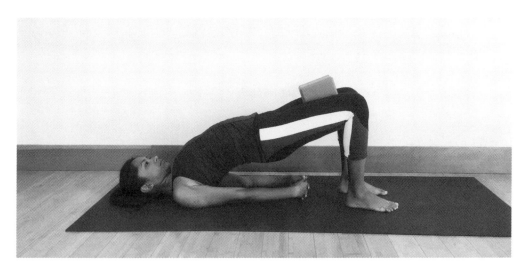

Restoring Rotational Capacity

To restore rotational capacity (and thus the ability to fully flex the knee with the thigh abducted, adducted, and in external rotation), it is important to develop flexibility in the muscles acting on the inner knee from above, including all hip rotators, the quadriceps, adductor longus and adductor brevis, semimembranosus, and semitendinosus hamstrings, gracilis, and sartorius. A challenge in doing so is that in stretching these muscles one might place excessive pressure on the inner knee. Along with using props as described in what follows, it is important to back off of any stretches that create even slight sharp pain in the inner knee.

THREAD THE NEEDLE   Lying supine with the feet positioned as for Setu Bandha Sarvanghasana (Bridge Pose), cross the right ankle to the left knee. If limited in the required range of motion to do this, lie supine near a wall, place the left foot on the wall about three feet off the floor, and then try to cross the right ankle onto the

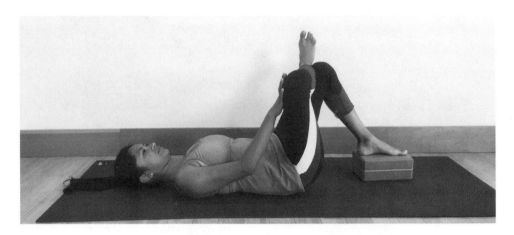

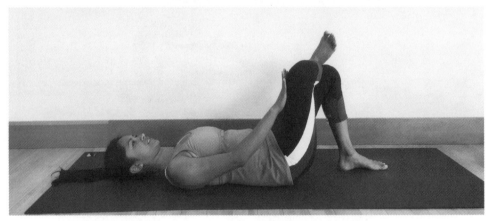

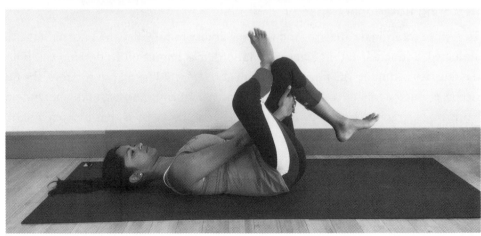

left knee. Clasp the hands behind the left knee, and alternately pull the left knee toward the left shoulder and release it away from the shoulder while keeping the hips on the floor. Explore using the right hand to press the right knee away from the right shoulder. Do several repetitions before holding at the maximum comfortable stretch for up to two minutes.

BADDHA KONASANA (BOUND ANGLE POSE) Lying supine with the soles of the feet together and knees apart, allow the inner thighs to relax and the knees to release toward the floor. If there is discomfort in the inner thighs or knees, place bolsters or blocks under the knees. Stay in this position for at least two minutes.

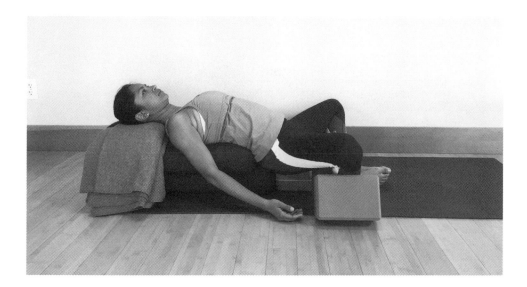

GOMUKHASANA (COW FACE POSE)
Sit for up to two minutes in Gomukhasana. If unable to sit upright and free of discomfort in the knees, then sit up on blocks.

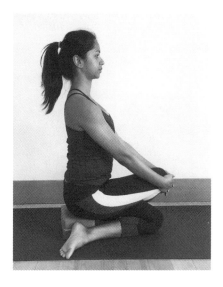

UPAVISTA KONASANA (WIDE-ANGLE SEATED FORWARD FOLD)   If when in the basic form of this asana there is any discomfort behind the knee, place a rolled blanket under it. If unable to sit comfortably upright, sit on a block or bolster. Hold for at least two minutes.

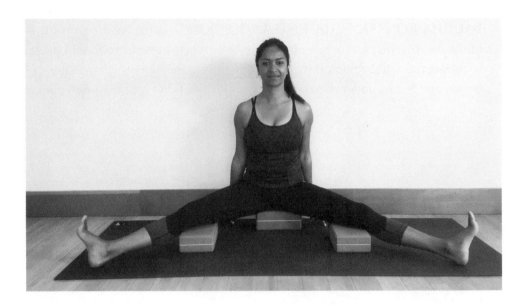

SUPTA PARIVARTANASANA (RECLINED TWIST)   Lying supine, clasp around the knee of the healing side to flex the hip, then draw that knee across the body, coming into the basic spinal twisting form of Supta Parivartanasana. With a strap looped around the foot of the healing leg, fully extend the knee of that leg while continuing to draw the leg across the body. Hold for two minutes.

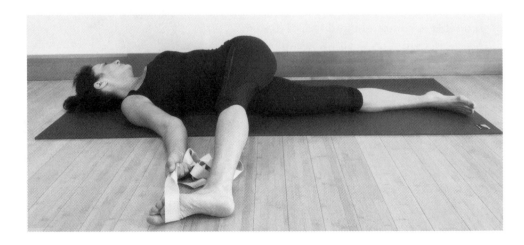

Medial Meniscus Tears

A meniscal tear is a break or rupture in the crescent moon–shaped pad of cartilage. It is a degenerative condition that will worsen without rest or (in the case of moderate to severe tears) treatment. Although tears can occur in several different parts of either or both menisci (flap tears, double flap tears, peripheral tears, horizontal flap tears, displaced flap tears, short and long longitudinal tears, repaired peripheral tears), the strong shearing or compressing forces that happen when the knee rotates while also flexing or extending are most likely to occur in the medial meniscus. (Due to its mobility, the lateral meniscus rarely tears, and when it does, it will often heal on its own due to the vascularization of the area—unlike its medial counterpart.) The medial meniscus is also more prone to tearing due to its structure being interwoven with the MCL, thus leading to meniscus damage when there is ACL or MCL injury.

THE PAINFUL EXPERIENCE

A tear in medial meniscus will produce sharp pain when internally rotating the tibia. Minor tears may produce slight pain and swelling, which typically diminishes within three weeks. There is typically tenderness at one point along the inner knee and more intense pain with either hyperextension or hyperflexion of the knee joint. There is also intense pain along the inner knee with external rotation of either the hip, lower leg, or foot.

THE KNOWN CAUSES

Most medial meniscus tears occur when the MCL and/or ACL tear. However, it also tears due to excessive compression (which can occur in Balasana [Child's Pose] or Virasana [Hero Pose]) or twisting through the joint (as occurs when positioning the leg for Padmasana [Lotus] and all other asanas in which the hip is abducted and externally rotated and the knee is flexed). With aging, the medial meniscus wears down and becomes more vulnerable to tears.

HOW IT HEALS

Where there is vascularity, there is the potential for self-healing. With minimal vascularity (none in its central portion), the medial meniscus does not heal well or at all. The physical therapy protocol for meniscus injury involves strengthening the various muscles that bear on the knee joint, as described for strengthening these muscles in relation to MCL repairs (described earlier).

HEALING WITH ASANA PRACTICES

See the practices given earlier for MCL repairs, focusing on those that help with strengthening the muscles that bear on the knee.

Iliotibial Band Syndrome

The tensor (from the Latin *tendere,* "to stretch") of the fascia lata (from the Latin *fasciae,* "of the band," and *latae,* "wide") is a long muscle that arises from the top of the pelvis (primarily at the ASIS and iliac crest). It is commonly called the TFL. It joins with gluteus medius and minimus fibers and then comes to be situated between two layers of fascia before inserting into the iliotibial (IT) band (or tract), which extends down the lateral thigh before crossing the knee and attaching to the lateral condyle of the tibia. In tensing the fascia lata and the IT band, this set of tissues stabilizes the femur on the tibia when standing and walking or running.

Iliotibial Band Syndrome (ITBS, also called Iliotibial Band Friction Syndrome, ITBFS) is the most common injury to the lateral knee among athletes,[12] and the most common overuse injury in the lower extremity among female athletes.[13] The syndrome refers to painful sensation at the lateral condyle of the femur or slightly lower that occurs with repetitive motion of the knee joint.

THE PAINFUL EXPERIENCE

ITBS causes a sharp and stinging sensation at the lateral condyle of the femur (just above the knee joint). The pain may be felt slightly lower or up along the IT band. It is typically felt during running or hiking when the foot contacts the ground or when placing twisting forces into the knee when changing directions in gait.

THE KNOWN CAUSES

Tightness in the IT band is widely held to be a leading cause of ITBS. However, no study to date has established this as a cause.[14] Until recently it was also thought that bursa inflammation caused ITBS. However, there is now considerable evidence that repetitive tightening of the lateral fascia increases tension in the IT band as it crosses the knee, not the swelling of bursa sacs.[15] Weak hip abductor muscles that cause increased hip adduction during the stance phase of gait are also a leading cause of ITBS.[16] Leg length discrepancy, foot arch pathologies, and some exercise habits (such as running on an uneven surface) are other factors. Runners with worn shoes or poor arch support and cyclists with the toe position even slightly internally rotated are more likely to experience ITBS.

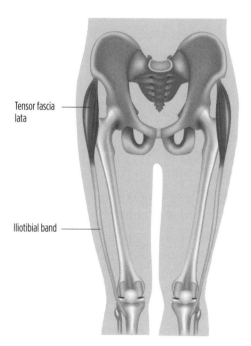

Tensor fascia lata

Iliotibial band

Figure 23.4: The Iliotibial Band

HOW IT HEALS

Difficulty in specific diagnosis creates difficulty in identifying beneficial treatments. To the extent that the friction is caused by tightness in the IT band, treatment should focus on stretching and reducing tension in the tensor fascia lata and the glutei (especially gluteus medius). If the cause is weak abductors, treatment should focus on strengthening the muscles of the lateral hip compartment.

HEALING WITH ASANA PRACTICES

Stretching and Reducing Tension

To stretch and reduce tension in the tensor fascia lata, follow these asanas:

SUPTA PARIVARTANASANA (RECLINED REVOLVED POSE) Lying supine, clasp around the knee of the healing side to flex the hip, then draw that knee across the body, coming into the basic spinal twisting form of Supta Parivartanasana. With a strap looped around the foot of the healing leg, fully extend the knee of that leg while continuing to draw the leg across the body. Hold for two minutes.

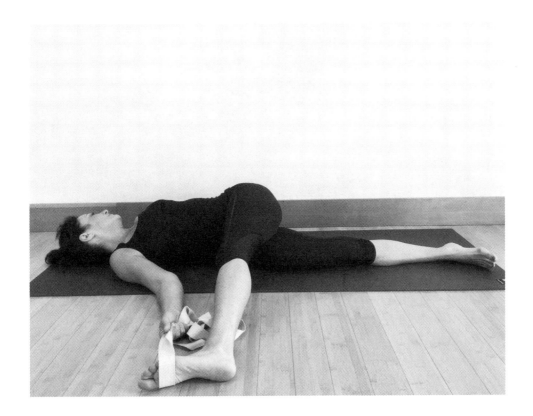

MARICHYASANA C (POSE DEDICATED TO THE SAGE MARICHI)   Sitting upright in Dandasana (Staff Pose), slide the foot of the healing leg in close to the hip. If it is difficult to sit upright on the front of the sitting bones and with the spine tall, place a block or other bolster under the sitting bones and modify how close the foot is drawn in toward the hip. Now cross the foot over the extended leg and place the foot on the floor. Turn toward the bent knee and clasp it with the hands or arms, twisting while keeping the sitting bones firmly rooted, keeping the extended leg engaged with isometric muscle contraction (especially in the quadriceps).

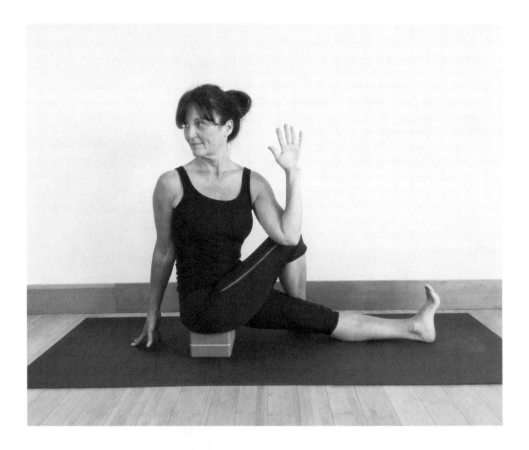

ARDHA MATSYENDRASANA (HALF LORD OF THE FISHES POSE)   Come into the basic form of Ardha Matsyendrasana. If unable to sit upright on the front of the sitting bones or if there is pressure in the knees, sit up on a prop. If it is difficult to draw the foot of the raised knee across to the floor, place it in front of the hip. Turn toward the lifted knee, clasping it with the hand or arm to pull it toward center while twisting toward it.

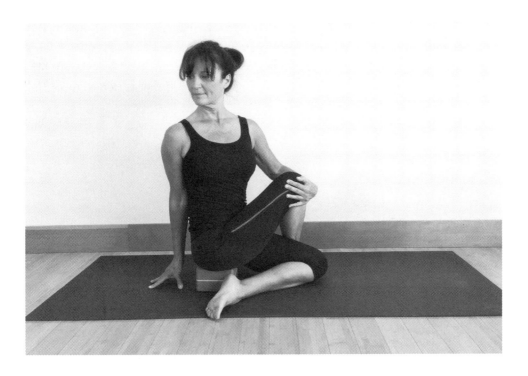

Strengthening the Hip Abductors

BIDALASANA (CAT POSE) Starting on all fours in Bidalasana, fully extend the healing leg straight back from the hip, then stretch it out laterally (abducting it) as far as comfortably possible without the hip lifting, then draw it back to center. Repeat up to twenty-five times, rest, and repeat two to three times.

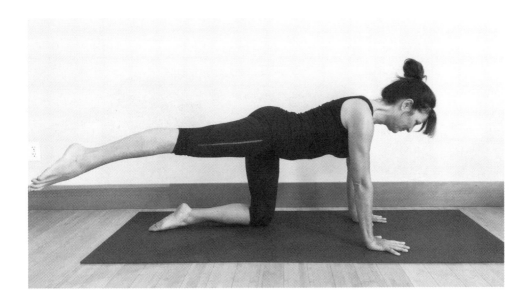

VASISTHASANA (SIDE PLANK) PREP POSE   Starting on all fours in Bidalasana, shift onto one hand and knee to come into Vasisthasana Prep Pose with the healing leg on top and fully extended with the foot on the floor. Slowly lift and lower the healing leg up to twenty-five times, rest, and repeat two to three times.

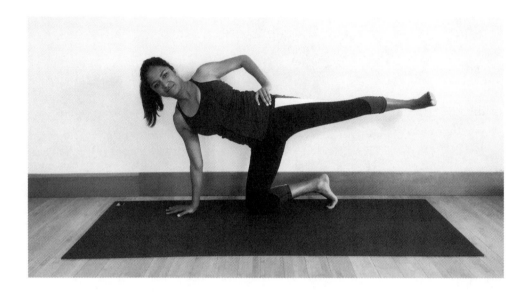

ARDHA CHANDRASANA (HALF MOON POSE)   Being sensitive to pressure in the hip, come into Ardha Chandrasana with the healing leg extending directly back from the upper hip. While maintaining the basic form of Ardha Chandrasana, slowly lower and lift the healing leg up to ten times before holding it in position level with the hip for five to ten breaths. If unstable, do this against a wall.

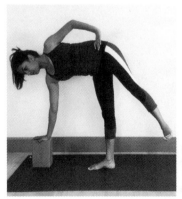 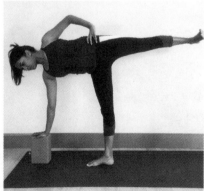 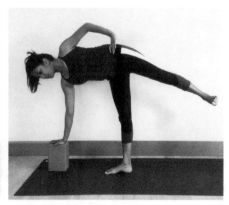

Upper Leg and Hip Issues

Hamstring Strains

The hamstrings are the principle flexors of the knee and extensors of the hip. They also co-contract with the quadriceps to stabilize the knee in isometric contraction, and they co-contract with the hip flexors to stabilize the thigh or pelvis, giving them an essential role in upright posture.

The hamstrings group consists of three muscles. The semimembranosus and the semitendinosus originate from the ischial tuberosity and run down to the medial side of the knee where they attach to the tibia, giving medial support to the knee as well as assisting in medial rotation. The biceps femoris originates on the back of the ischial tuberosity (long head) and the back of the femoral shaft (short head), merging along the way before crossing the lateral side of the knee and inserting via a common tendon on the lateral side of the head of the fibula, which allows it to externally rotate the lower leg at the knee. The partial origin of the biceps femoris (its short head) on the

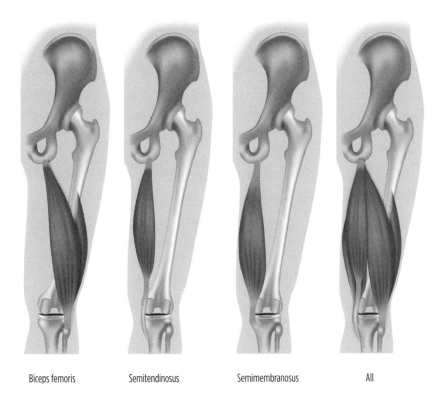

Biceps femoris   Semitendinosus   Semimembranosus   All

Figure 23.5: The Hamstrings

back of the femoral shaft also leads up to the attachment of the adductor magnus, giving the adductor magnus a "half hamstring" function that, when tight, adds further limitation to wide-angled forward bends such as Upavista Konasana. In crossing from the pelvis to the back of the thighs and lower legs, the hamstrings have a strong role in extending the hip.

The complex dynamic function of the hamstrings in gait predisposes them to strain: in a single stride, they concentrically contract to flex the knee, eccentrically contract to inhibit knee extension, then immediately concentrically contract to extend the hip. They are most stretched at the very moment they strongly contract eccentrically and change function, leading to a great propensity to be strained. Hamstring strains are the most common muscle injury in several sports (soccer, football, basketball, running),[17] and considerable anecdotal evidence from my observation finds that it is the most common muscle tear in yoga due to excessive, excessively fast, and repetitive stretching of the muscles.

Although hamstring injuries can occur at the tendinous insertion of the muscles on the lower leg or in the body of the muscles, the most common tear is at their tendinous origins at and immediately behind the sitting bones (ischial tuberosities). Here we will focus on this most common tear.

Hamstring origin tears have varying grades of severity:

Grade 1: Overstretching without a tear in the muscle, with slight pain that may not be felt until at rest. There is no loss of strength or flexibility although there is a sense of tightness when attempting to stretch through full range of motion.

Grade 2: A partial tear in the muscle, pain is felt with stretching or contracting, with slightly sharp sudden pain during use in certain positions. Use with resistance creates pain.

Grade 3: Severe or full rupture, sudden intense pain, inability to walk without pain.

THE PAINFUL EXPERIENCE

Pain varies from very mild cramping with use to sharp and persistent pain with or without use. The strain is often felt as a pinching sensation at the sitting bones.

THE KNOWN CAUSES

The primary risk factor in hamstring strain is a prior hamstring strain, especially in the absence of effective prior rehabilitation.[18] There are many other factors, including repetitive stress, age, peak torque of the quadriceps, weight, flexibility, ankle range of motion, proprioception, specific activity, and mental state.[19]

In yoga asana practices, the hamstrings are stretched in a wide array of postures and in dynamic movements when either transitioning between asanas or extending range of motion within an asana. Movement from Urdhva Hastasana (Upward Arms Pose) to Uttanasana (Standing Forward Fold Pose), one of the most common asana transitions in all flow styles of yoga, involves eccentric contraction of the hamstrings in resisting gravity. When eccentrically contracting, a muscle is lengthening (stretching) even as its fibers are contracting. When this transition is done too quickly and without effective stabilization through the quadriceps and other stabilizers, the body's natural neurological mechanism of reciprocal inhibition will not properly activate to allow the muscle to normally stretch, thereby causing injurious tension in the muscle—most commonly at its tendinous origin. This effect is called *stretch reflex*. Done slowly and consciously, this movement is among the very few in all yoga practices in which the hamstrings are significantly strengthened, which is particularly important given that the hamstrings are intensely stretched in most forward bends.

A second frequent cause of hamstring injury in yoga occurs in seated forward bends when students pull the flesh of the gluteus maximus out or back and away from the sitting bones, a common instruction given by teachers who want students to have their sitting bones firmly rooted to the floor. This causes the stretch in the hamstrings to be overly concentrated at their tendinous origins where there is greatest risk of strain rather than deeper into the body of the muscles as they run down the backs of the legs. Although firm rooting of the sitting bones is very important in all seated asanas, one can attain sufficient rooting without overexposing the hamstring tendons as just described.

A third frequent cause of hamstring injury in yoga occurs in standing and seated forward bends in which the students engage in ballistic stretching (bouncing) or in simply moving too far in their own safe range of motion given the relative health and flexibility of their hamstrings. These causes are exacerbated when holding asanas longer than necessary for the release of muscular tension. (The science of flexibility long ago established that muscle fibers attain their maximum release [stretch] within two minutes of being held in any given position. Thereafter, any further range of motion is due to muscle strain, deep stretching in the tendons, or stretching of ligaments, any of which can be injurious.)[20]

HOW IT HEALS

Specific risk factor analysis is important in designing an effective treatment plan. The RICE method is still generally recommended as the initial treatment. If rested, Grade 1 tears generally self-resolve within a few days to a few weeks. If not rested, Grade 1 tears can worsen. Grade 2 tears generally require longer-term treatment whereas Grade 3 tears generally require surgery followed by a treatment plan similar to that given for Grade 2 tears.

RICE is recommended immediately upon injury.[21] Other treatments can begin once normal pain-free gait is achieved. Anti-inflammatory drugs are not recommended because they inhibit three vitally important physiological healing processes: 1) the work of large specialized cells called *macrophages* that engulf and digest injured muscle fiber cells; 2) the proliferation of satellite cells that give rise to regenerated muscle; and 3) protein synthesis that must occur in the redevelopment of healthy muscle fibers.[22]

Further healing involves a combination of strengthening and stretching exercises. We will explore these exercises through healing asanas.

HEALING WITH ASANA PRACTICES

There is a vast difference in the use of—and effects on—the hamstrings when stretching them in standing forward bends such as Prasarita Padottanasana (Wide Angle Forward Fold), seated forward bends such as Paschimottanasana (Seated Forward Bend Pose), and supine forward bends such as Supta Padangusthasana (Reclined Big Toe Pose). As noted previously, slow movement from standing to a forward bent position eccentrically contracts and strengthens the hamstrings while they are being stretched. Although this is important in preventing injury to the hamstrings, it is part of treatment only *after* injured muscle and tendon fibers are fully functional. There is also a significant difference in strengthening exercises that utilize isometric versus isokinetic muscular contraction. Here we offer conservative treatment suggestions that honor how the hamstrings most effectively heal.

Restoring Strength

To help restore hamstring strength, begin with knee flexion movements before exploring the more intense leg extension movements. Use pain as a friend: if anything hurts, back off.

PRONE KNEE FLEXION When able to make pain-free flexion of the knee, slowly flex it to draw the heel toward the hip, at first using only the weight of the lower leg for resistance. Hold the lower leg in place every few degrees of movement for several breaths, using isometric contraction to engage the hamstrings muscles. Go only to 50 to 75 percent of intensity. As healing progresses to the subacute phase, add resistance by placing the foot of the healthy leg against the heel of the healing leg and begin exploring moving slowly through the full range of knee flexion motion. Transition to Balasana (Child's Pose) to allow the hamstrings to fully shorten and relax.

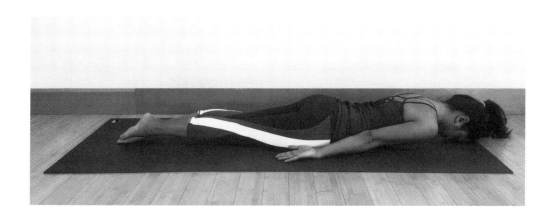

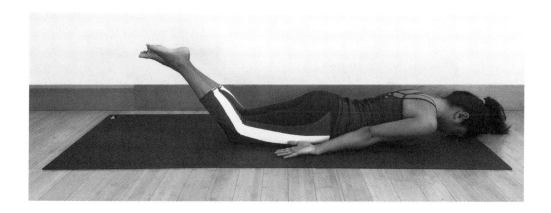

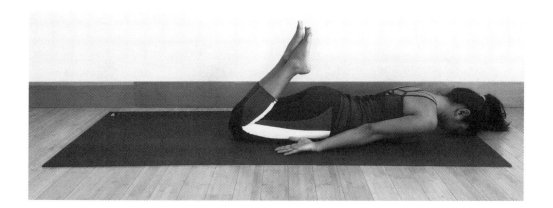

LEG LIFTS   When able to make pain-free full range of knee flexion movement against resistance, continue lying prone and slowly extend (lift) and lower the healing thigh while keeping the knee fully extended. Do up to three sets of fifteen repetitions before shifting into Balasana, allowing the hamstrings to fully shorten and relax.

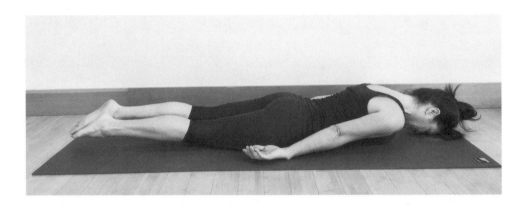

BIDALASANA (CAT POSE) LEG LIFTS   Positioned on all fours in Bidalasana, fully extend the healing leg with the toes curled under on the floor. Explore slowly lifting and lowering the healing leg while keeping the knee fully extended. Do up to three sets of fifteen repetitions before shifting into Balasana, allowing the hamstrings to fully shorten and relax.

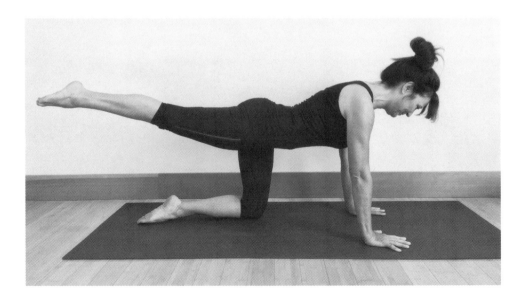

SETU BANDHA SARVANGHASANA (BRIDGE POSE)   Lying supine, position the feet near the hips hip-distance apart to prepare for Setu Bandha Sarvanghasana. Slowly lift the pelvis while focusing on pressing up into the sitting bones, pressing the hamstrings tendons into the ischial tuberosities while elongating the tailbone toward the knees. Hold for five to eight breaths before very slowly lowering down and resting for several breaths. If pain-free, repeat this two or three times daily.

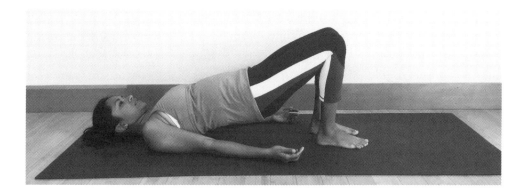

UTTANASANA (STANDING FORWARD FOLD POSE)   We build the greatest strength in the hamstrings when we use them in eccentric contraction. This is how the hamstrings work when swan-diving from standing upright into a standing forward bend. Do not attempt this until in the subacute phase of healing. Move slowly and at first with bent knees to better moderate tension in the hamstrings.

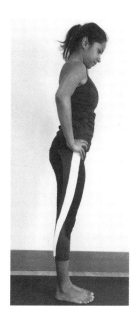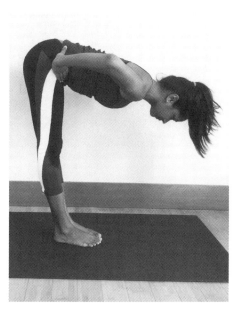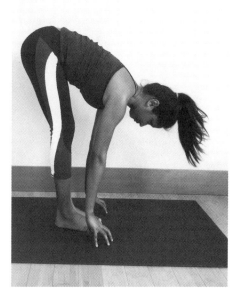

If comfortable, explore folding forward and down with the knees fully extended. As with all forward bends, try to initiate and maximize the movement through the forward (anterior) rotation of the pelvis before allowing the spine to flex. In rising back to standing upright, proceed in the same way: slowly, at first with bent knees, and gradually with fully extended knees.

Restoring Flexibility

To help restore hamstring flexibility, work lying supine so that the only tension in the hamstrings is that created by pulling on the knees or the foot using the clasp of a strap around the foot. This position allows the healing stretch to be as slight as can be and to very specifically target the hamstrings. Recall that the hamstrings are biarticular—they cross and thereby mobilize and stabilize two joints, creating knee flexion and hip extension. The practices given here are designed to prepare the hamstrings for even greater flexibility once healed. Practicing with patience, do not yet attempt Hanumanasana (Splits).

APANASANA (KNEES-TO-CHEST OR WIND-RELIEVING POSE)   Start with Apanasana, keeping the knees fully flexed while alternately drawing them toward and away from the chest. As the hips are fully flexed, this will introduce a slight stretch into the hamstrings.

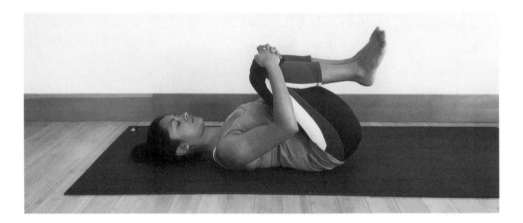

SUPTA PADANGUSTHASANA (RECLINED BIG TOE POSE)   Begin stretching with Supta Padangusthasana. Clasp a strap that is placed around the foot of the healing leg and flex both the knee and hip of the healing leg. With light resistance through the strap, slowly move toward fully extending the knee while reducing the degree of hip flexion as much as required to feel only a comfortable stretch in the hamstrings. Do three sets of fifteen repetitions. When this is entirely comfortable, begin increasing hip flexion while keeping the knee fully extended.

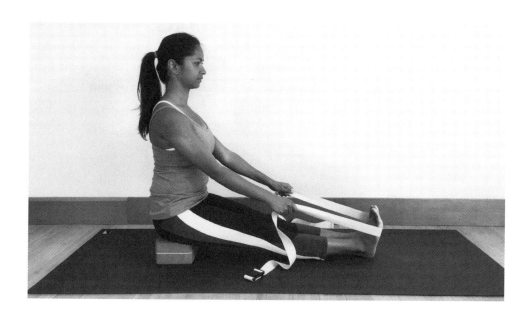

DANDASANA (STAFF POSE) AND PASCHIMOTTANASANA (SEATED FOR-WARD BEND POSE)   Sit upright in Dandasana and clasp a strap that is placed around the balls of the feet. If unable to sit fully and comfortably upright, place a block or firm bolster under the sitting bones, elevated as high as necessary to position the pelvis level with the legs fully extended. (If unable to attain this posture with props, stay with the prior stretching practice.) Firming the quadriceps muscles, slowly press more and more strongly out through the heels while slowly pointing and flexing the ankle joints (plantar flexion and dorsiflexion). Hold with dorsiflexion for five to ten breaths. Also explore slowly and gradually rotating the pelvis forward into Paschimottanasana while maintaining a neutral spine.

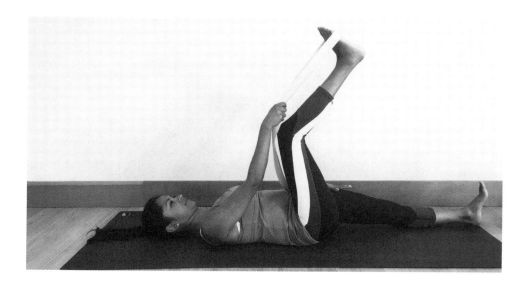

UPAVISTA KONASANA (WIDE-ANGLE SEATED FORWARD FOLD)   Sit upright with the legs separated wide apart in the preparatory position for Upavista Konasana. If unable to sit fully and comfortably upright, place a block or firm bolster under the sitting bones, elevated as high as necessary to position the pelvis level with the legs fully extended. Pressing out through the heels while firming the quadriceps muscles, explore slowly and gradually rotating the pelvis forward while maintaining a neutral spine.

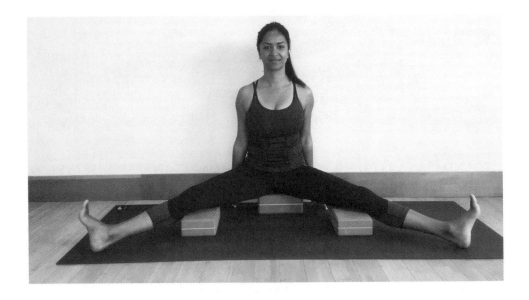

ADHO MUKHA SVANASANA (DOWNWARD FACING DOG POSE)   Begin to explore Adho Mukha Svanasana, initially keeping the knees slightly bent.

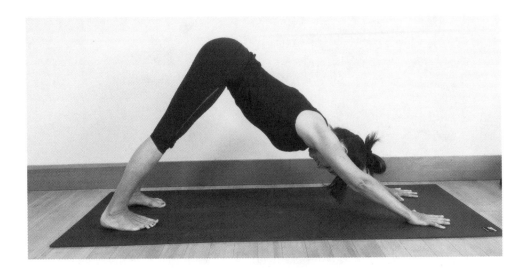

Femoral Neck Syndrome and Microfractures

The rounded head of the femur is attached to the femur by a small bridge called the neck of the femur. The length, girth, and angle of inclination of the neck in relation to the femur varies with age,[23] sex,[24] and development[25] (from around 115 degrees to 140 degrees). Although ordinarily a strong structure, in older children and adolescents this structure can be weakened by repetitive shearing stress on the epiphysis due to a weakened epiphyseal plate, especially with abduction and external rotation of the hip. In elderly people the femoral neck is often weakened due to osteoporosis.

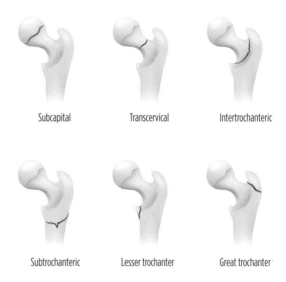

Subcapital Transcervical Intertrochanteric

Subtrochanteric Lesser trochanter Great trochanter

Figure 23.6: Femoral Neck Fractures

If the femoral neck is weak, it is more subject to microfractures.[26] Femoral neck syndrome describes the gradual accretion of microfractures. Due to the vascular anatomy of the femoral neck (i.e., inhibited flow of blood to the femoral head), a great concern with microfractures in the femoral neck is reduction of blood supply to the head due to ruptures of blood vessels, which leads to avascular necrosis (AVN) of the femoral head (compromising the already precarious circulation of blood in it).

THE PAINFUL EXPERIENCE

The mostly insidious nature of femoral neck fractures can create pain that ranges over time from a slightly irritating pinching sensation to pain of debilitating intensity.

THE KNOWN CAUSES

Minor femoral neck fractures are easily confused with hip bursitis or other conditions and thus worsen due to continued repetitive use and mistreatment. The cause often arises from stressful repetitive physical activity, including activity that places excessive biomechanical forces on the hip joint. Insufficiency fractures arise from compromised bone that occurs with osteoporosis, hyperparathyroidism, and menopause.[27] Many studies show the relatively high incidence of microfractures of the femoral neck in military recruits as well as in athletes involved in hip-intensive load carrying.[28]

Certain movements in yoga asana practices can create similarly intensive torqueing force on the femoral neck, as when transitioning directly from internally rotated to externally rotated hip standing balancing postures. To be more anatomically correct, the potentially injurious transition occurs when moving into or away from full hip abduction when the full weight of the body is bearing down through one hip, as in the direct transition from Virabhadrasana III (Warrior III Pose) to Ardha Chandrasana (Half Moon Pose) or the opposite transition.

A metabolic derangement may create an underlying susceptibility. Specifically, bone reabsorption (stimulated by greater mechanical loading) might not be counterbalanced by osteoblast-mediated metabolic repair, with bone reabsorption thus exceeding the bone's capacity to remodel (heal).[29]

HOW IT HEALS

Healing depends largely on the nature of the fractures and the condition of the person. If the fracture is displaced, treatment generally involves anatomical reduction followed by surgical internal fixation and several weeks or months of physical therapy along with the use of crutches. Many surgical repairs lead to misalignment of the joint and ongoing hip pain. In some cases, including those involving AVN, full hip replacement might be indicated (a very common orthopedic procedure with high success rates).

HEALING WITH ASANA PRACTICES

There is no evidence that postural practices or physical therapy can heal fractured bone. Rather, these tools can be effectively applied as part of postoperative care and rehabilitation in alignment with physical therapy protocols. This can begin the first day following surgery with moving from a bed to a chair and back to the bed. Two to three days post surgery one typically begins walking with the aid of crutches or a walker for a period of two to three months. During this time, specific exercises can be undertaken to restore overall posture, gait, balance, range of motion, and strength. Certain ranges of motion will be contraindicated if there was also a hip replacement, specifically adduction across the medial line and other postures that cause abductive pressure at the hip joint.

DANDASANA (STAFF POSE)

Supine Ankle Pumps: Lying supine, alternately point and flex the foot through the maximum range of motion. Do up to fifty repetitions several times every day.

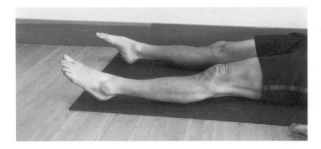
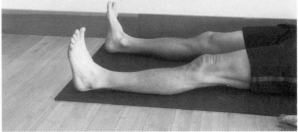

Supine Ankle Rotations: Lying supine, move the foot in circles in one direction five times, then the other direction five times, doing these sets in each direction four to five times per day.

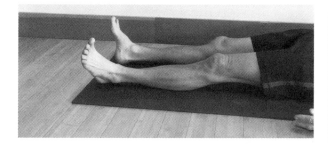
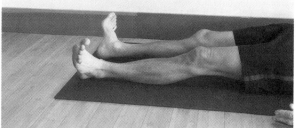

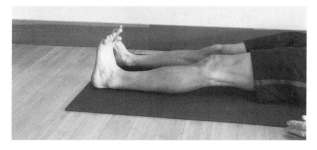

Heel Slides: Lying supine, press the heel of the foot down into the floor while slowly sliding the heel toward the hip. Use the downward pressure of the heel to create resistance in the movement. Do three sets of ten repetitions two to three times per day.

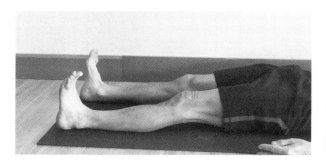
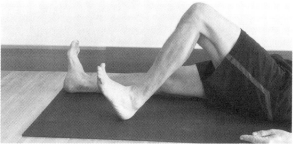

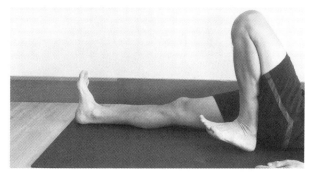

SAVASANA (CORPSE POSE)   Lying supine, at first relax and let everything settle.

Savasana Glutei Contractions: Lying supine, alternately squeeze and relax the buttocks ten to fifteen times. On the final contraction, hold firmly for up to thirty seconds.

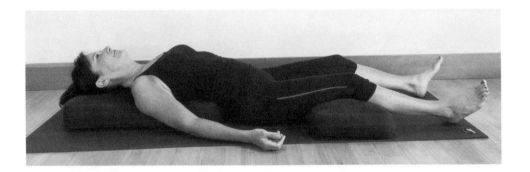

Savasana Quadriceps Contractions: Lying supine, alternately squeeze and relax the quadriceps ten to fifteen times. On the final contraction, hold firmly for up to thirty seconds.

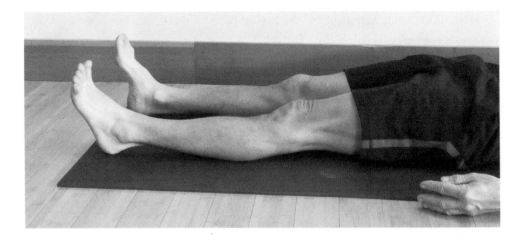

TADASANA (MOUNTAIN POSE)   Each of the following exercises are initiated standing in Tadasana.

Buttocks Squeeze: Standing in Tadasana, alternately squeeze and relax the buttocks ten to fifteen times. On the final contraction, hold firmly for up to thirty seconds.

Quadriceps Squeeze: Standing in Tadasana, alternately squeeze and relax the quadriceps ten to fifteen times. On the final contraction, hold firmly for up to thirty seconds

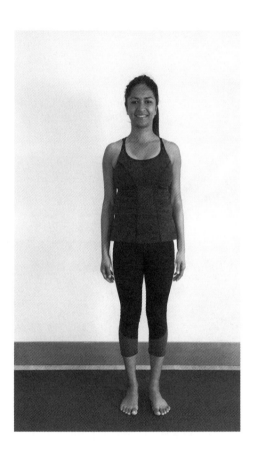

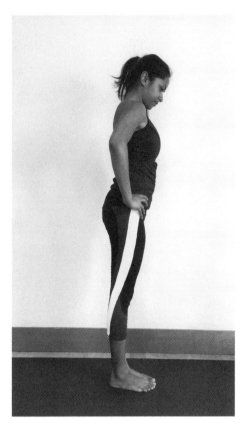

Utthita Hasta Padangusthasana A with Leg Lifts: Standing in Tadasana, alternately lift (flex) and lower the leg up to fifteen times while keeping the standing leg straight (knee fully extended) and stable, the pelvis neutral, and the spine in its natural form. On the final lift hold for as long as comfortably possible. Repeat two to three times per day.

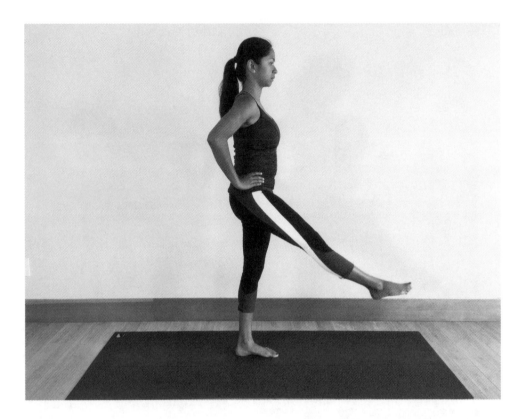

Utthita Hasta Padangusthasana B with Leg Lifts: Standing in Tadasana, alternately abduct and lower the leg up to fifteen times while keeping the standing leg straight (knee fully extended) and stable, the pelvis neutral, and the spine in its natural form. On the final lift hold for as long as comfortably possible. Repeat two to three times per day.

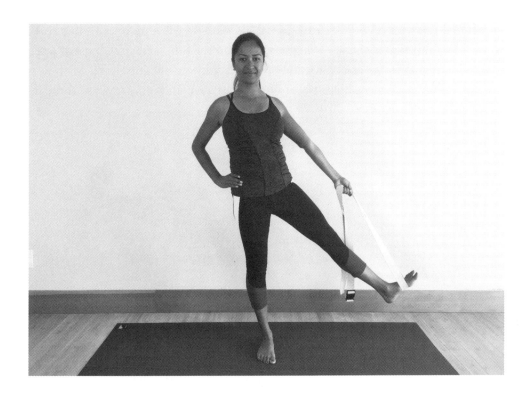

MALASANA (GARLAND POSE) SUPPORTED SQUATS Standing in Tadasana with the feet positioned hip-distance apart, alternately bend and extend the knees while aligning the kneepcaps with the centers of the feet. Gradually bend the knees more deeply, moving beyond Utkatasana and toward Malasana. Only lower as far as it is comfortable, pressing back to straight legs.

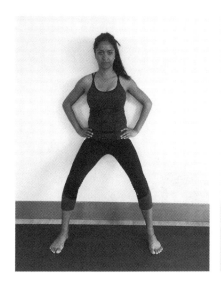
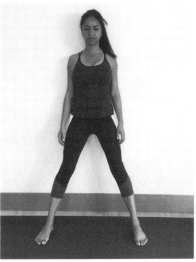
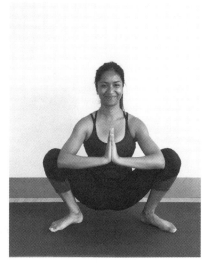

BIDALASANA (CAT POSE) LEG ABDUCTION   Starting on all fours in Bidalasana, fully extend the leg straight back from the hip, then stretch it out laterally (abducting it) as far as comfortably possible without the hip lifting, then draw it back to center. Repeat up to twenty-five times, rest, and repeat two to three times.

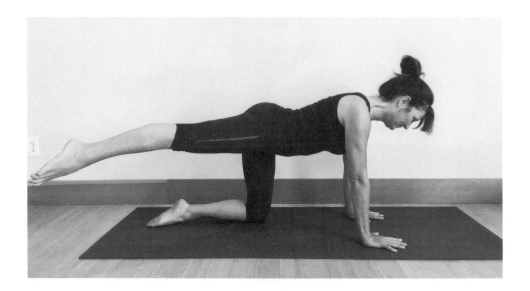

VASISTHASANA (SIDE PLANK) PREP POSE LEG ABDUCTION   Starting on all fours in Bidalasana, shift onto one hand and knee to come into Vasisthasana Prep Pose with the healing leg on top and fully extended with the foot on the floor. Slowly lift and lower the healing leg up to twenty-five times, rest, and repeat two to three times.

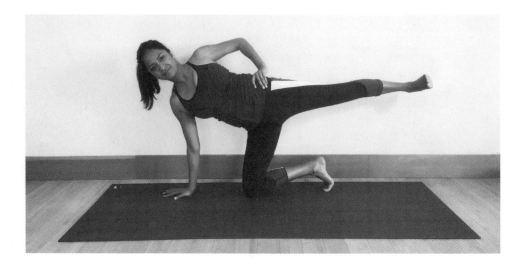

ARDHA CHANDRASANA (HALF MOON POSE) Being sensitive to pressure in the hip, come into Ardha Chandrasana with the healing leg extending directly back from the upper hip. While maintaining the basic form of Ardha Chandrasana, slowly lower and lift the healing leg up to ten times before holding it in position level with the hip for five to ten breaths. If you feel unstable, do this against a wall.

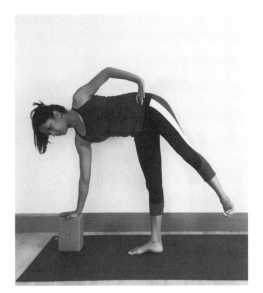
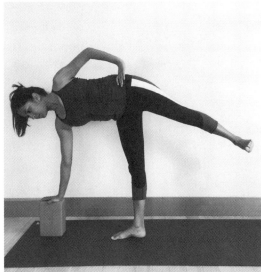

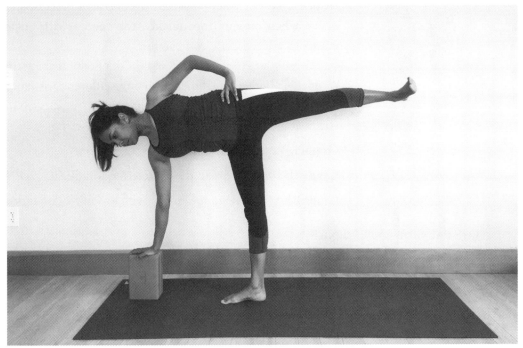

Hip Adductor Strains

Groin has the curious etymological root from Old English of *grunde*, "abyss," referring to the crease on the junction between the abdomen and thigh. Anatomists refer to this as the inguinal line, where the inguinal ligament runs from the pubic bone to the ASIS. But in popular parlance, groin refers both to that area—the site of inguinal hernias—and the area from the pubis to the inner thighs, with muscle pulls throughout these contiguous areas called sports hernias. Although some strains extend into both areas—they meet in the area around the pubic bone—when identifying specific injuries and related treatments, it is important to differentiate the two.

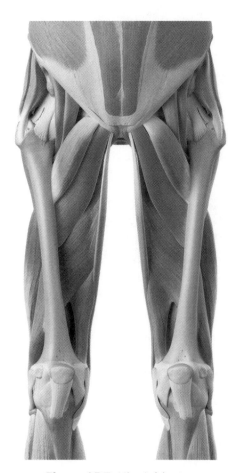

Here we focus on the lower area, where hip adductor strains occur. The hip adductor muscle group consists of the four named adductor muscles—magnus, minimus, brevis, and longus—plus the gracilis and pectineus. The named adductors originate at the inferior pubic ramus and insert on the linea aspera (a rough-surfaced ridge on the femur), whereas gracilis and pectineus originate at the pubic arch and pectineal line of the pubis, respectively, and insert at the medial tibia and pectineal line of the femur, respectively. These muscles act to pull the legs together when in concentric contraction and control the movement of the legs away from each other when in eccentric contraction. Most strains occur when moving too quickly, too far, or with unstable control with eccentric contraction.

Although tears can occur within the belly of the muscles or at their boney attachments, the musculotendous junction near to where these muscles originate is the most commonly strained area.[30] Adductor strains vary in severity:

Grade I: Very mild strain with no torn fibers.

Grade II: Minor tears in the muscle-tendon fibers.

Figure 23.7: Hip Adductors   **Grade III:** Moderate to severe tear with loss of tendon function.

THE PAINFUL EXPERIENCE

Pain varies depending on the severity of strain. With the initial strain there is usually sudden sharp pain in the upper inner thigh.[31] Grade I strains cause mild discomfort without causing limited activity. Grade II strains cause moderate discomfort and typically inhibit normal activity, including walking. Grade III strains involve severely torn fibers that cause muscle spasms and are painful in making any simple abductive or adductive movements of the thigh.

THE KNOWN CAUSES

Strain occurs when extreme force is placed on the adductor tendons, where the sarcomeres (a structural unit of muscle fiber) are less elastic than those in the belly of the muscle. This most commonly occurs with a rapid shift to adduction while the legs are moving apart, forced abduction that places an excessive stretching force on the tendons, and explosive acceleration.[32] Although previous adductor tendon injury is the leading risk factor, older age and weaker adductor muscles are significant risks factors.[33] Previous injury is particularly significant in causing a chronic condition due to the injured person choosing to ignore pain and resume vigorous activity amid even mild strain.

Tight and/or weak adductor muscles are significant factors. Strains in yoga asana practices often occur due to excessive force when moving into or holding standing postures that involve hip abduction such as Virabhadrasana II (Warrior II Pose), specifically with the abducted back leg, as well as asanas such as Upavista Konasana (Wide-Angle Seated Forward Fold) and Eka Pada Koundinyasana (Pose Dedicated to the Sage Koundinya) in which the legs are stretched apart. Overstretching is a less common cause than excessively forceful movement or holding, although holding abducted positions for long periods of time will introduce potentially excessive stretching forces into the tendons.

HOW IT HEALS

One should first be clear on the specific injury by having an orthopedic physician or physical therapist conduct differential diagnosis that rules out injuries with similar symptoms, including iliopsoas tendonitis or bursitis, sacroiliac (SI) joint dysfunction, nerve entrapment, hip joint pathologies, STDs, and gynecological complaints.[34] When acute, one should protect the strained muscles from further strain by avoiding activities that deeply stretch or engage the adductor muscles. Hot packs, soaking in a hot bath, and massage all help to promote blood flow to the area. With Grade I strains one can immediately begin pain-free progressive stretching and strengthening activities. If it's a Grade II or III strain, crutches are indicated if walking is painful, and one should continue with protection, rest, and warmth until pain-free stretching and strengthening is possible.

HEALING WITH ASANA PRACTICES

The primary focus of asana is on restoring a healthy range of motion with appropriate stretching and strengthening of the affected muscles and tendons.

Stretching the Adductors

To stretch the adductors, follow these asanas:

ANANDA BALASANA (HAPPY BABY POSE)   Begin lying supine and drawing the knees into alignment with the hips. Clasp the feet or the thighs and very slightly and gently pull the knees toward the shoulders while keeping the tailbone on the floor. Alternately release and go more deeply with this stretch only so far as to create a very slight stretch in the inner thighs. After several of these repetitive movements, hold at about an 80 percent stretch for up to two minutes.

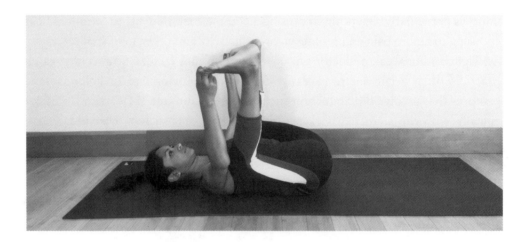

EKA PADA RAJAKAPOTASANA PREP (ONE-LEGGED KING PIGEON POSE PREP)   Begin lying supine with the feet placed on the floor as for Setu Bandha Sarvanghasana (Bridge Pose). Cross the ankle of the healing leg to the opposite knee, keeping the ankle joint in dorsiflexion. Clasp behind the knee of the

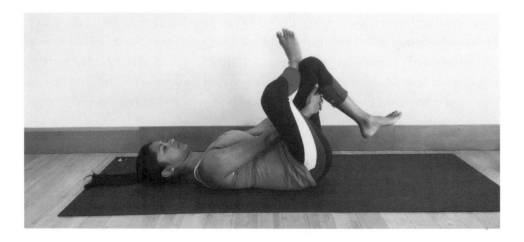

healthy leg and pull it toward the shoulder on that same side of the body while keeping the tailbone on the floor. Alternately release and go more deeply with this stretch only so far as to create a very slight stretch in the inner thighs. After several of these repetitive movements, hold at about an 80 percent stretch for up to two minutes.

BADDHA KONASANA (BOUND ANGLE POSE) Sitting upright, bend the knees and bring the soles of the feet together, allowing the knees to release toward the floor only as far as there is no pain or feeling of deep stretching in the inner thighs. Starting with the pelvis neutral (level) and maintaining the natural form of the spine, press the heels together while attempting to slightly rotate the pelvis forward. Hold at about an 80 percent stretch for up to two minutes.

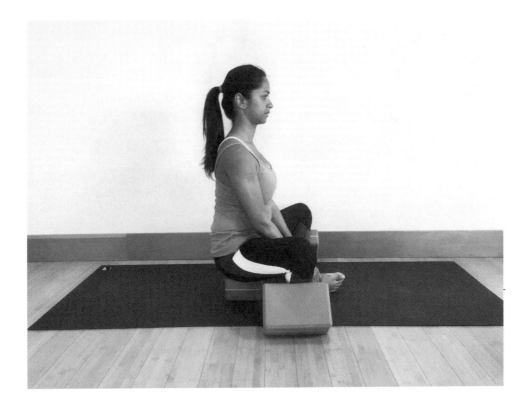

UPAVISTA KONASANA (WIDE-ANGLE SEATED FORWARD FOLD) Sitting upright, separate the legs only so far as there is only a very slight stretching sensation in the inner thighs. Press out through the heels and firm the quadriceps muscles. Maintaining the natural form of the spine, explore slowly and slightly rotating the pelvis forward. Alternately release and go more deeply with this stretch only so far as to create a very slight stretch in the inner thighs. After several of these repetitive movements, hold at about an 80 percent stretch for up to two minutes.

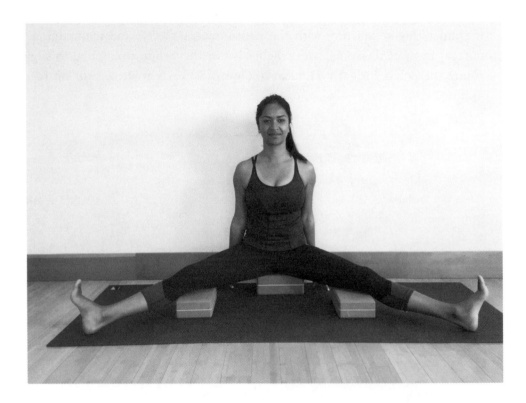

SUPTA PADANGUSTHASANA (RECLINED BIG TOE POSE) Lying supine with a strap looped around the foot of the healing leg, clasp the strap and extend the healing leg straight up from the hip. Keeping the opposite hip grounded to the floor, slowly and slightly abduct the leg (reach it out to the side), using the strap to control the range of motion and to assist in returning the leg to vertical position. Focus on gentle stretching while keeping the inner thigh muscles relaxed—assist both the abduction and adduction with the use of the strap. Alternately release and go more deeply with this stretch only so far as to create a very slight stretch in the inner thighs. After several of these repetitive movements, hold at about an 80 percent stretch for up to one minute.

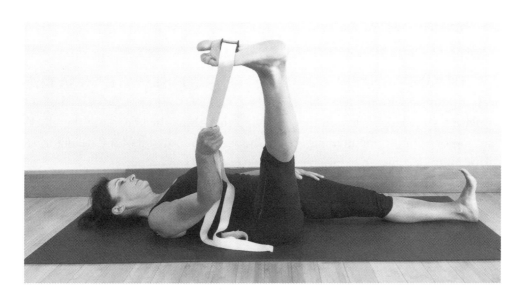

VIPARITA KARANI (ACTIVE REVERSAL POSE)   Lying supine with the legs positioned up against a wall, slowly slide the heels away from each other while using the hands to control the range of motion. Back slightly away from the maximum pain-free stretch and hold for two minutes.

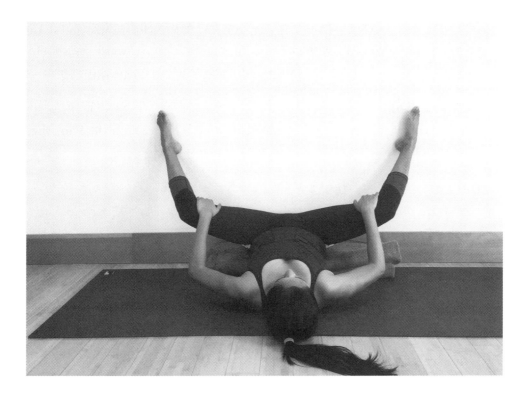

Strengthening the Adductors

To strengthen the adductors, follow these asanas:

SETU BANDHA SARVANGHASANA (BRIDGE POSE) WITH YOGA BLOCK
Lying supine with the feet placed on the floor as for Setu Bandha Sarvanghasana, place a yoga block between the knees and then press the knees into the block for up to one minute, maintaining steady isometric contraction of the adductors. Rest for up to one minute before repeating several times.

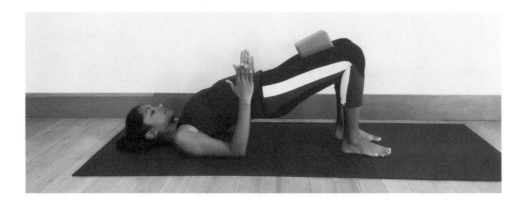

ANANDA BALASANA (HAPPY BABY POSE)   Begin lying supine and drawing the knees into alignment with the hips or slightly closer toward the shoulders. Place the hands on the outside of the knees to control movement of the knees away from each other, then place the hands on the inside of the knees and press the knees toward each other while giving pain-free resistance with the hands. Repeat this slow movement for one to two minutes, then place the feet on the floor slightly wider than hip-distance apart and let the knees rest together.

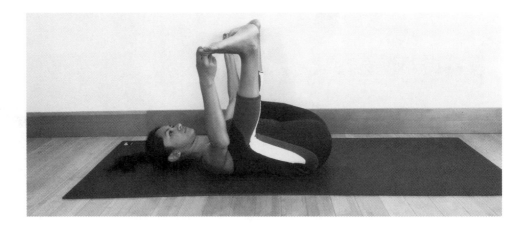

SUPTA PADANGUSTHASANA (RECLINED BIG TOE POSE) Lying supine with a strap looped around the foot of the healing leg, clasp the strap and extend the healing leg straight up from the hip. Keeping the opposite hip grounded to the floor, slowly and slightly abduct the leg (reach it out to the side), using the strap to assist with the abduction and adduction motions, utilizing the eccentric and concentric contraction of the adductor muscles only to the extent that there is no pain.

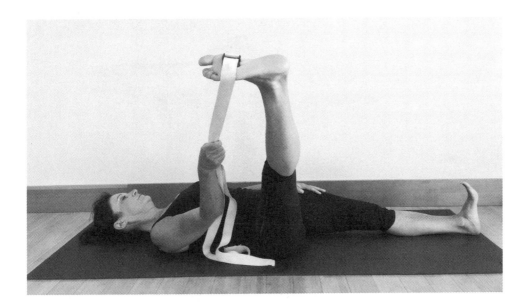

VIPARITA KARANI (ACTIVE REVERSAL POSE) Inverted in Viparita Karani, slowly abduct the legs into the shape of a lateral "V." Next, slowly adduct them back to center. Repeat up to fifteen times. If pain-free, explore dividing the movement into several stages, holding isometrically at each stage before very slowly transitioning to the next stage.

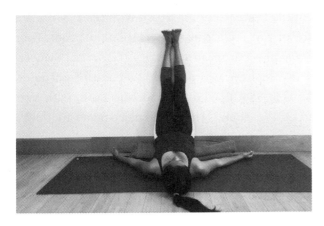
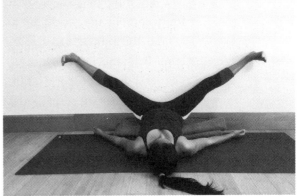

VIRABHADRASANA II (WARRIOR II POSE)   In Virabhadrasana II, create a feeling of pulling the feet toward each other to isometrically engage the adductors of the back leg. Explore very slowly deepening and then lessening the lunge by using the inner thigh muscles of the back leg to lift and lower.

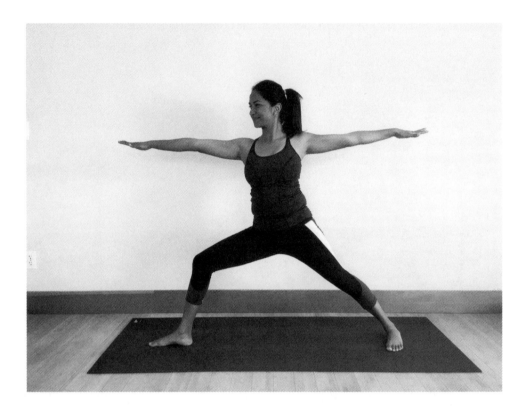

Hip Replacement

According to the Centers for Disease Control and Prevention (CDC), there were over 332,000 hip replacement surgeries in the United States in 2015, with the U.S. ranked fourteenth in the world in the rate of hip replacements per 100,000 people—far behind the leading rates found in wealthy European countries (Germany, Switzerland, Belgium, Denmark, and Norway lead the world). For comparative purposes, Germany had 296 per 100,000, the U.S. 184, Poland 44, and Mexico 8, with over 164 countries ranked behind Mexico.[35] The point is that hip replacements are now a common orthopedic procedure, this due to advances in successful surgical technique rather than higher rates of hip diseases such as osteoarthritis, an aging population, or the growing prevalence of obesity (all of which are risk factors in debilitating hip pathologies.

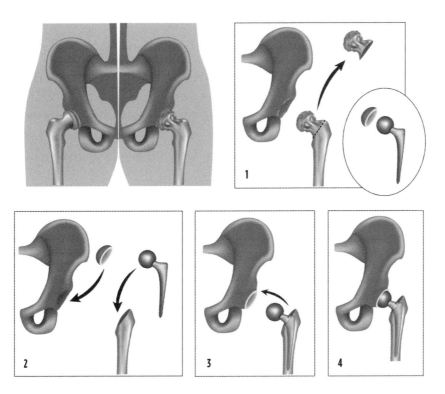

Figure 23.8: An Artificial Hip

Full hip replacement is an orthopedic procedure in which the femoral head and acetabulum are replaced with 1) a metal or ceramic femoral component that is cemented into the femoral shaft, 2) a polyethylene acetabular cup that is placed into the hip socket, and 3) an articular interface that is part of a metal or ceramic femoral head. The posterior approach (which is most common) provides easier surgical access and preserves the hip adductors but has a relatively high dislocation rate.[36] Lateral and anterolateral approaches have lower dislocation rates but often cause long-term instability due to weakened adductors,[37] while more recently developed anterior approaches have significantly lower rates of dislocation and easier rehabilitation.[38] Minimally invasive approaches are available with some conditions.[39]

Students with hip replacements in yoga classes are at high risk of dislocating the replaced hip in a wide array of standing, seated, and supine positions, particularly those involving hip adduction along with external pressure to the lateral side of the knee. Examples of this position and force include Parivrtta Parsvakonasana (Revolved Extended Side-Angle Pose), Ardha Matsyendrasana (Half Lord of the Fishes Pose), and Supta Padangusthasana B (Reclined Big Toe Pose).

THE PAINFUL EXPERIENCE

The greatest pain related to hip replacements comes prior to the replacement due to friction and pressure in the hip joint caused by osteoarthritis, rheumatoid arthritis, post-traumatic arthritis, avascular necrosis, and childhood hip diseases. These conditions involve chronic inflammation that increases pain. Short-term postsurgical pain is typically medicated with nonsteroidal anti-inflammatory drugs, with severe pain (rare) treated with opioids. With successful surgery, pain generally diminishes quickly, although there is often mild aching, especially with changes in weather.

THE KNOWN CAUSES

The conditions that lead to an indication of hip replacement include osteoarthritis, rheumatoid arthritis, post-traumatic arthritis, avascular necrosis, and childhood hip diseases.

HOW IT HEALS

Although hip replacement addresses the immediate conditions in the hip that indicated this surgical procedure, long-term health depends on treatments that restore range of motion, strength, endurance, and balance when standing on the healing leg only. If there are no other serious health conditions (such as cardiac atrophy or edema), physical therapy should begin on the first postoperative day.

One of the primary postoperative concerns with hip replacement is the risk of dislocation, which varies in relation to the approach (posterior, anterior, etc.) and unique health factors of the individual. Hip flexion with internal rotation and adduction beyond the midline is contraindicated with the posterior approach, while extension with external rotation and abduction is contraindicated with the anterior approach. It is important to note that these are common movements in many basic yoga asanas.

HEALING WITH ASANA PRACTICES

Although it is important to be attentive to the contraindications just described, healing can be enhanced through a combination of yoga asanas.

Restoring Strength and Weight-Bearing Capacity

To help restore strength and weight-bearing capacity, follow these asanas:

DANDASANA (STAFF POSE)   There are several healing activities one can do on the first postoperative day while sitting in Dandasana. If unable to sit upright, explore these exercises lying supine in bed. Start with isometric contraction of the quadriceps to reawaken muscles and stimulate circulation. Flex, extend, and rotate the ankles, feet, and toes to further stimulate circulation.

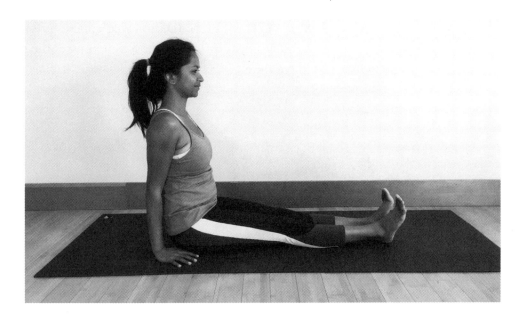

SVANASANA (CORPSE POSE) WITH PROGRESSIVE ENGAGEMENT AND RELAXATION Lying supine, first explore progressively relaxing every muscle. Then begin to alternately engage muscles isometrically before allowing them to more deeply relax. Start with the quadriceps, then the glutei, then the abdomen, gradually engaging and relaxing everywhere. Then come back to the quadriceps and glutei, more strongly squeezing them for five to ten seconds before letting them completely relax.

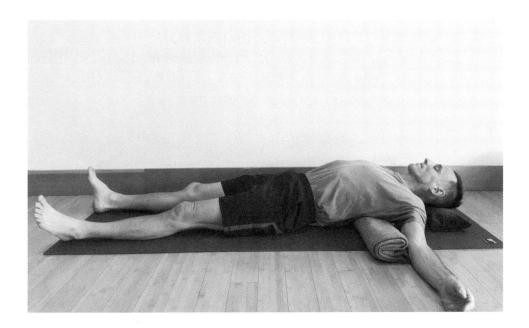

SVANASANA (CORPSE POSE) WITH HEEL SLIDES   Lying supine, pressing down through the heel of the healing side, slowly slide the heel in toward the hip, then slide it away to fully straighten the leg. Keep the kneecap pointing straight up. Do three sets of fifteen repetitions.

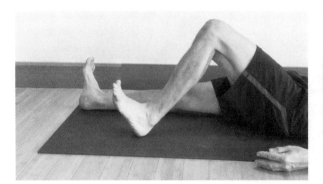
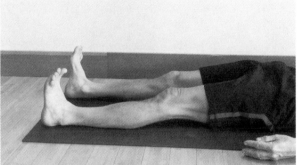
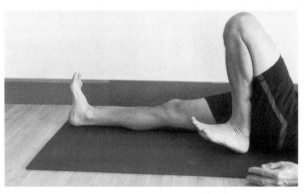

SETU BANDHA SARVANGHASANA (BRIDGE POSE)   Lying supine with the feet positioned near the hips hip-distance apart, slowly lift the hips while keeping the knees aligned with the hips. Lift and release down five times. On the fifth lift, hold for up to ten breaths. Repeat two to three times.

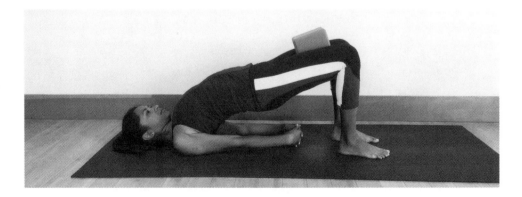

BIDALASANA (CAT POSE) AND SPINAL BALANCING On all fours, first move the pelvis forward and back several times while alternately moving the spine into extension and flexion (cat/cow movements). Then extend the healing leg straight back with the toes curled under on the floor. If comfortable in the low back, slowly lift and lower the extended leg up to twenty-five times, holding for five to ten breaths on the last lift. Repeat on the other side. Then once again

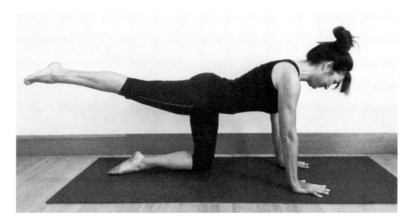

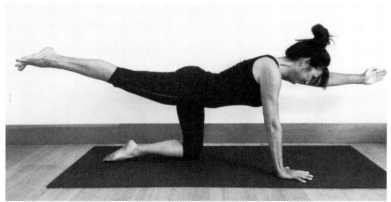

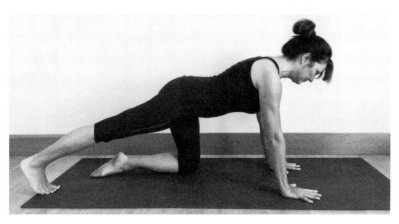

extend the healing leg back while reaching the arm on the opposite side forward (turn the palm of that hand toward center to create space around the neck and stabilize the shoulder). While stretching the fingers and toes of the lifted limbs away from each other, slowly abduct those limbs out only so far as possible while keeping the hips and upper back level with the floor before returning to a neutral position. Repeat up to twenty-five times and hold in abduction for five to ten breaths. Rest in Balasana (Child's Pose), which also stretches the hip abductors and extensors.

TADASANA (MOUNTAIN POSE) Standing with the feet positioned hip-distance apart and with weight primarily on the healthy hip, consider using crutches, a cane, or a wall for added support. Gradually place greater weight on the healing side until comfortable standing with equal weight on each leg.

UTKATASANA (AWKWARD POSE OR CHAIR POSE) Standing with the feet hip-distance apart and hands on the hips, slowly bend the knees while aligning them over the centers of the feet (be particularly aware of not allowing the knees to splay in toward each other). Rotate the pelvis forward and back to find where it

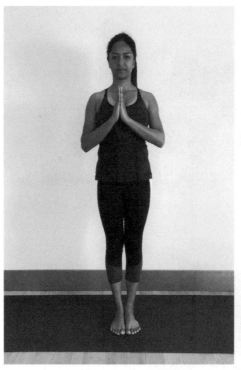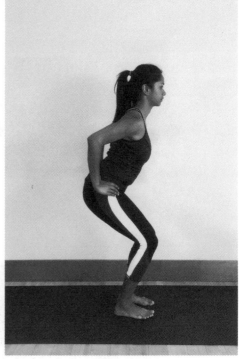

feels like the spine is drawing naturally up from the pelvis. Release the arms down, turn the palms out, and reach the arms overhead. Explore bending the knees up to ninety degrees and then press back to standing fully upright. Repeat five to ten times. On the last repetition, hold with the knees bent and arms overhead for up to ten breaths.

VIRABHADRASANA II (WARRIOR II POSE)   Start standing with the feet separated the length of one's leg plus one's foot, turn the foot of the healing side out ninety degrees (externally rotating at the hip). Place the hands on the hips to position the hips level with each other and the pelvis in neutrality (neither in anterior nor posterior rotation). Keeping the hands on the hips to maintain this position of the pelvis, slowly bend the externally rotated hip until the knee is aligned over the heel (no further; less far is okay). Lift the arms out level with the floor. Focusing on the feet and legs, firmly root down into the feet while creating a feeling of pressing the hip of the bent leg in toward the midline while pressing the knee toward the little-toe side of the foot. Alternately bend and straighten the leg several times before holding isometrically for five to ten breaths.

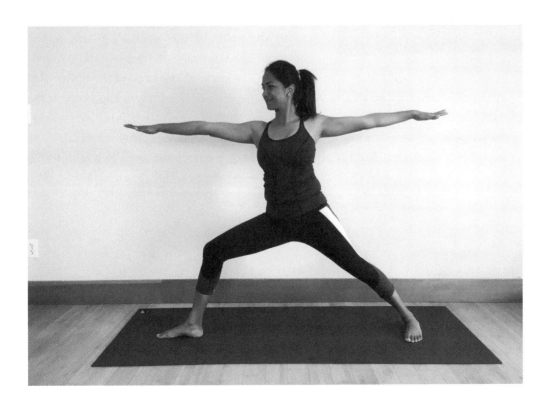

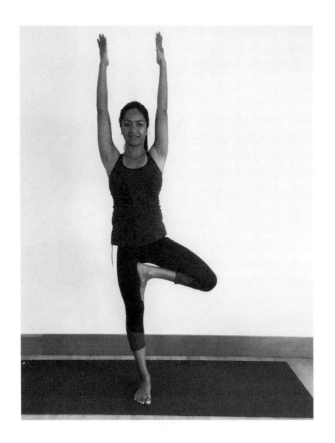

VRKSASANA (TREE POSE) Standing with the feet hip-distance apart, lift the heal of the fully healthy leg to explore what it feels like bearing weight through the healing side. If comfortable with the heel slightly lifted, explore flexing that hip to lift the foot entirely off the floor, bearing full weight down through the healing leg. Do not take the full form of Vrksasana (with the foot placed on the inner thigh) until feeling fully stable and strong around the outside of the standing hip.

Restoring Flexibility

To help restore flexibility, follow these asanas:

EKA PADA RAJAKAPOTASANA PREP (ONE-LEGGED KING PIGEON POSE PREP) Begin lying supine with the feet placed on the floor as for Setu Bandha Sarvanghasana (Bridge Pose). Cross the ankle of the healing hip side to the opposite knee, keeping the ankle joint in dorsiflexion. Clasp behind the knee of the healthy leg and pull it toward the shoulder on that same side of the body while keeping the tailbone on the floor. Alternately release and go more deeply with this stretch only so far as to create a very slight stretch around the healing hip. After several of these repetitive movements, hold at about an 80 percent stretch for up to two minutes.

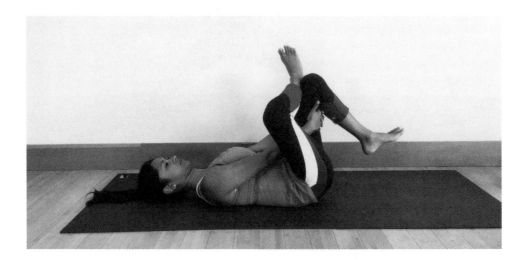

SUPTA PADANGUSTHASANA (RECLINED BIG TOE POSE)   Lying supine with a strap looped around the foot of the healing side, clasp the strap and extend the healing leg straight up from the hip. Keeping the opposite hip grounded to the floor, slowly and slightly abduct the leg, using the strap to control the range of motion and to assist in returning the leg to its vertical position. Focus on gentle stretching while keeping the inner thigh muscles relaxed—assist both the abduction and adduction with the strap. Alternately release and go more deeply with this stretch only so far as to create a very slight stretch in the inner thighs. After several of these repetitive movements, hold at about an 80 percent stretch for up to one minute.

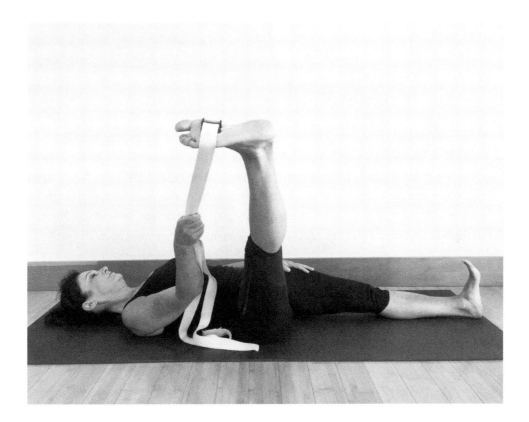

SUPTA PARIVARTANASANA (RECLINED REVOLVED POSE)   Lying supine, draw the knees together and into alignment with the hips (do not go beyond ninety degrees of hip flexion). Place a block between the knees and another block (or bolster) on the floor next to the healthy hip. Slowly release the knees to the side until they are resting on the block. Do not let the knee of the upper hip travel below the level of the hip (i.e., do not adduct toward the midline—add blocks if this occurs).

For a deeper stretch of the lateral hip compartment, straighten the upper leg, using a strap around the foot to pull and thereby deepen the stretch into the hip (and the entire IT band).

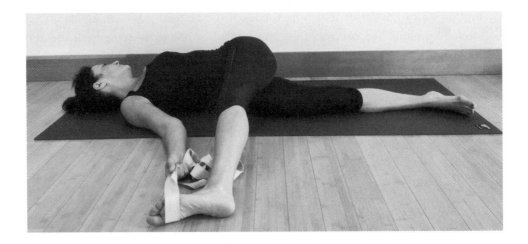

ANJANEYASANA (LOW LUNGE POSE)   From Tadasana, step one foot back about one leg length and release that knee to the floor. Draw the torso upright, place the hands on the hips to assist in positioning the pelvis neutrally, and then slowly and more deeply bend the front knee to stretch the hip flexors. **Note: This is contraindicated if the hip replacement was an anterior approach.**

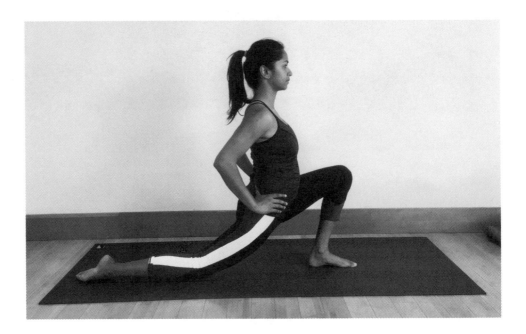

Piriformis Syndrome

The piriformis is a flat, pear-shaped muscle that originates on the anterior sacrum (S2–S4), posterior portions of the ishium, and the obturator foremen, where it then exits the pelvis through the greater sciatic foramen and inserts by a rounded tendon on the superior and posterior aspect of the greater trochanter. It externally rotates the hip when the hip is extended and abducts the hip when the hip is flexed.[40] Although innervated by branches from the L5, S1, and S2 nerve roots, part of the sciatic nerve

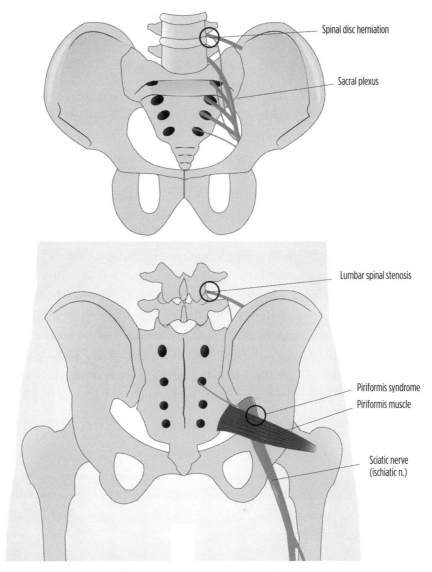

Figure 23.9: Piriformis Syndrome

passes close to or through the piriformis (in about 20 percent of people, the sciatic nerve divides the belly of the muscle).

When the piriformis muscle is tight or in spasm, it can entrap and compress the sciatic nerve and cause pain similar to that found with pressure on the sciatic nerve in the low back, leading to difficulty in precise diagnosis. (Nerve routing varies considerably, and related factors such as disc degeneration and vertebral segment instability all contribute to various patterns of cause and diagnostic challenge.)[41] Orthopedic physicians and physical therapists use the FAIR test (involving flexion, abduction, and internal rotation of the hip) as a primary diagnostic tool, and use electromyography to add a more specific diagnosis.[42] Women are twice as likely as men to develop this condition (often during pregnancy when the piriformis works more strongly to stabilize the pelvis).

THE PAINFUL EXPERIENCE

Piriformis syndrome causes a dull and persistent ache in the gluteal region that often radiates down the back of the thigh, calf, and foot. It often worsens after prolonged sitting or after walking or running with poor biomechanics (specifically with over-pronation of the feet).

THE KNOWN CAUSES

Piriformis syndrome (introduced as a controversial diagnosis in 1928 by William Yeoman)[43] is also referred to as pseudosciatica and hip socket neuropathy, reflecting contending theories of the underlying pathophysiology and etiology. The condition can be classified as Primary Piriformis Syndrome, in which symptoms arise from a pathology of the piriformis itself, or Secondary Piriformis Syndrome, in which symptoms arise from other causes such as leg length discrepancy, trauma, over-pronation of the foot (causing the piriformis to overwork in aligning the knee), or tightness or weakness of closely related muscles (particularly weak glutei and/or tight adductors). Diagnosis attempts to differentiate it from other sources of sciatic nerve entrapment and unrelated conditions with similar symptoms (such as ischial tuberosity bursitis).

HOW IT HEALS

Piriformis Syndrome responds well to stretching exercises, myofascial release, and massage along with avoiding causal activities such as sitting for long periods of time or walking with poor biomechanics. Strengthening the glutei muscles can help reduce the tendency of the piriformis to overwork.

HEALING WITH ASANA PRACTICES

The primary focus of asana in healing piriformis syndrome is on stretching and relaxing the piriformis and the hip rotators (internal and external), strengthening the hip abductors, establishing and supporting healthy spine alignment (primarily in the lumbar segment and softening the piriformis muscles), strengthening the hip abductors and adductors, and reducing tension around the sacroiliac (SI) joint.

Stretching and Relaxing

To stretch and relax the piriformis and hip rotators, follow these asanas:

EKA PADA RAJAKAPOTASANA PREP (ONE-LEGGED KING PIGEON POSE PREP) Begin lying supine with the feet placed on the floor as for Setu Bandha Sarvanghasana. Cross the ankle of the healing leg to the opposite knee, keeping the ankle joint in dorsiflexion. Clasp behind the knee of the healthy leg and pull it toward the shoulder on that same side of the body while keeping the tailbone on the floor. Alternately release and go more deeply with this stretch only so far as to create a very slight stretch in the inner thighs. After several of these repetitive movements, hold at about an 80 percent stretch for up to two minutes.

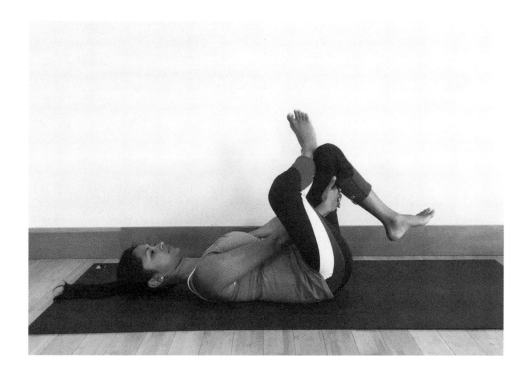

GOMUKHASANA (COW FACE POSE) Sitting upright with the legs positioned for Gomukhasana, turn the torso slightly to face the shin of the leg on top. (If unable to sit comfortably in basic Gomukhasana form while elevated on a block, stay with the prior asana.) While keeping the spine elongated, fold forward over the shin. Hold for up to two minutes, then to remove tension from the knees, shake out the legs for a few breaths while sitting in Dandasana.

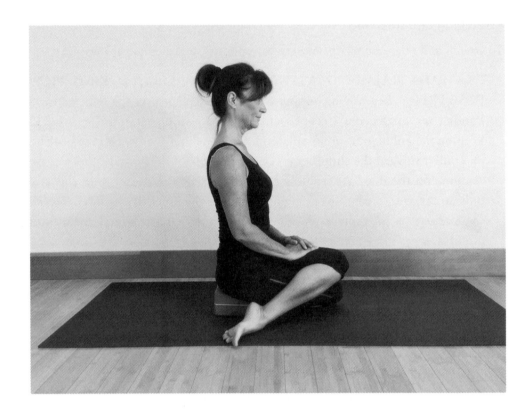

SUPTA PADANGUSTHASANA (RECLINED BIG TOE POSE) Lying supine, clasp around the knee of the healing side to flex the hip, then draw that knee across the body, coming into the basic spinal twisting form of Supta Padangusthasana. With a strap looped around the foot of the healing side, fully extend the knee of that leg while continuing to draw the leg across the body. Hold for two minutes.

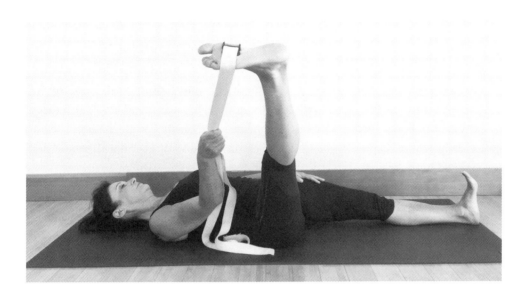

BADDHA KONASANA (BOUND ANGLE POSE)   Sitting upright, bend the knees and bring the soles of the feet together, allowing the knees to release toward the floor only as far as there is no pain or feeling of deep stretching in the knees or low back. Starting with the pelvis neutral (level) and maintaining the natural form of the spine, press the heels together while attempting to slightly rotate the pelvis forward. Hold for up to two minutes.

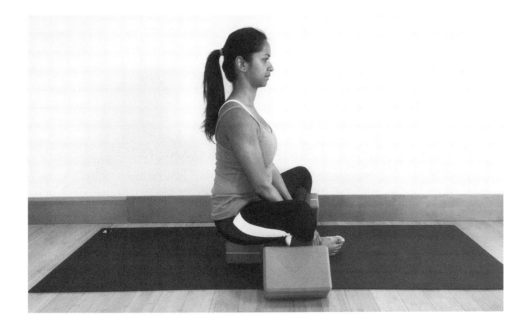

MARICHYASANA C (POSE DEDICATED TO THE SAGE MARICHI)   Sitting upright in Dandasana, slide the foot of the healing leg in close to the hip. If it is difficult to sit upright on the front of the sitting bones and with the spine tall, place a block or other bolster under the sitting bones and modify how close the foot is drawn in toward the hip. Now cross the foot over the extended leg and place the foot on the floor. Turn toward the bent knee and clasp it with the hands or arms, twisting while keeping the sitting bones firmly rooted, keeping the extended leg engaged with isometric muscle contraction (especially in the quadriceps).

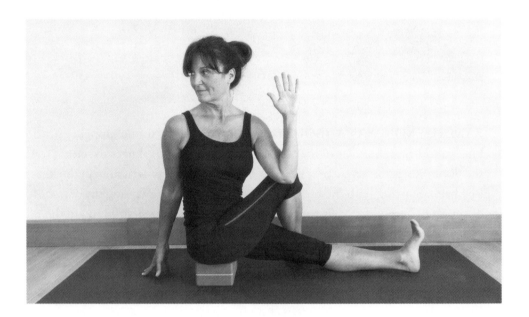

Strengthening the Hip Abductors

To strengthen the hip abductors, follow these asanas:

BIDALASANA (CAT POSE) AND SPINAL BALANCING   On all fours, first move the pelvis forward and back several times while alternately moving the spine into extension and flexion (cat/cow movements). Then extend the healing leg straight back with the toes curled under on the floor. If this is comfortable in the low back, slowly lift and lower the extended leg up to twenty-five times, holding for five to ten breaths on the last lift. Repeat on the other side. Then once again extend the healing leg back while reaching the arm on the opposite side forward (turn the palm of that hand toward center to create space around the neck and stabilize the shoulder). While stretching the fingers and toes of the lifted limbs away from each other, slowly abduct those limbs out only so far as possible while keeping the hips and upper back level with the floor before returning to a neutral position. Repeat up to twenty-five times and hold in abduction for five to ten breaths. Rest in Balasana, which also stretches the hip abductors and extensors.

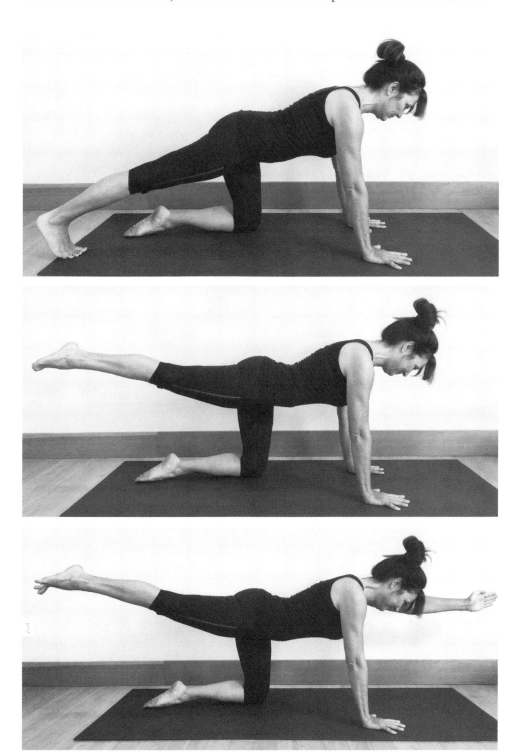

VIRABHADRASANA II (WARRIOR II POSE)   Start standing with the feet separated the length of one's leg plus one's foot, turn the foot of the healing side out ninety degrees (externally rotating at the hip). Place the hands on the hips to position the hips level with each other and the pelvis in neutrality (neither in anterior nor posterior rotation). Keeping the hands on the hips to maintain this position of the pelvis, slowly bend the externally rotated hip until the knee is aligned over the heel (no further; less far is okay). Lift the arms out level with the floor. Focusing on the feet and legs, firmly root down into the feet while creating a feeling of pressing the hip of the bent leg in toward the midline while pressing the knee toward the little-toe side of the foot. Alternately bend and straighten the leg several times before holding isometrically for five to ten breaths.

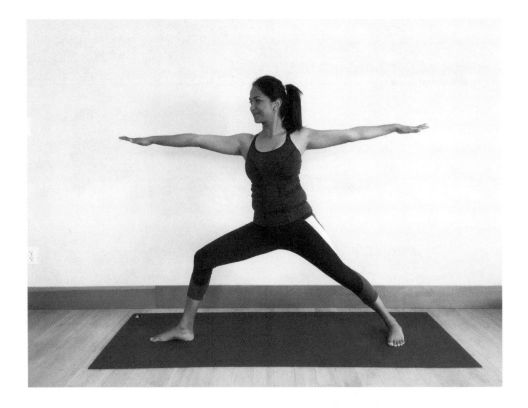

VASISTHASANA (SIDE PLANK) PREP POSE   Starting on all fours in Bidalasana, shift onto one hand and knee to come into Vasisthasana Prep Pose with the healing leg on top and fully extended with the foot on the floor. Slowly lift and lower the healing leg up to twenty-five times, rest, and repeat two to three times.

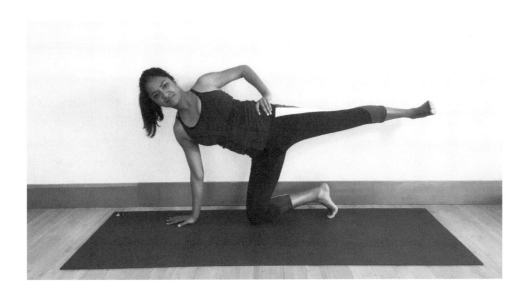

ARDHA CHANDRASANA (HALF MOON POSE) Being sensitive to pressure in the hip, come into Ardha Chandrasana with the healing leg extending directly back from the upper hip. While maintaining the basic form of Ardha Chandrasana, slowly lower and lift the healing leg up to ten times before holding it in position level with the hip for five to ten breaths. If unstable, do this against a wall.

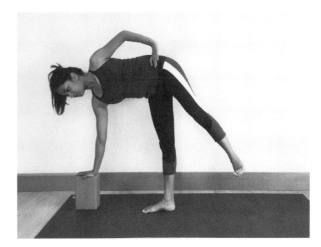

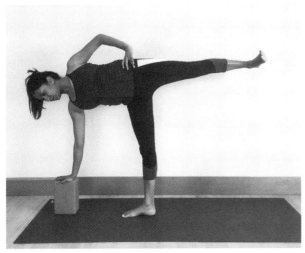

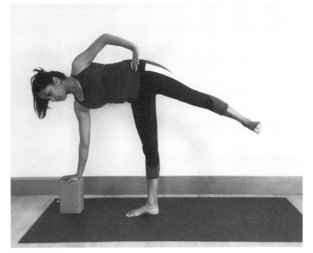

Strengthening the Hip Rotators

To strengthen the hip internal and external rotators, follow these asanas:

VIRABHADRASANA II (WARRIOR II POSE)   Start standing with the feet separated the length of one's leg plus one's foot, turn the foot of the healing side out ninety degrees (externally rotating at the hip). Place the hands on the hips to position the hips level with each other and the pelvis in neutrality (neither in anterior nor posterior rotation). Keeping the hands on the hips to maintain this position of the pelvis, slowly bend the externally rotated hip until the knee is aligned over the heel (no further; less far is okay). Lift the arms out level with the floor. Focusing on the feet and legs, firmly root down into the feet while creating a feeling of pressing the hip of the bent leg in toward the midline while pressing the knee toward the little-toe side of the foot. Alternately bend and straighten the leg several times before holding isometrically for five to ten breaths to further strengthen the hip external rotators.

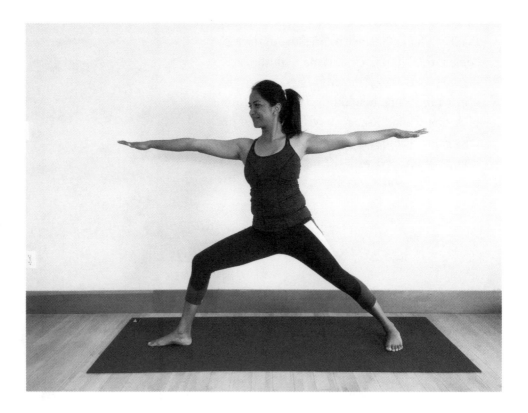

UTTHITA TRIKONASANA (EXTENDED TRIANGLE POSE)   Standing with the feet positioned parallel to each other one leg length apart, turn the right foot out ninety degrees. Position the arms level with the floor. Isometrically engaging the quadriceps muscles while creating a feeling of pressing the right sitting bone toward the left heel, reach the torso and right arm out to the right in alignment directly over the thigh without allowing the spine to fold forward. Place the right hand on a block, chair, or the shin and either place the left hand on the left hip or reach it straight up. Hold for up to two minutes while focusing on keeping the quadriceps muscles firm and pressing the right sitting bone toward the left heel. If it bothers the neck holding the head out horizontally from the spine, relax and ease the head down. This will strengthen the external rotators of the right hip.

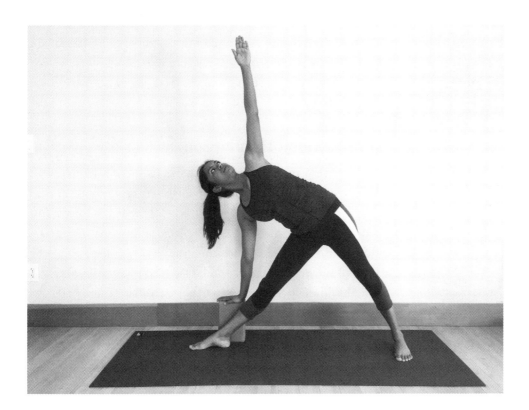

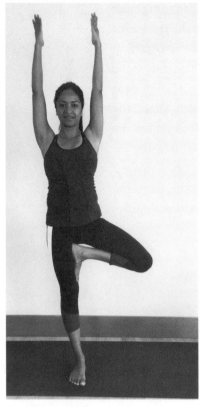

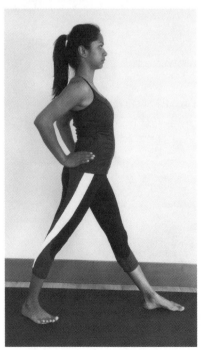

VRKSASANA (TREE POSE) Standing in Tadasana, consider using a wall for added stability in moving toward standing on one foot. Flex the right hip to clasp the knee and position the right foot along the inner right thigh. If unable to place the foot above the knee, place it below the knee, not against it at all. With the hands on the hips, bring the bent knee forward as far as necessary to position the hips even with each other. Keeping the hips evenly aligned, press the right knee back and hold for up to two minutes to strengthen the external rotators of the hip.

PARSVOTTANASANA (INTENSE SIDE STRETCH POSE) PREP From Tadasana, step one foot back slightly less than one leg length and bring that heel in toward the midline up to forty-five degrees while keeping the hips pointing evenly forward. If it is difficult to keep the hips even, reduce how far the back heel is drawn toward the midline and take a slightly wider lateral stance. Awaken pada bandha in the back foot and use that action to more directly spiral the inner thigh of the back leg back, thereby engaging the internal rotators of the hip.

Sacroiliac Joint Dysfunction

The sacrum, translated from the Latin *os sacrum* from the Greek *hieron osteon*, "sacred bone," is a large triangular bone at the base of the spine that has three articulations: 1) with the lowest lumbar vertebra (L5); 2) with the coccyx (the tailbone, a vestige of our primordial tail); and 3) with the ilium bones (the two ear-shaped bones of the pelvis). The articulation of the sacrum's alae (wings) with the ilium bones gives us the sacroiliac joints (SIJ), which transfer weight from the upper body to the pelvis and hips. Thus, there is force on the sacrum from above and below in movement of the torso and legs. The sacrum also accommodates the spinal nerves and is perforated by sacral foramina through which nerves transit into the pelvis and the lower body.

The sacrum is held very stably in place between the ilium bones by interosseous and sacroiliac ligaments. (Despite its very limited mobility, it is a synovial joint.) Its very slight normal gliding and rotary movements are further limited by the surrounding presence

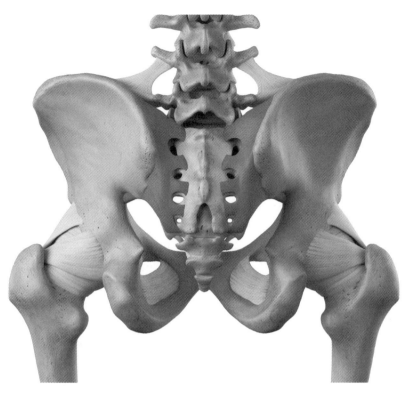

Figure 23.10: The Sacroiliac Joint

of strong and heavy muscle tissues as well as by the sacrotuberous and sacrospinous ligaments that limit upward movement of the sacrum and provide resilience amid activity such as landing from a jump. SIJ dysfunction refers to pain in the region that is due primarily to hypermobility or hypomobility, which can occur simultaneously on two sides. SIJ pain can also arise from arthritis, leg length discrepancy, pelvic fractures, and pregnancy.

THE PAINFUL EXPERIENCE

There is no debate about the SIJ as a significant source of chronic low back pain.[44] Common symptoms of SIJ dysfunction also include pain in the buttocks, groin, hips, and legs. Pain in the low back and hip are more associated with hypermobility whereas pain on one side of the low back, buttocks, and down into the leg are more associated with hypomobility. Pain varies from a dull ache to sharp and stabbing depending on the proximate cause, immediate activity (including prolonged sitting), posture, and physiological factors that include hormonal changes attendant to the menstrual cycle.[45]

THE KNOWN CAUSES

As noted earlier, the exact cause of SIJ dysfunction often cannot be determined as it can arise from a wide array of conditions, including arthritis, leg length discrepancy, lumbar spinal conditions, pelvic trauma, and pregnancy. Its primary causes are hypermobility and/or hypomobility in the SIJ itself.

SIJ hypermobility is caused by the inability of the supporting ligaments to stabilize the joints. In most cases the weakened ligamentous support is caused by a traumatic injury.[46] During pregnancy, heightened relaxin hormone levels relax (soften) ligaments throughout the body, functioning in this way to allow greater pelvic dilation during labor; in many women, the SIJ never restabilizes postpartum.[47] SIJ hypomobility can arise from a variety of causes but is most commonly associated with osteoarthritis, with abnormal adhesion and rigidity in the bones of the joints.

The unreliability of x-ray, CT scan, and MRI methods in discerning SIJ conditions has led to several clinical physical examination assessments for better determining the source of pain.

HOW IT HEALS

Treatment strategies depend on diagnosis. Most conditions are given conservative treatment that includes rest, anti-inflammatory medication, and physical therapy. In cases of severe pain that is not responsive to conservative treatment, surgical fusion is sometimes recommended.

HEALING WITH ASANA PRACTICES

Most SIJ dysfunction is associated with hypermobility and related asymmetrical torqueing forces on the joints. Yet while postural and action-oriented asymmetry may contribute to SIJ dysfunction, effective treatment can utilize asymmetrical asanas for realignment and stabilization.

SIJ dysfunction invites very patient and attentive asana practice. Many common asanas can exacerbate tension in the SIJ, particularly asymmetrical standing balance poses such as Virabhadrasana III (Warrior III Pose) and Parivrtta Ardha Chandrasana (Revolved Half Moon Pose), and asymmetrical hip openers such as Gomukhasana (Cow Face Pose) and the prone version of Eka Pada Rajakapotasana (One-Legged King Pigeon Pose) that can overstretch the external rotators.

Stabilizing and Restoring Balanced Functioning

To stabilize and restore balanced functioning of the SIJ, follow these asanas:

SALABHASANA A (LOCUST POSE) LEG LIFTS   Lying prone with the arms on the floor along the sides of the body and with the legs together, firmly press the feet down to awaken the legs while pressing the tailbone slightly toward the heels. Slowly lift the legs slightly off the floor and slowly release them back down. If pain-free, repeat several times, lifting slightly higher each time. Explore lifting the torso at the same time, eventually holding for five to ten breaths.

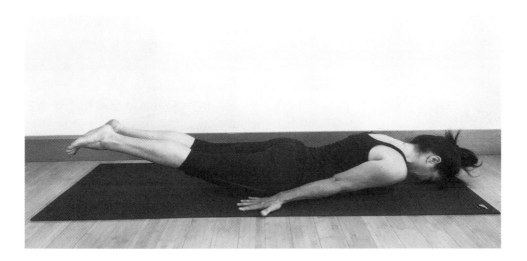

SETU BANDHA SARVANGHASANA (BRIDGE POSE)   Lying supine, position the feet near the hips and in line with the hips to prepare for Setu Bandha Sarvanghasana. Slowly lift the pelvis while focusing on pressing up into the sitting bones, pressing the hamstrings tendons into the ischial tuberosities while elongating the tailbone toward the knees. Hold for five to eight breaths before very slowly lowering down and resting for several breaths. Repeat two or three times.

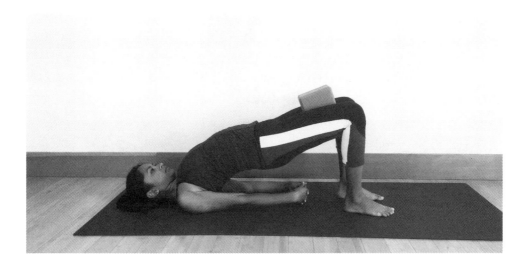

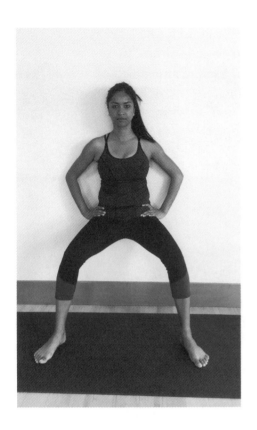

RIKSASANA (BEAR POSE) PREP   Standing with back against a wall and the feet positioned hip-distance apart about one-half leg length away from the wall, slowly slide the pelvis down the wall until the thighs are level with the floor (or less far if this is too difficult). Do not let knees travel beyond the heels. Hold for one to two minutes.

VIRABHADRASANA II (WARRIOR II POSE)   Start by standing with the feet separated by the length of one's leg plus one's foot, and turn the foot of the healing side out ninety degrees (externally rotating at the hip). Place the hands on the hips to position the hips level with each other and the pelvis in neutrality (neither in anterior nor posterior rotation). Keeping the hands on the hips to maintain this position of the pelvis, slowly bend the externally rotated hip until the knee is aligned over the heel (no further; less far is okay). Lift the arms out level with the floor. Focusing on the feet and legs, firmly root down into the feet while creating a feeling of pressing the hip of the bent leg in toward the midline while pressing the knee toward the little-toe side of

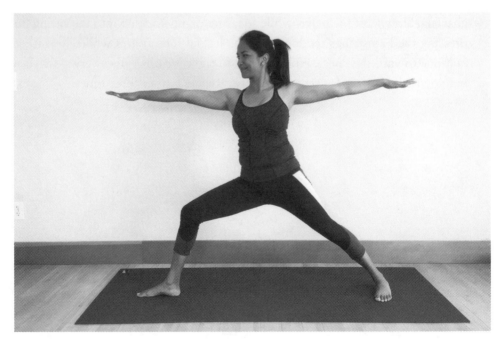

the foot. Alternately bend and straighten the leg several times before holding iso-metrically for five to ten breaths to further strengthen the hip external rotators.

UTTHITA TRIKONASANA (EXTENDED TRIANGLE POSE)   Standing with the feet positioned parallel to each other one leg length apart, turn the right foot out ninety degrees. Position the arms level with the floor. Isometrically engaging the quadriceps muscles while creating a feeling of pressing the right sitting bone toward the left heel, reach the torso and right arm out to the right in alignment directly over the thigh without allowing the spine to fold forward. Place the right hand on a block, chair, or the shin and either place the left land on the left hip or reach it straight up. Hold for up to two minutes while focusing on keeping the quadriceps muscles firm and pressing the right sitting bone toward the left heel. If it bothers the neck to hold the head out horizontally from the spine, relax and ease the head down. This will strengthen the external rotators of the right hip.

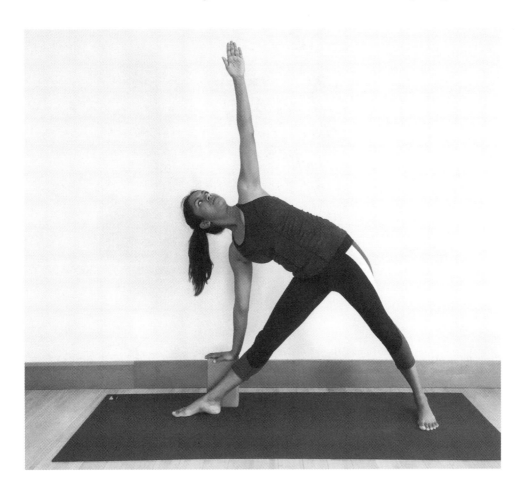

MARICHYASANA C (POSE DEDICATED TO THE SAGE MARICHI)   Sitting upright in Dandasana, slide the foot of the healing leg in close to the hip. If it is difficult to sit upright on the front of the sitting bones and with the spine tall, place a block or other bolster under the sitting bones and modify how close the foot is drawn in toward the hip. Now cross the foot over the extended leg and place the foot on the floor. Turn toward the bent knee and clasp it with the hands or arms, twisting while allowing the sitting bone on the side you are twisting toward to shift back, thereby allowing the lumbar segment to move with the pelvis.

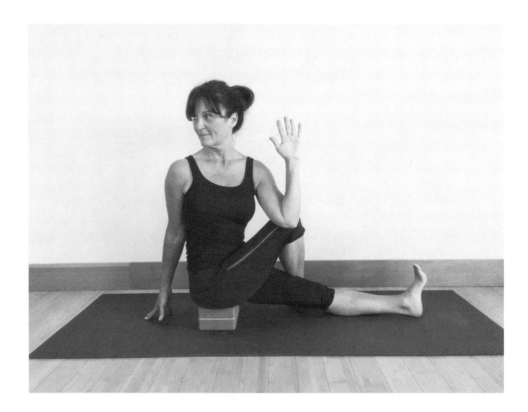

ARDHA MATSYENDRASANA (HALF LORD OF THE FISHES POSE)   Come into the basic form of Ardha Matsyendrasana. If unable to sit upright on the front of the sitting bones or if there is pressure in the knees, sit up on a prop. If it is difficult to draw the foot of the raised knee across to the floor, place it in front of the hip. Turn toward the lifted knee, clasping it with the hand or arm to pull it toward center while twisting toward it. Allow the sitting bone on the side you are twisting toward to shift back, thereby allowing the lumbar segment to move with the pelvis.

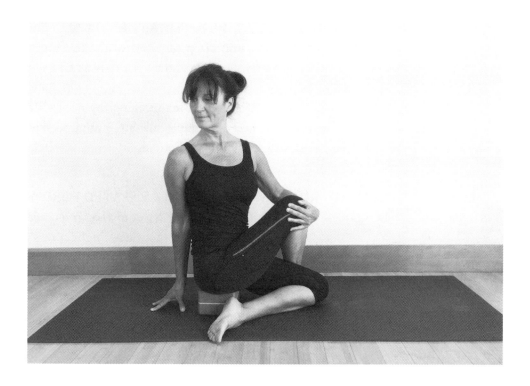

EKA PADA RAJAKAPOTASANA PREP (ONE-LEGGED KING PIGEON POSE PREP)   Begin lying supine with the feet placed on the floor as for Setu Bandha Sarvanghasana. Cross the ankle of the healing leg to the opposite knee, keeping the ankle joint in dorsiflexion. Clasp behind the knee of the healthy leg and pull it toward the shoulder on that same side of the body while keeping the tailbone on the floor. Alternately release and go more deeply with this stretch only so far as to create a very slight stretch in the inner thighs. After several of these repetitive movements, hold at about an 80 percent stretch for up to two minutes.

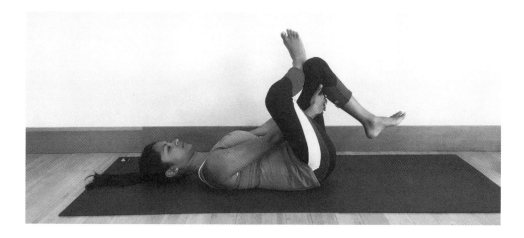

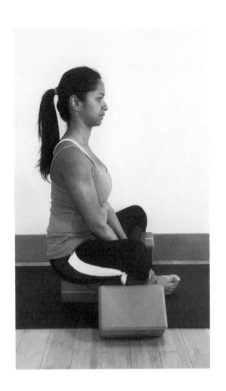

BADDHA KONASANA (BOUND ANGLE POSE) Sitting upright, bend the knees and bring the soles of the feet together, allowing the knees to release toward the floor only as far as there is no pain or feeling of deep stretching in the inner thighs. Starting with the pelvis neutral (level) and maintaining the natural form of the spine, press the heels together while attempting to slightly rotate the pelvis forward. Hold at about an 80 percent stretch for up to two minutes.

UPAVISTA KONASANA (WIDE-ANGLE SEATED FORWARD FOLD) Sitting upright, separate the legs only so far as there is a very slight stretching sensation in the inner thighs. Press out through the heels and firm the quadriceps muscles. Maintaining the natural form of the spine, explore slowly and slightly rotating the pelvis forward. Alternately release and go more deeply with this stretch only so far as to create a very slight stretch in the inner thighs. After several of these repetitive movements, hold at about an 80 percent stretch for up to two minutes.

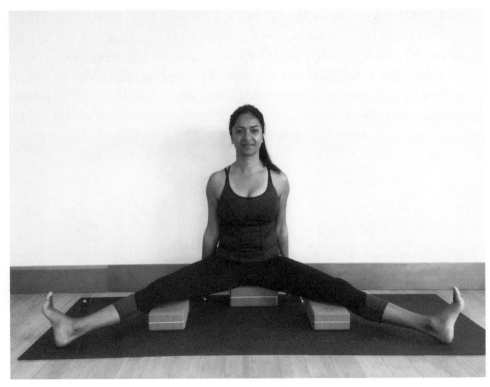

EKA PADA RAJAKAPOTASANA PREP (ONE-LEGGED KING PIGEON POSE PREP)   Begin lying supine with the feet placed on the floor as for Setu Bandha Sarvanghasana. Cross the ankle of the healing leg to the opposite knee, keeping the ankle joint in dorsiflexion. Clasp behind the knee of the healthy leg and pull it toward the shoulder on that same side of the body while keeping the tailbone on the floor. Alternately release and go more deeply with this stretch only so far as to create a very slight stretch in the inner thighs. After several of these repetitive movements, hold at about an 80 percent stretch for up to two minutes.

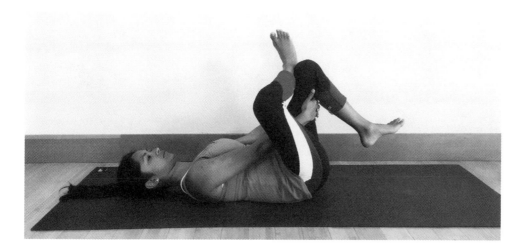

GOMUKHASANA (COW FACE POSE)   Sitting upright with the legs positioned for Gomukhasana, turn the torso slightly to face the shin of the leg on top. (If unable to sit comfortably in basic Gomukhasana form while elevated on a block, stay with the prior asana.) While keeping the spine elongated, fold forward over the shin. Hold for up to two minutes, then to remove tension from the knees, shake out the legs for a few breaths while sitting in Dandasana.

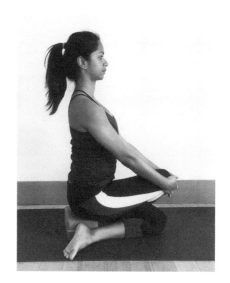

SUPTA PARIVARTANASANA (RECLINED REVOLVED POSE) Lying supine, clasp around the knee of the healing side to flex the hip, then draw that knee across the body, coming into the basic spinal twisting form of Supta Parivartanasana. With a strap looped around the foot of the healing side, fully extend the knee of that leg while continuing to draw the leg across the body. Hold for two minutes.

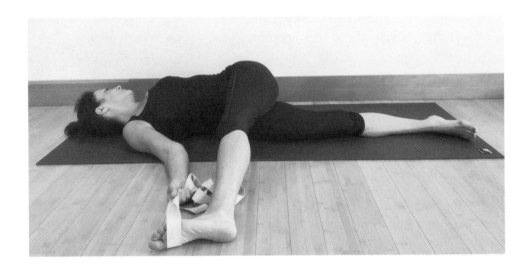

Spinal and Neck Conditions

Lumbar Hyperlordosis

The term *lordosis* (commonly called swayback) refers to the abnormal anterior rotation of the pelvis at the hip joints that produces an abnormal increase in the normal lordotic curvature of the lumbar spine segment.[48] Lordosis becomes hyperlordosis when the arch causes pain. Hyperlordosis causes uneven (wedging) pressure on the intervertebral discs, painful pressure on nerves, and the potential to herniate discs. It also affects the other spinal segments, increasing the natural curves in the thoracic and cervical spine segments.

THE PAINFUL EXPERIENCE

Lumbar hyperlordosis is one of the most common causes of pain in the lower back.[49] The pain can be moderate or severe and tends to increase with physical activity.

THE KNOWN CAUSES

Several factors can contribute to lumbar hyperlordosis. Imbalances in muscle strength and flexibility are the leading factors. Spinal and bone conditions, including spondylolisthesis (forward displacement of a vertebral body, most often L5) and osteoporosis, are

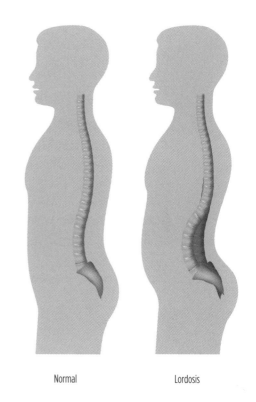

Normal   Lordosis

Figure23.11: The Lumbar Spine Segment

also common causes of hyperlordosis. Pregnancy (second and third trimesters) and obesity (when there is a potbelly) also cause excessive forward rotation of the pelvis. Here we focus on muscular imbalances.

Weak anterolateral abdominal muscles (rectus abdominus and transverse abdominus), weak or overstretched hamstring muscles, tight hip flexors (iliopsoas and rectus femoris), and tight posterolumbro muscles (especially quadratus lumborum [QL]) all cause the pelvis to rotate forward at the hip joints even when attempting to stand upright with normal posture.

HOW IT HEALS

If caused by muscular imbalance, hyperlordosis is corrected and pain generally resolves by attaining muscular balance. If caused by spondylolisthesis, lumbar hyperlordosis can be often treated with physical therapy, although severe cases are often treated pharmacologically and surgically. If caused by pregnancy, hyperlordosis generally self-resolves with restoration of the normal line of gravity. If caused by potbellied obesity, the condition is generally corrected by weight loss.

HEALING WITH ASANA PRACTICES

The primary focus of asana is on restoring muscular balance in support of pelvis neutrality in relation to the femurs and spine. This involves stretching and developing increased flexibility in the hip flexors and QLs while developing greater strength and tonicity in the anterolateral abdominal muscles and hamstrings.

Stretching and Lengthening the Hip Flexors

To stretch and lengthen the hip flexors, follow these asanas:

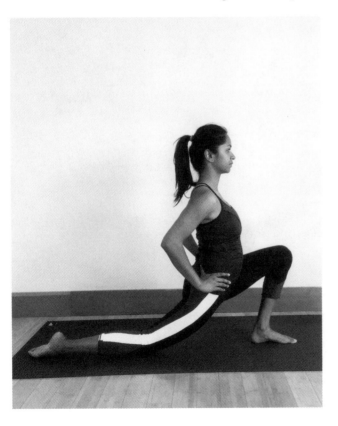

ANJANEYASANA (LOW LUNGE POSE)
From Tadasana, step one foot back about one leg length and release that knee to the floor. Position the torso upright and place the hands on the hips to assist in positioning the pelvis neutrally (where it feels level). Keep the hands on the hips with the thumbs pointing down near the SI joints. While slowly bending the front knee, use the hands to keep the pelvis from rotating forward. Unless one has acute knee issues, it is okay to let the knee travel beyond the heel, which will allow a deeper stretch in the hip flexors. Be more interested in keeping the pelvis level than in deepening the lunge. Inhaling, back away from the lunge, exhaling, lunge more deeply, moving repetitively in this way five to ten times before holding a comfortably deep lunge position for up to one minute. Do both sides equally.

ASHTA CHANDRASANA (EIGHT-POINT CRESCENT MOON POSE) From Tadasana, step one foot back about one leg length with the toes curled under on the floor. Position the torso upright and place the hands on the hips to assist in positioning the pelvis neutrally (where it feels level). Keep the hands on the hips with the thumbs pointing down near the SI joints. While slowly bending the front knee into alignment over the heel (not past it in order to keep stress away from the knee), use the hands to keep the pelvis from rotating forward. Be more interested in keeping the pelvis level than in deepening the lunge. Inhaling, back away from the lunge, exhaling, lunge more deeply, moving repetitively in this way five to ten times before holding a comfortably deep lunge position for up to one minute. Do both sides equally.

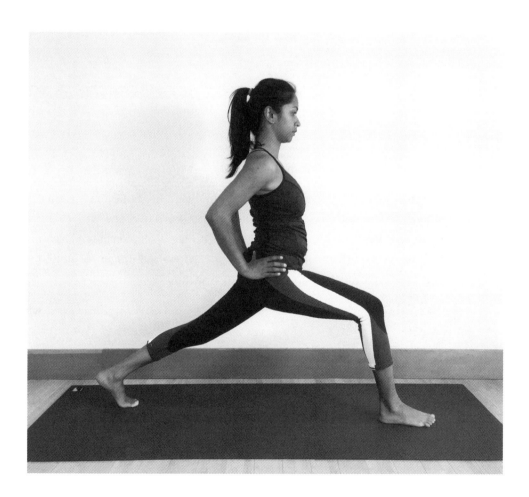

SUPTA VIRASANA (RECLINING HERO POSE)   Explore this only with healthy knees. Start in Virasana (Hero Pose) with a block placed under the sitting bones and at least one bolster placed behind the block. Slowly release back onto the bolster, going only as far as there is no intense pressure or pain in the knees or low back (if necessary add props or stay with the lunge poses). Keep the knees on the floor and let everything relax. Hold for up to two minutes.

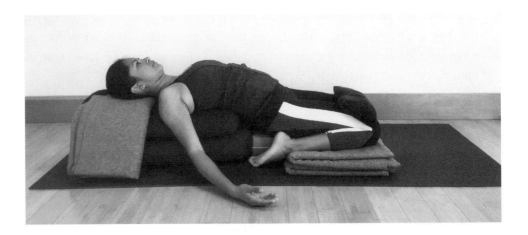

Stretching the QLs

To stretch the QLs, follow these asanas:

BALASANA (CHILD'S POSE) VARIATION   Begin in Balasana. Rather than folding forward over both thighs, fold obliquely forward over the right thigh while reaching the left arm forward from the shoulder. Play with alternately arching the left lower back up and then back down while stretching out longer through the left arm and hand. Explore both sides for one to two minutes.

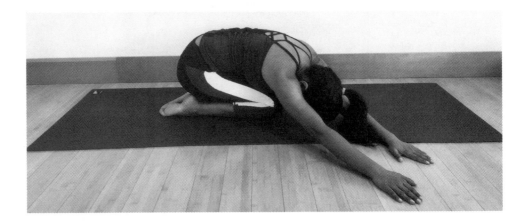

SUPTA PARIVARTANASANA (RECLINED REVOLVED POSE) Lying supine, clasp around the knee of the healing side to flex the hip, then draw that knee across the body, coming into the basic spinal twisting form of Supta Parivartanasana. With a strap looped around the foot of the crossed over leg, fully extend the knee of that leg while continuing to draw the leg across the body. Hold for two minutes. Explore on both sides.

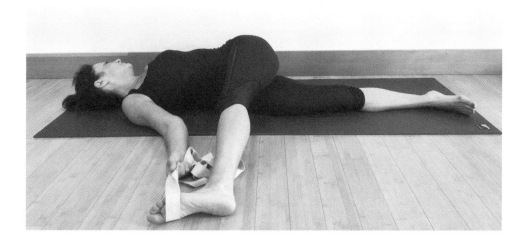

PARIVRTTA JANU SIRSASANA (REVOLVED HEAD-TO-KNEE POSE) VARIATIONS Start sitting upright with the legs positioned in the basic form for Parivrtta Janu Sirsasana with the left knee flexed and right leg fully extended. Twist to align the sternum with the bent left knee. While maintaining maximum length in the low back, extend the torso to the right (over the straight leg) while reaching

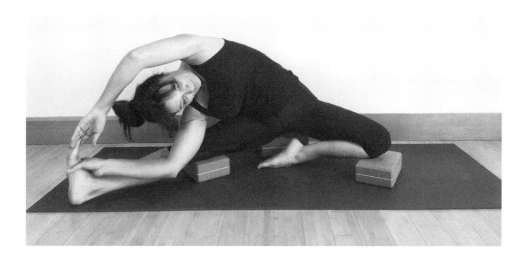

the left arm straight up from the shoulder (in flexion and external rotation). While keeping the left sitting bone firmly rooted to the floor, explore very slightly and sensitively turning the torso toward the floor while stretching from the back of the left hip through the left fingertips. Explore on both sides for up to two minutes.

Strengthening the Hamstrings

To strengthen the hamstrings, follow these asanas:

BIDALASANA (CAT POSE) VARIATION   Positioned on all fours in Bidalasana, fully extend the right leg with the toes curled under on the floor. Explore slowly lifting and lowering the right leg while keeping the knee fully extended. Do up to three sets of fifteen repetitions before switching sides.

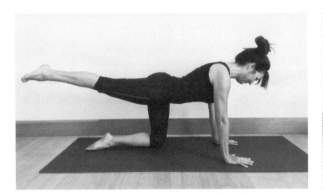 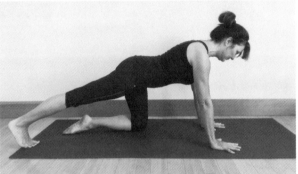

SETU BANDHA SARVANGHASANA (BRIDGE POSE) VARIATIONS   Lying supine, position the feet near the hips and in line with them to prepare for Setu Bandha Sarvanghasana. Slowly lift the pelvis while elongating the tailbone toward the knees, and while lifting reach the arms overhead to the floor. While at the

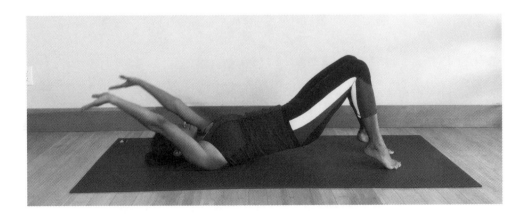

maximum elevation of the pelvis away from the floor, lift the heels to more easily lengthen the tailbone toward the heels while releasing the spine slowly to the floor one vertebra at a time from top to bottom. Repeat ten to fifteen times and then hold in Bridge Pose for five to eight breaths before very slowly lowering down and resting for several breaths. If pain-free, repeat two or three times.

TADASANA (MOUNTAIN POSE) TO UTTANASANA (STANDING FOR-WARD FOLD) AND BACK We build the greatest strength in the hamstrings when using them in eccentric contraction. This is how the hamstrings work when swan-diving from standing upright into a standing forward bend. Do not attempt this until in the subacute phase of healing. Move slowly and at first with bent knees to better moderate tension in the hamstrings. If comfortable, explore folding forward and down with the knees fully extended. As with all forward bends, try to initiate and maximize the movement through the forward (anterior) rotation of the pelvis before allowing the spine to flex. In rising back to standing upright, proceed in the same way: slowly, at first with bent knees, and gradually with fully extended knees.

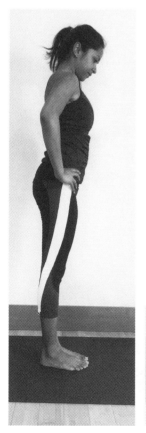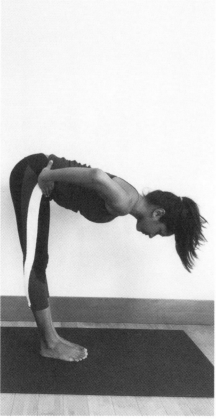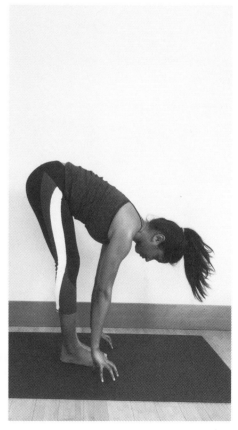

Strengthening the Anterolateral Abdominal Muscles

To strengthen the anterolateral abdominal muscles, follow these asanas:

DWI CHAKRA VAHANASANA (YOGIC BICYCLES)   From Apanasana, interlace the fingers and cup the head in the hands. With the exhalation, curl the torso up, drawing the elbows toward the knees while extending the right leg straight out about one foot off the floor and extending the right arm out over

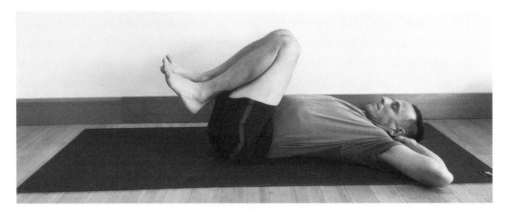

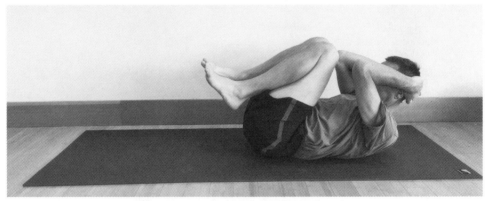

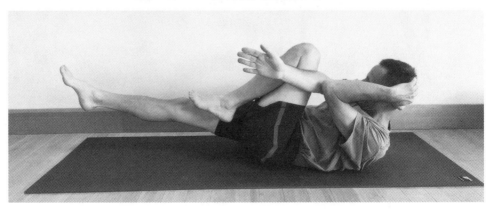

the right leg. Complete the exhalation while drawing the right arm across the left knee and drawing the elbows together. Inhaling, release down, drawing the knees toward the chest and head and elbows to the floor. Move slowly and work as low, deep, and broadly through the belly as possible. Be more interested in moving slowly yet steadily rather than seeing how many you can do with a timed sequence. Move with the breath. Repeat on the other side, continuing for one to three minutes.

PELVIC TILTS From Apanasana, extend the legs straight up, interlace the fingers, and cup the head in the hands. Keeping the legs vertical, on the exhalation draw the elbows toward the knees without changing the position of the legs. Keeping the upper back and shoulders lifted, with each exhale very slowly and smoothly curl the tailbone up, releasing it down as the breath flows out. Be more interested in slow and smooth movement than in maximizing the pelvic tilt by jerking the tailbone up. Repeat five to twenty-five times.

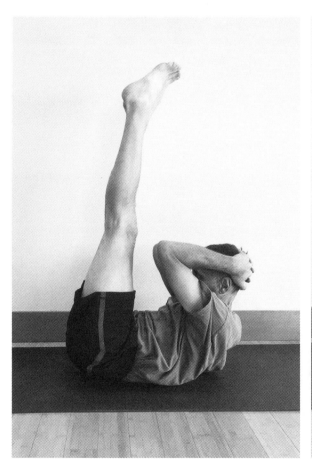
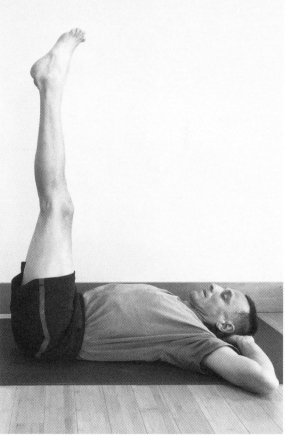

JATHARA PARIVARTANASANA (REVOLVING TWIST POSE) The basic form of this asana can be either a held twist (Supta Parivartanasana) or an abdominal core strengthening movement. With the arms extended out like a cross and palms pressing down, alternately move the legs (or bent knees) back and forth to the left and right while gazing in the opposite direction of the legs, keeping the knees or legs from touching the floor. Inhaling, extend the legs over; exhaling, draw them back up to center.

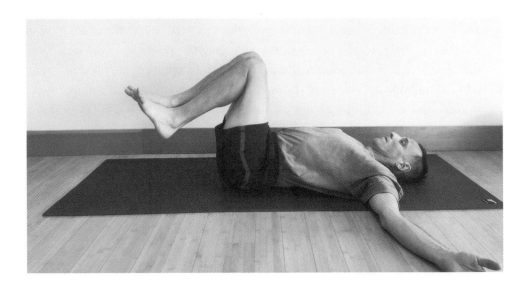

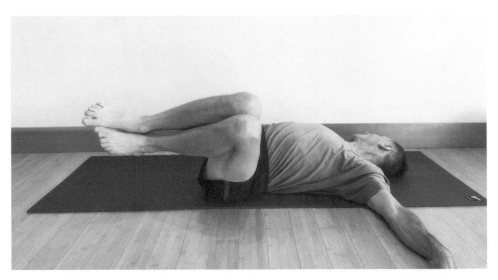

Degenerative Disc Disease

The vertebral column (spine) generally consists of 33 vertebrae (rarely 32 or 34) arranged in five regions: cervical (C1–C7), thoracic (T1–T12), lumbar (L1–L5), sacral (S1–5), and coccygeal (four that are not ordinarily numbered). Although vertebrae in the sacral and coccygeal regions are fused, fibrocartilaginous intervertebral discs separate, bind, and provide shock absorption between all but two of the other twenty-four vertebrae—the atypical C1 and C2 (Atlas and Axis, respectively), with C1 resting on the facets of C2. Thus, the most superior disc is between C2 and C3, and the most inferior disc is between L5 and S1.

The varying shapes of the intervertebral discs give curvature to the spine. All have a common structure: the *annulus fibrosus*, several thin fibrocartilaginous layers that form an outer ring (thinner posteriorly) and that is bonded to the articular surfaces of the vertebral bodies, and the *nucleus pulposus*, an inner fibrogelatinous pulp that is the cushioning mechanism. The discs broaden when weighted. When excessively weighted, they can herniate or protrude in ways that press on nerve roots and cause pain. Due to the structure of the discs (the pulp is located relatively posteriorly where there is less ligamentous support), excessively strong spinal flexion (forward folding)—especially when combined with spinal rotation—is the leading cause of bulging and herniated discs placing pressure on nerve roots.[50]

The intervertebral discs naturally and progressively degenerate across the lifespan, albeit differently depending on conditions discussed in the following text.[51] They also degenerate and regenerate daily, losing height due to compressive loading forces during the day that expel fluid from the disc, then gaining height at low loading pressure as osmotic pressure imbibes fluid back into the disc.[52] As a result we literally shrink and grow in height in every diurnal cycle (i.e., daily, which is why car drivers need to adjust their rear-view mirror every morning and night), while across the lifespan we shrink: every ninety-year-old is slightly shorter than when he or she was twenty-five years old.

These natural processes of disc degeneration combine with individual genetic endowments and lifestyle choices (and accidents) to determine the rate and extent of degenerative disc disease. Specific degenerative conditions vary, including the location and extent of disc space narrowing (stenosis), herniation, extent

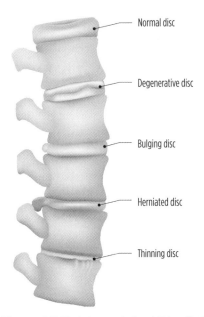

Normal disc

Degenerative disc

Bulging disc

Herniated disc

Thinning disc

Figure 23.12: Intervertebral Disc Pathologies

of end plate sclerosis, development of bone spurs, and the consequent narrowing of the foramina that places more pressure on nerve roots.[53]

THE PAINFUL EXPERIENCE

There is a vast range of degenerative disc-related pain experiences. When symptomatic (often it is not), it is most often experienced as chronic low back pain that may or may not vary depending on position or activity (sitting, standing, walking, folding, etc.). Whereas low back pain is the most common, one can also experience chronic pain in the neck. Pressure on sciatic nerve roots can cause tingling and pain through the buttocks, thighs, and lower legs. The degree of pain varies from very mild to debilitating.

THE KNOWN CAUSE

The primary cause of intervertebral disc degeneration is the relationship between disc structure and force on the disc. Age is the leading factor in loss of disc fluid.[54] Repetitive and excessive spinal movement, obesity, repetitive heavy lifting, acute injury, and smoking cigarettes exacerbate natural disc degeneration.[55]

HOW IT HEALS

Conventional medical practices call for progressive treatments, starting with ice or heat in combination with anti-inflammatory medications, physical therapy, and surgery that ranges from removal of a damaged disc to spinal fusion to placement of an artificial disc. There is growing interest in biological treatment approaches in which various cell therapy techniques show promise in reversing disc degeneration, including protein injection, gene therapy, and platelet-rich plasma cocktails.[56]

HEALING WITH ASANA PRACTICES

The general asana strategy for degenerative disc disease is to develop the balance in muscular strength and flexibility that supports healthy posture, this in conjunction with neuromuscular re-education that refines the use of muscles that affect pressure in and around the spine. It is important to understand that while current research shows promise for biological treatments with the potential to reverse certain degenerative conditions, at present we must proceed with the awareness that there is not a cure for disc degeneration. Here we offer postural practices that focus on healthy postures and help to reduce compressive pressure in the spine due to disc degeneration.

The suggestions offered here are informed in part by the patient-centered self-help-oriented treatment methods developed by Robert McKenzie and known in physical therapy as the McKenzie Protocol or McKenzie exercises. We also draw from the Alexander Technique.

Establishing an Inner Foundation

To establish an inner foundation for healthy upright posture, practice these asanas:

UTKATASANA (CHAIR POSE) MODIFIED   Begin sitting in a chair the height of which allows the thighs to be level and the feet firmly placed on the floor hip-distance apart. With the hands on the hips, rotate the pelvis forward and back to find where it feels like the weight of the body is centered very slightly to the front of the sitting bones. This establishes a level pelvis and will help in positioning the spine in its natural form. With the fingers placed on the lowest front ribs, alternately press the ribs into and away from the fingers to find where it feels like they are in their natural place. Elevate the shoulders toward the ears, draw them back, and then draw the shoulders lightly down against the back ribs. Rest the hands comfortably on the thighs. Position the head level, where it feels like it is effortlessly floating on top of the spine. The spine is now in (or close to) its natural form (all conditions notwithstanding, particularly pathological ones that affect spinal posture).

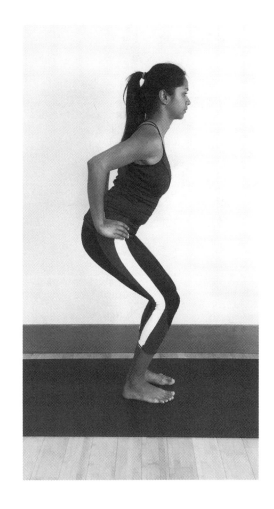

Changing as little as possible, root the sitting bones firmly into the seat of the chair. Breathing slowly and fully in and slowly and completely out, feel the natural ways the body moves through the cycles of breath. Focusing on keeping the spine in its neutral and natural alignment, with each inhalation consciously extend taller while minimizing disturbance to the form of the spine. With the completion of each exhalation, feel how the abdominal muscles lightly engage and girdle in toward the spine; without squeezing the belly, try to maintain this light abdominal muscular engagement while next inhaling and while maintaining the position of the pelvis, spine, shoulder girdle, and head. Stay with this practice for up to five minutes. With the completion of the exhalations, explore holding the breath out for two to ten seconds while more strongly engaging the abdominal muscles. Be sure to let the abdominal muscles slightly soften before inhaling.

TADASANA (MOUNTAIN POSE)   Begin with the cultivation of pada bandha described on page 107. With pada bandha active, firm the quadriceps while pressing the femurs back (try to point the kneecaps straight forward). Rotate the pelvis forward and back to find where it feels level (use the prior practice of Utkatasana to get a better feeling for this.) With the fingers placed on the lowest front ribs, alternately press the ribs into and away from the fingers to find where it feels like

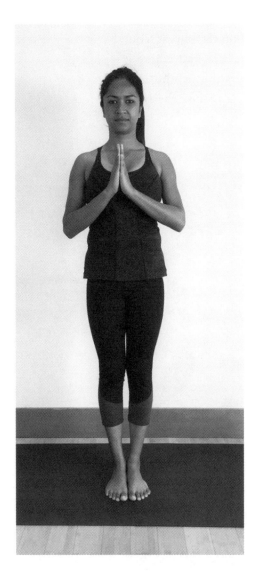

they are in their natural place. Elevate the shoulders toward the ears, draw them back, and then draw the shoulders lightly down against the back ribs. Relax the arms down by the sides of the thighs or hips. Position the head level, where it feels like it is effortlessly floating on top of the spine with the ears aligned with the shoulders. The spine is now in (or close to) its natural form (all conditions notwithstanding, particularly pathological ones that affect spinal posture). With pelvic neutrality, the spine will come into its natural curvature (neutral extension), unless there is significant muscular imbalance or a pathological condition such as scoliosis or kyphosis.

Breathing slowly and fully in and slowly and completely out, feel the natural ways the body moves through the cycles of breath. Focusing on keeping the spine in its neutral and natural alignment, with each inhalation consciously extend taller with a feeling of the crown of the head reaching up while minimizing disturbance to the form of the spine. With the completion of each exhalation, feel how the abdominal muscles lightly engage and girdle in toward the spine; without squeezing the belly, try to maintain this light abdominal muscular engagement while next inhaling and while maintaining the position of the pelvis, spine, shoulder girdle, and head. Stay with this practice for up to two minutes. With the completion of the exhalations, explore holding the breath out for two to ten seconds while more strongly engaging the abdominal muscles. Be sure to let the abdominal muscles slightly soften before inhaling.

SETU BANDHA SARVANGHASANA (BRIDGE POSE) PREP—LOW BACK PRACTICE 1   Here we take the preparatory form of Bridge Pose to explore the connection between breathing and developing muscular support for a neutral lumbar spine. Lying supine with the feet positioned by the hips hip-distance apart, slide one hand under the low back area. Rotate the pelvis to create just enough space for the hand. With each exhalation, feel how the abdominal muscles engage and cause the low back to press toward the floor. Rather than allowing the spine to change form with the exhalations, focus on maintaining the neutral position of the pelvis in relation to the low back and try to maintain the natural lumbar curve. With the completion of each exhalation, hold the breath out for up to five seconds while more firmly engaging the abdominal muscles that naturally contract when exhaling out all of the breath. This practice will help to train the abdominal muscles to contract in support of a healthy natural spinal form.

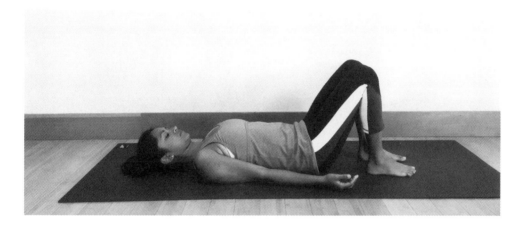

SETU BANDHA SARVANGHASANA (BRIDGE POSE) PREP—LOW BACK PRACTICE 2   Building on Low Back Practice 1, on each exhalation try to draw one knee in toward the same side shoulder without disturbing the natural form of the spine (keep the normal lumbar curve). Then try to draw in both knees at the same time without affecting the spine.

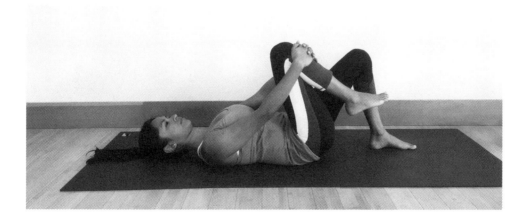

SETU BANDHA SARVANGHASANA (BRIDGE POSE) PREP—LOW BACK PRACTICE 3 Building on Low Back Practice 1, place a strap around one foot, extend that leg toward the sky, and alternately bend and straighten the knee of that leg to stretch the hamstrings without disturbing the neutral position of the spine and pelvis.

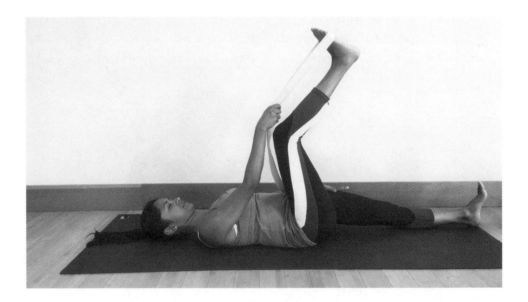

SALABHASANA A (LOCUST POSE) DYNAMIC STRENGTHENING PRACTICE 1 Lying prone with the arms on the floor along the sides of the body and the legs together, firmly press the feet down to awaken the legs while pressing the tailbone slightly toward the heels. With the inhalation, very slowly and slightly lift the chest and head off the floor while maintaining the natural shape of the neck (do not try to lift the ears higher than the shoulders). With the exhalation very

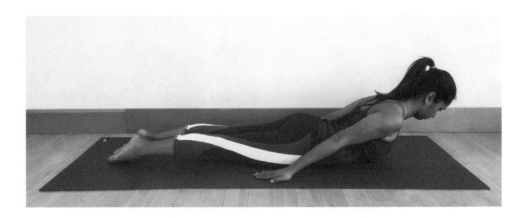

slowly release the chest and head to the floor. Take a few breaths to rest and completely relax, then repeat several times. Explore lifting slightly higher each time. Move very slowly to move more consciously (especially with greater conscious awareness of sensation in the low back). Slow movements will also help to establish more refined neuromuscular action in this movement and thus help develop better muscular support for the lumbar spine.

SALABHASANA A (LOCUST POSE) DYNAMIC STRENGTHENING PRACTICE 2   Explore doing the Dynamic Strengthening Practice 1 while lifting the legs and torso simultaneously. Focus on keeping space and comfort in the low back by pressing the tailbone toward the heels and extending long through the legs with a feeling of sending energy out through the toes. This practice adds strength to the hamstrings, which helps to keep the pelvis from excessive anterior rotation.

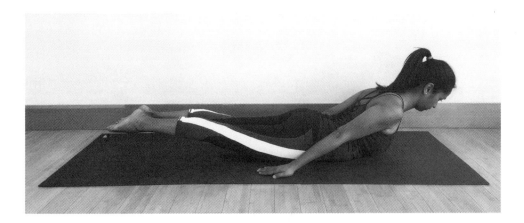

BIDALASANA (CAT POSE) WITH SPINAL BALANCING   On all fours, first move the pelvis forward and back several times while alternately moving the spine into extension and flexion (cat/cow movements). Then extend the healing leg straight back with the toes curled under on the floor. If comfortable in the low back, slowly lift and lower the extended leg up to twenty-five times, holding for five to ten breaths on the last lift. Repeat on the other side with the other leg. Again extend the healing leg back while reaching the arm on the opposite side forward (turn the palm of that hand toward center to create space around the neck and stabilize the shoulder). While stretching the fingers and toes of the lifted limbs away from each other, slowly abduct those limbs out only so far as possible while keeping the hips and upper back level with the floor before returning to a neutral position. Be very sensitive to the low back, neck, and wrist of the grounding hand. Repeat up to twenty-five times and hold in abduction for five to ten breaths. Rest in Balasana, allowing the low back to slightly round. If this basic form of Child's Pose causes strong stretching or discomfort in the low back (or knees), separate the knees slightly wider than hip-distance apart so there is less pressure in the low back.

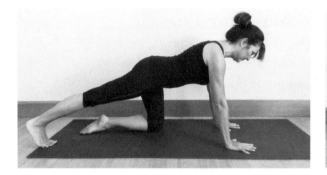
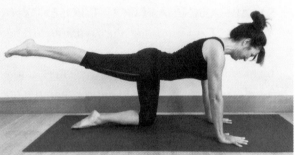

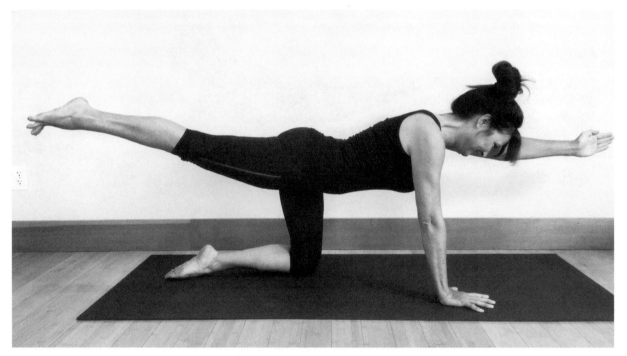

SUPTA PADANGUSTHASANA (RECLINED BIG TOE POSE) Lying supine with a strap looped around the foot, clasp the strap and extend the leg straight up from the hip. Keep the opposite hip grounded to the floor. Maintaining slight tension in the strap, slowly bend and straighten the lifted leg several times while keeping the pelvis and low back stable (keep the natural lumbar curve). Focus on gently stretching the hamstrings. After several of these repetitive movements, hold at about an 80 percent stretch for up to one minute.

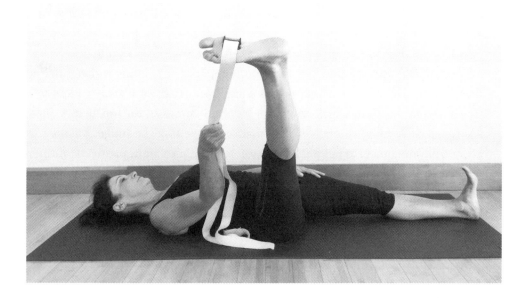

EKA PADA RAJAKAPOTASANA PREP (ONE-LEGGED KING PIGEON POSE PREP) Begin lying supine with the feet placed on the floor as for Setu Bandha Sarvanghasana. Cross the ankle of the right leg to the opposite knee, keeping the ankle joint in dorsiflexion. Clasp behind the knee and pull it toward the shoulder on that

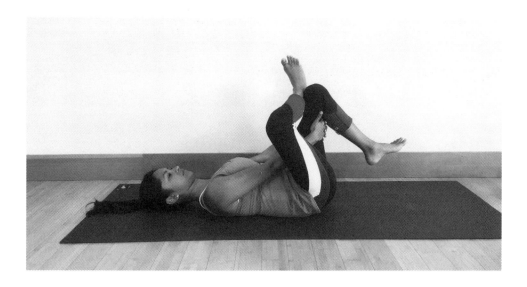

same side of the body while keeping the tailbone on the floor (maintain a neutral pelvis and a natural lumbar curve). After several of these repetitive movements, hold at about an 80 percent stretch for up to two minutes.

ANJANEYASANA (LOW LUNGE POSE)   From Tadasana, step one foot back about one leg length and release that knee to the floor. Position the torso upright and place the hands on the hips to assist in positioning the pelvis neutrally (where it feels level). Keep the hands on the hips with the thumbs pointing down near the SI joints. While slowly bending the front knee, use the hands to keep the pelvis from rotating forward. Unless one has acute knee issues, it is okay to let the knee travel beyond the heel, which will allow a deeper stretch in the hip flexors. Be more interested in keeping the pelvis level than in deepening the lunge. Inhaling, back away from the lunge, exhaling, lunge more deeply, moving repetitively in this way five to ten times before holding a comfortably deep lunge position for up to one minute. Do both sides equally.

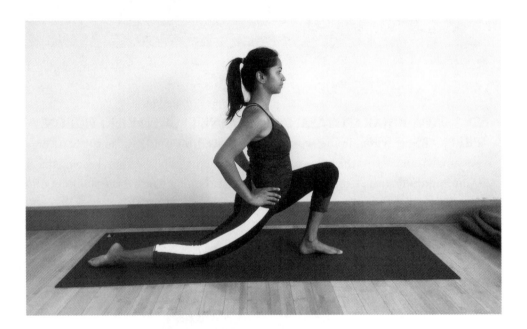

BALASANA (CHILD'S POSE) VARIATION   Begin in Balasana. Rather than folding forward over both thighs, fold obliquely forward over the right thigh while reaching the left arm forward from the shoulder. Play with alternately arching the left lower back up and then back down while stretching out longer through the left arm and hand. Explore both sides for one to two minutes.

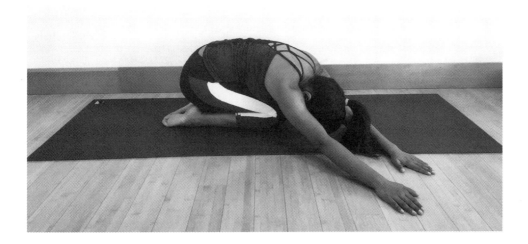

SUPTA PARIVARTANASANA(RECLINED REVOLVED POSE)   Laying supine, clasp around the knee of the healing side to flex the hip, then draw that knee across the body, coming into the basic spinal twisting form of Supta Parivartanasana. With a strap looped around the foot of the crossed over leg, fully extend the knee of that leg while continuing to draw the leg across the body. Hold for two minutes. Explore on both sides.

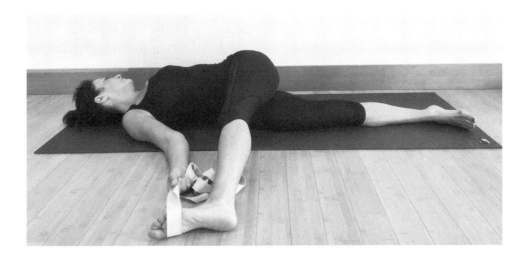

**PARIVRTTA JANU SIRSASANA (REVOLVED HEAD-TO-KNEE POSE) VARI-
ATIONS**   Start sitting upright with the legs positioned in the basic form for
Parivrtta Janu Sirsasana with the left knee flexed and right leg fully extended.
Twist to align the sternum with the bent left knee. While maintaining maximum
length in the low back, extend the torso to the right (over the straight leg) while
reaching the left arm straight up from the shoulder (in flexion and external
rotation). While keeping the left sitting bone firmly rooted to the floor, explore
very slightly and sensitively turning the torso toward the floor while stretching
from the back of the left hip through the left fingertips. Explore on both sides
for up to two minutes.

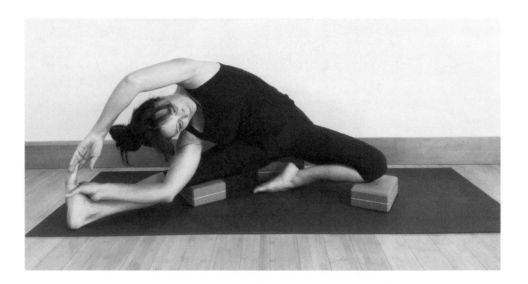

DWI CHAKRA VAHANASANA (YOGIC BICYCLES)   From Apanasana, interlace the fingers and cup the head in the hands. With the exhalation, curl the
torso up, drawing the elbows toward the knees while extending the right leg
straight out about one foot off the floor and extending the right arm out over
the right leg. Complete the exhalation while drawing the right arm across the
left knee and drawing the elbows together. Inhaling, release down, drawing the
knees toward the chest and head and elbows to the floor. Move slowly and work
as low, deep, and broadly through the belly as possible. Be more interested in
moving slowly yet steadily rather than seeing how many you can do with a timed
sequence. Move with the breath. Repeat on the other side, continuing for one to
three minutes.

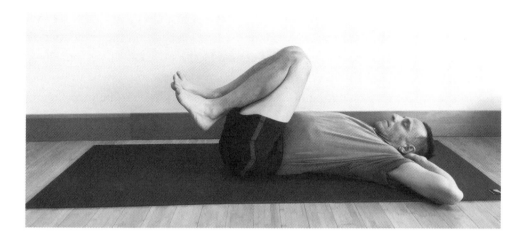

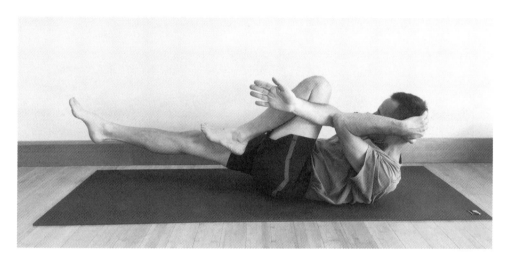

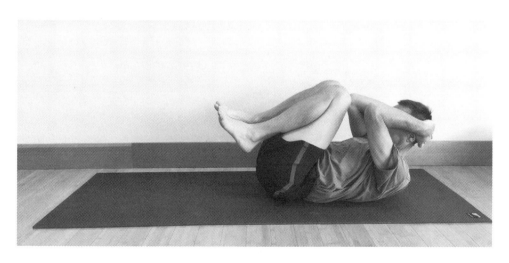

PELVIC TILTS   From Apanasana, extend the legs straight up, interlace the fingers, and cup the head in the hands. Keeping the legs vertical, on the exhalation draw the elbows toward the knees without changing the position of the legs. Keeping the upper back and shoulders lifted, with each exhale very slowly and smoothly curl the tailbone up, releasing it down as the breath flows out. Be more interested in slow and smooth movement than in maximizing the pelvic tilt by jerking the tailbone up. Repeat five to twenty-five times.

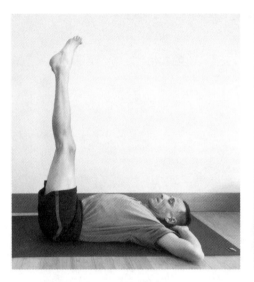 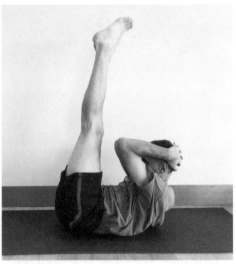

JATHARA PARIVARTANASANA (REVOLVING TWIST POSE)   The basic form of this asana can be either a held twist (Supta Parivartanasana) or an abdominal core strengthening movement. With the arms extended out like a cross and palms

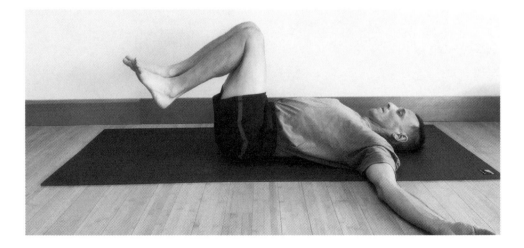

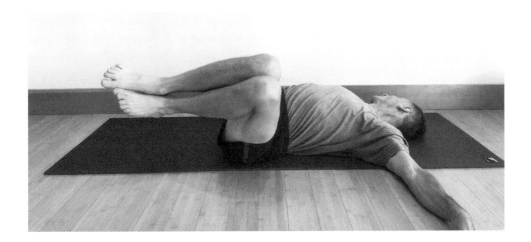

pressing down, alternately move the legs (or bent knees) back and forth to the left and right while gazing in the opposite direction of the legs, keeping the knees or legs from touching the floor. Inhaling, extend the legs over; exhaling, draw them back up to center.

Postural Kyphosis (Hunchback)

Kyphosis, from the Greek *kyphos*, "hump," is an abnormal increase in the posterior curvature of the spine. It most commonly refers to exaggerated posterior curvature in the thoracic segment of the spine where it produces a hunchback appearance (cervical and lumbar kyphosis also occur). It is also called Dowager's hump, "dowager" from the Latin root word *dotis*, "dowry," this coinage reflecting the greater propensity for elderly women with osteoporosis to develop kyphosis and hyperkyphosis (in which the angle is greater than forty degrees).[57]

Here we focus on postural kyphosis, which typically starts in childhood and is possibly associated with underlying feelings of sadness and hopelessness.[58] As the upper back rounds, muscles across the upper back are stretched and weakened due to lack of balanced engagement. As the chest collapses, muscles and ligaments anterior to the spine become shorter and breathing becomes more habitually shallow. Kyphosis also introduces a greater lordotic curve to the cervical

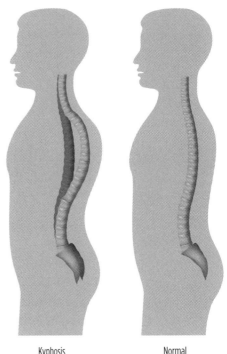

Kyphosis   Normal

spine, increasing chronic tension in the neck as it is held in excessive extension. In older age and particularly with osteoporosis, kyphosis is increasingly debilitating and associated with spinal fractures.

Thus, kyphosis is a self-reinforcing postural tendency with significant health consequences, including pain and nerve damage from nerve root entrapment, across the span of life. It complicates many of the simplest yoga asanas, especially backbends and twists, and makes many other activities, from sitting to cycling to gardening, more difficult.

THE PAINFUL EXPERIENCE

Pain varies depending primarily on the severity of abnormal curvature. It tends to be in the area of curvature. One is just as likely to experience fatigue and, in the lower limbs, weakness, as pain. With hyperkyphosis there is a greater likelihood of chronic nerve pressure as well as difficulty in breathing.

THE KNOWN CAUSES

Although kyphosis can arise from degenerative diseases such as arthritis and osteoporosis, childhood Scheuermann's disease (wedging of vertebrae), plasma cell cancer (multiple myeloma), or trauma, it most commonly arises from habitual slouching.[59]

HOW IT HEALS

Postural kyphosis and hyperkyphosis generally respond well to specific stretching and strengthening exercises, including yoga asanas.[60] In cases of hyperkyphosis, especially among the elderly, surgical treatment might be indicated.[61]

HEALING WITH ASANA PRACTICES

The primary focus of asana in healing postural kyphosis is reducing tension in the upper back, increasing strength in the back extensors, and establishing better postural alignment through thoracic rotation, thoracic extension, shoulder flexion, and hip extension. These healing practices are given in an ordered sequence with several asanas addressing more than one of these focus areas.

Reducing Tension in the Upper Back

SAVASANA (CORPSE POSE)   Fold or roll up a blanket to around one to three inches of thickness when compressed. Lie supine (as in Savasana) with the blanket positioned under the shoulder blades crosswise. Place a cushion under the head to ensure comfort in the neck (there should be no more pressure in the

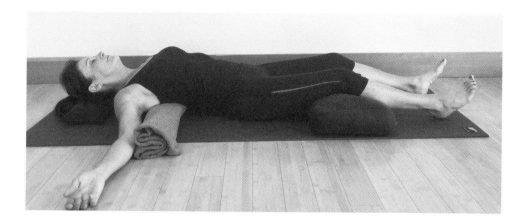

neck than with lying supine without the blanket under the shoulder blades). Breathe deeply with a focus in each exhalation on expanding in the area over the blanket. With the exhalations, allow everything to relax and release. After two minutes of deep breathing, simply relax and stay in this position for as long as it is comfortable.

SUPTA PARIVARTANASANA (RECLINED REVOLVED POSE) Lying supine, clasp around one knee to flex the hip, then draw that knee across the body, coming into the basic spinal twisting form of Supta Parivartanasana. With a strap looped around the foot of the crossed over leg, fully extend the knee of that leg while continuing to draw the leg across the body. Hold for two minutes. Explore on both sides.

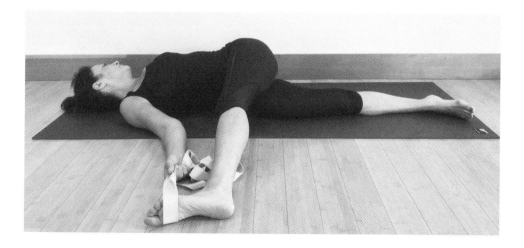

Strengthening Back Extensors and Decreasing Their Length

BIDALASANA (CAT POSE) AND SPINAL BALANCING On all fours, first move the pelvis forward and back several times while alternately moving the spine into extension and flexion (cat/cow movements). Then extend one leg straight back with the toes curled under on the floor. If comfortable in the low back, slowly lift and lower the extended leg up to twenty-five times, holding for five to ten breaths on the last lift. Repeat on the other side. Then once again extend one leg back while reaching the arm of the opposite side forward (turn the palm of that hand toward the center to create space around the neck and stabilize the shoulder).

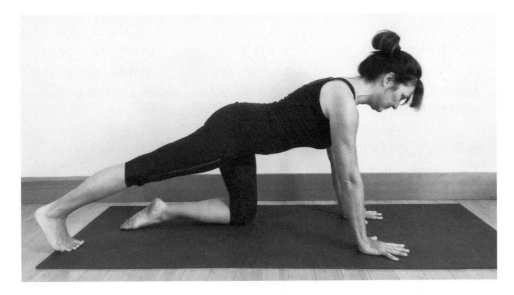

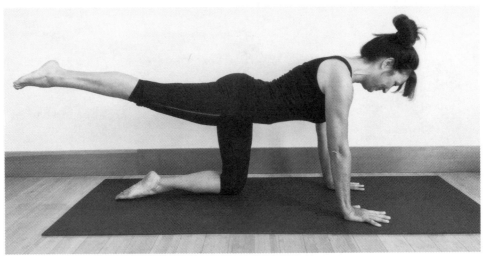

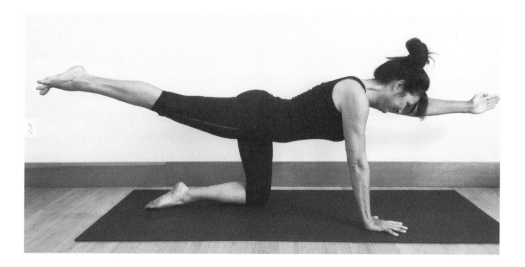

While stretching the fingers and toes of the lifted limbs away from each other, slowly abduct those limbs out only so far as possible while keeping the hips and shoulders level with the floor before returning to a neutral position. Repeat up to twenty-five times. Rest in Balasana.

ANAHATASANA (PUPPY DOG OR MELTING HEART POSE)   Begin on all fours in Bidalasana. Reach the arms forward from the shoulders and press the hands firmly and evenly into the floor. Try to rotate the shoulder blades out away from the spine. With each inhalation lift the chest up away from the floor. With each exhalation stretch the chest toward the floor. Repeat ten to fifteen times before holding the chest toward the floor for up to two minutes.

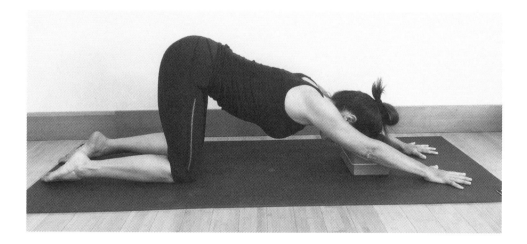

SALABHASANA A (LOCUST POSE) DYNAMIC STRENGTHENING PRACTICE 1 Lying prone with the arms on the floor along the sides of the body and the legs together, firmly press the feet down to awaken the legs while pressing the tailbone slightly toward the heels. With the inhalation, very slowly and slightly lift the chest and head off the floor while maintaining the natural shape of the neck (do not try to lift the ears higher than the shoulders). With the exhalation very slowly release the chest and head to the floor. Take a few breaths to rest and completely relax, then repeat several times. Explore lifting slightly higher each time.

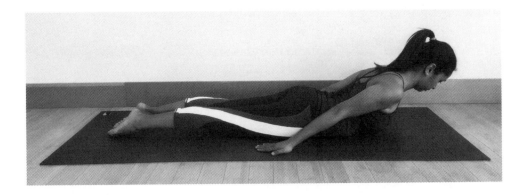

SALABHASANA A (LOCUST POSE) DYNAMIC STRENGTHENING PRACTICE 2 Explore doing the Dynamic Strengthening Practice 1 while lifting the legs and torso simultaneously. Focus on keeping space and comfort in the low back by pressing the tailbone toward the heels and extending long through the legs with a feeling of sending energy as though out through the toes.

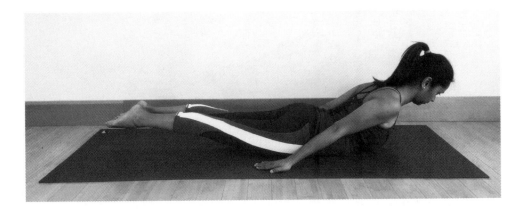

ARDHA MATSYENDRASANA (HALF LORD OF THE FISHES POSE)   Position the legs for Ardha Matsyendrasana. If necessary, sit on a block to position the pelvis level and to feel free of tension in the knees. Clasp the lifted knee with both hands to help draw the pubis down and the sternum up with each inhalation. Pressing the thoracic spine forward as if into the center of the sternum, begin rotating the torso toward the side with lifted knee. With each inhalation release slightly away from the twist in order to more easily relengthen up through the spine. With each exhalation explore twisting further around. Explore for one to two minutes before switching sides.

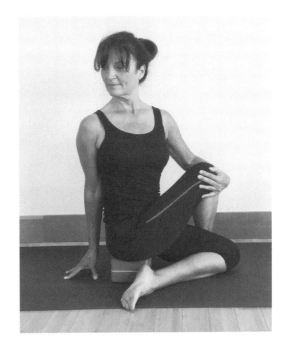

SETU BANDHA SARVANGHASANA (BRIDGE POSE) VARIATIONS   Lying supine, position the feet near the hips and in line with them to prepare for Setu Bandha Sarvanghasana. Slowly lift the pelvis while elongating the tailbone toward the knees, and while lifting, reach the arms overhead to the floor. While at the maximum elevation of the pelvis away from the floor, lift the heels to more easily lengthen the tailbone toward the heels while releasing the spine slowly to the floor one vertebra at a time from top to bottom. Repeat ten to fifteen times and then hold in Bridge Pose for five to eight breaths before very slowly lowering down and resting for several breaths. Repeat two or three times.

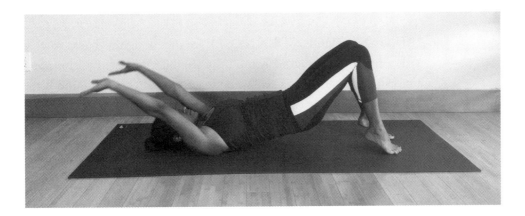

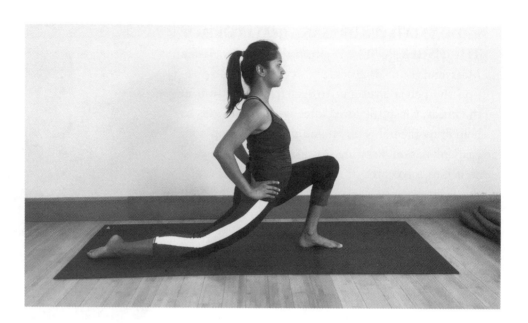

ANJANEYASANA (LOW LUNGE POSE) From Tadasana, step one foot back about one leg length and release that knee to the floor. Position the torso upright and place the hands on the hips to assist in positioning the pelvis neutrally (where it feels level). Keep the hands on the hips with the thumbs pointing down near the SI joints. While slowly bending the front knee, use the hands to keep the pelvis from rotating forward. Unless one has acute knee issues, it is okay to let the knee travel beyond the heel, which will allow a deeper stretch in the hip flexors. Be more interested in keeping the pelvis level than in deepening the lunge. Inhaling, back away from the lunge, exhaling, lunge more deeply, moving repetitively in this way five to ten times before holding a comfortably deep lunge position for up to one minute. Do both sides equally.

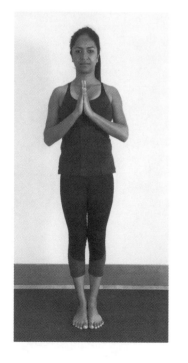

TADASANA (MOUNTAIN POSE) Stand with the back to a wall with a foam block placed behind the shoulder blades. Position the feet hip-distance apart, bring pada bandha actions to the feet, and firm the thighs. Align the pelvis neutrally over the thighs. Lift the shoulders toward the ears, draw them back, and then draw the shoulder blades down the back. Pressing the back into the block while breathing deeply, with each inhalation consciously draw taller through the spine while lifting the sternum. With each exhalation try to keep the sternum lifted and draw the shoulder blades more down the back while pressing the lower tips of the shoulder blades in toward the spine. Explore for two to three minutes.

SUPTA PARIVARTANASANA (RECLINED REVOLVED POSE) Repeat the same practice described for this asana in the earlier "Reducing Tension in the Upper Back" section.

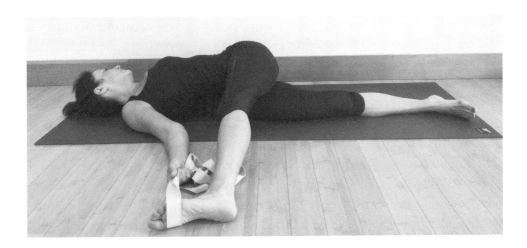

SVANASANA (CORPSE POSE) Repeat the same practice described for this asana in the earlier "Reducing Tension in the Upper Back" section.

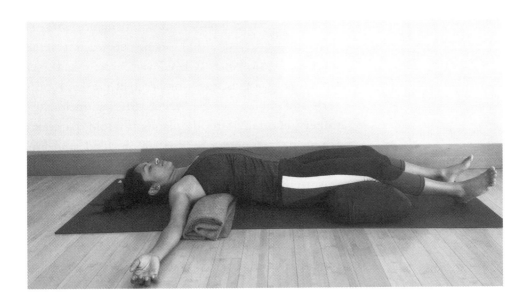

Neck Pain

The colloquial euphemism "pain in the neck" refers to a persistent source of interpersonal annoyance.[62] Looking more closely at the association of these two terms reveals a curious irony. "Pain," rooted in the Greek *poine*, "retribution, penalty," and Old French *peine*, "woe, suffering, punishment," is generally undesirable and may hurt. "Neck," rooted in the Old Germanic *hals*, "column," gave rise to the Middle English *halsen*, "to embrace or caress affectionately," which by the early nineteenth century in northern English dialect came to mean "to kiss, embrace," a generally desirable experience that may feel good. Pain and desire thus come together, albeit in a different way than is found in the heart of ancient yoga philosophies in which pain and suffering are posited as the inspiration for yoga and in which yoga is the path to freedom.

The neck is thus a place where one might experience much pleasure yet also a place perhaps most vulnerable to sudden trauma.[63] In yoga asana practice, it is often in the hot pursuit of intensifying pleasure or joy arising in deep backbends, twists, forward bends, and inversions that the neck is taken too quickly or too far in its safe ranges of motion or intrinsic pressure. In larger life, there is a vast array of sources of neck pain,[64] including sleeping posture, prolonged posture, repetitive actions, spinal pathologies, emotional stress, arthritis, carotid artery dissection, thyroid cancer, esophageal trauma, and whiplash.

The neck is a highly complex structure with many different vital tissues and organs crowded together—muscles, fascia, bones (C1–C7 vertebrae, hyoid), nerves (spinal cord, vagus, superior brachial plexus, local sensory and motor nerves), veins, arteries (including the rather important carotid), glands (thyroid, parathyroid, lymph nodes), plus tubes for lymph, food, and breath. Although the neck muscles are relatively simple in contrast to the other very complex neck organs, the array of neck muscles that can gather tension is itself complex: superficial and lateral muscles (platysma, sternocleidomastoid, trapezius), posterior triangle muscles (splenius capitis, levator scapulae, middle and posterior scalenes), anterior triangle muscles (four suprahyoid muscles, four infrahyoid muscles), four paired suboccipitals, prevertebral muscles (logus colli, longus capitis, rectus capitis anterior, rectus capitis lateralis), and the semispinalis and multifidi attached to the spine.

Here we focus on muscular tension that most likely arises from postural conditions or from anxiety, the latter given the euphemistic expression of being "uptight"—with the shoulders lifted toward the ears, muscles holding them firmly there, there is often chronic pain in the neck. The muscles most likely implicated in this tension—either directly or through a myofascial source of referred pain[65]—are the levator scapulae, upper trapezius, sternocleidomastoids (SCMs), semispinalis, multifidi, splenii, suboccipitals, and the rhomboids, all except the rhomboids with direct attachment to the neck.

THE PAINFUL EXPERIENCE

Neck pain symptoms vary widely from a deep and persistent ache in any structure to very specific areas of extremely sharp sensation that can be stimulated with the slightest of movements.

THE KNOWN CAUSES

Muscular tension as a source of neck pain arises primarily from postural problems, including while sleeping. The postural problems may originate as far away as the feet (causing postural pathologies up through the legs, pelvis, torso, and shoulder girdle) or from much closer, including habitual ways of holding the head. Lordosis, kyphosis, scoliosis, and other distortions in the curvature of the spine will cause misalignment of the cervical spine segment, causing muscular imbalance and tension in and around the neck. Emotional conditions such as stress and depression can also result in muscular tension around the neck.

HOW IT HEALS

Most cases of muscular neck tension can be effectively healed through targeted exercises, relaxation practices, and massage. Medications (muscle relaxants and anti-inflammatories) are often prescribed for neck tension. Heat patches or creams and cold packs are often found to reduce pain in the neck.[66] Some conditions (such as nerve entrapment) may require surgery.

HEALING WITH ASANA PRACTICES

The primary focus of asana in healing muscular neck pain is to reduce muscular tension through proper skeletal alignment and the muscular stretching and strengthening that support it. A regular well-balanced general asana, pranayama, and meditation practice will help reduce the emotional stress often at the root of muscular neck tension. Most involve sitting upright in Sukasana (Simple Seated Pose) or any comfortable sitting position, including in a chair, standing in Tadasana (Mountain Pose), or lying supine.

Sitting comfortably, consider placing a bolster under the sitting bones and back against a wall in exploring the following neck stretches. (Some require being away from the wall.)

SHOULDER ROLLS   Roll the shoulders forward, up, back, and down several times, then go the opposite direction. Be very sensitive to pain; back off the movement if painful.

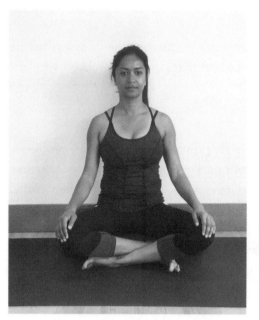 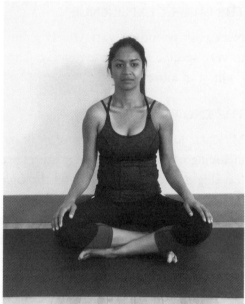

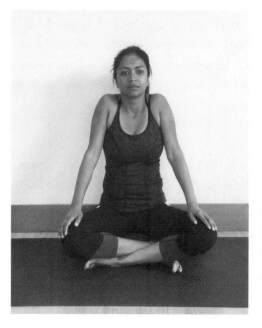 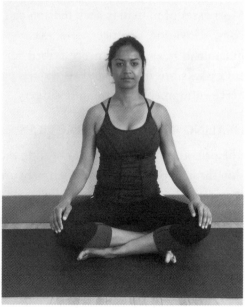

ROTATION AND FLEXION WITH ARM CLASP—PRACTICE 1   Reach the right hand around the back to clasp the left arm above the elbow. Use the right hand to pull the left shoulder slightly back and down. Turn the head toward the right shoulder. On the inhalations slightly lift the chin, on the exhalations draw the chin closer to the right shoulder. Hold for several breaths with the chin toward the shoulder and explore very slightly tilting the head left and right. Repeat several times before switching sides.

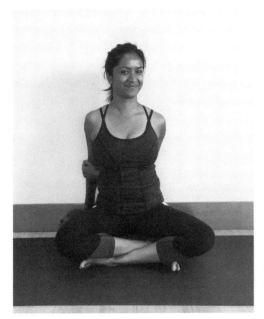
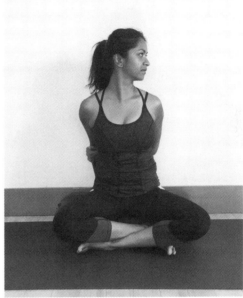
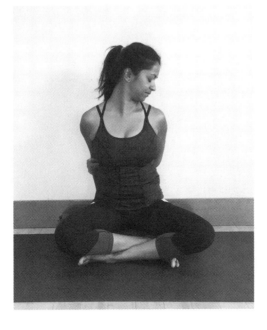

ROTATION AND FLEXION WITH ARM CLASP—PRACTICE 2   Clasp the arm, turn the head toward the right shoulder, and draw the chin toward the shoulder as described in Practice 1. Very slowly and sensitively draw the chin toward the distal right collarbone and then all the way across toward the distal left collarbone. Lift the chin slightly, then draw it toward the distal left collarbone and across to the right. Repeat several times before switching sides.

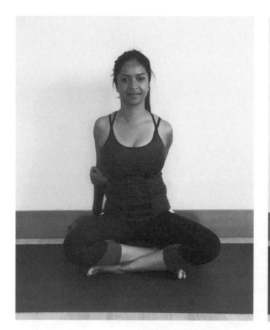
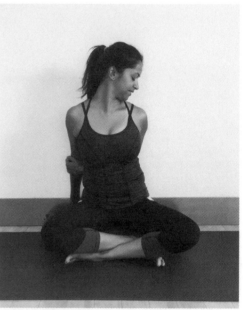
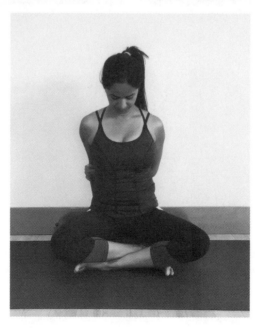

ROTATION AND FLEXION WITH ARM CLASP—PRACTICE 3 Clasp the arm as described in Practice 1. Slowly and sensitively tilt the head to the right, drawing the right ear toward the right shoulder. Slow lift the head back to the starting position. Repeat several times before switching sides.

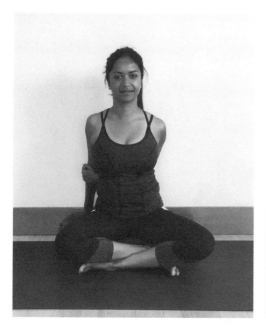
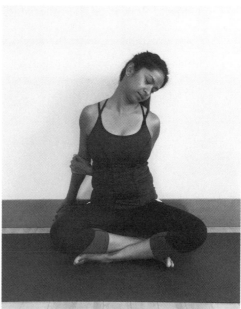

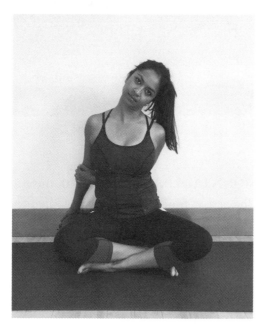

GARUDASANA (EAGLE POSE) ARMS   Position the arms as in Garudasana. If unable to cross the elbows, use one arm to help draw the opposite arm directly across the upper chest. Draw the shoulder blades down away from the neck and against the back ribs. Hold this position while breathing deeply and exploring very slight movements of the head in every direction except back. Do not hyperextend the neck. Repeat on the other side.

Come to standing with the feet positioned hip-distance apart in the basic form of Tadasana.

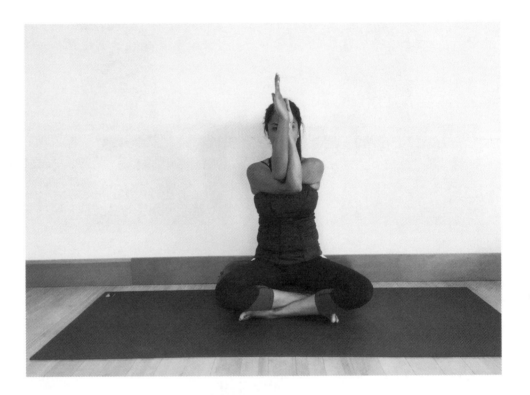

TADASANA (MOUNTAIN POSE)   Begin with the cues given for pada bandha. With pada bandha active, firm the quadriceps while pressing the femurs back (try to point the kneecaps straight forward). Rotate the pelvis forward and back to find where it feels the pelvis is level (use the prior practice of Utkatasana to get a better feeling for this). With the fingers placed on the lowest front ribs, alternately press the ribs into and away from the fingers to find where it feels like they are in their natural place. Elevate the shoulders toward the ears, draw them back, and then draw the shoulders lightly down against the back ribs. Relax the arms down by the sides of the thighs or hips. Position the head level, where it feels like it is effortlessly floating on top of the spine with the ears aligned with the shoulders. The spine is now in (or close to) its natural form (all conditions notwithstanding, particularly pathological ones that affect spinal posture). With pelvic neutrality, the spine will come into its natural curvature (neutral extension), unless there is significant muscular imbalance or a pathological condition such as scoliosis or kyphosis.

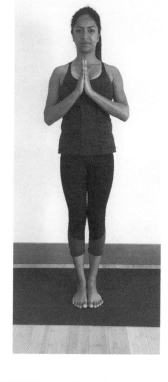

Breathing slowly and fully in and slowly and completely out, feel the natural ways the body moves through the cycles of breath. Focusing on keeping the spine in its neutral and natural alignment, with each inhalation consciously extend taller with a feeling of the crown of the head reaching up while minimizing disturbance to the form of the spine. With the completion of each exhalation, feel how the abdominal muscles lightly engage and girdle in toward the spine; without squeezing the belly, try to maintain this light abdominal muscular engagement while next inhaling and while maintaining the position of the pelvis, spine, shoulder girdle, and head. Stay with this practice for up to two minutes. With the completion of the exhalations, explore holding the breath out for two to ten seconds while more strongly engaging the abdominal muscles. Be sure to let the abdominal muscles slightly soften before inhaling.

URDHVA HASTASANA (UPWARD HANDS POSE) WALL STRETCH
Standing in Tadasana, position the arms with the elbows at shoulder height and flexed to ninety degrees with the palms touching the wall. On each inhalation bring the upper body (torso and head) slightly away from the wall. With each exhalation, bring the upper body toward the wall, stretching the levator scapulae muscles. Repeat ten to fifteen times.

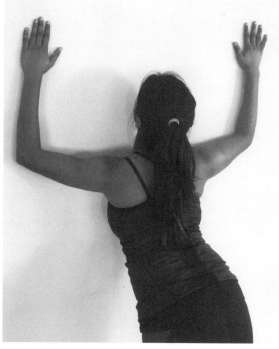

TADASANA WITH PRASARITA C ARMS   Standing in Tadasana, interlace the fingers behind the back. If it is difficult to interlace the fingers, hold a strap between the hands behind the back. Lift the arms away from the back only as far as the chest does not collapse and the shoulders do not lift toward the neck. Explore moving the head, first very slowly forward and back to center, then to each side and back to center, then with rotation and back to center. Explore moving the head more intuitively, tuning in to sensations in the neck to better guide the movements.

Now come to the floor.

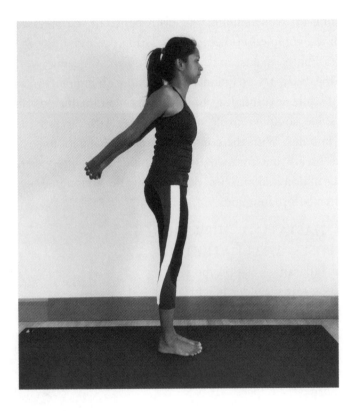

BIDALASANA (CAT POSE) MOVEMENTS   Tune in to sensations in the neck. If this basic position is uncomfortable in the neck, stay with the upright sitting practices described earlier, or go on to the following upright standing practices. If comfortable here, pull the shoulder blades down the back, away from the neck. Keeping the gaze down and the back of the neck long, with each inhalation slowly rotate the pelvis forward while drawing the sternum forward. With each exhalation reverse these movements, arching the spine up while drawing the forehead and pubis toward each other. Repeat ten to fifteen times. Rest in Balasana. If Balasana is not comfortable on the neck, place a cushion under the forehead to ensure the neck is in its natural form.

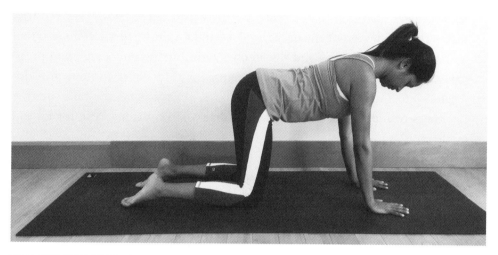

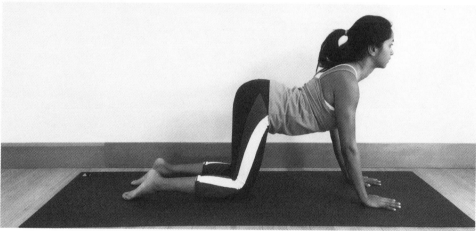

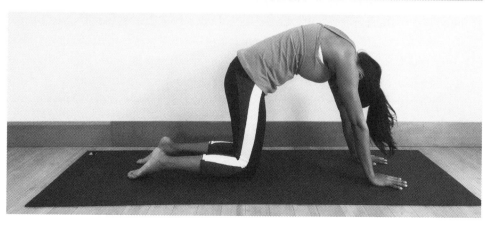

SETU BANDHA SARVANGHASANA (BRIDGE POSE) Although Bridge Pose is generally classified as a backbend, it creates a forward bend (flexion) in the neck. Place a folded blanket (two to three inches thick when compressed) under the back and shoulders with the head on the floor and space under the neck. Slowly lift the hips to create the backbend while being very sensitive to the increasing flexion of the neck. Look straight up toward the ceiling so there is no rotation in the neck. Bend the elbows, pointing the fingers up, and press the elbows more firmly down to explore expanding the chest without introducing tension into the neck. While in Bridge Pose, always press the tailbone toward the knees to reduce pressure in the low back. Hold Bridge Pose for up to two minutes.

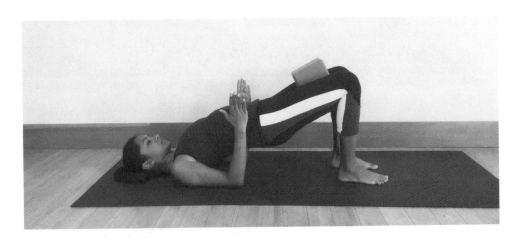

BHARADVAJRASANA A (SIMPLE NOOSE POSE A) From Dandasana, leaning to the left, bend both knees to draw both heels back to the right, keeping the left ankle under the right thigh. If unable to sit tall on the front of the sitting bones or if there is pressure in the knees, sit on a firm bolster. Twisting to the left, reach the left hand behind the back and clasp a piece of clothing or the right inner thigh. Rooting the sitting bones, elongate the spine with each inhale, using the handclasps to leverage the twist with each exhale. Create a feeling of drawing the upper spine in toward the heart center, drawing the shoulder blades down the back and spreading the collarbones. While twisting the torso to the left, turn the head toward the right shoulder. Explore slowly and slightly lifting and lowering the chin, tilting the head side to side, and rotating the head side to side. Do both sides for one to two minutes.

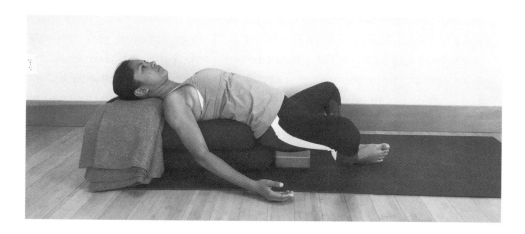

SUPTA BADDHA KONASANA (RECLINED BOUND ANGLE POSE) From the preparatory (upright) position for Baddha Konasana, place a bolster (or two) behind the pelvis before slowly reclining back onto it. If the neck is not comfortable in this position, place a blanket under the head. Release the arms to the sides either onto the floor or onto bolsters. If there is discomfort in the inner knees or inner thighs, place blocks under the knees. Rest here for five to ten minutes, letting go of tension breath by breath.

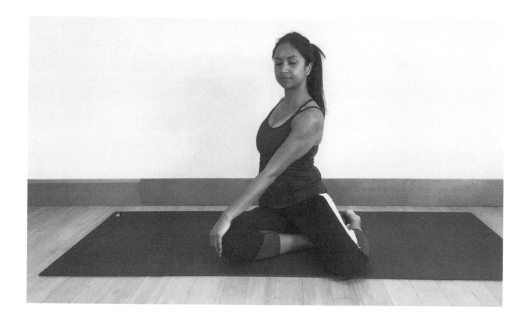

VIPARITA KARANI (ACTIVE REVERSAL POSE)   Sitting sideways next to a wall, slowly recline onto the back while swiveling the hips toward the wall and extending the legs up the wall. If tight hamstrings do not allow the legs to extend up with the buttocks touching the wall, slide the hips out away from the wall. Place a folded blanket under the lower back to create more ease through the lower back and sacrum. The palms can rest on the belly and heart, or drape the arms onto the floor, palms turned up. The legs can be held together with a strap, and a sandbag can be placed on the feet for stability. Play with positioning the legs as for Baddha Konasana (Bound Angle Pose) or Upavista Konasana (Wide-Angle Seated Forward Fold). Rest here for five to ten minutes, letting go of tension breath by breath.

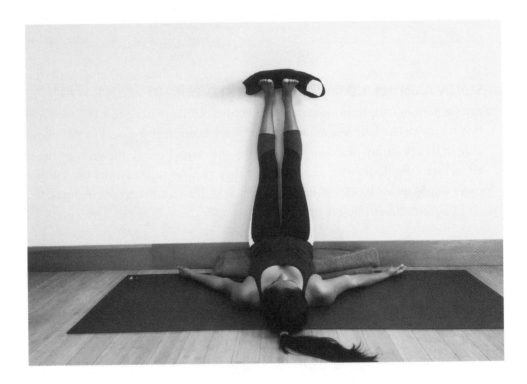

SAVASANA (CORPSE POSE)   Savasana (from sava, "corpse") is the ultimate asana for reintegration after practicing other asanas and pranayama. Lying supine, spread out as comfortably as possible with the arms draped onto the floor and palms facing up. If there is any discomfort in the lower back, place a rolled blanket under the knees. Lift the chest a little to let the shoulder blades relax slightly toward each other, then lie back down with more spaciousness across the heart center. Take one last deep inhale, then with the exhalation, let everything go, starting with allowing the breath to flow however it naturally will. There is no need for the muscles to do anything at all. Simply let it all be with a sense of all the muscles and bones letting go of each other, a sense of detachment all through the body. Stay in Savasana for at least five minutes.

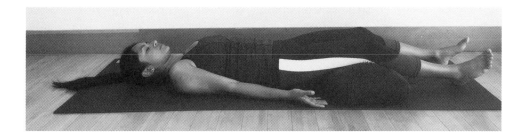

Structural Idiopathic Scoliosis

Most general models of the human skeleton shown in anatomy textbooks and online sources depict a perfectly symmetrical structure: the feet and legs are the same length, the pelvis is neutral, the spine has its four curves, the shoulders are level, everything is in balance and perfectly aligned. Then there is reality. In over 2,000 postural observations done in my yoga teacher workshops dating back to 1998, not a single participant has been found with such so-called perfect posture. Not one. Put differently, we are anything but perfectly symmetrical beings. Yet in some individuals we find significant deviation from idealized symmetry or an increasing tendency for such deviation to develop, with potentially serious impacts on general health and well-being.

Scoliosis is the mostly mysterious abnormal lateral curvature and rotation of the spine. In the most common type of scoliosis, *structural idiopathic scoliosis*, the mystery resides in the unknown origin and potential progression (including physiological mechanisms of progression) of the pathological curvature.[67] Structural idiopathic scoliosis most commonly arises in adolescence, primarily among girls.[68] In all cases it is impossible to predict how far and for what time the deviation will progress, and in many cases progression intermittently stops and resumes. In extreme cases the progression is life-threatening if it progresses into later adulthood.[69]

Other types of scoliosis have clearer pathophysiology and etiology. In *functional scoliosis*, lateral deviation arises from leg length discrepancy (also referred to as *static scoliosis*), repetitive asymmetrical activities

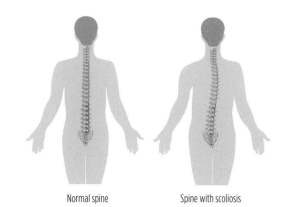

Normal spine   Spine with scoliosis

(such as daily golf swings on one side or daily long-distance driving with a wallet elevating one side of the pelvis), or muscle spasm due to trauma or habitually poor posture (also referred to as *habitual scoliosis*). In *myopathic scoliosis*, there is asymmetrical weakness of the intrinsic spinal muscles, and in *hemivertebra scoliosis* one lateral half of the vertebra did not properly develop.

Here we focus on structural idiopathic scoliosis, even as many of the practices given here can be beneficial to all types of scoliosis. Although specific individual deviations vary, four patterns of curvature are most prevalent: right thoracic convexity, left lumbar convexity, right thoracolumbar convexity, and right thoracic convexity combined with left lumbar convexity. Most thoracic and double curves are right convexity and most lumbar curves are left convexity. Many cases of thoracic convexity also involve kyphosis.

THE PAINFUL EXPERIENCE

Mild scoliosis can be undetected and pain-free. During adolescence, the deviation generally does not place pressure on internal organs or nerves, resulting in little or no pain. As abnormal lateral curvature and rotation of the spine progress, there is increasing muscular tension in the back, shoulders, and neck due to postural compensation. Extreme deviation can compress the lungs (and thereby inhibit breathing) and cause persistent painful pressure on nerves along the spine, including in the low back and down the legs (due to pressure on the sciatic nerves).

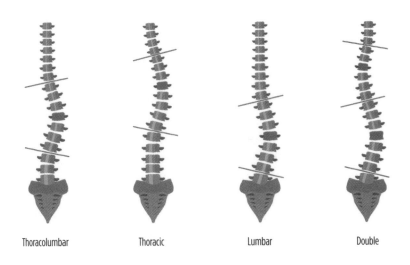

Thoracolumbar   Thoracic   Lumbar   Double

Figure 23.13: Four Common Types of Curve

THE KNOWN CAUSES

As previously discussed, it is possible to identify causes of functional scoliosis (leg length discrepancy, poor posture, etc.). Although structural scoliosis is idiopathic[70]—there is no well-established body of evidence of a disorder such as partial paralysis, congenital malformation, or metabolic—there is growing evidence that aberrations in the vestibular apparatus (which provides information about spatial orientation and equilibrium) may play a role in the development and progression of structural idiopathic scoliosis.[71] Some congenital diseases such as cerebral palsy and spinal bifida are associated with scoliosis but not known to be fundamentally causative.

HOW IT HEALS

Treating scoliosis starts with measured observation over a period of time to determine progression. Where there is evidence of significant progression in childhood or adolescence, preventative bracing is generally used. If bracing is not successful, surgical installation of a rod attached to the spine is often recommended; in some cases spinal fusion is indicated.

There is growing evidence of the efficacy of physical therapy methods that address specific deviations with stretching and strengthening exercises. Although there is little evidence that curvature can be corrected, there is evidence that progression can be slowed or stopped and that discomfort can be alleviated.[72] There is also some evidence of a specific yoga pose (modified Vasisthasana [Side Plank Pose]) in developing asymmetrical muscular strength that results in reducing primary scoliotic curves.[73]

HEALING WITH ASANA PRACTICES

Recent research and practices have generated deepening insight into healing scoliosis with yoga. There is not common agreement about some of the most fundamental questions, including whether yoga can reverse scoliosis (most say no) and whether to even attempt going against the socoliotic tendencies with postural practices (which is widely debated). All teach the importance of improving postural alignment, beginning in the feet, legs, and pelvis, all recognize the critical importance of stretching and strengthening the iliopsoas and other muscles that act directly on the lumbar spine in relation to the pelvis, and all recognize the importance of correct diagnosis prior to prescribing particular asana practices.

Rather than attempting to summarize or synthesize this work, here we provide reference to three exceptionally insightful sources. Elise Browning Miller, whose 2003 book *Yoga for Scoliosis* remains a basic resource on this topic, has produced a variety of media offering specialized practices for different types of curves. Rachel Krentzman's 2016 book *Scoliosis, Yoga Therapy, and the Art of Letting Go* provides an insightful discussion of the anatomy of scoliosis as well as practices for reducing related back pain.

Loren Fishman and his associates recently completed a systematic study of the effects of Vasisthasana (Side Plank Pose) on right thoracic scoliosis, offering a fine example of how scientific research methods can provide deeper insight into the benefits of yoga (he claims to have found that Vasisthasana can reduce the curvature).

Thoracic Outlet Syndrome

The thoracic cavity is the chamber in the upper torso that contains the organs of the cardiovascular system (heart and great vessels), respiratory system (lungs, diaphragm, trachea, bronchi), digestive system (esophagus), endocrine glands, nervous system (including the vagus nerves), and lymphatics (including the thoracic duct). The cavity is enclosed by the ribs, spine, and sternum and has two openings, the superior thoracic aperture (or thoracic inlet) and the inferior thoracic aperture (or thoracic outlet, which is closed by the diaphragm). In confusing nomenclature, the superior thoracic aperture, located between the collarbone and first rib, is referred to as the thoracic *outlet* when discussing the nerves, arteries, and veins that pass through it from the thorax to the neck and arms.

Thoracic Outlet Syndrome (TOS) refers to compression of these nerves, arteries, or veins. Here we focus on the most common type of compression (95 percent of cases):[74]

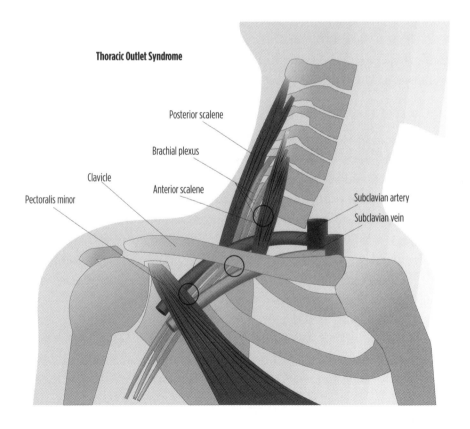

Thoracic Outlet Syndrome

Posterior scalene

Brachial plexus

Clavicle

Pectoralis minor

Anterior scalene

Subclavian artery

Subclavian vein

neurogenic[75]—the compression of C8 and T1 nerve roots, which are part of the brachial plexus nerve network. However, it is important to note that pure neurogenic TOS is considered rare because other structures are typically involved, leading to continued debate of whether neurogenic TOS is underdiagnosed or overdiagnosed.[76] When the brachial plexus is compressed, one experiences pain, tingling, numbness, and weakness in the shoulders, neck, arms, and hands.

THE PAINFUL EXPERIENCE

Neurogenic TOS causes numbness or tingling in the arms, hands, or fingers and deep aching, burning, or sharp pain in the neck, shoulders, or hands. The pain is often intermittent. It can also occur along with ulnar nerve compression at the elbow or medial nerve compression (manifesting as carpal tunnel syndrome).[77]

THE KNOWN CAUSES

Although there are multiple causes of neurogenic TOS (including tumors and cysts), most are due to congenital abnormalities, trauma, or repetitive stress. Congenital abnormalities include 1) a set of supernumerary (extra) ribs (cervical ribs) that attach to C7 and may compress the brachial plexus, 2) excessive tightness in the fibrous band connecting the ribs and spine, and 3) structural deviation in the scalene muscles.[78]

Trauma to the neck, shoulders, or arms can cause neurogenic TOS, especially where there is congenital predisposition. Trauma can occur due to a traumatic event such as whiplash in a rear-end car crash or long-term postural misalignment, especially slouching.

Neurogenic TOS is also caused by repetitive activities that compress the neck and upper back.[79] Such compression is common in the repetitive actions involved in moving from Phalakasana (Plank Pose) to Chataranga Dandasana (Four-Limbed Staff Pose) to Urdhva Mukha Svanasana (Upward Facing Dog Pose), especially when the shoulder blades are not drawn down away from the neck and against the back ribs; and repetitive activities with the arms overhead, including swimming, throwing a ball, or holding the arms in full flexion in Virabhadrasana III (Warrior III Pose).

HOW IT HEALS

Healing neurogenic TOS depends on the structure(s) compressing the brachial plexus (cervical rib? anterior scalene? prolonged transverse process? acromionclavicular joint injury? cervical disc injuries? shoulder impingement?). Although surgical treatment might be indicated (and is often successful),[80] targeted postural exercises that stretch and strengthen shoulder and upper back muscles can relieve pressure on the thoracic outlet and reduce or eliminate the symptoms associated with TOS.[81]

HEALING WITH ASANA PRACTICES

The primary focus of asana is on postural exercises that support normal upright sitting and standing and that stretch and strengthen shoulder and upper back muscles.

SHOULDER ROLLS Roll the shoulders forward, up, back, and down several times, then go the opposite direction. Be very sensitive to pain; back off the movement if painful.

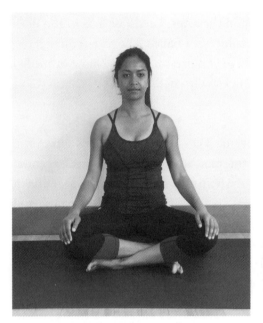
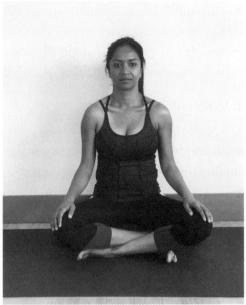
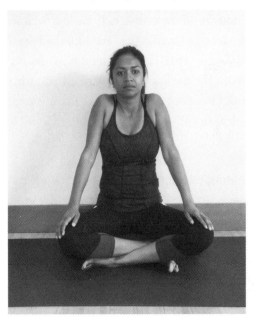
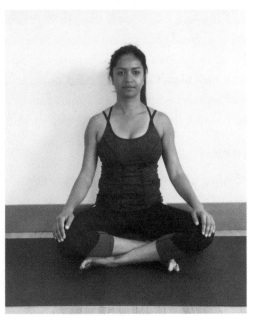

ROTATION AND FLEXION WITH ARM CLASP—PRACTICE 1 Reach the right hand around the back to clasp the left arm above the elbow. Use the right hand to pull the left shoulder slightly back and down. Turn the head toward the right shoulder. On the inhalations slightly lift the chin, on the exhalations draw the chin closer to the right shoulder. Hold for several breaths with the chin toward the shoulder and explore very slightly tilting the head left and right. Repeat several times before switching sides.

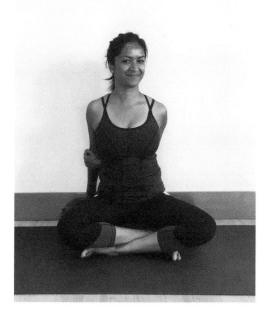
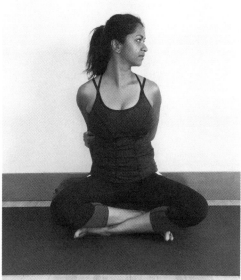
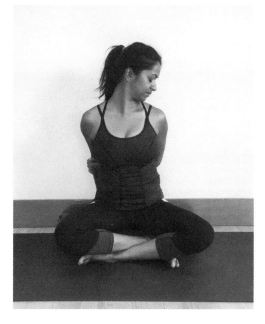

ROTATION AND FLEXION WITH ARM CLASP—PRACTICE 2   Clasp the arm, turn the head toward the right shoulder, and draw the chin toward the shoulder as described in Practice 1. Very slowly and sensitively draw the chin toward the distal right collarbone and then all the way across toward the distal left collarbone. Lift the chin slightly, then draw it toward the distal left collarbone and across to the right. Repeat several times before switching sides.

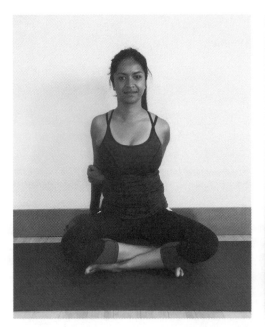
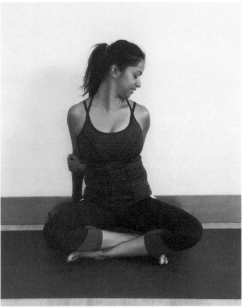
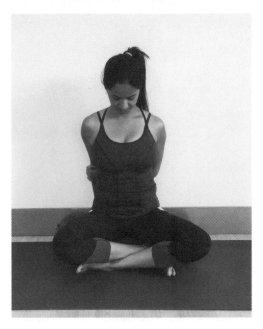

ROTATION AND FLEXION WITH ARM CLASP—PRACTICE 3   Clasp the arm as described in Practice 1. Slowly and sensitively tilt the head to the right, drawing the right ear toward the right shoulder. Slow lift the head back to the starting position. Repeat several times before switching sides.

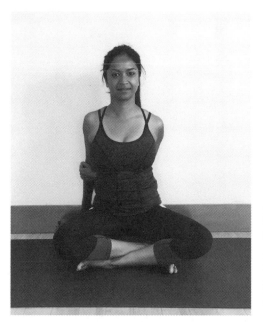
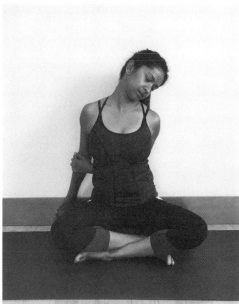

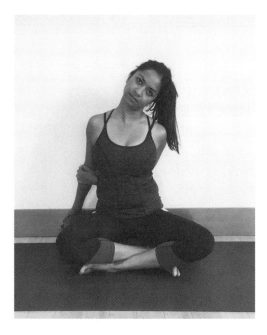

GARUDASANA (EAGLE POSE) ARMS   Position the arms as in Garudasana. If unable to cross the elbows, use one arm to help draw the opposite arm directly across the upper chest. Draw the shoulder blades down away from the neck and against the back ribs. Hold this position while breathing deeply and exploring very slight movements of the head in every direction except back. Do not hyperextend the neck. Repeat on the other side.

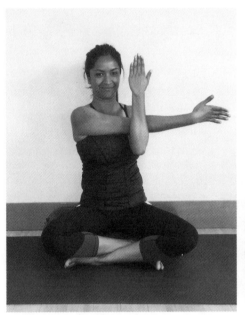 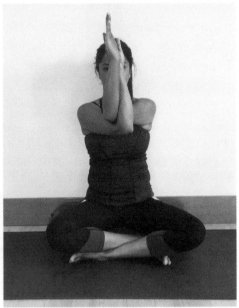

VIRABHADRASANA II (WARRIOR II) ARM PRACTICE   Sitting (or standing) in the form of Warrior II, slowly abduct the arms until level with the floor, then slowly release the arms back to the sides. Repeat this "nerve gliding" exercise ten to fifteen times to help restore the ability of nerves to stretch through this range of motion.

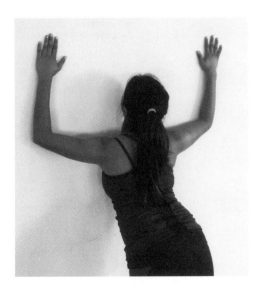

URDHVA HASTASANA (UPWARD HANDS POSE) WALL STRETCH
Standing in Tadasana (Mountain Pose), position the arms with the elbows slightly below shoulder height and flexed to ninety degrees with the palms touching the wall. On each inhalation bring the upper body (torso and head) slightly away from the wall. With each exhalation, bring the upper body toward the corner, stretching the levator scapulae muscles. Repeat ten to fifteen times.

TADASANA WITH PRASARITA C ARMS Standing in Tadasana, interlace the fingers behind the back. If it is difficult to interlace the fingers hold a strap between the hands behind the back. Lift the arms away from the back only as far as the chest does not collapse and the shoulders do not lift toward the neck. Explore moving the head, first very slowly forward and back to center, then to each side and back to center, then with rotation and back to center. Explore moving the head more intuitively, tuning in to sensations in the neck to better guide the movements.

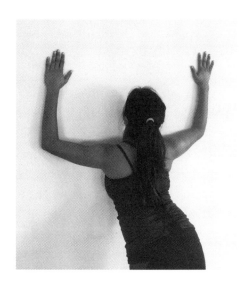

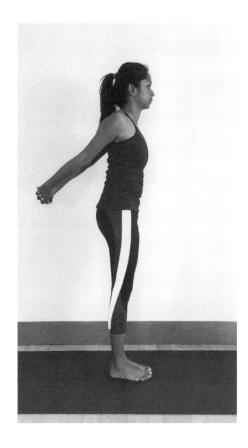

ANAHATASANA (PUPPY DOG OR MELTING HEART POSE)   Begin on all fours in Bidalasana (Cat Pose). Reach the arms forward from the shoulders and press the hands firmly and evenly into the floor. Try to rotate the shoulder blades out away from the spine. With each inhalation lift the chest up away from the floor. With each exhalation stretch the chest toward the floor. Repeat ten to fifteen times before holding the chest toward the floor for up to two minutes.

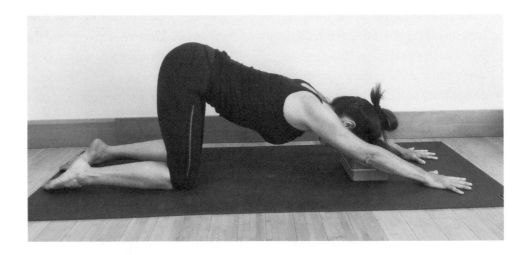

SALABHASANA A (LOCUST POSE) DYNAMIC STRENGTHENING PRACTICE 1   Lying prone with the arms on the floor along the sides of the body and the legs together, firmly press the feet down to awaken the legs while pressing the tailbone slightly toward the heels. With the inhalation, very slowly and slightly lift the chest and head off the floor while maintaining the natural shape of the neck (do not try to lift the ears higher than the shoulders). With the exhalation very slowly release the chest and head to the floor. Take a few breaths to rest and completely relax, then repeat several times. Explore lifting slightly higher each time.

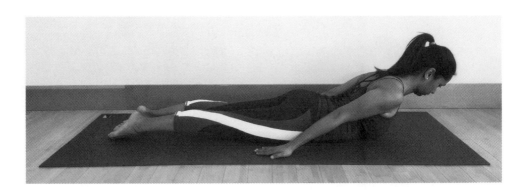

SETU BANDHA SARVANGHASANA (BRIDGE POSE) VARIATIONS Lying supine, position the feet near the hips and in line with them to prepare for Setu Bandha Sarvanghasana. Slowly lift the pelvis while elongating the tailbone toward the knees, and while lifting, reaching the arms overhead to the floor. While at the maximum elevation of the pelvis away from the floor, lift the heels to more easily lengthen the tailbone toward the heels while releasing the spine slowly to the floor one vertebra at a time from top to bottom. Repeat ten to fifteen times and then hold in Bridge Pose for five to eight breaths before very slowly lowering down and resting for several breaths. Repeat two or three times.

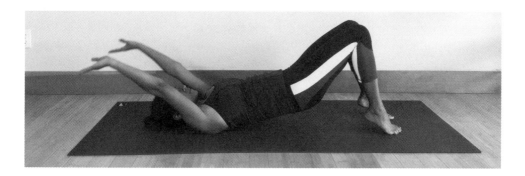

SAVASANA (CORPSE POSE) Fold or roll up a blanket to around one to three inches of thickness when compressed. Lie supine (as in Savasana) with the blanket positioned under the shoulder blades. Place a cushion under the head to ensure comfort in the neck (there should be no more pressure in the neck than when lying supine without the blanket under the shoulder blades). Breathe deeply with a focus in each exhalation on expanding in the area over the blanket. With the exhalations allow everything to relax and release. After two minutes of deep breathing, simply relax and stay in this position for as long as it is comfortable.

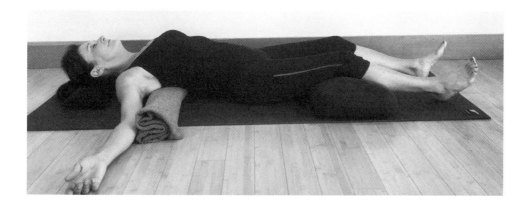

Shoulder, Arm, and Hand Conditions

Shoulder Joint Adhesive Capsulitis

Adhesive capsulitis, colloquially called "frozen shoulder," is a painful shoulder condition that makes it difficult to abduct the arm. Widely considered idiopathic (of unknown or unclear cause), the condition involves fibrous adhesions (scarring) and inflammation between the articular capsule of the glenohumeral joint (commonly called the shoulder joint), the rotator cuff, the subacromial bursa, and the deltoid muscle.[82] The inflammation and adhesions cause chronic pain and greatly limit range of motion. Although not actually frozen, the shoulder with adhesive capsulitis is in fact very warm due to inflammation, yet it is able to move, albeit painfully. But because the pain inhibits movement, there is less movement, and with less movement there is greater adhesion and more pain.

THE PAINFUL EXPERIENCE

Part of the insidious nature of adhesive capsulitis is that it involves intensely sharp pain when moving the arm in certain directions (particularly abduction) and often even greater dull aching pain when lying still or in a restricted position. Simple movements, especially those involving external rotation, can be extremely painful. The gradual onset of pain and restricted movement over a period of several weeks to several months typically gives way to less pain yet improved range of motion for around six months. The condition usually resolves in six months to two years. As it resolves, the pain may diminish even without improvement in range of motion.

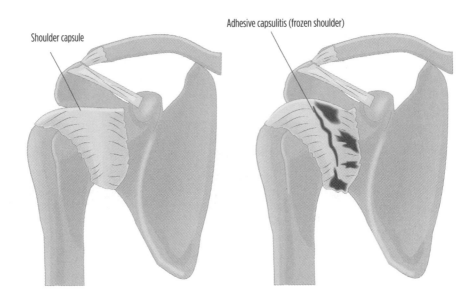

Shoulder capsule

Adhesive capsulitis (frozen shoulder)

THE KNOWN CAUSES

Although specific causes are unclear, there are several risks for the adhesions that create frozen shoulder.[83] The leading risk factor is age.[84] A sedentary lifestyle and a job involving little physical activity also places one at greater risk of developing this condition. Other risk factors include accidents (starting with glenohumeral dislocations), supraspinatus tendinitis, partial tearing of the rotator cuff, diabetes, and connective tissue diseases. Once there is some adhesion, movement becomes painful. With greater pain when attempting to move the joint, one typically moves it less. The less it is moved the greater the development of adhesions.

HOW IT HEALS

Although time may heal most ailments, it is not the primary source of healing adhesive capsulitis. Unlike most musculoskeletal disorders, which require rest to heal, a frozen shoulder benefits from the full range of movements in the glenohumeral joint. An MRI can help identify specific areas of adhesion one can address with physical therapy.

HEALING WITH ASANA PRACTICES

The primary focus of asana is on restoring pain-free range of motion though targeted stretching. We also focus on strengthening the rotator cuff.

Restoring Range of Motion

To restore range of motion in the gleno-humeral joint, follow these asanas:

TADASANA (MOUNTAIN POSE) WITH ARM SWINGS Standing in Tadasana next to a chair, place the hand of the healthy side on the chair and lean slightly forward to allow the healing arm to dangle down from the shoulder joint. Slowly swing the arm like a pendulum, then around in circles, for one to two minutes. Repeat several times every day.

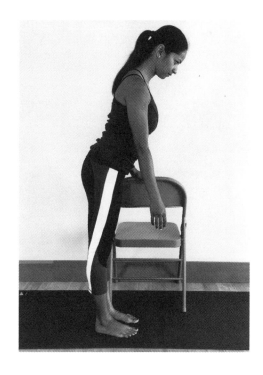

GARUDASANA (EAGLE POSE) SHOULDER PREP POSITION Standing in Tadasana, use the healthy arm to help gently lift and pull the healing arm across the chest in adduction. Explore alternately rotating the arm into external and internal rotation. Hold and explore for one to two minutes several times every day.

PRASARITA PADOTTANASANA C (WIDE ANGLE FORWARD FOLD C) ARM STRETCH POSITION Standing in Tadasana, clasp a strap in the hands behind the back shoulder-distance apart. Use the healthy arm to gently pull the healing arm farther behind the back. Hold for one to two minutes. Repeat several times every day.

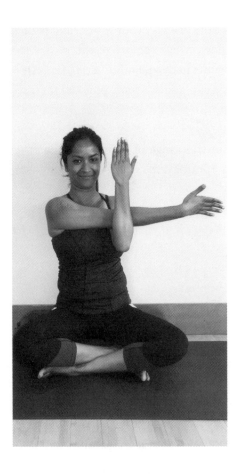

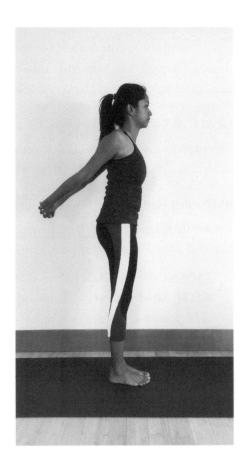

GOMUKHASANA (COW FACE POSE) ARM STRETCH POSITION   If Prasarita Padottanasana C Arm Stretch Position is comfortable, explore positioning the arms for Cow Face Pose with the healthy arm overhead and the healing arm behind the back. Clasp a strap and explore pulling the hands toward each other. Hold for one to two minutes. Repeat several times every day.

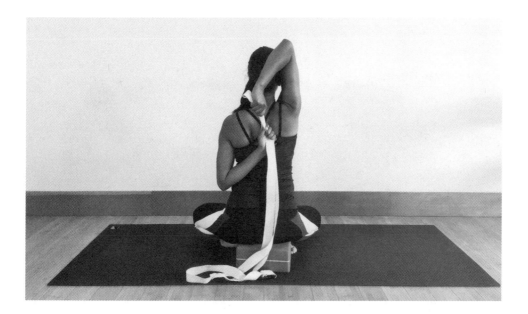

TADASANA FINGER WALK Stand facing a wall with the fingers on the wall at hip height. Slowly walk the fingers up the wall as far as comfortable. Repeat several times every day.

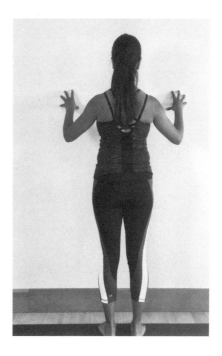

BIDALASANA (CAT POSE) TO UTTHITA BALASANA (EXTENDED CHILD'S POSE)   If comfortable in the healing shoulder while on all fours in Bidalasana, draw in a deep breath with a feeling of breathing more space into the shoulder. On the exhalation slowly draw the sitting bones toward the heels while keeping the hands in place, going only so far as is comfortable. On each inhalation rise slightly away from the maximum stretch, and on each exhale explore stretching farther. Continue to explore in this way for one to two minutes. Repeat several times every day.

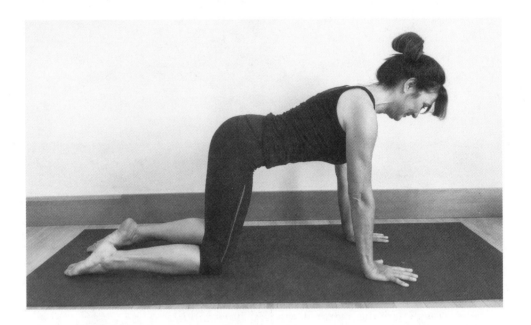

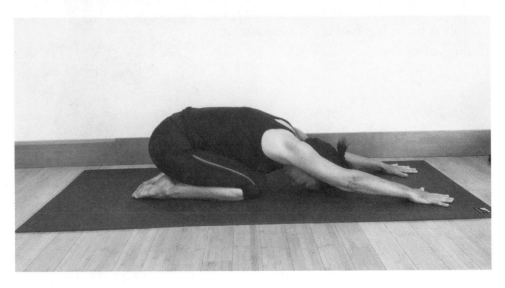

Strengthening the External Rotators

To strengthen the external rotators, follow these asanas:

SUKASANA (SIMPLE POSE)   Sitting comfortably (if necessary, sit on a bolster and/or against a wall), flex the elbows to ninety degrees with the thumbs pointing up. Keeping the elbows by the sides and the forearms level with the floor, slowly externally rotate the arms as far as possible without pain and hold in this position for five to ten breaths. Slowly release back to the starting position. Repeat ten to fifteen times.

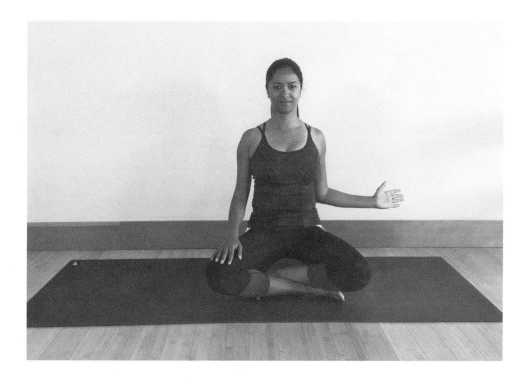

PARSVA SAVASANA (SIDE CORPSE POSE) SHOULDER ROTATIONS   Lying on the side of the healthy shoulder, place the elbow of the healing shoulder on that same side hip with the hand on the floor. Keeping the elbow on the hip, slowly externally rotate the arm as far as possible without pain, and then slowly release the hand back to the floor. Explore holding in the lifted position (externally rotated) for five to ten breaths. Repeat ten to fifteen times. When this is relatively easy, do the same movements with a very light weight in the hand.

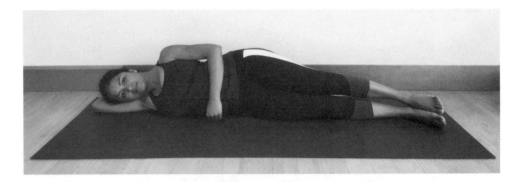

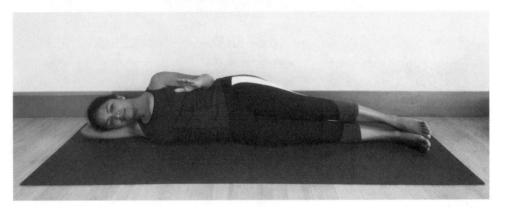

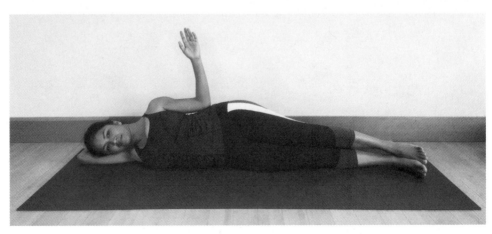

ANAHATASANA (PUPPY DOG POSE) SHOULDER ROTATIONS   Explore this once there is sufficient range of motion to position the arms overhead free of pain. Begin on all fours in Bidalasana. Reach the arms forward from the shoulders and press the hands firmly and evenly into the floor. Slowly rotate the shoulder blades in toward the spine (internally rotating the arms), then reverse this movement, externally rotating the shoulder blades out away from the spine. Focus on slow and steady movement. Explore holding the externally rotated position for five to ten breaths.

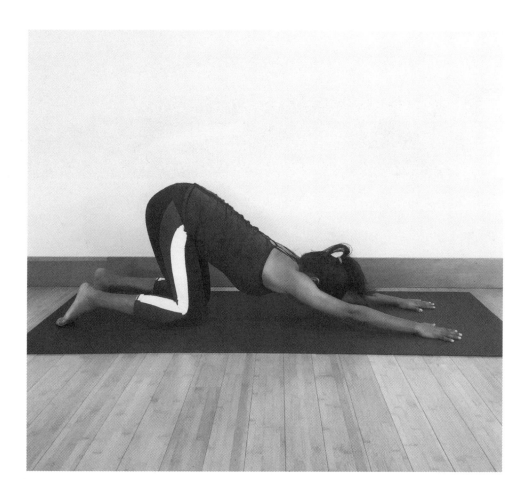

Strengthening the Internal Rotators

To strengthen the internal rotators, follow these asanas:

SAVASANA (CORPSE POSE) SHOULDER ROTATIONS   Lying supine, flex the elbow on the healing side ninety degrees with the fingers pointing up. Keeping the elbow at the side, slowly externally rotate the arm only as far as comfortable. More slowly raise the arm back (internally rotating back to the starting position). Repeat ten to fifteen times.

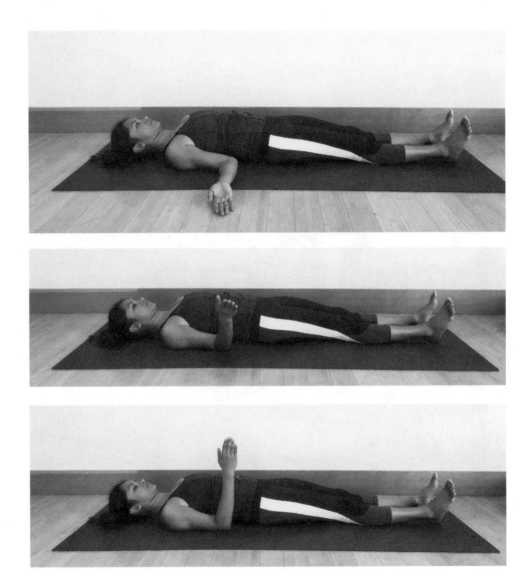

PARSVA SAVASANA (SIDE CORPSE POSE) SHOULDER ROTATIONS Lying on the side of the healing shoulder on a bench or a stack of bolsters with the shoulder and elbow at the edge of the elevated prop, flex the elbow to ninety degrees. Keeping the elbow on the prop, slowly externally rotate the arm as far as possible without pain, and then slowly internally rotate the arm to bring the hand across the torso (keeping the elbow on the prop). Repeat ten to fifteen times. When this is relatively easy, do the same movements with a very light weight in the hand.

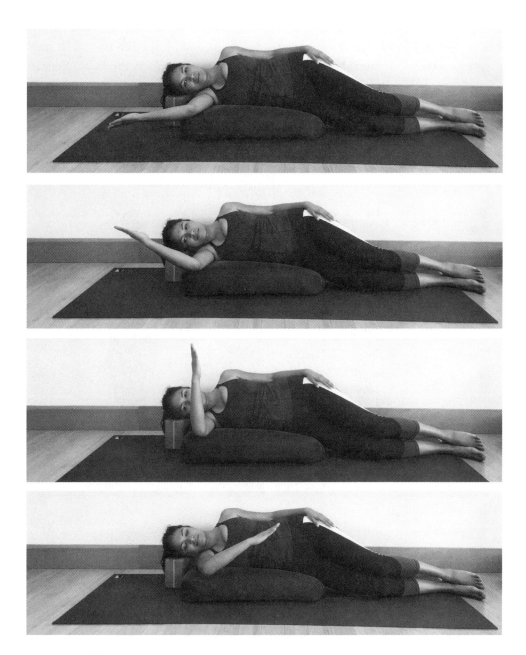

Strengthening the Abductors

To strengthen the abductors, follow these asanas:

ARDHA URDHVA HASTASANA (HALF UPWARD HAND POSE)   Standing in Tadasana, slightly internally rotate the arms until the thumb tips point toward the hips. (Note that this is the opposite rotation generally done in preparation for reaching the arms out and up overhead.) Keeping the shoulder blades lightly rooted down against the back ribs and the tops of the shoulders level with each other, fully extend through the arms, elbows, and fingers. Very slowly lift the arms out laterally (abduction) and up toward being level with the floor. Lift only so far as there is no pain. Very slowly lower the arms back to the sides. Repeat ten to fifteen times. Explore holding the arms in abduction for as long as doing so is pain-free. If this is very easy and the shoulders do not elevate, explore the same movements with very light weights in the hands. Explore this same set of movements with all asanas in which the arms are abducted to ninety degrees, such as in Virabhadrasana II (Warrior II Pose).

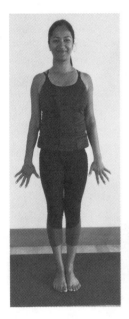
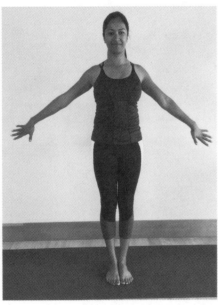
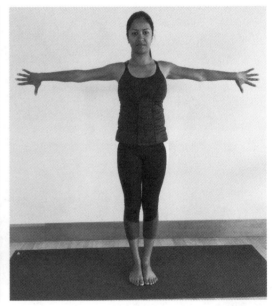

Rotator Cuff Tears

The shoulder girdle (also called the pectoral girdle) is a complex of three joints, one of which, the ball-and-socket glenohumeral joint, is commonly called the shoulder joint. The glenohumeral joint, where the proximal humeral bone joins the glenoid fossa of the scapula, is where most movement occurs when moving the upper arm. Movements in this joint involve movements in the other two joints of the shoulder girdle (steroclavicular and acromioclavicular). All are mobilized and stabilized by a complex set of ligaments, muscles, and tendons.

The rotator cuff is a musculotendinous structure that surrounds, mobilizes, and stabilizes the glenohumeral joint, securing ("cuffing") the relatively large

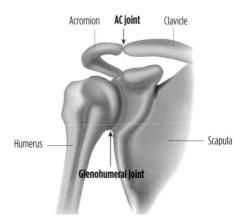

Figure 23.14: The Glenohumeral Joint

head of the arm bone in the very shallow golf tee–shaped glenoid fossa. It consists of four muscles—supraspinatus, infraspinatus, teres minor, and subscalularis—referred to as SITS. The tendons of these muscles interweave with the fibrous articular capsule of the glenohumeral joint, cuffing the humeral bone from the direction of its origin and thus reinforcing the joint's stability anteriorly, posteriorly, and superiorly.

Supraspinatus: Abducts the arm to ninety degrees (level with the ground), comes from across the top of the scapula (along the supraspinous fossa), securing the joint superiorly.

Infraspinatus: A strong external rotator of the humerus, covers most of the posterior scapulae and attaches to the middle facet on the greater tubercle of the humerus, securing the joint posteriorly (along with the teres minor).

Teres Minor: Also an external rotator of the humerus, originates on the inferior angle of the scapulae and attaches to the inferior facet on the greater tubercle of the humerus, securing the joint posteriorly (along with the supraspinatus).

Subscapularis: An internal rotator and adductor of the humerus, pulls from its origin on the anterior surface of the scapulae to its attachment on the lesser tubercle of the humerus, securing the joint anteriorly.

Injury and disease and associated muscular weakness or tightness compromises the stabilizing and mobilizing functions of the rotator cuff muscles, often causing painful movement and increasing the propensity for subluxation or dislocation of the glenohumeral joint.[85] It is the most frequently dislocated joint in the body, with most dislocations occurring inferiorly as there is not a rotator cuff muscle with an inferior attachment or cuffing. Rotator cuff tears (partial and full) can occur due to acute trauma, repetitive movement (especially in sports such as volleyball in which the arms are involved in powerful overhead movements), or disease (particularly degenerative tendonitis in menopausal women and elderly people).[86]

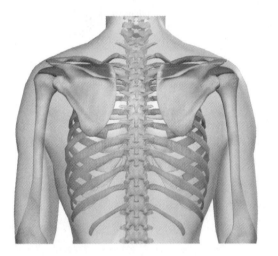
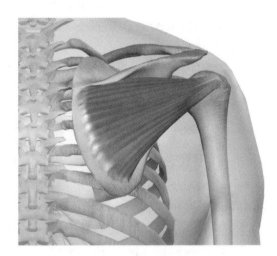
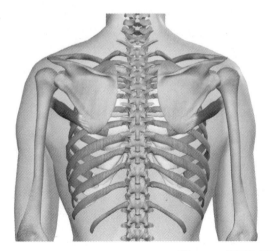
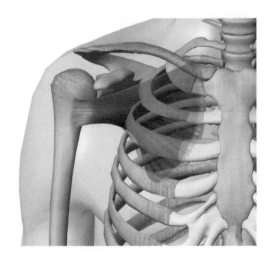

Figures 23.15–23.18: The Rotator Cuff

THE PAINFUL EXPERIENCE

Most rotator cuff injury and disease cause a dull deep ache in the shoulder, especially with overhead activities and abduction of the arm. The pain tends to be isolated to the shoulder and not refer down to the elbow (if it does there may be a compressed nerve in the neck or larger shoulder girdle). An acute tear that occurs with subluxation or dislocation immediately causes intense sharp pain, and when the joint is reset, there is a deep dull ache for at least a few days. If there is a chronic tendon tear—which increases the likelihood of subluxation—pain will gradually increase along with a growing feeling of weakness and increasingly limited range of motion (especially in trying to bring the arm behind the back).

THE KNOWN CAUSES

There are several risk factors associated with rotator cuff tears. Dominant hand repetitive arm movement, advancing age, sex, smoking, and kyphotic-lordotic postures all predispose one to tears.[87] Traumatic force is the leading cause of full tears, subluxation (a partial dislocation), and dislocation.

HOW IT HEALS

There are widely varying medical opinions regarding rotator cuff injuries and how they best heal, and uncertainty regarding the advice one should give concerning specific exercises as treatment options.[88] The general health of one's rotator cuff muscles and tendons—their tissue quality—significantly affects healing. Full and many partial rotator cuff tears require immobilization by placing the arm in a sling before and after surgical or nonsurgical treatment. Full tears require surgical treatment, whereas even some unreconstructed partial tears that are not surgically treated can lead to complications, including more likely full tears.[89] Many partial tears can be effectively treated with physical therapy,[90] involving daily exercises with range of motion and flexibility practices and alternate day strengthening practices.[91]

HEALING WITH ASANA PRACTICES

Asana practices can be tailored to strengthen, stretch, and tone the rotator cuff muscles once torn tendons have healed and a physical therapist has given assistance in regaining partial range of motion using passive mobilization of the glenohumeral joint. The asanas should focus on the balanced restoration of strength and flexibility. Here we look at asanas for strengthening each of the four rotator cuff muscles and for restoring healthy range of motion.

Strengthening Muscles

To strengthen the supraspinatus muscle, follow this asana:

ARDHA URDHVA HASTASANA (HALF UPWARD HAND POSE)   Standing in Tadasana, slightly internally rotate the arms until the thumb tips point toward the hips. (Note that this is the opposite rotation generally done in preparation for reaching the arms out and up overhead.)

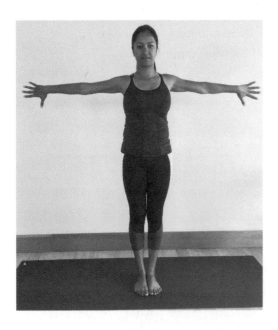

Keeping the shoulder blades lightly rooted down against the back ribs and the tops of the shoulders level with each other, fully extend through the arms, elbows, and fingers. Very slowly lift the arms out laterally (abduction) and up toward being level with the floor. Lift only so far as there is no pain. Very slowly lower the arms back to the sides. Repeat ten to fifteen times. Explore holding the arms in abduction for as long as doing so is pain-free. If this is very easy and the shoulders do not elevate, explore the same movements with very light weights in the hands. Explore this same set of movements with all asanas in which the arms are abducted to ninety degrees, such as in Virabhadrasana II (Warrior II Pose).

To strengthen the infraspinatus and teres minor muscles, follow these asanas:

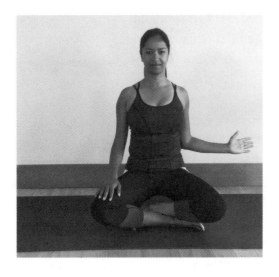

SUKASANA (SIMPLE POSE) SHOULDER ROTATIONS   Sitting comfortably (if necessary sit on a bolster and/or against a wall), flex the elbows to ninety degrees with the thumbs pointing up. Keeping the elbows by the sides and the forearms level with the floor, slowly externally rotate the arms as far as possible without pain and hold in this position for five to ten breaths. Slowly release back to the starting position. Repeat ten to fifteen times.

PARSVA SAVASANA (SIDE CORPSE POSE) SHOULDER ROTATIONS   Lying on the side of the healing shoulder on a bench or a stack of bolsters with the shoulder and elbow at the edge of the elevated prop, flex the elbow to ninety degrees. Keeping the elbow on the prop, slowly externally rotate the arm as far as possible without pain, and then slowly internally rotate the arm to bring the hand across the torso (keeping the elbow on the prop). Repeat ten to fifteen times. When this is relatively easy, do the same movements with a very light weight in the hand.

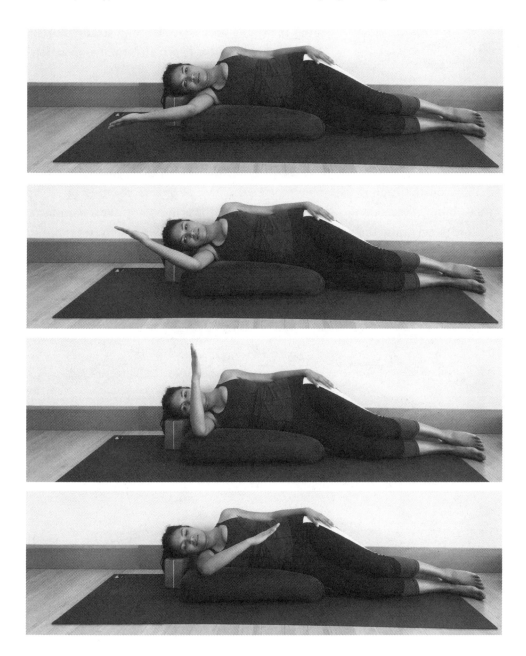

ANAHATASANA (PUPPY DOG POSE) SHOULDER ROTATIONS Explore this once there is sufficient range of motion to position the arms overhead free of pain. Begin on all fours in Bidalasana (Cat Pose). Reach the arms forward from the shoulders and press the hands firmly and evenly into the floor. Slowly rotate the shoulder blades in toward the spine (internally rotating the arms), then reverse this movement, externally rotating the shoulder blades out away from the spine. Focus on slow and steady movement. Explore holding the externally rotated position for five to ten breaths.

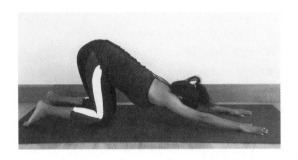

There is very little one can do to strengthen the subscapularis muscle in basic asanas. It generally acts with the latissimus dorsi and teres major muscles in pulling activities such as rock climbing or pull-ups.

SAVASANA (CORPSE POSE) SHOULDER ROTATIONS Lying supine, flex the elbow on the healing side ninety degrees with the fingers pointing up. Keeping the elbow at the side, slowly externally rotate the arm only as far as comfortable. More slowly raise the arm back (internally rotating back to the starting position). Repeat ten to fifteen times.

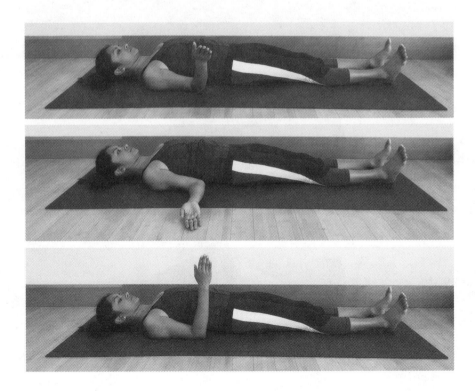

PARSVA SAVASANA (SIDE CORPSE POSE) SHOULDER ROTATIONS   Lying on the side of the healing shoulder on a bench or on a stack of bolsters with the shoulder and elbow at the edge of the elevated prop, flex the elbow to ninety degrees. Keeping the elbow on the prop, slowly externally rotate the arm as far as possible without pain, and then slowly internally rotate the arm to bring the hand across the torso (keeping the elbow on the prop). Repeat ten to fifteen times. When this is relatively easy, do the same movements with a very light weight in the hand.

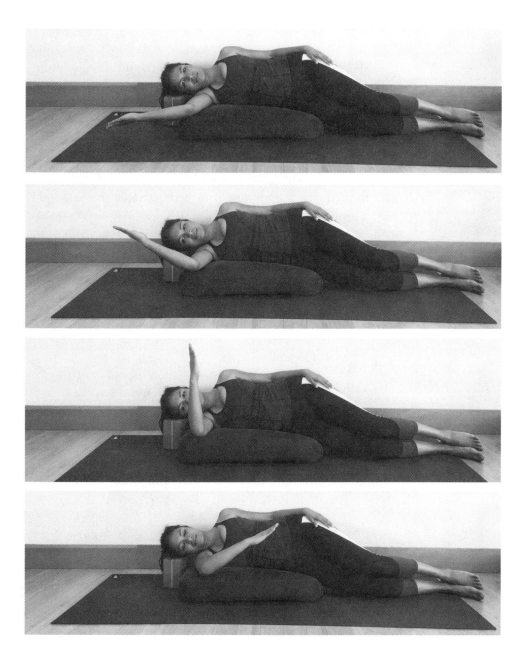

Restoring Range of Motion

To restore range of motion in the glenohumeral joint, follow these steps:

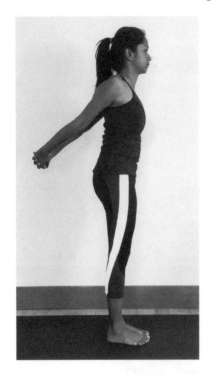

TADASANA (MOUNTAIN POSE) WITH PRASARITA C ARMS
Standing in Tadasana, interlace the fingers behind the back. If it is difficult to interlace the fingers hold a strap between the hands behind the back. Lift the arms away from the back only as far as the chest does not collapse and the shoulders do not lift toward the neck. Explore moving the head, first very slowly forward and back to center, then to each side and back to center, then with rotation and back to center. Explore moving the head more intuitively, tuning in to sensations in the neck to better guide the movements.

GARUDASANA (EAGLE POSE) ARMS PREP POSITION   Position the arms as in Garudasana. If unable to cross the elbows, use one arm to help draw the opposite arm directly across the upper chest (in adduction). Try to internally rotate the arm (turning the arm to point the thumb down) to better stretch the external rotators. Draw the shoulder blades down away from the neck and against the back ribs. Hold this position while breathing deeply and exploring very slight movements of the head in every direction except back. Do not hyperextend the neck.

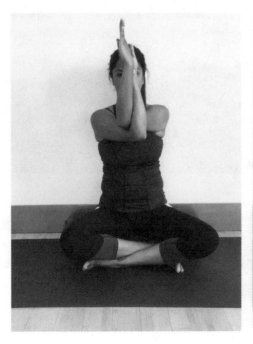
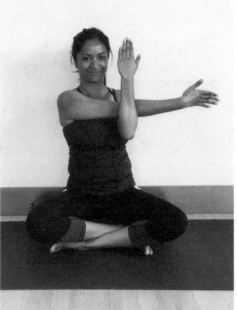

ANAHATASANA (PUPPY DOG OR MELTING HEART POSE)   Begin on all fours in Bidalasana (Cat Pose). Reach the arms forward from the shoulders and press the hands firmly and evenly into the floor. Try to rotate the shoulder blades out away from the spine. With each inhalation lift the chest up away from the floor. With exhalation stretch the chest toward the floor. Repeat ten to fifteen times before holding the chest toward the floor for up to two minutes.

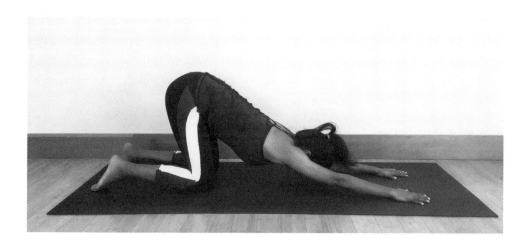

Shoulder Impingement Syndrome

Shoulder Impingement Syndrome (SIS) is the most common shoulder ailment: among the one-third of adults who complain of shoulder problems, fully half have this condition.[92] It is common because the supraspinus tendon crosses over the subacromial bursa with very little space to spare. When this bursa sac is inflamed (subacromial bursitis), the space between the coracoacromial arch of the scapula and the humeral head can compress the subacromial bursa, rotator cuff tendons, and the biceps tendon. Alternately called subacromial impingement syndrome or painful arch syndrome, SIS causes pain when abducting the arm and in overhead positioning of the arm.

When abducting the arms to an overhead position, the gap between the humeral head and the acromion process diminishes. If attempted with the arms internally rotated,

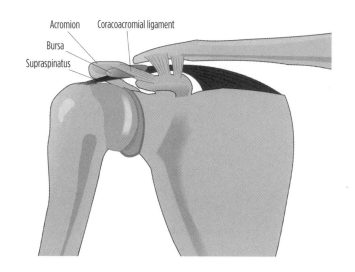

the gap more immediately closes, inhibiting further abduction. Simply externally rotating the arms prior to abduction positions the humeral head in a way that allows impingement-free movement—unless there is something else closing the gap. Inflammation of the subacromial bursa is one of the prime suspects in narrowing the gap; the other is faulty glenoscapular rhythm.

THE PAINFUL EXPERIENCE

Although with SIS there can be persistent pain amid normal daily activity, acute pain is felt around the top of the shoulder, lateral to the acromion, when abducing, flexing overhead, or extending the arm (especially when trying to reach it around behind the back). Pain may radiate along the outside of the arm and can also be present when lying on that shoulder when sleeping.

THE KNOWN CAUSES

The principle causes of SIS are interrelated—poor posture, rotator cuff weakness, faulty scapulohumeral rhythm (particularly with repetitive movements such as doing Sun Salutations in flow-style yoga classes), and scapular instability. In healthy glenohumeral and scapulohumeral rhythm, which starts with healthy posture and a healthy rotator cuff, externally rotated arms abduct and the scapulae elevate in a coordinated rhythm. This causes the acromion process (the pointed boney structure at the most lateral-superior aspect of the scapulae—the top outer part of the shoulder) to lift, thereby creating more space for the humeral head to move.[93] Weakness in the rotator cuff muscles inhibits proper external rotation; tightness in the lower trapezius, serratus anterior, and rhomboids inhibits scapular elevation; and weakness in the levator scapulae further limits scapular elevation. With tight or dysfunctional deltoids, this combination of musculoskeletal factors disturbs healthy glenohumeral and scapulohumeral rhythm, with the subacromial bursa being among the primary structures affected. Other factors can be involved in SIS, including acromioclavicular arthritis, calcified ligaments, and structural abnormalities.

HOW IT HEALS

SIS can generally be treated with physical therapy, although in some cases arthroscopic surgery is recommended. Corticosteroids are often given for persistent impingement. There is growing interest and some supportive evidence of the efficacy of therapeutic taping, acupuncture, and therapeutic massage.

HEALING WITH ASANA PRACTICES

Yoga asana practices can help support many of the physical therapy treatments indicated for SIS. This begins with postural correction. Several asana practices can improve scapular movement and rhythm, increase range of motion in the shoulder joint, and strengthen the rotator cuff.

Reducing Tension and Increasing Range of Motion

To reduce muscular tension and increase range of motion, follow these asanas:

TADASANA (MOUNTAIN POSE)   Explore all of the elements of Tadasana to help in developing or restoring basic upright standing posture in which there is a relatively straight line (gravitational line) from the ankle (later malleolus) to the knee to the hip (greater trochanter) to the shoulder to the ear. Start with pada bandha in the feet, engage the legs, establish pelvic neutrality in the spine with its natural curves, and keep the head positioned level on top of the spine. Considering any deviations from this posture, gradually stretch, strengthen, and comfortably stabilize in this form when standing. Explore the following practices to move into greater postural integrity with primary focus on the spine and shoulder girdle.

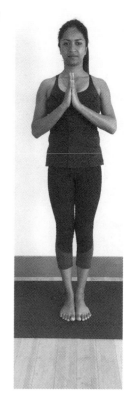

TADASANA WITH ARM SWINGS   Standing in Tadasana next to a chair, place the hand of the healthy side on the chair and lean slightly forward to allow the healing arm to dangle down from the shoulder joint. Slowly swing the arm like a pendulum, then around in circles, for one to two minutes. Repeat several times every day.

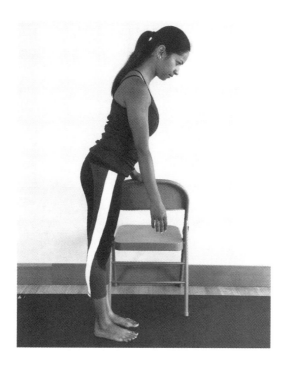

GARUDASANA (EAGLE POSE) SHOULDER PREP POSITION Standing in Tadasana, use the healthy arm to help gently lift and pull the healing arm across the chest in adduction. Explore alternately rotating the arm into external and internal rotation. Hold and explore for one to two minutes several times every day.

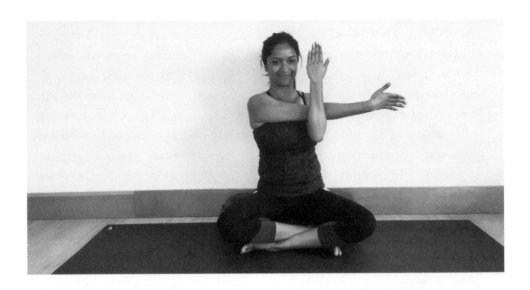

PRASARITA PADOTTANASANA C (WIDE ANGLE FORWARD FOLD C) ARM STRETCH POSITION Standing in Tadasana, clasp a strap in the hands behind the back shoulder-distance apart. Use the healthy arm to gently pull the healing arm farther behind the back. Hold for one to two minutes. Repeat several times every day.

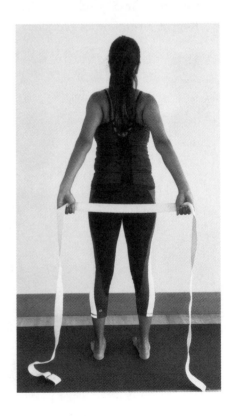

GOMUKHASANA (COW FACE POSE) ARM STRETCH POSITION   If Prasarita Padottanasana C Arm Stretch Position is comfortable, explore positioning the arms for Cow Face Pose with the healthy arm overhead and the healing arm behind the back. Clasp a strap and explore pulling the hands toward each other. Hold for one to two minutes. Repeat several times every day.

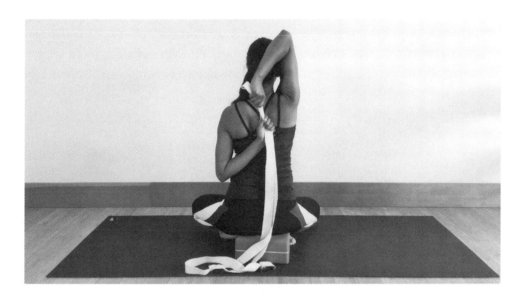

TADASANA FINGER WALK   Stand facing a wall with the fingers on the wall at hip height. Slowly walk the fingers up the wall as far comfortable. Repeat several times every day.

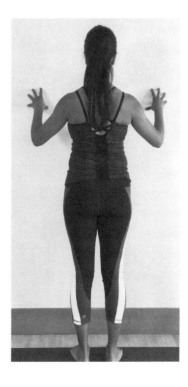

Strengthening and Stabilizing

To strengthen and stabilize through the shoulder girdle, follow these asanas:

BIDALASANA (CAT POSE) TO UTTHITA BALASANA (EXTENDED CHILD'S POSE)   If comfortable in the healing shoulder while on all fours in Bidalasana, draw in a deep breath with a feeling of breathing more space into the shoulder. On the exhalation slowly draw the sitting bones toward the heels while keeping the hands in place, going only so far as is comfortable. On each inhalation rise slightly away from the maximum stretch, and on each exhale explore stretching farther. Continue to explore in this way for one to two minutes. Repeat several times every day.

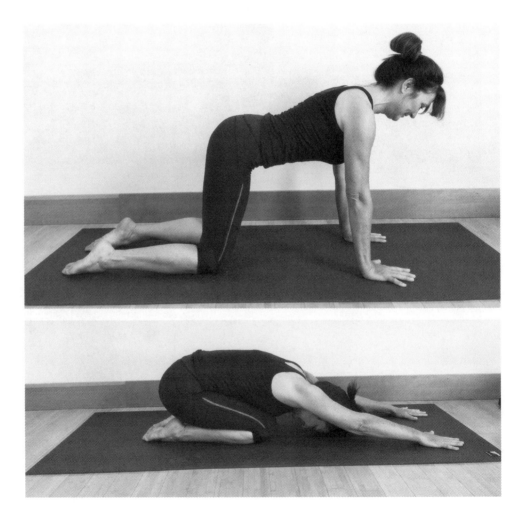

SUKASANA (SIMPLE POSE) SHOULDER ROTATIONS   Sitting comfortably (if necessary sit on a bolster and/or against a wall), flex the elbows to ninety degrees with the thumbs pointing up. Keeping the elbows by the sides and the forearms level with the floor, slowly externally rotate the arms as far as possible without pain and hold in this position for five to ten breaths. Slowly release back to the starting position. Repeat ten to fifteen times.

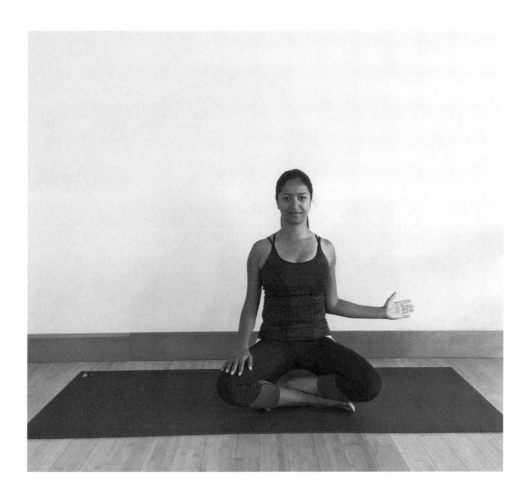

PARSVA SAVASANA (SIDE CORPSE POSE) SHOULDER ROTATIONS   Lying on the side of the healing shoulder on a bench or on a stack of bolsters with the shoulder and elbow at the edge of the elevated prop, flex the elbow to ninety degrees. Keeping the elbow on the prop, slowly externally rotate the arm as far as possible without pain, and then slowly internally rotate the arm to bring the hand across the torso (keeping the elbow on the prop). Repeat ten to fifteen times. When this is relatively easy, do the same movements with a very light weight in the hand.

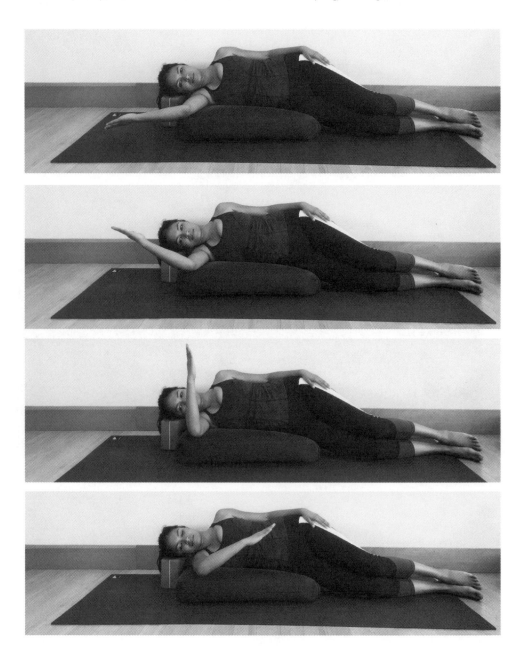

ANAHATASANA (PUPPY DOG POSE) SHOULDER ROTATIONS Explore this once there is sufficient range of motion to position the arms overhead free of pain. Begin on all fours in Bidalasana. Reach the arms forward from the shoulders and press the hands firmly and evenly into the floor. Slowly rotate the shoulder blades in toward the spine (internally rotating the arms), then reverse this movement, externally rotating the shoulder blades out away from the spine. Focus on slow and steady movement. Explore holding the externally rotated position for five to ten breaths.

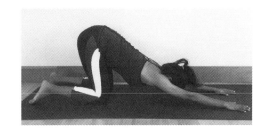

SAVASANA (CORPSE POSE) SHOULDER ROTATIONS Lying supine, flex the elbow on the healing side ninety degrees with the fingers pointing up. Keeping the elbow at the side, slowly externally rotate the arm only as far as is comfortable. More slowly raise the arm back (internally rotating back to the starting position). Repeat ten to fifteen times.

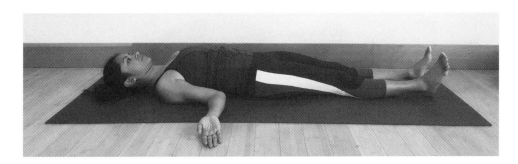

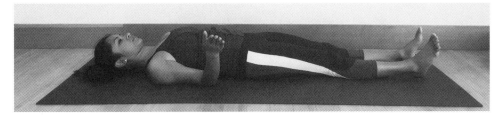

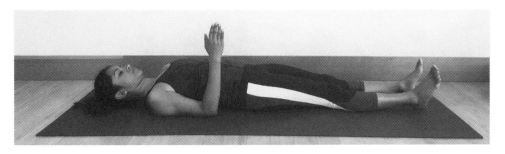

PARSVA SAVASANA (SIDE CORPSE POSE) SHOULDER ROTATIONS   Lying on the side of the healing shoulder on a bench or on a stack of bolsters with the shoulder and elbow at the edge of the elevated prop, flex the elbow to ninety degrees. Keeping the elbow on the prop, slowly externally rotate the arm as far as possible without pain, and then slowly internally rotate the arm to bring the hand across the torso (keeping the elbow on the prop). Repeat ten to fifteen times. When this is relatively easy, do the same movements with a very light weight in the hand.

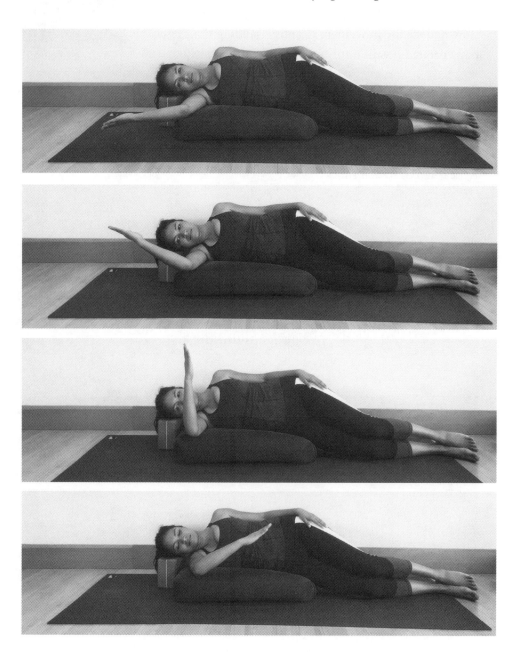

ARDHA URDHVA HASTASANA (HALF UPWARD HAND POSE)   Standing in Tadasana, slightly internally rotate the arms until the thumb tips point toward the hips. (Note that this is the opposite rotation generally done in preparation for reaching the arms out and up overhead.) Keeping the shoulder blades lightly rooted down against the back ribs and the tops of the shoulders level with each other, fully extend through the arms, elbows, and fingers. Very slowly lift the arms out laterally (abduction) and up toward being level with the floor. Lift only so far as there is no pain. Very slowly lower the arms back to the sides. Repeat ten to fifteen times. Explore holding the arms in abduction for as long as is pain-free. If this is very easy and the shoulders do not elevate, explore the same movements with very light weights in the hands. Explore this same set of movements with all asanas in which the arms are abducted to ninety degrees, such as in Virabhadrasana II (Warrior II Pose).

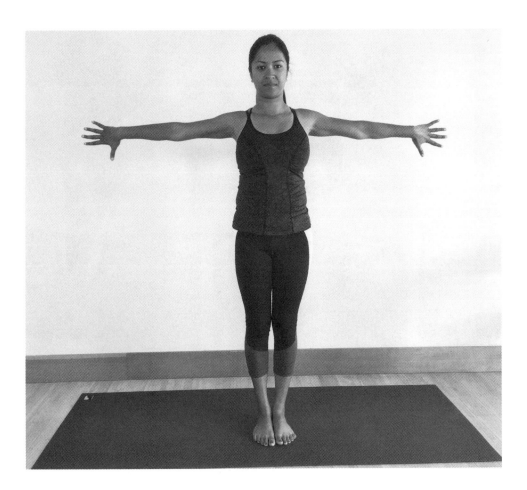

WALL PHALAKASANA (WALL PLANK POSE) Start standing facing a wall (have the feet an arm-length away from the wall) in Tadasana and place the hands on the wall one hand-length lower than the shoulders with the elbows fully extended. Slowly bend the elbows to bring the upper body closer to the wall, and then reverse this movement, pressing away from the wall until the arms are fully extended. Keeping the shoulder blades rooted down the back, repeat ten to fifteen times before holding in the fully extended elbow position for up to one minute.

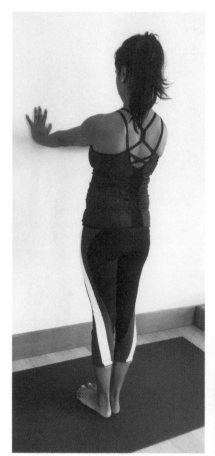 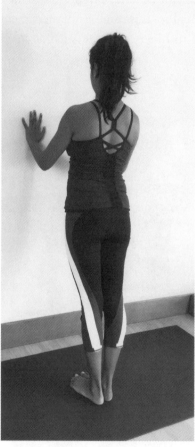 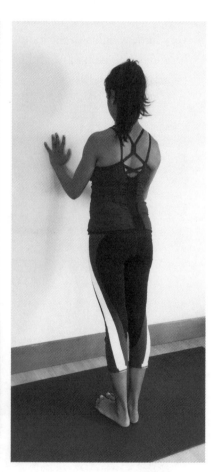

BIDALASANA SCAPULAE ENGAGEMENT   Starting in the basic form of Bidalasana with the elbows fully extended, slowly draw the chest toward the floor without bending the elbows, then slowly reverse this movement by pressing the chest up away from the floor. Try to keep the shoulder blades rooted against the back ribs and as far down the back (away from the neck) as possible. Continue with this very slow movement ten to fifteen times. Next, come to the halfway point in this movement and hold for up to one minute while continuing to focus on holding the shoulder blades down and away from the neck.

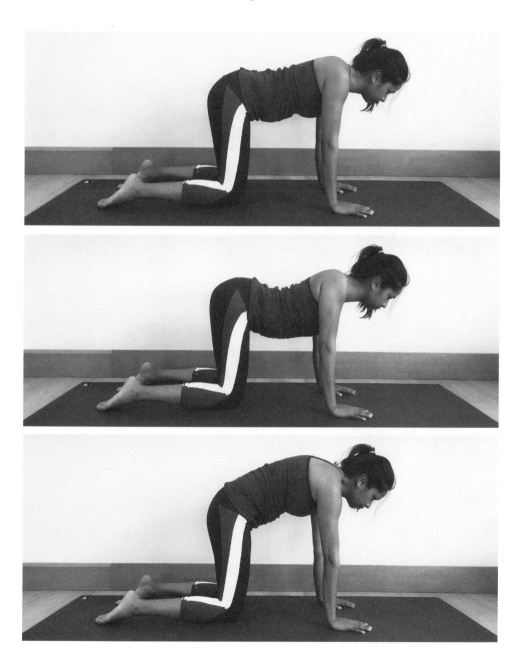

PHALAKASANA (PLANK POSE)   Come into the basic form of Phalakasana. If uncomfortable, stay with the Bidalasana Scapulae Engagement practice just described. If comfortable, slowly draw the chest toward the floor without bending the elbows, then slowly reverse this movement by pressing the chest up away from the floor. Keep the arms straight and the shoulder blades rooted down and against the back ribs. Continue with this very slow movement ten to fifteen times. Next, come to the halfway point in this movement and hold for up to one minute while continuing to focus on holding the shoulder blades down away from the neck.

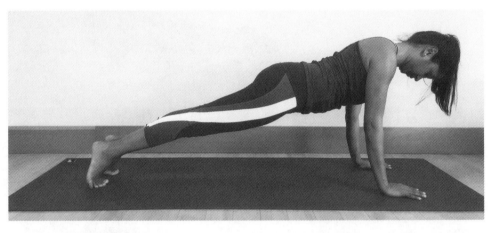

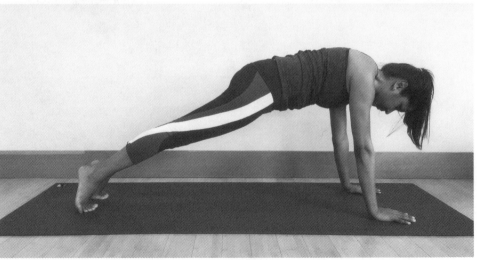

URDHVA HASTASANA (UPWARD HANDS POSE) WALL STRETCH Standing in Tadasana, position the arms with the elbows slightly below shoulder height and flexed to ninety degrees with the palms touching the wall. On each inhalation bring the upper body (torso and head) slightly away from the wall. With each exhalation, bring the upper body toward the wall, stretching the levator scapulae muscles. Repeat ten to fifteen times. If comfortable, explore stretching the arms fully overhead into full Urdhva Hastasana, then reroot the shoulder blades down the back while trying to rotate the shoulder blades away from the spine.

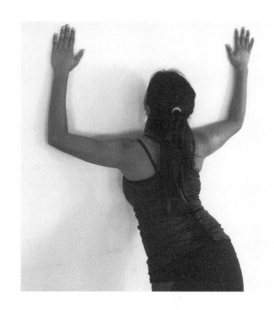

Elbow Tendinopathy ("Tennis Elbow")

Commonly called "tennis elbow" and sometimes erroneously referred to as elbow tendonitis (inflammation), elbow tendinosis—more technically epicondylosis—is a misuse and overuse injury to the lateral or medial elbow common in sports and yoga.

Lateral epicondylosis is found far more frequently than medial epicondylosis and is our focus here. It is often diagnosed as tendonitis. However, close examination of this condition does not reveal signs of inflammation.[94] Rather, microscopic examination shows degeneration within a substance (angiofibroblasts) of the elbow extensor (triceps brachii and anconeus) and/or wrist extensor (extensor carpi radialis brevis and longus) tendons, destabilizing and weakening them.[95] Although a common pathology among athletes, it also occurs in about 1 to 3 percent of the general population and is more common among carpenters than tennis players.[96]

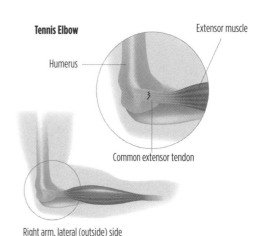

Right arm, lateral (outside) side

THE PAINFUL EXPERIENCE

Elbow tendinopathy is experienced as sharp pain at or around the lateral elbow, especially when lifting, resisting gravity in movements such as the transition from Phalakasana (Plank Pose) to Chataranga Dandasana (Four-Limbed Staff Pose) to Urdhva Mukha

Svanasana (Upward Facing Dog Pose), or gripping with the hand. There might be point tenderness at the lateral epicondyle even when at rest, and the pain can radiate into the forearm or upper arm. There can also be swelling and stiffening.

THE KNOWN CAUSES

The primary causes of elbow tendinopathy are misuse—poor biomechanics[97]—and overuse, both of which I frequently observe among yoga students, especially in dynamic-style yoga practices. Its popular "tennis elbow" name arises from an improper backhand hitting technique in tennis in which power is generated from the forearm rather than the shoulder and rotation through the torso. Although it can be caused by a traumatic event, it is generally a misuse injury or a repetitive stress injury involving wear and tear on the relatively avascular tendons. Gradually increasing stress on the tendons causes their degeneration, which in turn leads to disarray of their collagen fibers (not their inflammation).[98]

HOW IT HEALS

Elbow tendinopathy heals very slowly, typically taking several weeks to many months to self-resolve. It is important to limit causative activities while developing healthier biomechanics in hand, forearm, and arm use. Hand and wrist splinting as well as bracing immediately below the elbow only during significant activity are found to help heal the ailing tendons.[99] Deep massage in and around the affected tissues, including the active release technique of soft tissue mobilization, has been found to be effective, as has acupuncture.[100] Steroid injections and surgery are used in some chronic conditions.[101]

HEALING WITH ASANA PRACTICES

The primary focus of asana is on developing greater flexibility and strength in the wrist extensor and flexor muscles, strengthening the shoulder girdle in ways that support healthier biomechanics in arm and elbow use, and developing those healthier biomechanics.

Developing Greater Strength and Flexibility

To develop greater flexibility and strength in the wrist extensor and flexor muscles, begin with general wrist therapy practices. Those practices can help develop flexibility in the forearm muscles.

SHISHULASANA (DOLPHIN POSE) PREP FOREARM MOVEMENTS   Starting on all fours in Bidalasana (Cat Pose), bring the elbows to the floor under the shoulders with the forearms aligned straight forward from the elbows. Press the shoulders away from the hands and root the shoulder blades down against the back ribs. Very slowly rotate the forearms to turn the palms up, then reverse this movement to slowly press the palms onto the floor. Alternating back and forth in this supination–pronation movement, after ten to fifteen repetitions, hold in each fully rotated position for up to one minute. Finally, shake out the wrists and self-massage throughout the forearms and into the bones of the wrists.

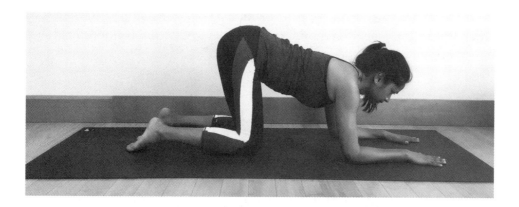

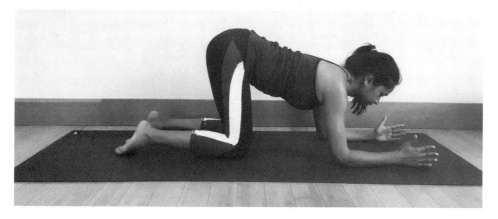

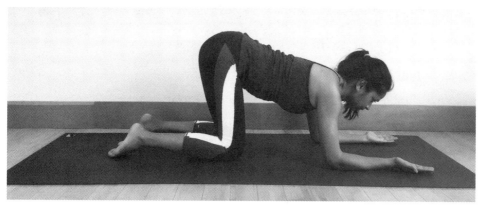

ANAHATASANA (PUPPY DOG POSE) FOREARM MOVEMENTS   Begin on all fours in Bidalasana. Reach the arms forward from the shoulders and press the hands firmly and evenly into the floor. Slowly rotate the shoulder blades in toward the spine (internally rotating the arms), then reverse this movement, externally rotating the shoulder blades out away from the spine. Holding the externally rotated position of the upper arms, proceed as described above for Shishuasana Prep in very slowly rotating the forearms to turn the palms up, then reversing this movement to slowly press the palms onto the floor. Alternating back and forth in this supination–pronation movement, after ten to fifteen repetitions hold in each fully rotated position for up to one minute.

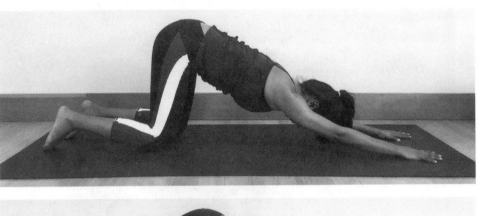

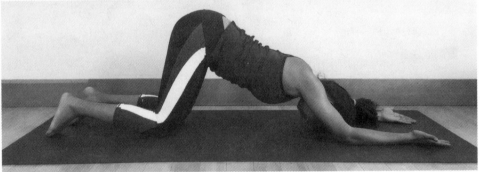

Strengthening the Shoulder Girdle

To strengthen the shoulder girdle, follow these asanas:

BIDALASANA (CAT POSE) SCAPULAE ENGAGEMENT   Starting in the basic form of Bidalasana with the elbows fully extended, slowly draw the chest toward the floor without bending the elbows, then slowly reverse this movement by pressing the chest up away from the floor. Try to keep the shoulder blades rooted against the back ribs and as far down the back (away from the neck) as possible. Continue with this very slow movement ten to fifteen times. Next, come to the halfway point in this movement and hold for up to one minute while continuing to focus on holding the shoulder blades down away from the neck and holding the torso stably in the halfway position.

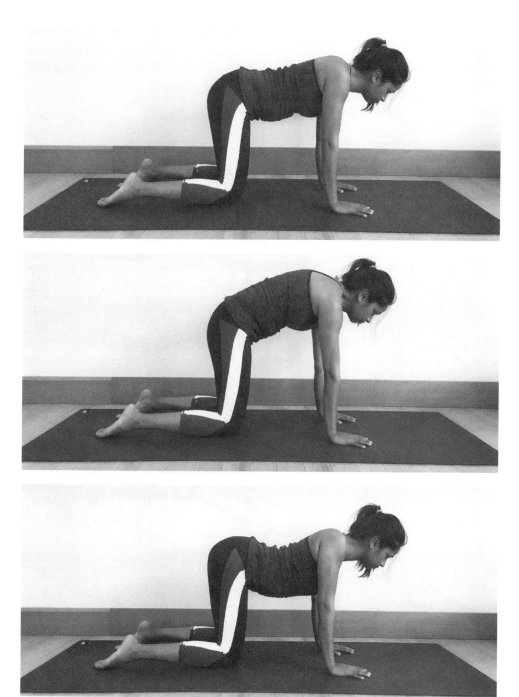

PHALAKASANA (PLANK POSE)   Come into the basic form of Phalakasana. If uncomfortable, stay with the Bidalasana Scapulae Engagement practice just described. If comfortable, slowly draw the chest toward the floor without bending the elbows, then slowly reverse this movement by pressing the chest up away from the floor. Keep the arms straight and the shoulder blades rooted down and against the back ribs. Continue with this very slow movement ten to fifteen times. Next, come to the halfway point in this movement and hold for up to one minute while continuing to focus on holding the shoulder blades down away from the neck.

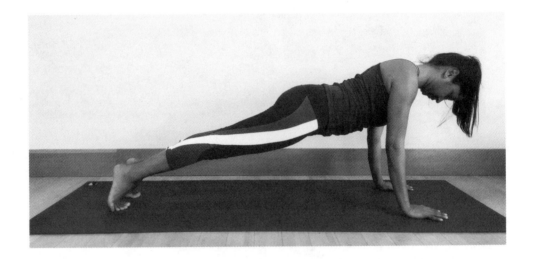

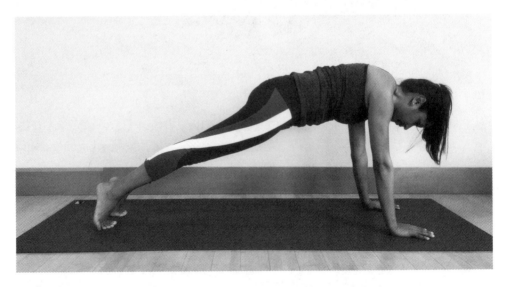

ADHO MUKHA SVANASANA (DOWNWARD FACING DOG POSE) Coming into the basic form of Adho Mukha Svanasana, bend both knees and begin to slowly bicycle the legs, very gradually drawing the heels closer to the floor. Gradually stabilize the legs; consider the option of keeping the knees bent so it is easier to hold this position amid tight hamstrings and hips. Root evenly through the hands, pressing firmly down through the knuckles of the index fingers, and spiral the shoulder blades out broadly from the spine. Hold for as long as is comfortable, and then rest in Balasana (Child's Pose).

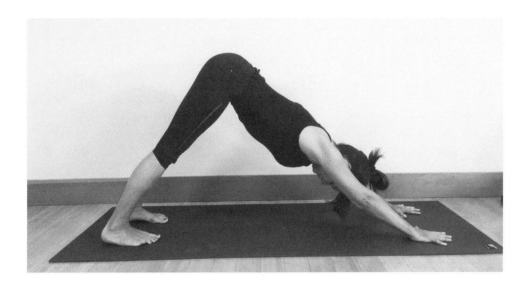

Developing Healthier Biomechanics

To develop healthier biomechanics in elbow movement (and further strengthen the shoulder girdle), follow these asanas:

PHALAKASANA (PLANK POSE) TO CHATARANGA DANDASANA (FOUR-LIMBED STAFF POSE) In exploring this movement, consider keeping the knees on the floor unless stable and comfortable with straight and active legs. The essential elements in this movement with respect to the elbow joints are to ensure that they a) align directly with the shoulders and wrists rather than splaying in or out, and b) do not waver both in and out. Place a thick, firm bolster (at least six inches thick) under the chest in the basic form of Phalakasana. If the legs are straight, press the heels as if into a wall while keeping the shoulder blades rooted down against the back ribs and creating a feeling of drawing the sternum forward. Keep the ears level with the shoulders rather than either extending or flexing the neck. On an exhalation slowly bend the elbows until the shoulders are just level with them—this is Chataranga Dandasana—and try to hold for one to two breaths before releasing onto the bolster. Try not to ever let the shoulders go lower than the elbows in Chataranga Dandasana because doing so causes excessive force into the front (anterior) shoulder joint capsule and with such repetitive movement can cause tears in the labrum. With greater strength, hold for longer before pressing back up into Phalakasana.

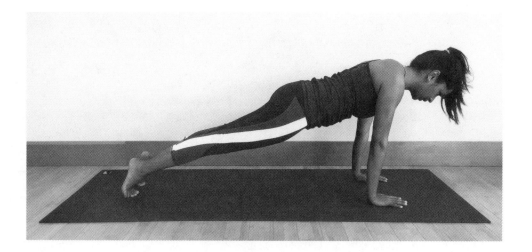

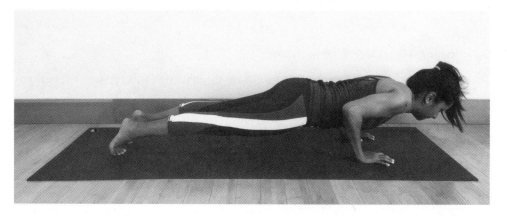

Wrist Pain and Carpal Tunnel Syndrome

Although wrist pain is clearly an overly general description and carpal tunnel syndrome (CTS) is a specific diagnosis, we discuss these together because of the various interrelated factors involved in them. Wrist pain almost invariably extends beyond the wrist, especially into the hand, and even when it does not, its cause can derive from factors extrinsic to the wrist itself.[102] The pain can also manifest in different parts of the wrist, offering some clues as to the cause. CTS occurs when the median nerve is entrapped in the small passageway on the palmar side of the wrist joint through which several tendons and the medial nerve pass.[103] Inflammation of the tendons places pressure on the nerve, causing pain or discomfort in the wrist, outer fingers (thumb, index finger, and middle finger), and sometimes up the forearm. Wrist and hand pain can also manifest in the fourth and fifth fingers due to pressure on the ulnar nerve.[104]

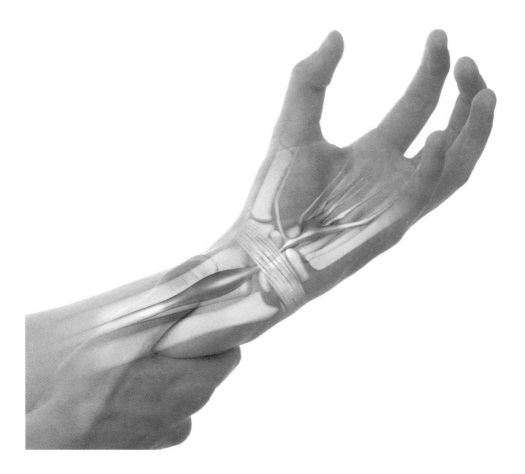

THE PAINFUL EXPERIENCE

CTS is generally experienced as a tingling, burning, pins and needles sensation, often at night when the wrist and hand are not in use. Ulnar nerve entrapment causes more of a tingling and numbing in the affected fingers, along with possible disruption of motor function. More acute pain in the wrist from a traumatic event involving bone fracture or ligament tears is experienced as sharp pain in the wrist itself along with numbing in the hand due to inflammation and related nerve pressure.

THE KNOWN CAUSES

Acute or chronic pain in the wrists and hands can arise from a variety of sources and thus can make diagnosis difficult. A traumatic event such as falling and landing on the wrist can cause bone fractures, ligament sprains and tears, and contusions.[105] Gradually increasing chronic pain is far more common and typically arises from repetitive stress, including in yoga classes in which there is tremendous pressure in the wrist joints while in extension (such as occurs in Plank Pose, Chaturanga Dandasana, Upward Facing Dog Pose, and Downward Facing Dog Pose, also in all arm balances except those with the forearms on the floor). Parents of infants and toddlers often develop wrist symptoms related to the repetitive stress involved in how they hold their child.[106]

Medical diagnostics can generally identify specific causes of wrist pain. Chronic, nontraumatic pain is by far most common and is most commonly caused by tendinopathy or nerve entrapment. Technical classification as CTS requires indentifying medial nerve entrapment in the carpal tunnel itself, this despite all of the symptoms of CTS arising just as much from medial nerve entrapment in the brachial plexus or at the elbow as from the inflammation of flexor tendons in the carpal tunnel. The elbow is also the likeliest location of ulnar nerve entrapment, which in yoga can be caused or exacerbated by misalignment of the elbows when bearing weight, especially in dynamic movements.[107] When the pain is experienced primarily at the base of the thumb or when using the thumb, one should have it evaluated for possible De Quervain's tenosynovitis by holding the thumb inside the fingers and abducting the right joint to determine if it produces pain at the base of the thumb, which is a positive test.[108]

HOW IT HEALS

Healing depends on the condition and its cause. Persistent wrist tenderness or strain usually benefits from ice, splints worn during sleep (due to the ways we tend to flex the wrist and otherwise place pressure on it during natural movement while sleeping), and anti-inflammatory agents (including turmeric and ginger). Repetitive stress injuries invite one to reduce or stop the repetitive actions and to assess the dynamics of posture and movement that are involved. In practicing yoga, there are several ways to play with slight modification of position and energetic action to variably affect pressure in the wrists, while props minimize the pressure from wrist extension. Acute injuries often require medical attention, and many chronic conditions also indicate receiving medical attention.

HEALING WITH ASANA PRACTICES

Students experiencing chronic wrist pain or CTS can benefit from warming up their fingers, hands, arms, and shoulders before beginning their practice. Wrist and forearm massage are also effective in helping reduce pain. So long as the pain is mild, the following practices can be healing.

Wrist-Specific Practices:

TADASANA WRIST THERAPY:　　Gently rotate the wrists through their full range of circular motion, repeatedly changing direction; then gently shake out the wrists for around thirty seconds. This can be incorporated in brief form into every Sun Salutation.

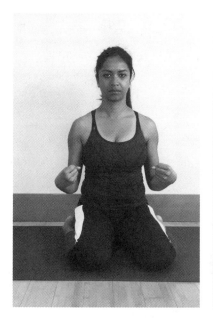 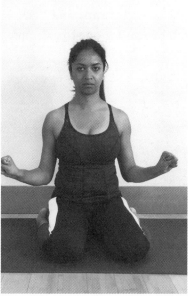 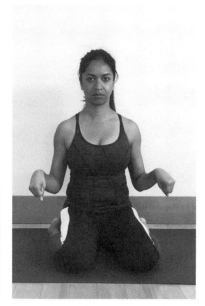

UTTANASANA WRIST PRATIKRIYASANA: Whenever folding into Uttanasana amid Sun Salutations, place the backs of the wrists toward or onto the floor and make an easy fist. This is less intense on the wrists than Pada Hastasana (also, more students can do it and it can be easily done with the exhale into Uttanasana).

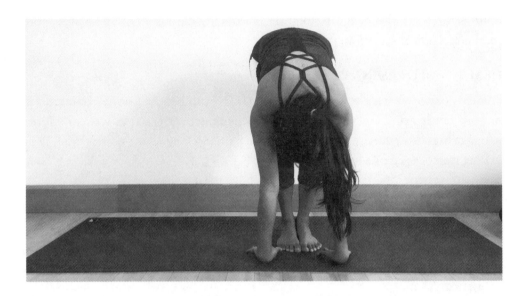

WRIST PUMPS: Holding the fingers of one hand with the fingers of the other hand, move the wrist forward and back while resisting the movement with the opposing hand. Repeat for one to two minutes if pain-free.

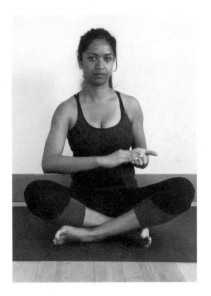 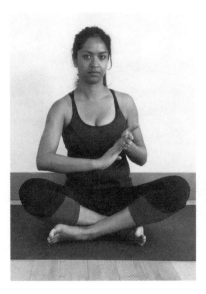 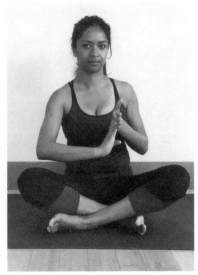

ANJALI MUDRA (REVERENCE SEAL): Press the palms and fingers (from the knuckles to the fingertips) firmly together at the chest in a prayer position for one to two minutes. This is also known as reverse Phalen's test; if there is a burning sensation inside the wrist joint within thirty seconds, this could indicate CTS. Reverse the position of the hands, placing the backs of the wrists and hands together, and press firmly for up to a minute (Phalen's test).

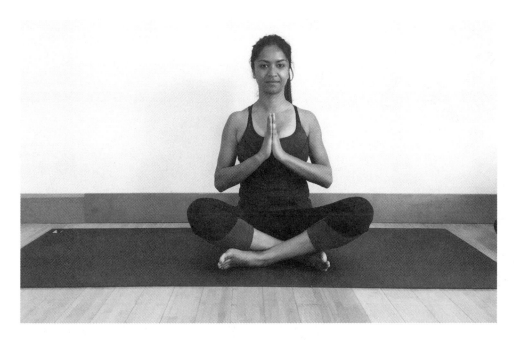

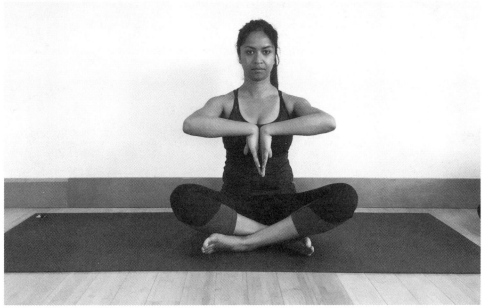

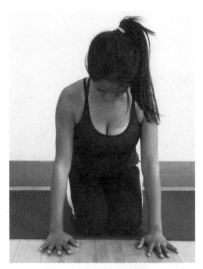

HAND DANCE: Kneeling comfortably, place the hands down on the floor with the fingers pointed forward, then turn the palms up, then down with the fingers out, up with the fingers in, down with the fingers back, up with the fingers back, continuing in this fashion with every permutation of palms up and down with the fingers forward, back, in, and out.

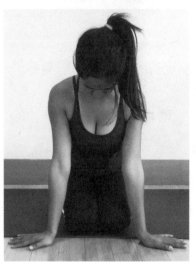
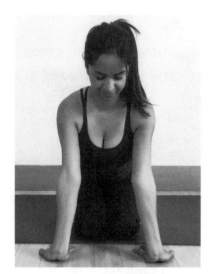
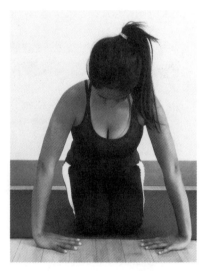

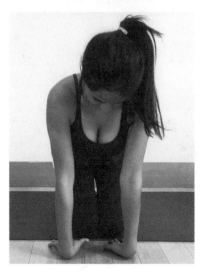
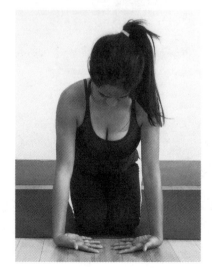
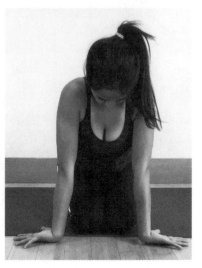

BASIC WRIST THERAPY

Students and clients experiencing mild wrist pain can benefit from warming up their fingers, hands, arms, and shoulders before beginning their practice. Wrist and forearm massage are also effective in helping reduce pain. So long as the pain is mild, the following exercises can be healing:

Tadasana Wrist Therapy: Gently rotate the wrists through their full range of circular motion, repeatedly changing direction, then gently shake out the wrists for around thirty seconds. This can be incorporated in brief form into every Sun Salutation.

Uttanasana Wrist Pratikriyasana: Whenever folding into Uttanasana amid Sun Salutations, place the backs of the wrists toward or onto the floor and make an easy fist. This is less intense on the wrists than Pada Hastasana (also, more students can do it and it can be easily done with the exhale into Uttanasana).

Wrist Pumps: Holding the fingers of one hand with the fingers of the other hand, move the wrist forward and back while resisting the movement with the opposing hand. Repeat for one to two minutes if pain-free.

Anjali Mudra: Press the palms and fingers (from the knuckles to the fingertips) firmly together at the chest in a prayer position for one to two minutes. This is also known as reverse Phalen's test; if there is a burning sensation inside the wrist joint within thirty seconds, this could indicate CTS. Reverse the position of the hands, placing the backs of the wrists and hands together, and press firmly for up to a minute (Phalen's test).

Hand Dance: Kneeling comfortably, place the hands down on the floor with the fingers pointed forward, then turn the palms up, then down with the fingers out, up with the fingers in, down with the fingers back, up with the fingers back, continuing in this fashion with every permutation of palms up and down with the fingers forward, back, in, and out.

Persistent wrist tenderness or strain usually benefits from ice, splints worn during sleep, anti-inflammatory agents (including turmeric and ginger), acupuncture, and other alternative treatments. Encourage students and clients to explore all possible measures and to consult a doctor for additional guidance.

Neck and Shoulder Girdle Practices

To address nerve pressure in the brachial plexus and shoulder girdle, follow these steps:

SHOULDER ROLLS   Roll the shoulders forward, up, back, and down several times, then go the opposite direction. Be very sensitive to pain; back off the movement if painful.

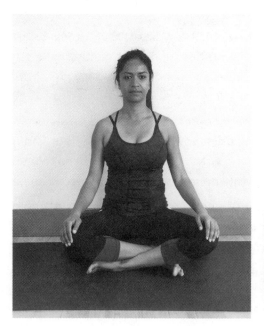
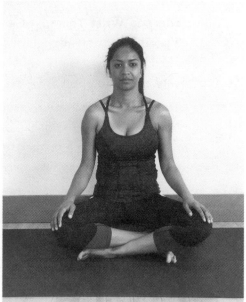
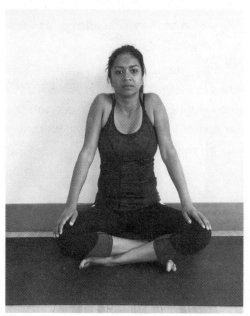
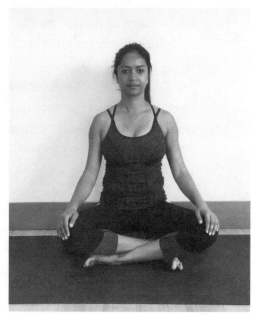

ROTATION AND FLEXION WITH ARM CLASP—PRACTICE 1   Reach the right hand around the back to clasp the left arm above the elbow. Use the right hand to pull the left shoulder slightly back and down. Turn the head toward the right shoulder. On the inhalations slightly lift the chin, on the exhalations draw the chin closer to the right shoulder. Hold for several breaths with the chin toward the shoulder and explore very slightly tilting the head left and right. Repeat several times before switching sides.

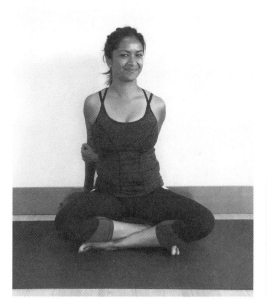
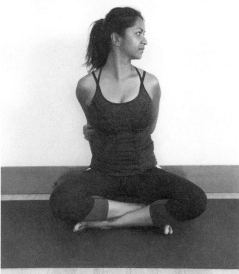

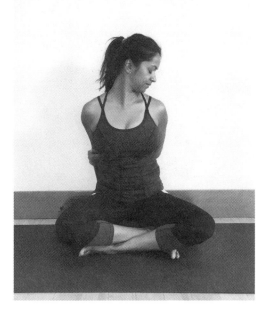

ROTATION AND FLEXION WITH ARM CLASP—PRACTICE 2   Clasp the arm, turn the head toward the right shoulder, and draw the chin toward the shoulder as described in Practice 1. Very slowly and sensitively draw the chin toward the distal right collarbone and then all the way across toward the distal left collarbone. Lift the chin slightly, then draw it toward the distal left collarbone and across to the right. Repeat several times before switching sides.

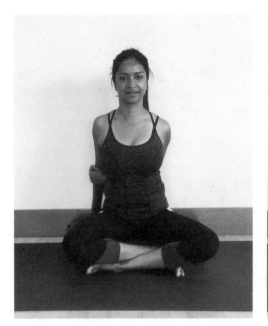
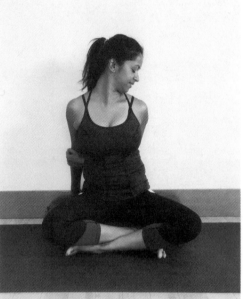
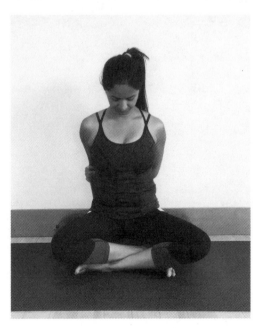

ROTATION AND FLEXION WITH ARM CLASP—PRACTICE 3 Clasp the arm as described in Practice 1. Slowly and sensitively tilt the head to the right, drawing the right ear toward the right shoulder. Slow lift the head back to the starting position. Repeat several times before switching sides.

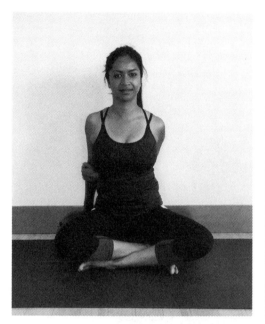
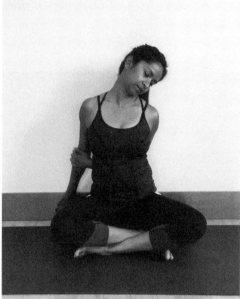

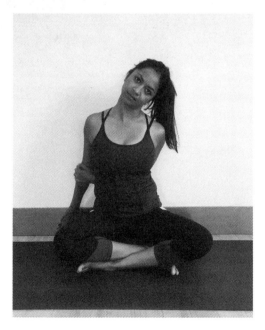

GARUDASANA (EAGLE POSE) ARMS   Position the arms as in Garudasana. If unable to cross the elbows, use one arm to help draw the opposite arm directly across the upper chest. Draw the shoulder blades down away from the neck and against the back ribs. Hold this position while breathing deeply and exploring very slight movements of the head in every direction except back. Do not hyperextend the neck. Repeat on the other side.

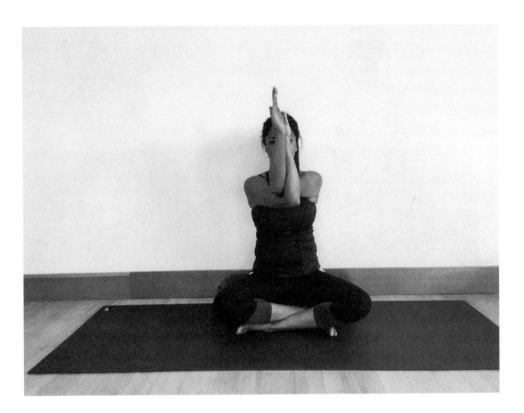

24

Mental, Emotional, and Behavioral Conditions

This happiness consisted of nothing else but the harmony of the few things around me with my own existence, a feeling of contentment and well-being that needed no changes and no intensification.
—HERMAN HESSE

LOSS OF CONTACT WITH REALITY is called psychosis. Without using this term, the ancient yogis described this condition in spiritual terms as existential suffering rooted in delusion. The lost reality was a spiritual one—one's essence as a spiritual being; the delusion arose from thinking that anything nonspiritual fundamentally matters. All of one's personal problems were considered spiritual issues to be resolved in spiritual practice or ritual. This theme is found throughout the history of yoga and is frequently seen as the *raison d'etre* of yoga.

The *Yoga Sutra of Patanjali* focuses on thinking itself as the basic problem, with the solution announced in its first and cardinal aphorism as *chitta vrtti nirodha*, "to still the fluctuations of the mind." The "true self" is said to reside beyond all thought, much as related by Lao Tzu in the first stanza of the *Tao Te Ching*: "the essential tao is the tao that cannot be told."[1] Thought is considered inherently problematic because it is seen as abstracted from reality rather than being real in and of itself. The ego-based, reactive, imaginary, and grasping mind is considered both cause and effect of an underlying ignorance—*avidya*—not merely of mundane matters but of reality itself. The interwoven veils of illusion and ignorance inhibit or disturb true perception and self-understanding; consequently, we suffer.

But there is hope: We are offered methods and practices for stilling the fluctuations of the mind. An essential part of the practice involves *pratyahara*, sensory isolation ("to relieve the senses of their external distractions"), for the initial purpose of attaining *dharana*, a more inwardly and singularly focused awareness. With greater meditative focus, the mind settles into a pure meditative condition called *dhyana*, which leads to the initial fruit of practice: a state of pure consciousness originally coined as *samadhi* in the *Maitri Upanishad*. As promised by Patanjali in the fourth century CE, the greater fruits of staying in the methods and practices of this yoga include bliss, various paranormal superpowers, spiritual ascendance, and even transcendence of this mortal coil.

Modern psychology both entertains and disregards these ideas. Although approaches such as Jungian psychology tap into the concept of removing veils of illusion in order to see oneself more clearly in the self-reflective mirror of consciousness, much of clinical psychology aims to strengthen the ego and one's self-concept for living with mental clarity and emotional ease in this world.[2] Both can make life better and more whole while living in the realities of this world, and both yoga and tantra offer a variety of concepts that can be applied in working with a wide range of difficulties that arise from the conditions of one's mental and emotional health.

For example, asanas offer a rich symbolism for reflecting on the qualities of one's life experience. *Tadasana* (Mountain Pose) can serve as a mirror into how we embody grounding in our lives, and the relationship between the conditions of our grounding and how we create space in our lives. Warrior poses invite us to experience the intensity of staying with challenging circumstances without losing a sense of calm, and a focused, steady awareness. Seated forward bends, in which we fold into ourselves, open us to deeper and quieter self-reflection, including within the shadows that manifest as a part of normal life rhythms. Inversions turn our world upside down, offering a different perspective on being on the Earthly plane.

We also have a rich array of yoga *mudras*, gestures (such as bowing), that can signify letting go of things that are obstacles while opening to new possibilities. *Jnana mudra*, the popular hand/finger position with the tips of the thumbs and forefingers touching, can signify opening to a greater sense of wholeness or oneness while the three extended fingers represent letting go of the obstacles to that feeling in daily life. In all of this there is an infinite universe of visualizations one can explore, embodying in consciousness the visions or intentions one has about living a more free and liberated life, or *jivanmukti*. We are invited by the concept of *tapas* to stay with the practice, to persevere even amid the intensity of whatever is revealed, while opening to deeper contentment, *santosa*, no matter what else is happening.

All of this is experienced uniquely in the unique lives of those doing these practices. Each and every asana, breath, and instance of self-awareness is an opportunity to discover what one gravitates toward, resists, enjoys, or dislikes, with an opportunity for gaining deeper insight in discerning patterns of mental, emotional, and physical reaction. Going deeper yet, one can consider the general effects of asanas on energy, mood, and mental tendency, and then explore asana, pranayama, and meditation practices that can enhance one's sense of being more fully awake, in balance, and at ease in life.

Here we will focus on several of the most common mental and emotional health challenges, explaining what they are and how yoga practices can be done to cultivate better psychological health. These conditions are explained in the American Psychiatric Association's *Diagnostic and Statistical Manual of Mental Disorders,* Fifth Edition (DSM-V), which is a classification and diagnostic tool that is not without controversy.[3] Without losing awareness of the controversies, DSM-V provides the most updated and unified Western understanding of all known mental and emotional disorders, including the most advanced insights into the neuroscience of psychology. We can utilize it for better understanding how people with mental health issues are generally understood and treated by mental health professionals while recognizing that its very strengths—primarily its systematic review and presentation of the most advanced research—can also be its chief weakness as some conditions are distorted by scientific pretention, professional bias, or financial interest.

Cultivating Emotional and Mental Health

We live in a world in which stress and anxiety are increasingly commonplace. According to the 2009 Stress in America Study by the American Psychological Association 42 percent of American adults reported an increase in stress over the previous year, with a total of 75 percent of adults experiencing moderate to high stress levels.[4] (Of course this statistic is very likely higher given that it is for the year of the greatest economic crash in over seventy-five years.) The top three stress responses are trouble sleeping (47 percent), irritability or anger (45 percent), and fatigue (43 percent). Even kids—twenty-four percent of teens and fourteen percent of younger children—are reporting stress, with forty-five percent of kids overall reporting trouble sleeping and thirty-six percent reporting stress-related headaches. And while the proximate causes are not surprising—money, work, family responsibilities, relationship issues, and personal health concerns top the adult list—the means of managing it are disturbingly stressful themselves, even if not entirely surprising: thirty-five percent surf the internet, twenty-six percent eat, and thirteen percent smoke tobacco to reduce stress. Many of these and other short-term solutions are ultimately sources of further stress and anxiety.

Not surprisingly, the pharmaceutical industry sees and exploits a market opportunity in this (or, put differently, humanely responds to human crises by offering ostensibly stabilizing medications), selling over $10 billion in antipsychotic and antidepressant prescription drugs to Americans in 2010 alone, nearly twice the amount of money spent by nearly twenty million Americans on yoga in the same year.[5] Although prescription drugs are vitally necessary for some people experiencing symptoms of emotional or mental imbalance, many others might find a more wholesome and sustainable solution through such bodymind awareness practices as are offered by yoga. Indeed, the American Psychological Association study finds that seven percent of Americans do turn to yoga to reduce stress. The question is this: Are they getting a stress-reducing yoga practice?

Before addressing this question, it is important to consider the other side of the emotional and mental health coin: depression. Although anxiety and depression are often closely associated, many people are depressed or "feeling down" yet not anxious (or vice versa). Meanwhile, it is important to note that feeling sad or down, usually thought of negatively, can be subtly beneficial in helping a person cope with certain circumstances. The perceived sadness attracts social support, can help calm a person suffering from other ailments, and can have a "sadder but wiser" effect as the person comes to see the world more realistically.[6] Yet surely with chronic depression we want to find a healthy way to cultivate steadier emotions and a deeper sense of contentment in life.

In the traditional yogic perspective, the tendencies toward anxiety and depression are symptomatic of an underlying energetic imbalance reflecting either a rajasic or tamasic state: *rajasic* when restless or anxious, *tamasic* when lethargic or depressed. Each of these conditions can be given a very general yogic prescription.

- If rajasic, we can offer students and clients the following:
  - A slower asana practice that includes long holds in forward bends
  - A long Savasana (Corpse Pose)
  - Calming forms of pranayama such as *nadi shodhana* (simply breathing consciously is calming)
  - Meditation practices in which the eyes are closed and students explore the slowing rhythms of thought
- If tamasic, we can offer students and clients the following:
  - A more vigorous, flowing style of asanas that includes a sustained series of stimulating backbends, arm balances, and twists
  - Invigorating forms of pranayama such as kapalabhati and bastrika
  - Guided meditation practices in which the eyes remain open with clear *dristi* (focused gaze) and a quality of mindfulness oriented toward being fully awake.

In the following pages we explore several human ailments that are generally referred to as emotional, mental health, or behavioral conditions, all of which occur in a bodymind in which other health-related conditions can be significant in their manifestation and relative intensity. Even a sprained ankle, let alone a life-threatening disease, can trigger depression. We can further apply these very general yoga practice prescriptions with adaptations that make them appropriate for a variety of specific mental/emotional conditions, offering practices that tap into traditional yogic theory and practice while recognizing and applying modern insights and practices found beyond the yoga realm.

Alzheimer's Disease

As best we understand it, the cognitive functions of the mind occur in the brain, an organ not recognized as significant (most often not recognized at all) in the ancient yoga literature, this despite Patanjali's yogic maxim, *chitta vrtti nirodoha*, "to still the fluctuations of the mind," being a leitmotif of yoga. This preeminent mammalian organ can have conditions that are far more consequential in daily life than the "monkey mind"—which certainly arises mostly from within it—that yoga aims to tame, harness, or direct in conscious ways. Among the most common brain ailments is dementia, a group of symptoms that disrupt and disturb normal cognitive function and that are often mistakenly thought to be exclusively associated with aging. Yoga may have a significant role to play in reducing the incidence and reducing the symptoms of dementia and its most common form, Alzheimer's disease, known as such from the early twentieth-century work of German psychiatrist Alois Alzheimer.

Alzheimer's disease, a chronic and progressive neurological disorder involving cognitive and functional disability, causes most cases of dementia.[7] Part of the insidious nature of Alzheimer's is its quiet yet gradual and persistent manifestation, which worsens over time.[8] The pathophysiological process of Alzheimer's begins to develop prior to experiencing the mild cognitive impairment that defines its earliest diagnosed stage. In its predementia (or preclinical) stage, symptoms include a generalized apathy, lack of attentiveness in basic daily activities, irritability, and weakened relational memory.[9] As this mild cognitive impairment increases, there are greater problems with memory, particularly regarding new experiences. In some there are difficulties with the memory, use of written and spoken language that inhibits basic communication, as well as with what were easy functions such as driving a car.[10] As the condition worsens, it may become difficult to remember even the closest friends and loved ones, there can be delusional expressions, and there can be physiological problems such as urinary incontinence. These conditions can worsen in its most advanced stage, even as there are passing moments of apparent recollection and recognition, although one is now completely dependent upon the care of others.

Its Painful Experience

There is as much written about the caregiver's experiences with another's Alzheimer's as there is about the subjective experience of this condition. There is a wide range of feelings described by those with Alzheimer's, including a growing sense of loss—loss of everything most meaningful in life, starting with a sense of losing connection with those held most dear in life, and with this a sense of isolation and loneliness. The worsening condition involves deep sadness, confusion, and anxiety, and with these emotions fear, paranoia, and anger.

The Known Causes

Although genetic factors appear significant in many cases of Alzheimer's, the causes remain largely mystifying, this despite billions of dollars of research into its etiology and pathophysiology. The most promising theories involve protein synthesis that affects neurotransmitters in ways that are described as "tangles" inside the brain, a pathology that appears to have genetic markers. There is presently research exploring many other factors, including vascular and metabolic conditions, diet, exercise, social relationships, and lifelong mental stimulation (i.e., new learning, which the promising fields of neuroplasticity and psychoneuroimmunology are presently exploring).

How It Heals

Steven Sabat provides an insightful prism for peering into the complexities of Alzheimer's subjective experience.[11] The profundity of his work is in highlighting that there can be beauty and value amid even the most disturbing human dysfunctions, an antidote to the stigmatizing judgments that can further beset one with Alzheimer's as well as his or her caregivers. Although medical science is progressing in its understanding of Alzheimer's disease in ways that may lead to treatments that slow its progression, yoga and other complementary healing modalities offer practices that can help prevent Alzheimer's and benefit the lives of those living with Alzheimer's today as well as their caregivers.[12]

Healing with Yoga

Several recent studies purport to show promise for yoga in healing for those with Alzheimer's and their caregivers. Unfortunately, most of the studies are poorly designed. One of the strongest studies gives evidence supporting the benefit of yoga for Alzheimer's caregivers.[13] For example, verbal nerve performance was found to have improved functional connectivity after twelve weeks of Kundalini yoga classes and Memory Enhancement Training (MET) in a study conducted at the UCLA Longevity Center.[14] Whether certain elements of the yoga classes (tuning in, warming up, pranayama, kriya, and meditation) or only their combination had specific efficacy, and the efficacy of these techniques separate from or in conjunction with the MET training, was not studied. The study also had a very small sample size (fourteen). A more promising and better designed study of The Sit "N" Fit Chair Yoga Program has shown efficacy in improving function across several physical measures among older adults, including gait and balance.[15] The primary limitation of this study is its very small sample size and absence of a control group.

Attention Deficit Hyperactivity Disorder (ADHD)

Living in a fast-paced world filled with attractive stimuli can make it difficult to focus. Add a tendency to be extremely active and impulsive and one has the three leading symptoms of Attention Deficit Hyperactivity Disorder (ADHD): inattentiveness, hyperactivity, and impulsivity. Although all such tendencies occur across a continuum of significance and can be sources of tremendous creativity and productivity, they can equally well cause personal and interpersonal problems. We now find that around eleven percent of children in the U.S. (plus four percent of adults) are diagnosed with ADHD, a proportion that is increasing by fifteen to twenty percent per year, with males being three times as likely as females to have this diagnosis. It is also critically important to appreciate how ADHD is among many conditions in which social construction can confuse a variety of natural human tendencies with an illness, leading certain behaviors to be stigmatized in ways that cause or complicate matters.[16]

ADHD typically begins in childhood—it is classified as a neurodevelopmental disorder of children and adolescents—and can extend well into adulthood. In many cases, ADHD is benign, with symptoms of impulsiveness, hyperactivity, and/or weak attention close to typical for one's age. ADHD reaches a problematic level when these tendencies cause significant functional impairment in school, work, and other activities.

The Painful Experience

ADHD negatively impacts classroom learning and can lead to problematic social relationships. With difficulty in paying attention, it is very difficult to learn, which can lead to low self-esteem and difficulty in peer relationships. With hyperactivity and impulsivity, it is very difficult to be still and patient, which can lead to behavioral difficulties and a tendency to violate accepted norms of interaction in the classroom, workplace, or home. Behavioral difficulties in turn lead to more challenging social interaction, with less acceptance by others and feelings of shame, social anomie, alienation, self-doubt, and depression. Most children with ADHD are diagnosed with other disorders,[17] including learning disabilities, and disorders tied to mood, sleep, and substance abuse.

The Known Causes

As with most health conditions, internal and external variables are at play with ADHD.[18] We know that epidemiology is a factor.[19] We also know that environmental factors are increasingly significant, especially with the ubiquitous presence of televisions, computers, and handheld electronic devices.[20]

How It Heals

Prescriptions for healing or living more easily with ADHD vary depending on whether treating a child or adult, and depending on the known causes and the severity of symptoms. In many cases, particularly among adults, medication is the leading form of treatment, often in conjunction with behavioral therapies. Pharmacological interventions are also common with children and adolescents, and are generally made in conjunction with various forms of behavioral therapy (interpersonal counseling, family therapy, social skills training, support groups).[21] There is increasing evidence in support of physical exercise in reducing the symptoms of ADHD[22] as well as with modalities drawn from alternative and complementary medicine.

Healing with Yoga

Perhaps the cardinal benefit of yoga is how it helps us to be calm. It can also help us focus and control our natural impulses. Part of the potential efficacy of yoga in healing or managing ADHD is that it invites and even requires focused attention and slow movement in activities that can be exciting. Just as we might begin most yoga practices with ujjayi pranayama, the power of *ujjayi* (controlled breathing) for those with ADHD gives them a sense of being more in control of their thoughts and behaviors, which is at the heart of healing with ADHD. Here we recommend guiding clients in ujjayi, viloma, sama/visma vritti, and nadi shodhana pranayamas in each practice session, focusing on keeping awareness in the breath. This greater concentration on the breath can contribute to being more focused and in control amid other activities such as work, homework, and social activities.

Asana practices also contribute to self-control, especially those postures that cannot be done well without focusing. Balancing postures are perfect in this regard as without focused awareness one has great difficulty balancing. Offering a variety of standing balancing asanas—starting with Tadasana (Mountain Pose), Garudasana (Eagle Pose), Ardha Chandrasana (Half-Moon Pose)—can help keep the client interested and focused. If the client has healthy wrists and shoulders, offer arm balances, starting with Bakasana (Crane Pose) and Adho Mukha Svanasana (Handstand).

Although these practices get one more out of his or her head and into one's body, they also invite mindful presence to one's immediate experience, which can help to calm the mind and reduce impulsivity. Going further, one can explore with the meditation tools presented in Chapter 22 to cultivate a quieter mind and open to living more calmly.

Substance Abuse

There are very different ideas about what constitutes substance abuse. To some, any use of certain substances is considered self-abuse because the substance is considered inherently harmful. Some consider age, asserting that any use of certain substances is self-abuse among those below the age of legal use while viewing the same use among legal adults as simple use.[23] There are also very different ideas about which substances, or quantities of certain substances, are considered harmful.[24] Other factors include a person's condition or activities, with pregnancy, certain medical conditions, and certain skill requirements—such as driving a car or operating other machinery—elevating what might otherwise be considered acceptably moderate consumption levels to that of substance abuse or high-risk behavior.

These issues are reflected in the guidance provided by the U.S. Centers for Disease Control (CDC) regarding moderate drinking.[25] While emphasizing that alcohol consumption is associated with several health risks (car crashes, violence, risky sexual behavior, high blood pressure, and some cancers), the identified risks vary across distinct populations, including by age and medical condition. The CDC acknowledges that many studies show that moderate alcohol consumption can reduce the risk of heart disease, yet balances this by pointing out that there are contrary findings in other studies. The CDC also points out that excessive alcohol consumption is responsible for 88,000 deaths in the United States each year.

In the minds of some, substance abuse is any illicit drug use, with illicit largely defined in legal terms. Thus, the United Nations World Drug Report indicates that about five percent of people worldwide, or 230 million people, have used an illicit substance, including 27 million for whom there is recurrent use that causes health problems.[26] In addressing only illicit drugs, these data do not include the most commonly used drugs, some of which have the most severe health consequences, including tobacco and alcohol. It does include cannabis, which is increasingly found to have a wide array of potentially beneficial effects for those experiencing a variety of health conditions ranging from cancer and HIV/AIDS to insomnia and anxiety, even as it can also be associated with health problems.[27]

We are thus left with a far less than precise definition of what constitutes substance abuse. At the risk of overgeneralizing, we can usefully consider substance abuse as occurring when the patterned use of a substance causes harm to oneself or others, leaving aside the fact that many so-called foods, such as GMO corn starch or refined sugar, could fall into this definition. Even this rough definition is not without challenge, especially as the entire discussion is value-laden.[28]

The Painful Experience

A person abusing a substance versus someone observing the abusing person's actions typically perceives the behavior very differently. When under the influence of a substance, one's perception can be distorted to the point of not thinking that he or she is impaired, one can be impulsive, or one can put himself or herself or others at risk of harm. Even when under the influence, there is often denial of the possibly abusive behavior or its consequences. Many people who smoke tobacco deny its health consequences despite overwhelming evidence that tobacco is extremely toxic, and that smoking leads to pulmonary disorders and causes cancer.

Nonetheless, where patterns of intoxicating substance use reach the level of risking harm, we find several painful experiences: a variety of systemic health problems, problems in social interaction, a tendency to socially isolate, automobile crashes, risky sexual behaviors, suicidal ideation and suicide, child abuse, domestic violence, panic attacks, mood disorders, and the physical and psychological effects of chemical dependency and withdrawal.

The Known Causes

Use is widely considered the starting point of abuse. Although this might be true (almost tautologically so), most people who use intoxicating substances do not abuse them. Thus, use cannot be considered the cause of abuse, but only an associated factor that becomes precipitous or causal in conjunction with other factors. Although tobacco, alcohol, and other drug use typically begins in adolescence, the larger conditions of one's life experience—the interrelated effects of certain aspects of early childhood development, family dynamics such as a chaotic or emotionally abusive home, lack of healthy social relationships, lack of a healthy self-concept, poor school performance, unhealthy peer relationships, traumatic experiences— all come into play in the tendency to go from use to abuse. With many substances, repeated use causes changes in neurotransmitters that create dependence on the substance for pleasure. There are also genetic factors than can affect addictive tendencies.

How It Heals

Here healing has two meanings: stopping the use or abuse, and addressing the health impacts caused by abuse. Substance abuse can have serious health consequences, with the impact of excessive alcohol and other drugs on the brain and other organs being well documented. The first step in healing is to stop using the substance. Depending on the substance and the overall condition of the person, there are seemingly infinite methods offered for this behavioral change, including self-discipline, participation in a self-help recovery program such as Alcoholics Anonymous or Narcotics Anonymous, psychotherapy (particularly cognitive behavioral therapy and family therapy), and in-patient treatment that may involve medications (such as methadone in treating opiate addiction).

As the bodymind is a whole organism, one cannot fully address substance abuse without addressing the physical, mental, and emotional aspects of this disease. The physical health toll of substance abuse often involves serious impact on internal organs, especially the brain, liver, and heart. Healthy nutrition, which may require nutrition counseling and assistance, is an essential component of restoring healthy function to these organs and to one's overall physiology. So is exercise, with which yoga has much to offer. Most high-quality in-patient and residential substance abuse treatment programs also offer fully integrated mental health treatment services along with other services, including a twelve-step group process, nutrition, exercise, and planning for a healthy future. Mental health treatment services can involve individual and group counseling, medication, and support services such as case management. These services are increasingly provided within a recovery model in which there is high confidence—some would say hope—that the recovering individual can fully heal. Thus, along with addressing matters of home (having a safe and stable place to live) and health, one also addresses one's larger life purpose, including having meaningful daily activities and a healthy network of community support. Yoga practices can be part of these recovery strategies.

Healing with Yoga

Yoga is increasingly part of the mainstream of recovery services, even in relatively conservative institutions such as the U.S. Veterans Administration, where until recently, yoga was considered a purely alternative therapy but is more and more considered as an integral component in recovery services, particularly for those involving the comorbidities of substance abuse and PTSD.[29] Yoga asana practices give recovering individuals a healthy way of being in their bodymind with self-acceptance and self-affirmation, to feel the intensity of their physicality free of harmful substances, and to discover anew (or for the first time) a sense of wholeness and vitality free of substance abuse.

Yoga and recovery programs are now widely available, including in U.S. Veterans Administration centers as well as in venerable yoga institutions such as Kripalu Center for Yoga and Health, Esalen Institute, and *Yoga Journal* conferences. Just as those free of substance abuse issues find in yoga a means for living relatively free of stress amid stressful conditions, it provides those in recovery a way to more easily tolerate the impulses that can lead back to substance abuse.[30] Rather than a narrowly prescribed set of asana practices for all individuals in recovery, yoga for recovery should draw from the full palette of yoga to offer practices that resonate with the unique conditions of an individual student or client, considering particularly asana and pranayama practices that are indicated or contraindicated for other conditions and intentions of the individual. Self-affirming holistic visualizations can be integrated into these practices as active tools for further engendering the healing qualities that can help with recovery.

Depression and Anxiety

As human beings, we share a wide range of emotional states, including qualities of sadness, melancholia, and existential crises that are typically labeled as depression, and as such considered unhealthy, even when they are normal responses to life events. The same life events can also lead to a state of deep uneasiness and apprehension characteristic of anxiety, giving us the entwined condition of dysthymic disorder. The clinical diagnosis of depression considers the severity and persistence of specific symptoms such as sadness, overarching hopelessness or pessimism, irritability, loss of interest in what were once pleasant activities, suicidal ideation, or difficulty sleeping, eating, or working. The technical definition of depression given in DSM-V distinguishes persistent depressive disorder, a depressed mood that lasts at least two years, from perinatal depression (also known as postpartum melancholia), psychotic depression (involving some form of psychosis), and seasonal affective disorder (winter depression brought on by diminished sunlight). There is a vast array of conditions and experiences within each of these psychological categories. DSM-V also distinguishes between episodic and habitual depression that can come to form a core part of someone's sense of self. These conditions are often comorbid with anxiety, which can be a generalized anxiety disorder, panic disorder, or social anxiety disorder.

The Painful Experience

Although acute or chronic depression can be debilitating and lead to harmful behaviors, mild depression can be an effective coping strategy; a means of deep self-reflection that ultimately opens someone to a clearer and healthier sense of self, others, and one's life situation; and a call for help. When acute or chronic, depression is, well, depressing: the otherwise vital ways of living one's life give way to self-defeating and self-destructive behaviors. Social isolation, substance abuse, and neglect of self-care are typical effects.

With anxiety—also a normal part of life as we feel anxious in anticipation of something—our fear and apprehension can easily come to interfere with our normal life, detracting from our work, relationships, and sense of wholeness. Generalized anxiety disorder manifests as restlessness, mental and physical fatigue, irritability, obsessive worry, muscle tension, and sleep problems. Panic disorder involves sudden feelings of fear and being out of control, while social anxiety disorder involves fear of social situations, especially when there is a sense of being judged.

The Known Causes

Depression can be caused by a wide array of conditions, starting with the conditions of one's life during childhood, particularly abandonment, physical abuse, and sexual abuse.[31] Many life events—some of which are less "events" than lifelong conditions—can trigger a depressive reaction: illness; major life changes; the experience of living in a racist, sexist, ageist, or otherwise discriminatory society; financial difficulty; violence; loss; social isolation; and difficult social relationships.[32] Drug abuse—even simple use of some substances and certainly the use of a wide array of FDA-approved medications—can cause or exacerbate mood disorders. There are also physiological factors that can create chemical imbalances in the brain that cause emotional depression. These same variables often lead to anxiety, particularly among those who are generally shy, feel weak, or are exposed to stressful life events.

How It Heals

Most depression passes with time, especially when one is capable of trying to be active, to share time with and confide in others, and to avoid known triggers. When depression is persistent or is experienced with other conditions such as acute anxiety or substance abuse, this may indicate the value of treatment. The most usual treatments for depression and anxiety are some form of psychotherapy, particularly cognitive behavioral therapy, and antidepressant medication, sometimes in combination.[33] In cases of severe chronic depression in which medications are not effective, electroconvulsive therapy is often recommended.

Seemingly every form of alterative and complementary therapy offers something for healing depression and anxiety.[34] Mindfulness-based meditation as a tool in cognitive therapy has gained significant traction as an effective method for reducing depression (and anxiety) across a wide spectrum of settings. Now, thirty-five years since Jon Kabat-Zinn's pioneering work, we have significant evidence of its efficacy.[35] We also find increasing evidence for the efficacy of other Buddhist-based meditation practices, including vipassana, in healing depression and anxiety.[36]

Healing with Yoga

As noted at the beginning of this chapter, many ancient to modern yoga theories and practices focus on mental health, including the *Yoga Sutra* by Patanjali, which sets out the basic purpose of yoga as *chitta vrtti nirodha*, "to calm the fluctuations of the mind." In the late twentieth century and to the present we find numerous elaborations and refinements of this idea,[37] and very recently evidence of efficacy from well-designed studies, each of which offer insight into specific yoga practices for healing depression and anxiety.[38]

The heart of yoga therapy for healing depression and anxiety rests in opening to self-acceptance while walking a path of life-changing practices. The embodiment practices of asana can help bring us into the present moment, thereby reducing the tendency to dwell on earlier life events or to obsess about something that has not yet happened. As discussed earlier regarding somatics and consciousness, yoga asana can be a tool for re-experiencing the bodymind in affirmative ways, rooting out embodied negative emotions while rendering a more peaceful and joyful bodymind. The basic idea here is that each moment in any asana is experienced as though we are opening so many different windows onto our tendencies in life, which allows us to see ourselves more clearly through the various thoughts and feelings that arise in reaction to an asana in that immediate moment.

When we add breathing practices, starting with basic ujjayi amidasana, we can play with the ways in which qualities of breathing affect qualities of self-awareness. While taking in breath, we tend to sense more expansive awareness, a greater and lighter space inside in which there is great potential for deeper personal insight. As we release the breath, we tend to settle, calm, and quiet down inside, especially in the natural pause that occurs when empty of breath. Staying in the simple meditation practice of breath-as-mantra can gradually allow us to let go of self-limiting and self-destructive patterns of mental and emotional reaction to life events, even as we might still find ourselves exposed to the very triggers that otherwise cause anxious or depressive episodes. Thus, it is in the blended practices of asana, pranayama, and meditation that we most come to the healing effects of yoga for depression and anxiety. You can refer to my book, *Yoga Sequencing: Designing Transformative Yoga Classes*, for specific practices designed to help with depression and anxiety.[39]

Insomnia

Insomnia—sleeplessness—is a common sleep disorder that includes difficulty falling asleep, difficulty sleeping soundly, or both. These conditions are more technically described as sleep onset insomnia (SOI) and sleep maintenance insomnia (SMI).[40] In addition to these types of insomnia, DSM-V adds early morning awakening with the inability to fall back to sleep, along with disturbance of normal daily activities, and difficulty sleeping at least three nights per week for a duration of three or more months to the broader definition. Short of the DSM-V criteria, we find many people with transient insomnia, which contrasts with the acute and chronic conditions that lead to severe sleep deprivation and a host of problems in daily functioning but is nonetheless disturbing. We also find misperception of sleep patterns in which someone thinks they have insomnia despite having nether SOI or SMI.[41]

The Painful Experience

Insomnia causes stress both in attempting to sleep and as due to sleep deprivation, which leads to daytime fatigue, clumsiness, irritability, and weakened cognitive function.[42] It also exacerbates various comorbid conditions, particularly depression and anxiety,[43] and can cause many other health problems, including heightened stress hormone levels, diabetes, muscle ache, headache, tremors, and memory lapses.[44]

The Known Causes

As with many health conditions, insomnia can be both cause and effect of other conditions. There is strong evidence of the comorbidity of insomnia and other health conditions and behaviors, ranging from depression to diabetes to wound healing.[45] Drug consumption (including alcohol and caffeine), hormonal shifts, pain, heart disease, arthritis, unbalanced exercise regimens, and a variety of mental health disorders, including PTSD, ADHD, bipolar disorder, and depression and generalized anxiety disorder are all associated with insomnia.

There are two main contending theories of insomnia: cognitive, in which rumination and hyperarousal are at play, and physiological, in which urinary cortisol levels, glucose utilization, and/or metabolic factors are at play.[46] Hormonal factors also appear to be significant, with postmenopausal women experiencing significantly greater insomnia than men.[47]

How It Heals

Although never studied scientifically, considerable anecdotal evidence points to reading my printed books (not eBooks) as among the effective antidotes to insomnia.

Sedatives are commonly prescribed in most cases of clinical insomnia, this despite medications being a secondary treatment.[48] Melatonin, antihistamines, antidepressants, and antipsychotics are commonly prescribed, as are herbs such as valerian root, cannabis, and passion flower. The primary medical treatment involves sleep hygiene, which includes a regular sleep schedule, nonstimulating presleep activity, moderate exercise well prior to attempting sleep, avoiding stimulants, and creating a conducive sleep environment (quiet, dark, and comfortable). Research shows that cognitive behavioral therapy is equally effective as medications in short-term treatment, even as they are often given in combination.[49]

Healing with Yoga

There is considerable evidence that yoga helps with sleep, including among those with other far more serious health conditions.[50] As with many other health conditions, the benefits of yoga derive from a well-rounded and consistent practice. Asana practices that are highly stimulating—flow styles, multiple linked standing postures, backbends, intense abdominal core movements, and arm balances—are ideally done in the early part of the day. Seated and supine forward bends and hip openers are calming, especially when held for at least several minutes with minimal or no effort. Propped forms of Paschimottanasana (Seated Forward Bend Pose), Viparita Karani (Active Reversal Pose), Supta Baddha Konasana (Reclined Bound Angle Pose), and Savasana (Corpse Pose) are all deeply calming. Nadi shodhana pranayama is also calming. The counting method of meditation described in Chapter 22 is among the most calming meditation techniques.

25

Practices for a Healthy Reproductive System

THE CONDITIONS OF MEN AND WOMEN change considerably across the broad span of their lives. Most of the changes are similar when considering the broad scope of human physical, emotional, and mental development from early childhood to the latest moments of life. Yet along the way there are several factors that bring us to give the conditions of women in yoga special consideration in crafting yoga sequences. Although there is no question that the onset of puberty is very significant in boys, the changes in boys pale in comparison with the hormonal and larger physical and physiological changes experienced by girls with menarche (the onset of menstruation) and the cyclical recurrence of menstruation until menopause. Although sharing in the experience of pregnancy and childbirth can be very significant to men, this experience pales even more in contrast to the experience of being pregnant, giving birth, breast-feeding, and healing in the postpartum period. And although men often have a variety of emotional and physical challenges in midlife, the hormonal changes that occur with menopause can greatly amplify the sense of dramatic change that signifies moving into a new phase of life.

Until the late twentieth century most writings on yoga practice did not differentiate between men and women primarily because yoga was largely the province of men (and mostly men of the upper castes in India's hierarchical social system). Indeed, across the broad span of yoga history, women were largely excluded from yoga, reflecting the "oppressive social and cultural context out of which the yoga tradition arose" in India, particularly during the Brahmanic period in which women, as Janice Gates reminds us, were defined as "impure" and thus pronounced by male yoga gurus as being ill-fit for the spiritually enlightening practices of yoga.[1] It is only much later that, with the development of yoga in the West, we begin to find specific guidance that addresses the special needs and conditions of women in yoga, albeit still often adhering to age-old patriarchal and sexist assumptions about women.

Even when not sexist, we find that many of the yoga practice prescriptions for women—often given by women—are based less on science than anecdotal assumption, superstition, or unfounded supposition that is repeatedly passed from teacher to student. For example, in the leading book on yoga for women, *Yoga: A Gem for Women,* Geeta Iyengar reiterates her father's admonition against doing yoga during menstruation, as follows: "During the monthly period (48–72 hours) complete rest is advisable. Asanas should not be practiced. Normal practice may be resumed from the fourth or fifth day."[2] She goes on to say that a few forward bends may be done during menstruation to reduce tension. More recently, in *The Women's Book of Yoga: Asana and Pranayama for All Phases of the Menstrual Cycle*, Bobby Clennell allows certain practices during the menstrual cycle while following the teachings on B. K. S. Iyengar, Geeta Iyengar, and other leading teachers in making this questionable assertion regarding the relationship between inversion and menstruation:

> *If the body is turned upside down, this process [of menstrual discharge] is disturbed and may force the menstrual flow back up into the menstrual cavity and up through the fallopian tubes, causing the uterus to perform an adapted function instead of its normal function.... Since the menstrual process is one of discharge, it is a commonsense precaution to avoid these poses. Do not practice any inversions until the menstrual flow has completely stopped.*[3]

This is now a "commonsense" notion in the yoga community if only because it has been repeated *mutatis mutandis, ad nauseam* for the past two generations. Yet menstrual flow is no more affected by one's relationship to gravity than the passage of food or water through the body. Try swallowing a mouthful of water when in Adho Mukha Svanasana (Downward-Facing Dog Pose) or Sirsasana (Headstand); does the water stay in your mouth, flood your sinuses, or move through your throat and into your stomach? As the NASA Medical Division has confirmed through studies of women in microgravity environments, medical science in general has established that menstrual egress is caused by hormonally induced intrauterine and intravaginal pressure along with the peristaltic action of muscles, which are not measurably influenced by gravity.[4] This is also why four-legged females have no problem with healthy menstrual flow despite not having a vertical orientation to gravity, and why a menstruating woman will flow just as normally whether sleeping on her belly or back despite her uterus and vagina being turned in opposite relation to gravity.[5]

This question of inversion and menstruation is often presented not as a matter of gravity but of subtle energy, specifically *apana-vayu*, which is said to be the energetic force responsible for "downward" movement. Thus, it is asserted that being upside down disturbs apana-vayu's function in eliminatory processes, disturbing healthy menstrual flow and causing retrograde menstruation. Despite no evidence to support this idea, it is particularly curious because subtle energy suddenly is subject to the gross material energy of gravity. Note that urination, which can be done inverted, is also governed by apana-vayu (one might try this in a bathtub for personal anecdotal confirmation).

We use this as one example of misinformation becoming urban yoga myth and then parading as fact in informing yoga sequences for women and others. Whether, how, or to what degree this and other fallacies are rooted in patriarchal or sexist assumptions would make for an interesting study that is far beyond the scope and purpose of this book. Rather, for our purposes, it points to the value of always asking "Why?" or "Why not?" when told that something must not be done or must be done only in a certain way or at a certain time. Whether the various admonitions about women in yoga (indeed, about everyone in yoga) are valid deserves to be studied, discussed, and ultimately considered through one's personal yoga experience. It is with these sensibilities—evidence combined with personal and shared understandings and experiences—that women (and men) ideally make decisions for what to do or not do in their personal yoga practice throughout the larger cycle of life. In advising students on the question of menstruation and inversion, longtime yoga teacher Barbara Benagh says that since "no studies or research make a compelling argument to avoid inversions during menstruation, and since menstruation affects each woman differently and can vary from cycle to cycle, I am of the opinion that each woman is responsible for her own decision."[6]

Practices for Women's Reproductive System Health

I am not afraid. I was born to do this.

—JOAN OF ARC

Practicing Yoga During Menstruation

Just as each student comes to the practice in a unique way, women experience their menstrual cycle in different ways. For some women, menstruation is simple and easy, while for others it can be painful and distressing. As just discussed, most of the literature on yoga for women advises a modified practice emphasizing basic restorative poses, no inversions, or no practice at all. Yet many active yoga students have maintained their regular practice while menstruating—including doing inversions—across the span of decades with no signs of ill effects. This suggests that the best guide to practice when menstruating is each student's personal experience and intuition. The basic question to ask is, "How do I feel?" It is entirely possible that cramps, bloating, fatigue, or other discomfort will be present, indicating a relaxing practice that helps to reduce pressure in the uterus and abdomen, as described in the following sequence.

BASIC ASANA PRACTICE SEQUENCE FOR EASING MENSTRUAL DISCOMFORT

1. **Supta Baddha Konasana:** Prop the back and head onto a set of bolsters or folded blankets and allow the thighs and arms to release toward the floor. Stay in this position for five to ten minutes.

2. **Apanasana:** Gently draw the knees toward the chest and move them around in increasingly large circles for one to two minutes.

3. **Ananda Balasana:** Clasp the feet to draw the knees toward the floor, slightly and gently rocking from side to side for one minute.

4. **Supta Padangusthasana:** Extend one leg out to the side, resting it on a bolster. Stay in this position for one minute, switch sides, and then repeat.

5. **Supta Virasana:** Propped as for Supta Baddha Konasana, place a strap around the thighs to keep them from splaying out and to reduce pressure in the lower back. Stay in this position for two to five minutes.

6. **Bidalasana:** Hold for one minute, alternately extending the legs back to release tension through the knees.

7. **Adho Mukha Svanasana:** Hold for one minute before resting in Balasana for five breaths. Repeat two to four times.

8. **Setu Bandha Sarvangasana:** Keep the tailbone very slightly tucked to maintain ease in the lower back while focusing the backbend more up the spine and into the heart center. Repeat once or twice.

9. **Supta Parivartanasana:** Press the upper hip away from the shoulder while pressing the lower leg back to reduce pressure in the lower back and sacroiliac joints. Hold for one minute, switch sides, and repeat two times.

10. **Gomukhasana:** Hold for one to three minutes on each side.

11. **Upavista Konasana:** Hold for two to five minutes. Consider placing a stack of bolsters under the torso and head.

12. **Paschimottanasana:** Hold for one to three minutes. Consider placing a stack of bolsters under the torso and head.

13. **Viparita Karani:** Elevate the pelvis on bolsters, release the arms overhead onto the floor, and stay for five to ten minutes.

Practicing Yoga During and After Pregnancy

Which yoga asana sequences are beneficial or possibly risky during pregnancy and in the early postpartum period (and during extended periods of lactation)? Which asanas are indicated and contraindicated during each trimester? How do these prescriptions vary depending on the unique woman and specific conditions such as age, number of previous pregnancies, and other factors?

These and other questions pertaining to working with pregnant students did not appear in the yoga literature until the late twentieth century. Looking more broadly to the general question of exercise and pregnancy, we find very different views in the modern historical literature, starting with Alexander Hamilton's 1781 "Treatise on Midwifery," which encouraged moderate exercise avoiding "agitation of the body from violent or improper exercise, as jolting in a carriage[,] riding on horseback, dancing, and whatever disturbs the body or mind."[7] Nineteenth-century scientific examination of exercise and birth outcomes all have similar findings showing an association between robust activity and lower birth weight, leading to legislation in several countries (but not the United States) prohibiting employment of women in the weeks preceding and following delivery.

By the early twentieth century we find a growing list of arbitrary restrictions on activity, derived more from cultural and social biases than scientific study. A 1935 issue of *Modern Motherhood* says to "bathe, swim, golf, and dance, but no excessive walking, horseback riding, or tennis," while noting that some expectant mothers experience no ill effects from such activities. Yet also in the 1930s, British writer and maternal advocate Kathleen Vaughan advocated improving joint flexibility through squats to widen the pelvic outlet as well as Baddha Konasana–like positions and pelvic floor exercises to prevent tears of the perineum. Still, during the 1940s and 1950s, most of the literature suggested very moderate activity and no sports, giving way in the 1950s to Vaughan's criticism of the sedentary life of English women in *Exercises Before Childbirth,* which presents both physical and psychological benefits of regular group exercise during pregnancy.[8]

In the 1970s and early 1980s, we find the emphasis shifting to control over the body and a sense of well-being, but the advice typically ignores basic physiological changes such as aortal compression syndrome, laxity of joints and ligaments, exaggerated lumbar lordosis, and abdominal compression issues. We also start to find the unexamined assumption that some minor dietary error or failure to engage in some specific regimen of prenatal exercises could damage the unborn child or mother, motivating many pregnant women to quickly immerse themselves in exercise programs, often predisposing them (and their babies) to injury. In the past thirty years we have come to much greater insights into the relationship between exercise and pregnancy, including clear evidence that normal daily activities in no way compromise the mother or baby unless there's some significant pathological condition. The emergent conventional wisdom offers several suggestions regarding exercise during pregnancy: it should be regular, not intermittent, and not competitive; if vigorous, it should not be in intense heat or humidity or with high fever; ballistic and jarring movements as well as deep flexion and extension of joints should be avoided; and if starting from a sedentary lifestyle, begin with very simple exercises.

These insights come largely through the lens of a Western medical and scientific model, which still mostly assumes the separation of body and mind. Taken to the extreme, this perspective considers thoughts and feelings largely irrelevant to physical welfare, addressing physical anomalies and problems with purely physical therapy, drugs, or surgery. Yet we find considerable evidence that emotion is a highly significant factor in pregnancy and delivery; holding on to a secret fear or having commitment issues and other emotional complexes can have a direct effect on the physiology of the body.[9] An increasing number of hospitals and birthing centers recognize that discharging emotions eases the way in labor, and so they offer a more peaceful environment and even encourage conscious breathing and meditation practices to ease labor and delivery.

All pregnant students can benefit from bringing greater awareness and support to the structure, muscles, and organs of their pelvis. This ideally begins well before pregnancy with a more focused practice of mula bandha as a tool for toning and refining one's awareness of the lower pelvic muscles and organs. Mula bandha helps to develop a stronger and more flexible set of perineal muscles, more awareness of the lower pelvic organs and their surrounding support structure, greater ease in the delivery process, and a reduction in several physical risks that often naturally occur during pregnancy, labor, and delivery, including perineal tears (or reduced indication of episiotomy), urinary incontinence, and vaginal prolapse. Building on the basic mula bandha practice, women can develop more subtle awareness and control of all of the superficial muscles of the perineal floor and higher up into the layers of deep pelvic muscles that surround and give support to the bladder, vagina, and rectum, as well as the ability to differentiate and differentially engage or release muscles acting on the pelvis from above and below.[10] With this awareness, women can participate in their birthing process in a safer and more conscious fashion.

We can usefully divide pregnant students into two general categories: (1) those with sedentary lifestyles, poor physical health, or high-risk pregnancy, and (2) those with active lifestyles, good overall health, and minimal pregnancy risks. Women in the first category should be encouraged to attend yoga classes designed specifically for pregnant students, typically referred to as prenatal yoga. Women in the second category should be encouraged to explore practicing in regular yoga classes with teachers who are prepared to give them informed guidance on when and how to modify their practice. Women in the second category and already regularly practicing yoga should be encouraged to do a maintenance practice along with the modifications discussed that follow; pregnancy is not the time to begin a vigorous yoga practice, nor is it the time to attempt new or more complex asanas.[11] In the following pages we offer separate sequences for these two relatively distinct groups of pregnant women in each trimester of pregnancy.

Yoga Practices by Stage of Pregnancy

GENERAL GUIDELINES AND PRACTICES FOR THE FIRST TRIMESTER

- During the early period of pregnancy up to around the thirteenth week, pregnant students should take it easy as they adjust to changing hormones and energy during an often intense and delicate period of transformation. This is a time for getting more grounded, slowing down a bit, focusing more inside, and creating a favorable environment for the ovum to grow into a healthy fetus.

- Stay with ujjayi pranayama. Do not do kapalabhati pranayama or other breathing techniques that involve pumping action in the belly.

- Do not jolt the body by jumping into asanas (if the student has a well-developed floating practice, she might feel comfortable staying with it).

- Minimize twisting (to minimize pulling on the broad ligament that attaches to the uterus); when twisting, focus the movement in the upper thoracic spine.

- Do basic pelvic awareness exercises.

- The fetus is very small and the uterus well protected inside the pelvis, so students can lie on their belly (until they are "showing").

- Develop more pelvic awareness by doing Bridge Rolls (undulating the pelvis and spine slowly in and out of Setu Bandhasana [Supported Bridge Pose]), Supta Baddha Konasana (Reclined Bound Angle Pose), Swastikasana (The Auspicious Pose), Vajrasana (Thunderbolt Pose), Virasana (Hero Pose), Upavista Konasana (Wide-Angle Seated Forward Fold), Gomukhasana (Cow Face Pose), Ananda Balasana (Happy Baby Pose),and Eka Pada Rajakapotasana Prep (One-Legged King Pigeon Pose Prep). Become very familiar with Malasana (Garland Pose).

- Do a variety of shoulder strengtheners and openers (see the discussion on shoulders earlier in Chapter 23).

- Explore Utthita Trikonasana (Extended Triangle Pose), Virabhadrasana II (Warrior II Pose), and Utthita Parsvakonasana (Extended Side Angle Pose) as hip openers that stimulate circulation in the legs and contribute to strong feet and legs, creating a more stable foundation for the off-kilter weight distribution soon to come.

- While still in the first trimester, begin to explore asanas and props that are used in the second and third trimesters.

Basic Asana Practice for the First Trimester of Pregnancy—New to Yoga

1. **Sukhasana:** One to two minutes. Welcome, set intention, begin guiding.
2. **Bidalasana:** Two minutes, moving through the spine and pelvis with Cat and Dog Tilts.
3. **Virasana:** Explore mula bandha.
4. **Bidalasana:** Five breaths.
5. **Adho Mukha Svanasana:** Ten breaths. Explain basic alignment and energetic actions.
6. **Classical Surya Namaskara:** Three times.
7. **Virabhadrasana II:** Five breaths on each side. Set up from Prasarita Padottanasana stance.
8. **Utthita Parsvakonasana:** Five breaths on each side.
9. **Utthita Trikonasana:** Five breaths on each side, then step to Tadasana.
10. **Malasana:** One to two minutes. Use props to make it accessible.
11. **Supta Padangusthasana:** Five breaths on each side.
12. **Apanasana:** Five breaths.
13. **Ananda Balasana:** Ten breaths.
14. **Setu Bandha Sarvangasana:** Five breaths. Repeat once or twice.
15. **Bharadvajrasana A:** Five breaths on each side; a 60 percent twist focused up the spine.
16. **Gomukhasana:** Five breaths on each side.
17. **Dandasana:** Five breaths.
18. **Upavista Konasana:** Two minutes.
19. **Baddha Konasana:** Two minutes.
20. **Paschimottanasana:** Two minutes.
21. **Viparita Karani:** Five minutes.
22. **Savasana:** Five to ten minutes.
23. **Sukhasana:** Meditation.

Asana Practice for the First Trimester of Pregnancy—Healthy and Experienced Yogini

1. **Sukhasana:** Three to five minutes. Welcome, set intention, begin guiding.

2. **Bidalasana:** Five rounds of Cat and Dog Tilts.

3. **Adho Mukha Svanasana:** Ten breaths.

4. **Classical Surya Namaskara:** Two times.

5. **Malasana:** Hold for one minute while repeatedly engaging and releasing mula bandha.

6. **Surya Namaskara A:** Two times.

7. **Malasana:** Hold for one minute while repeatedly engaging and releasing mula bandha.

8. **Surya Namaskara B:** Two times.

9. **Balasana:** Rest for one minute, then come to Tadasana.

10. **Vrksasana:** Ten breaths on each side.

11. **Virabhadrasana II:** Five breaths on each side. Set up from Prasarita stance.

12. **Utthita Parsvakonasana:** Five breaths on each side.

13. **Utthita Trikonasana:** Five breaths on each side.

14. **Ardha Chandrasana:** Five breaths on each side.

15. **Garudasana:** Five breaths on each side.

16. **Prasarita Padottanasana A:** Ten breaths.

17. **Prasarita Padottanasana C:** Ten breaths.

18. **Malasana:** Two minutes.

19. **Dandasana:** Five breaths.

20. **Setu Bandha Sarvangasana:** Five breaths. Repeat three or four times.

21. **Apanasana:** Ten breaths. Move the knees around in circles.

22. **Bharadvajrasana A:** Five breaths on each side.

23. **Gomukhasana:** Five breaths on each side.

24. **Upavista Konasana:** Ten breaths.

25. **Baddha Konasana:** Ten breaths.

26. **Dandasana:** Five breaths.

27. **Paschimottanasana:** Two minutes.

28. **Halasana (Plow Pose):** Five breaths.

29. **Salamba Sarvanghasana:** Two to three minutes.

30. **Karnapidasana:** Five breaths.

31. **Uttana Padasana (Extended Leg Pose):** Five breaths.

32. **Savasana:** Five to ten minutes.

33. **Sukhasana:** Five minutes of guided heart-to-belly meditation.

GENERAL GUIDELINES AND PRACTICES FOR THE SECOND TRIMESTER

- With the placenta fully functional, hormone levels balance out and the pregnancy is generally well established. This is the perfect time to focus on cultivating strength and stamina, to refine awareness of the pelvis and spine, and to build more internal support for the inevitable challenge to balance and ease that will happen as the baby grows. The size of the belly varies greatly in the second trimester; different women show at different points in time. As a woman's pregnancy starts to show, the pelvis no longer protects the uterus, so it is time to start adapting asanas accordingly. Toward the middle of the second trimester, students should tune in more to any sense of numbness while lying on their back as the increasing weight of the baby may place pressure on the vena cava, restricting the flow of blood back to the mother's heart.

- Avoid jarring movements, intense abdominal work such as Yogic Bicycles and Navasana (Boat Pose), and kapalabhati pranayama. It is important to avoid pressure on the abdomen and to develop a supple belly; female athletes with tight abdominal muscles are at highest risk of perineal tears and urinary incontinence arising from downward pressure.

- Use pelvic neutrality exercises in Tadasana (Mountain Pose)and Urdhva Hastasana (Upward Hands Pose) to cultivate alignment of the spine, and stay with the Bridge Roll practice.

- Practice Surya Namaskara (Sun Salutations) with the feet apart in Tadasana, step back to Phalakasana (Plank Pose), and use folded blankets to support the ribs and hips when lying prone in preparation for either Salabhasana (Locust Pose) or Urdhva Mukha Svanasana (Upward-Facing Dog Pose). Integrate squats into the salutations.

- Practice standing asanas to develop or maintain leg strength and to open the hips and pelvis (modify and use a wall or chair for support as needed): Vrksasana (Tree Pose), Garudasana (Eagle Pose), Anjaneyasana (Low Lunge Pose), Ashta Chandrasana (Crescent Pose), Virabhadrasana I and II (Warrior I and II Poses), Utthita

Trikonasana (Extended Triangle Pose), Parsvottanasana (Intense Extended Side Stretch Pose), and Utthita Parsvakonasana (Extended Side Angle Pose).

- Explore a variety of seated hip openers and forward folds: Baddha Konasana (Bound Angle Pose), Upavista Konasana (Wide-Angle Seated Forward Fold), Parivrtta Janu Sirsasana (Revolved Head-to-Knee Pose), Bharadvajrasana (Sage Bharadvaj's Pose), Eka Pada Rajakapotasana Prep (One-Legged King Pigeon Pose Prep), Gomukhasana (Cow Face Pose), Dandasana (Staff Pose), Paschimottanasana (Seated Forward Bend Pose), and with legs apart, Marichyasana A (Sage Marichi's Pose), and Janu Sirsasana (Head-to-Knee Forward Bend). Release pressure in the sacroiliac joint with the knees wide apart in Balasana (Child's Pose).

- For relaxation, explore Viparita Karani (Active Reversal Pose) with legs straight up the wall, apart, and with the feet together and knees apart; elevate the feet in Baddha Konasana; raise the hips and legs onto a long bolster in Savasana.

- From around the twenty-fifth week of pregnancy, become more aware of any numbness or tingling sensations when lying on your back as this may be an indication of the baby pressing down on the vena cava, the "vein of life" that returns blood to the heart from the lower extremities. Increasingly prop up your back, shoulders, and head when on your back, eventually you need to be propped to about forty-five degrees when close to term.

Asana Practice for the Second Trimester of Pregnancy—New to Yoga

1. **Sukhasana:** One to two minutes. Welcome, set intention, begin guiding.

2. **Parivrtta Sukhasana:** Hold each side for ten breaths, focusing on creating the twist from the midthoracic spine upward, keeping the belly soft and spacious.

3. **Bidalasana:** Five times of Cat and Dog movements.

4. **Virasana:** Hold for two minutes, alternately engaging and releasing mula bandha.

5. **Bidalasana:** Stretch one leg back at a time, pressing back through the heel to release tension in the knees.

6. **Adho Mukha Svanasana:** One minute.

7. **Classical Surya Namaskara:** Three times, pausing for several breaths in Tadasana between each time.

8. **Balasana:** One minute.

9. **Virabhadrasana II:** Set up from Prasarita stance and hold each side five to ten breaths.

10. **Utthita Parsvakonasana:** Five to ten breaths on each side.

11. **Utthita Trikonasana:** Five to ten breaths on each side. Practice at a wall for added support.

12. **Vrksasana:** Encourage use of a wall for added support. Hold each side for one minute.

13. **Prasarita Padottanasana C:** One minute.

14. **Malasana:** Two minutes.

15. **Salabhasana A:** Place props under the hips, legs, chest, and forehead to ensure the belly is free. Lift and release five times before holding for five breaths. Repeat three times.

16. **Setu Bandha Sarvangasana:** Keep the tailbone tucked to bring the arch up the spine and minimize pressure in the belly. Hold for five breaths and repeat once or twice.

17. **Ananda Balasana:** One minute, gently rocking side to side on the sacrum.

18. **Bharadvajrasana A:** Five to ten breaths on each side, focusing the twist in the upper thoracic area.

19. **Dandasana:** One minute, concentrating on rooting the sit bones to fully extend the legs and spine.

20. **Upavista Konasana:** Two minutes.

21. **Paschimottanasana:** Two minutes.

22. **Supta Baddha Konasana:** Do a deep heart-centered breathing practice for three to five minutes.

23. **Viparita Karani:** Five to ten minutes with a bolster under the sacrum. Alternate leg positions (basic form, wide apart, knees apart, with feet together).

24. **Sukhasana:** Five minutes of guided heart-to-belly meditation.

Asana Practice for the Second Trimester of Pregnancy—Healthy and Experienced Yogini

1. **Sukhasan:** Three to five minutes. Welcome, set intention, begin guiding.

2. **Bidalasana:** Five times of Cat and Dog stretches.

3. **Classical Surya Namaskara:** Two times.

4. **Malasana:** Hold one minute while repeatedly engaging and releasing mula bandha.

5. **Surya Namaskara B:** Three times.

6. **Malasana:** Two minutes while repeatedly engaging and releasing mula bandha.

7. **Vrksasana:** One minute on each side.

8. **Virabhadrasana II:** Five to ten breaths on each side. Set up from Prasarita stance.

9. **Utthita Parsvakonasana:** Five to ten breaths on each side.

10. **Utthita Trikonasana:** Five to ten breaths on each side.

11. **Ardha Chandrasana:** Five breaths on each side. Practice next to a wall if uncertain of balance.

12. **Garudasana:** One minute on each side.

13. **Prasarita Padottanasana A:** Five breaths.

14. **Prasarita Padottanasana C:** Five breaths.

15. **Malasana:** One minute while repeatedly engaging and releasing mula bandha.

16. **Uttanasana:** Five breaths. Step back to Adho Mukha Svanasana.

17. **Adho Mukha Svanasana:** One minute.

18. **Balasana:** One minute.

19. **Salabhasana A:** Place props under the hips, legs, chest, and forehead to ensure the belly is free. Lift and release five times before holding for five breaths. Repeat three times.

20. **Ustrasana:** Five to ten breaths. Repeat once or twice.

21. **Balasana:** Five to ten breaths.

22. **Supta Parivartanasana:** One minute on each side.

23. **Ananda Balasana:** One minute.

24. **Dandasana:** One minute, cultivating mula bandha.

25. **Upavista Konasana:** One to two minutes.

26. **Baddha Konasana:** One to two minutes.

27. **Parivrtta Janu Sirsasana:** Five to ten breaths on each side.

28. **Paschimottanasana:** Hold for one minute, separating the legs wider to accommodate the belly.

29. **Balasana:** Five breaths.

30. **Halasana:** Five breaths.

31. **Salamba Sarvangasana:** Two to three minutes. Explore leg variations.

32. **Karnapidasana:** Five breaths.

33. **Uttana Padasana Prep:** Five breaths.

34. **Savasana:** Five to ten minutes.

35. **Sukhasana:** Five minutes of guided heart-to-belly meditation.

GENERAL GUIDELINES AND PRACTICES FOR THE THIRD TRIMESTER

This is the time to refocus on cultivating energy, especially by resting amid the flow of asanas to allow the body to integrate the practice more fully. It is increasingly important to limit time lying supine as the weight of the baby puts greater pressure on the vena cava. Relaxin hormone levels are now sufficiently high to cause the softening of ligaments throughout the body (not just in the pelvis), potentially causing fallen arches (as the calcaneonavicular ligaments stretch), weakness in the knees, and instability in the sacroiliac and other joints throughout the body.

- Continue working on postural alignment to give support to the spine.

- Become increasingly familiar with using a chair to support a variety of standing and sitting asanas (including Virabhadrasana and Malasana).

- Become increasingly aware of any numbness or tingling sensations when lying on your back as this may be an indication of excessive pressure on the vena cava.

- After the thirty-fourth week, be aware that Adho Mukha Svanasana and other inversions can cause (or reverse!) breech presentation.

- Begin doing birthing visualizations in squatting and other abducted hip-opening positions.

- Explore using a high bolster for long holds in Supta Baddha Konasana.

- Increasingly rest in Savasana, lying on the side of the body with props between the knees, under the head, and under the upper arm for easy comfort and relaxation.

Asana Practice for the Third Trimester of Pregnancy—New to Yoga

1. **Supta Baddha Konasana:** Five to ten minutes. Prop the back at a forty-five-degree angle, and give ample support to the head and arms.

2. **Upavista Konasana:** Five minutes. Prop the chest and forehead.

3. **Marichyasana A Variation:** Two minutes on each side. Sit tall and use one hand to pull on the lifted knee, the other hand to pull on the opposite knee, and relieve pressure on the pubic symphysis.

4. **Parivrtta Janu Sirsasana:** Five to ten breaths on each side, then repeat.

5. **Bidalasana:** Ten times of Cat and Dog tilts, then rest in Balasana with the knees wide apart.

6. **Anahatasana:** Ten breaths.

7. **Malasana:** One to two minutes. Use a wall for added support.

8. **Tadasana:** Five breaths.

9. **Vrksasana:** One minute on each side, then repeat. Use a wall for added support.

10. **Virabhadrasana II:** One to two minutes. Place a chair under the sitting bone of the bent leg.

11. **Utthita Parsvakonasana:** Five to ten breaths on each side.

12. **Dandasana:** One minute.

13. **Paschimottanasana:** Two to three minutes.

14. **Uttana Padasana Prep:** One minute.

15. **Viparita Karani:** Five to ten minutes.

16. **Sukhasana:** Five minutes of guided heart-to-belly meditation.

Asana Practice for the Third Trimester of Pregnancy—Healthy and Experienced Yogini

1. **Supta Baddha Konasana:** Five to ten minutes. Prop the back at a forty-five-degree angle.

2. **Upavista Konasana:** Five minutes. Prop the chest and forehead.

3. **Marichyasana A Variation:** Two minutes on each side. Sit tall and use one arm to press out on the lifted knee, the other hand to pull on the opposite foot (use a strap to keep the spine extended).

4. **Parivrtta Janu Sirsasana:** Five to ten breaths on each side.

5. **Bidalasana:** Ten times of Cat and Dog tilts, then rest in Balasana.

6. **Anahatasana:** Ten breaths.

7. **Adho Mukha Svanasana:** One minute. *Discontinue this inverted asana starting at 33 weeks.*

8. **Uttanasana:** Two minutes.

9. **Malasana:** Two to three minutes. Use a wall for added support.

10. **Tadasana:** Five breaths.

11. **Vrksasana:** One minute on each side. Use a wall for added support.

12. **Virabhadrasana II:** Five to ten breaths on each side.

13. **Utthita Parsvakonasana:** Five to ten breaths on each side.

14. **Utthita Trikonasana:** Five to ten breaths on each side.

15. **Garudasana:** Two minutes on each side.

16. **Prasarita Padottanasana C:** One minute. Slowly roll up to standing to minimize light-headedness.

17. **Dandasana:** One minute.

18. **Upavista Konasana:** One to two minutes.

19. **Parivrtta Janu Sirsasana:** Two minutes on each side.

20. **Baddha Konasana:** Two minutes.

21. **Paschimottanasana:** Two to three minutes.

22. **Uttana Padasana Prep:** One minute.

23. **Viparita Karani Variation:** Five to ten minutes.

24. **Sukhasana:** Five minutes of guided heart-to-belly meditation.

Asana Practice for the Third Trimester of Pregnancy—During Labor

Standing Pelvic Rocking: Stand with the feet mat-width apart about two feet from a wall, extend the hands up the wall, and move the hips side to side in a circular motion to encourage labor and reduce discomfort.

Bidalasana: Sway the hips from side to side while arching the spine like a cat during contractions.

Anahatasana: Explore Anahatasana if the labor is moving fast and too intensely.

Balasana: Modify by positioning the knees wide apart, keeping the torso relatively upright, placing the hands on the floor, and leaning slightly forward.

Malasana: Sit on a bolster and recline slightly back against an exercise ball. Have a partner sitting behind to lift the shoulders and help relieve pressure in the pelvis.

Parivrtta Janu Sirsasana: Keeping the bent knee lifted, press it outward while pulling on the opposite foot or leg to reduce pressure in the pubic symphysis.

Anjaneyasana: With a wide lateral yet short stance, shift the hips forward and back, first on one side and then the other to reduce pressure at the pubic symphysis.

GENERAL GUIDELINES AND PRACTICES FOR POSTPARTUM REINTEGRATION

It is important for new mothers to slowly increase energy, redevelop muscle strength, and cultivate more endurance after giving birth. There should be no abdominal pressure from core work or kapalabhatipranayama for at least six weeks (longer if there was an episiotomy or perineal tear, allowing complete healing before starting pelvic floor exercises); gradually move back into toning the abdominal core. There are heightened levels of relaxin hormone until around two months postpartum or post-lactation if breastfeeding, so encourage students to stay with an 80 percent practice when doing deep stretches (especially forward folds and backbends).

Asana Practice for Postpartum Reintegration

1. **Anahatasana:** One minute, moving the joined knees in circles.

2. **Jathara Parivartanasana:** Keep the knees bent and move them slowly and slightly side to side to gently stretch and strengthen the abdominal muscles.

3. **Bidalasana:** Rotate the pelvis forward and back while undulating up along the spine for two to three minutes.

4. **Urdhva Mukha Pasasana:** One to two minutes on each side.

5. **Balasana:** Five breaths.

6. **Anahatasana:** Breathe deeply while stretching the shoulders and chest.

7. **Salabhasana A:** Move in and out with the flow of the breath for five cycles of breath, then release and rest.

8. **Salabhasana C:** Five to ten breaths.

9. **Adho Mukha Svanasana:** Five breaths, then rest in Balasana.

10. **Prasarita Padottanasana C:** One minute.

11. **Virabhadrasana II:** Five breaths on each side. Use a shorter than usual stance, and don't lunge so deeply.

12. **Utthita Parsvakonasana:** Five breaths. Keep a shorter than usual stance, and still don't lunge so deeply.

13. **Utthita Trikonasana:** Five breaths on each side, be sensitive to overstretching in the groins and lower pelvis.

14. **Tadasana:** Refocus on clear intention.

15. **Garudasana:** Five to ten breaths on each side.

16. **Surya Namaskara A:** Move slowly, step to Phalakasana, and consider using knees-chest-chin to the floor and Salabhasana A rather than Urdhva Mukha Svanasana. Hold Adho Mukha Svanasana for five breaths.

17. **Balasana:** One minute.

18. **Gomukhasana:** One to two minutes on each side.

19. **Apanasana:** Five breaths.

20. **Pelvic Tilts:** Ten times.

21. **Yogic Bicycles:** One minute.

22. **Dandasana:** Five breaths.

23. **Paschimottanasana:** Two minutes.

24. **Viparita Dandasana:** Five minutes.

25. **Savasana:** Five minutes.

26. **Sukhasana:** Heart-centered calming meditation.

Yoga Practices for Menopausal Comfort

Just as menarche and pregnancy signal potentially profound life changes, the transition to menopause is a powerful cause for pause and reflection in a woman's life. Contrary to popular misconception, menopause is not a disease but rather a natural transition that every fertile woman experiences in her life cycle, normally between the ages of forty-five and fifty-five, with symptoms lasting for five or more years after her last period.[12] The ovaries are gradually reducing their production of estrogen and progesterone, which causes changes in a woman's entire reproductive system. The vagina gradually shortens, its walls become thinner and less elastic, lubricating secretions become watery, and the labia atrophy. Menstruation becomes irregular for a period of up to three years before ending completely.

Along the way, common symptoms include hot flashes, night sweats, insomnia, flushed skin, an irregular heartbeat, mood swings, headaches, forgetfulness, diminished libido, urinary incontinence, and aches and pains in the joints. Many women describe feeling misunderstood or unappreciated by their partner, children, and friends, exacerbating feelings of loneliness, anxiety, depression, and other emotional and mental imbalances. Many women with severe symptoms turn to hormone therapy, which is contraindicated for some women, while many others take other prescription drugs to alleviate specific symptoms such as depression and hot flashes. One of the long-term effects of decreased estrogen levels may be bone loss and eventual osteopenia or osteoporosis, which can lead to several further health challenges.

The surest path to reducing or eliminating some of the symptoms of menopause is to maintain one's overall health, starting with not smoking, maintaining regular exercise, and maintaining a nutritious diet. There are also many alternative health practices such as acupuncture and yoga that have proven helpful in making the symptoms of menopause more tolerable. Here we focus on yoga asana sequences that can help maintain overall comfort and health by reducing the effects of hot flashes, osteoporosis, and emotional fluctuations.[13]

ASANA PRACTICE FOR SYMPTOMS OF HOT FLASHES

1. **Viparita Karani:** Place a bolster under the sacrum and stay in the pose five to ten minutes. Play with alternating leg position to reduce tension in the legs.

2. **Apanasana:** One minute.

3. **Ananda Balasana:** One minute, and then come onto all fours.

4. **Adho Mukha Svanasana:** One to two minutes. If too intense, do Anahatasana.

5. **Balasana:** One minute.

6. **Uttanasana:** Two minutes. *Note: Contraindicated if one has advanced osteoporosis.*

7. **Halasana:** Three to five minutes with the shoulders and back propped on blankets and the legs resting on a chair. *Note: Contraindicated if one has advanced osteoporosis.*

8. **Salamba Sarvangasana:** Three to five minutes.

9. **Karnapidasana:** Five to ten breaths. *Note: Contraindicated if one has advanced osteoporosis.*

10. **Uttana Padasana Prep:** Stay in the prep position with the legs on the floor.

11. **Viparita Karani:** Rest for five minutes with bolster and alternative positions as in the first pose in this sequence.

ASANA PRACTICE FOR BONE HEALTH—PREVENTING OSTEOPOROSIS

1. **Sukhasana:** Three to five minutes.

2. **Bidalasana:** Alternately extend the opposite arm and leg and hold for five breaths on each side. Alternatively, extend the lifted arm and leg out and back to center five times.

3. **Phalakasana:** Five to ten breaths.

4. **Balasana:** Five breaths.

5. **Adho Mukha Svanasana:** Ten breaths.

6. **Ardha Uttanasana:** Five breaths.

7. **Uttanasana:** Five breaths.

8. **Tadasana:** Ten breaths.

9. **Utkatasana:** Five breaths. Press to standing and repeat twice.

10. **Virabhadrasana II:** Five to ten breaths on each side. Set up from Prasarita stance.

11. **Utthita Parsvakonasana:** Five to ten breaths on each side.

12. **Utthita Trikonasana:** Five to ten breaths on each side.

13. **Prasarita Padottanasana A:** One minute, come up slowly, and step to Tadasana.

14. **Vrksasana:** Hold each side for one minute.

15. **Garudasana:** One minute on each side. Step back into Adho Mukha Svanasana.

16. **Adho Mukha Svanasana:** One to two minutes. Stronger students can come to a wall and explore Handstand for up to one minute, rest, and repeat.

17. **Phalakasana:** Five breaths, then release to the floor and rest.

18. **Salabhasana A:** Five breaths each for three times.

19. **Setu Bandha Sarvangasana:** Five breaths each repeated two to three times. Either rest in Apanasana, Supta Baddha Konasana, or do the following asana.

20. **Urdhva Dhanurasana:** Five breaths each repeated one to three times.

21. **Supta Parivartanasana:** Five breaths on each side.

22. **Supta Padangusthasana B:** Ten breaths on each side.

23. **Ananda Balasana:** Five breaths.

24. **Apanasana:** Five breaths.

25. **Dandasana:** Five breaths.

26. **Upavista Konasana:** Ten breaths.

27. **Baddha Konasana:** Ten breaths.

28. **Paschimottanasana:** Two minutes.

29. **Viparita Karani:** Five minutes.

30. **Savasana:** Five to ten minutes.

31. **Sukhasana:** Meditation.

ASANA PRACTICE FOR REDUCING MOOD SWINGS

easy 1. **Sukhasana:** Three to five minutes.

2. **Supta Baddha Konasana:** Five to ten minutes, propped comfortably.

cross legged 3. **Swastikasana:** Two to three minutes on each side.

Cat/cow 4. **Bidalasana:** Five times of Cat and Dog stretches.

Downdog 5. **Adho Mukha Svanasana:** One to two minutes.

childs 6. **Balasana:** Five to ten breaths.

Warrior II 7. **Virabhadrasana II:** Five to ten breaths on each side.

extended triangle
8. **Utthita Trikonasana:** Five to ten breaths on each side.
Revolved Wide Leg Standing Forward Fold
9. **Parivrtta Ardha Prasarita:** Five to ten breaths on each side.

10. **Malasana:** One minute, then come to Tadasana.
tree pose
11. **Vrksasana:** One minute on each side.
Sun Salutation A's
12. **Surya Namaskara A:** One minute, then lie prone.
locust
13. **Salabhasana A:** Three times for one, three, and then five breaths.
bow
14. **Dhanurasana:** Five to ten breaths; repeat two or three times.
child's
15. **Balasana:** Five to ten breaths.
Reclined Spinal Twist
16. **Supta Parivartanasana:** Five breaths on each side. Repeat twice.
staff
17. **Dandasana:** One minute.
Seated Forward Fold
18. **Paschimottanasana:** One to two minutes.
Plough Pose
19. **Halasana:** Five breaths, or do Viparita Karani until Savasana.
shoulderstand
20. **Salamba Sarvangasana:** Two to three minutes.
Ear Pressure Pose
21. **Karnapidasana:** Five breaths.
Fish
22. **Uttana Padasana:** Five breaths.

23. **Savasana:** Five to ten minutes.
easy
24. **Sukhasana:** Do nadi shodhana pranayama for five minutes, then settle into heart-centered meditation.

Infertility

There are different definitions of infertility, with most being applied only to women despite men having fertility issues. The epidemiological concept of infertility refers to the inability to conceive and/or carry a pregnancy to term. Although the underlying conditions are primarily biological (and related to the overall health of the reproductive and endocrine systems), psychological and environmental factors can be significant.[14] All factors combined give us approximately five percent infertility globally.[15] Sexually transmitted diseases, particularly chlamydia and gonorrhea, appear to be the leading cause, while diabetes, thyroid disorders, celiac disease, and certain environmental toxins are all known causes.[16]

The yoga therapy perspective on infertility starts with cultivating overall health through a well-balanced yoga practice and lifestyle choices, particularly eating nutritious food, sleeping well, and engaging in life-affirming activities. This general statement is made in the context of vast new insight into the pathophysiology of infertility that increasingly draws from genomic science and is increasingly pinpointing the variety of courses infertility can take, and with it a variety of new drug-based therapies.

Infertility is most often addressed as a matter for couples, even as many individuals pursue fertility independently. With both women and men, yoga can be beneficial, especially as medical assistance in fertilization can be exorbitantly expensive and is not covered in many health insurance plans.[17] One unfortunate irony in this is that fertility assessments and treatments often reveal other underlying health conditions, yet due to lack of resources, they are not discovered until symptomatic.[18]

Yoga asana practices for women's fertility focus on a holistic practice complemented by specific asanas that may increase circulation to and awareness of the reproductive organs. These asanas include Baddha Konasana (Bound Angle Pose), Supta Baddha Konasana (Reclined Bound Angle Pose), Malasana (Garland Pose), Ananda Balasana (Happy Baby Pose), Gomukasana (Cow-Face Pose), and externally-rotated hip standing asanas such as Virabhadrasana II (Warrior II Pose) that involve significant engagement and release of muscles bearing on the inferior pelvis. Each of these asanas can be practiced in ways that use mula bandha actions to bring greater stimulation and awareness to the muscles in the lower pelvis.[19] More general asana practice—a well-balanced practice that includes asanas from every asana family—can aid hormonal balance by enhancing the functioning of the endocrine system.

Male infertility is due primarily to low sperm count, which in turn is caused primarily by endocrine system dysfunctions that are often rooted in lifestyle choices.[20] As with women, the primary yoga practice is a general, well-balanced set of asanas that brings strength, flexibility, and vitality to the entire bodymind. Meditation and visualization practices can embody a sense of vitality and contribute to a more positive outlook on life, which in turn can reinforce healthy lifestyle choices that emphasize nutrition, rest, and balanced exercise.

Endometriosis

Endometriosis is a common gynecological disorder in which uterine lining tissue develops outside the uterus, primarily on the ovaries and fallopian tubes.[21] In rare cases, it can develop elsewhere in the body, most commonly in the abdominal wall but also in the lungs, pleura, kidneys, brain, and extremities.[22] With severe uterine endometriosis, women are at risk of ovarian tissue damage, which can lead to reduced ovarian reserve and, in about half of all cases, infertility. Endometriosis affects around ten percent of women, mostly in their thirties and forties, although it can affect prepubescent girls.

Endometriosis typically comes to one's awareness due to pelvic pain, although the condition can be relatively asymptomatic (around twenty-five percent of women with endometriosis are asymptomatic) and consequently may remain undetected. It is often associated with recurring or chronic pelvic pain and painful sexual intercourse, although in seventy-five percent of women there is related pain only when menstruating. There is no association between the extent of endometriosis and pain, with some women experiencing severe cramping or stabbing pain while others do not experience any pain. It can be associated with ovarian cancer.[23]

Although generally considered idiopathic, retrograde menstruation may explain many cases, leading medical researchers to point to genetic factors and environmental conditions in explaining its pathophysiology.[24] Along with being of unknown specific cause, there is no known cure for this condition. Treatment generally focuses on nonsurgical pain management, although surgery is used to alleviate pain by removing the endometriosis, or, in severe cases, by hysterectomy. Another strategy involves hormone treatments designed to block production of estrogen.

Nonsurgical pain management is approached in several ways, including with pain-killing NSAIDs (nonsteroidal anti-inflammatory drugs) that block the production of protaglandin, and pain-modifying medications that alter the perception of pain.[25] Some women find that a hot water bottle or hot bath helps to reduce pain and reduce related stress. Yoga-based practices and other forms of physical exercise can be utilized to help manage or reduce stress and anxiety, to strengthen and relax the pelvic floor, and, in postoperative care, to restrengthen compromised abdominal and low back muscles.[26] To explore pelvis floor exercises, see Blandine Calais-Germain's *The Female Pelvis*.[27] Refer to the low back exercises given in Chapter 23 for strengthening abdominal and low back muscles. Simple breathing exercises, particularly the basic form of nadi shodhana, can help in relaxing, especially when done in conjunction with visualization practices that focus on softening and relaxing.

Male Prostatitis

As discussed earlier, the male prostate gland tends to become inflamed in men after forty years of age, causing an often-painful condition that is the most common health complaint in older men. The gland wraps around the urethra just below the bladder. With prostatitis, the urethra is compressed. Most prostatitis (95%) is a benign prostatic hyperplasia, which inhibits urination while creating the need to urinate more often, hesitancy in starting urination, and a feeling of not completely evacuating the bladder. The gland inflames due to an increase in aromatase and 5-alpha reductase enzyme activity, leading to a decrease in testosterone and increase in estrogen, which is the major factor that causes growth in the prostate.

A physical rectal exam is the basic procedure for estimating the condition of the prostate. Rather than evaluating only for prostatis, this procedure is also used to identify lumps that could indicate the presence of prostate cancer. Blood tests and other forms of urological examination can differentiate conditions. The severity of prostatitis suggests the appropriate treatment, with severe conditions generally treated with alpha-blockers, reductase inhibitors, and even phosphodiesterase-5 inhibitors that are more commonly prescribed for erectile dysfunction.

Yoga postural practices that stimulate circulation in the lower pelvic region are commonly suggested as helping to reduce the incidence or severity of prostatitis. Without citing any evidence of efficacy, *Yoga Journal* recommends Paripurna Navasana (Full Boat Pose), Baddha Konasana (Bound Angle Pose), Supta Padangusthasana (Reclined Big Toe Pose), Salambha Sirsasana I (Supported Headstand I), and Salambha Sarvanghasana (Supported Shoulderstand),[28] curiously omitting mula bandha practices in which the muscles of the pelvic floor are directly engaged. The Wise-Anderson Protocol, also called the Stanford Protocol, utilizes simple asanas such as Baddha Konasana (Bound Angle Pose) in conjunction with paradoxical relaxation exercises that in yoga would be described as the repetitive engagement and release of mula bandha, which is found to help reduce pressure on the prostate gland.[29]

A significant factor affecting men's prostate health and other reproductive system issues involves the common reticence among men to seek medical or alternative treatments for health conditions they perceive as related to their sense of masculinity, the other side of which is treatment providers who are not sensitive to this sensitivity among many men.[30] Yoga can reduce this inhibition by helping men to cultivate self-acceptance for who they are.

Erectile Dysfunction

Erectile dysfunction (ED) is the inability to develop or maintain a sufficiently firm erection for successful sexual intercourse. It has a significant effect on men's quality of life and that of their partner(s).[31] Erection occurs as the effect of blood engorging the penis, usually as a result of sexual arousal arising from direct physical stimulation of the penis (reflex erection) and/or emotional or erotic stimulation (psychogenic erection).[32] Nicotine use is one of the leading causes of ED due to arterial restriction,[33] while diabetes, depression, heart disease, neurological disorders, the effects of prostate surgery, and kidney failure are additional causes (and, with depression, a mutual causality).[34]

Oral medications, in particular phosphodiesterase-5 inhibitors known by their brand names as Viagra, Cialis, and Levitra, are among the most widely used treatments for ED. All can have a variety of side effects, including headache, diarrhea, muscle cramps, sinus congestion, and redness in the face and neck. In extreme cases, surgical procedures are used, including prosthetic implants. In cases caused by inhibited psychogenic erection, psychological treatment is recommended.

There are no studies on yoga practices and ED, although there are common claims among yoga practitioners that doing yoga is associated with stronger or more sustained erections. The mental relaxation and emotional calming effects of some yoga practices might assist with psychogenic erection, while practices that bring more awareness to the pelvic floor and lower pelvic organs might help with both reflex and psychogenic erection.

Part VI

Epilogue: The Promising Future of Yoga Therapy

ALTHOUGH FUTURISTS BRING RICH COMPLEXITY to visions of what might be, with yoga therapy we attempt to stand simply yet stably on the shoulders of ancient-to-contemporary yoga to suggest and encourage realistic possibilities for practices that might serve us well as we move further along on this ecologically challenged planet spinning and wobbling through space and time with a vast array of challenges and opportunities for the conditions of our health. We join the ancient yogis, wrapped as we are in certain veils of illusion and mystification, even in the twenty-first century, while doing the best we can to understand the nature of life, our conditions, and how to make our lives better with the clearest and healthiest intentional actions, some of which are discovered intuitively, even as they might be informed by scientific discovery.

With whatever sources of insight we have, we make what might be fateful choices in attempting to cure or heal what ails us. We are potentially vital beings possessed of self-healing capacities that can be enhanced by practices that cultivate more radiant well-being or terribly compromised by disease and dysfunctional behavior. There may always be imbalance, various pathologies, and mysterious disorders, yet with deepening insights that accrue with open-minded exploration and systematic study, we are making great gains in global health.

There are healthy discussions and debates within the yoga community regarding the efficacy of yoga practices in treating ailments. The conversation covers the very definition of yoga therapy, the role of the yoga therapist, the standards of training and experience for competence in offering therapeutic yoga, the relationship between yoga therapy and other healing modalities, and the quality of studies that make claims about the benefits and contraindications of various yoga techniques for different conditions. The International Association of Yoga Therapists (IAYT) publishes peer-reviewed articles reporting the findings of increasingly well-designed studies of yoga's vast therapeutic applications and sponsors an annual conference that brings the yoga therapy community together to share knowledge and further develop yoga therapy as a model for healing. We also find more and more high-quality books that provide focused consideration of yoga for various ailments ranging from asthma and cancer to arthritis and substance abuse.

As discussed in Chapter 17, we are finding greater clarity in the very concept of yoga therapy and differentiation in the overlapping roles of the yoga teacher and yoga therapist. This bodes well for all concerned—yoga teachers and their students, yoga therapists and their clients. This clarity can only help in the further integration of yoga's therapeutic benefits in the larger health care system, especially because when we are listening to one another, we can further ensure less iatrogenesis among those whose intentions or methods are less than pure or properly informed, while we highlight and support those who do have pure intentions and methods.

As we continue rooting our practices in the root motivations of yoga—to reduce suffering, to live more awakened lives, to make life better—and remain open to new discoveries, yoga therapy will be more and more a source of healing and creating heaven on earth. This is our promise, one we can best fulfill one conscious breath at a time.

Notes

Introduction

1. *Yoga Journal* (2015).

2. See D. G. White (2012).

3. Although we generally think of yoga as a healing practice, there are also many students who are injured doing yoga or whose health conditions are made worse, not better, in doing certain yoga practices. See Broad (2012a, 2012b) for more information.

4. See Grad (2002, 982).

5. Both definitions honor the etymological root of the term *health*, from the Old English *health*, meaning "wholeness," and the earlier Proto-Germanic *hailitho*, from Proto-Indo-European *kailo*, meaning "whole." See Wiktionary (2017).

6. World Health Organization (2016).

7. Throughout this book I use the neologism *bodymind* in keeping with the view that the body and mind are not separate but rather a whole—and in my view (and that of many other nondualists) sensing this whole is at the heart of yoga practice and healing. This view stands in contrast to the dominant dualist views found in both Eastern and Western philosophy and forms a central theme of this book and the healing modalities explored here, which are primarily concerned with most easily cultivating the healthiest life.

8. From the earlier times of yoga to the present, from India to the entire world, the founders and purveyors of nearly every yoga method (or lineage or brand) have claimed that their way is the most true or beneficial, asserting some notion of *orthopraxy*—correct practice—that only they or their designated progeny of teachers can offer. We reject this arrogance.

9. IAYT (2012).

Part I

1. To explore, see Sjoman (1999), De Michelis (2004), Singleton (2010), and D. G. White (2000; 2012).

Chapter 1

1. Pervasive suffering as described in the *Bhagavad-Gita* is rooted in *maya*, "illusion," while for Patanjali the basic problem is *avidya*, "ignorance." Both sources consider liberation and clear consciousness as synonymous.

2. Merriam-Webster (2017).

3. In *The Yoga Tradition*, Feuerstein (2001) reveals plurality and diversity across the ages while positing a singular tradition.

4. To more deeply explore this point and what follows here, see D.G. White (2012).

5. See Monier Williams (1899).

6. Prabhavananda and Isherwood (1944).

7. David G. White (2012, 4). The other five branches of Indian philosophy are Yoga, Nyaya, Vaisheshika, Mimamsa, and Vedanta.

8. Vivekananda (1956). See David G. White (2014) on the historicity of the *Yoga Sutra* and how its many quite different interpretations and commentaries are rooted in the real lives of its translators and commentators.

9. Most readings and discussions of the *Yoga Sutra* ignore the last two of these chapters, perhaps because they test credulity in a modern age that wants evidence for paranormal claims.

10. David G. White (2012, 7).

11. The paradigmatic instance of such assertion is found in Choudhury (2000, 3).

12. A prime example is Frawley (1999, 3). Although stating that yoga has "maintained an unbroken line of development," on the next page he says nearly the opposite, noting that, "Yoga is a distillation of wisdom from the myriad sages across the ages … as adapted to the particular requirements of each age and each person." Which is it: unbroken or adapted? He is anything but alone: Burgin (2016), in *Yoga Basics'* "History of Yoga," mentions 5,000 and 10,000 years old.

13. Cushman (2007) gives us "5,000 years of innovation." See also Crangle (1994, 4–7) for as early as 3300 BCE, Zimmer (1951, 21) for prevedic, and Samuel (2008) on the Sramana movement.

14. These styles typically reject the label *style*, which suggests it is one of many, and instead use the turn of phrase *the practice*, implying that it's *the* practice.

15. Krishnamacharya and his main biographers (or hagiographers)—his son T.V.K. Desikachar, grandson Kausthab Desikachar, and student A.G. Mohan—variously give this and other explanations for Krishnamacharya's knowledge of yoga, adding the myth that he and Pattabhi Jois discovered the Ashtanga Vinyasa system in an ancient manuscript they found in the Calcutta Library (said to have since been eaten by ants) and the story that Krishnamacharya experienced seven years in Tibet where he learn the extant knowledge of yoga from the last remaining living source, one Sri Bramacharya. To learn more, see Sjoman (1999), Singleton (2010), and David G. White (2014), especially White's chapter on "The Strange Case of Tirimulai Krishnamacharya."

16. See Eliade (1969), Feuerstein (2001), Stephens (2010), and David G. White (2009; 2012).

17. The specious assertion that such a culturally significant practice somehow escaped the early writings and iconography is betrayed by the mention or portrayal of every other culturally significant practice. Why would yoga be unique in its exclusion?

18. Witzel (1997).

19. Michaels (2004).

20. Feuerstein (2001).

21. Our primary source for transliteration of the classical Upanishads is Roebuck (2000).

22. Aiyar (1914).

23. Malinar (2008, 207).

24. Vivekananda (1956).

25. Bouanchaud (1999).

26. Feuerstein (2001, 341).

27. David G. White (2000).

28. Tigunait (1999, 104–105).

29. Davidson (2003).

30. Feuerstein (2001, 343).

31. Odier (2004).

32. To explore the diverse worlds of tantra, see David G. White (1996; 2000; 2003; 2009).

33. Muktibodhananda (1985, 190–227).

34. Ibid., verse 17.

35. Iyengar (1985, 10).

36. Muktibodhananda (1985, verse 44).

37. Ibid., verse 150.

Chapter 2

1. For examples regarding both yoga and ayurveda, see Singh et al. (2002), Mackenzie and Rakel (2006, 215), Lad (1985, 3), and Frawley (1999, 3).

2. Zysk (1998).

3. Zimmer (1948, 2–3) and Wujastyk (2003, xxviii–xxix).

4. Frawley (1999, 5) appears to be the first to make this unsupported assertion and the source to which others later point for validating reference.

5. Wujastyk (2003, 260). To explore further, see Zysk (1998) and Chattopadhyaya (1979), noting that these sources predate the publication of many works making the spurious claims.

6. See Bolling (1962, 762–772), Zimmer (1948).

7. On sources, for the Caraka Samhitā we use P. V. Sharma (1992); for the Suśruta Samhitā we use P. V. Sharma (2001).

8. P. V. Sharma (1992, 185–190). This development is closely coincident with developments in Greek medicine in the fifth century BCE, in which Hippocrates exchanges divine notions of medicine for rational observation as the basis for medical knowledge, with prayers and sacrifices giving way to treatments based on keeping the body in balance.

9. Wujastyk (2012, 32).

10. Wujastyk (2003, 193–196 *passim*).

11. Vagbhata's (1999) *Ashtangasamgraha* covers much of the same material but due to textual issues has only recently become incorporated into ayurvedic curricula. For more on this, see Zysk (1991, 114–116).

12. With the *Bower Manuscript* we find evidence of ayurvedic knowledge and practice in sixth century CE western China that may predate Vagbhata's work. See Hoernle (1987) and Wujastyk (2012, 149–151).

13. Wujastyk (2003, 168).

14. This passage summarizes the ultimate expression of prakriti as the material force of the universe becomes manifest in the human being. See Chapter 3 for details on this process. Zimmer (1948, 164) discusses how in many traditions—from the Greeks' Homer to a Pueblo chief in discussion with Carl Jung (and we could add the Indians' *Surya*)—the heart is considered the seat of emotions and consciousness.

15. Wujastyk (2003, 272).

16. In both appreciating and assessing the efficacy of ayurveda, one might consider weighing certain measurable realities such as life expectancy. Although life expectancies in India and Europe are similar prior to the rise of Western scientific medicine (around thirty years of age in 1500), by 1900 life expectancy in Europe has risen to forty-nine while in India it is still around thirty.

17. More specific definitions of *kaivalya* include "isolation" (in the *Vamana Puranas*), "absolute unity" (in the *Bhagavata Puranas*), and "detachment of the soul from matter or further transmigrations" (in the *Mahabharata*) (Monier-Williams 1899, 311).

18. Chapter 4 of Patanjali's *Yoga Sutra* is titled "Kaivalya Pada." There is some evidence—specifically the form of Sanskrit in which it is written—that this may have been composed by a different author hundreds of years after Patanjali in an attempt to bring a different philosophical congruence to the larger work. See David G. White (2014) to further explore this question of philology in correct identification of authorship.

19. See Larson and Bhattacharya (2008, 32–51) for an introduction to Samkhya philosophy that attempts to clarify its historical development and key concepts, including the salient differences between and commonalities of Samkhya and Yoga philosophy.

20. Larson and Bhattacharya (2008, 89).

21. Other views of purusha such as those found in Advaita Vedanta assert that purusha is a singular, not plural, consciousness (Arvind Sharma 1997, 155–157).

22. Monier-Williams (1899, 1135).

23. Ibid., 863.

24. Ibid., 438.

25. Wujastyk (2003, 277–8).

26. Larson and Bhattacharya (2008, 80).

27. P. V. Sharma (1992, 59).

28. Mehta (2002, 313).

29. Wujastyk (2003, 274).

30. Lad (2001, 29).

31. Tiwari (1995, 5). Looking at original ancient source materials for further insight into the concept of dosha, the *Rigveda* uses the term to mean "darkness" and "night," whereas in the Upanishads and *Mahabharata* it means "fault," "vice," "deficiency," "want," and "disadvantage." In Susruta's *Compendium*, in which the term is applied to ayurveda, we find "alteration," "affection," "morbid element," and "disease," each applied to the three humors themselves (along with doshabheda, a particular disease of the three humors). See Monier-Williams (1899, 498) on etymology and use.

32. Wujastyk (2003, 74).

33. Ibid., 116–17.

34. Ibid., 206.

35. Ibid., 274.

36. As we discuss further in this chapter, nearly every source from the ancients to contemporaries gives somewhat (sometimes very) different delineations of the doshas and element manifestations of prakriti. For a discussion of the original sources, see Kutumbiah (1969), especially on the doctrine of Tridosha, and Svoboda (1988) and Svoboda and Lad (1995).

37. Lad (2001, 45).

38. Tiwari (1995, 7).

39. Pole (2013).

40. There are also five lesser vayus: *naga* (burping), *kurma* (blinking), *krekara* (coughing and sneezing), *devadatta* (yawning), and *dhanamjaya* (the air that bloats a corpse). The earliest discussion of prana-vayu is in the *Artharaveda*.

41. Lad (2001, 46, 48) and Remski (2012, 39).

42. In my own earlier writing (Stephens 2010, 52), I share in what I now think is the confusing suggestion that the vayus (or for that matter, the chakras) have certain clearly identifiable physical locations. Put differently, these associations are mysterious, metaphoric, and/or mistaken.

43. Lad (2001, 51).

44. Wujastyk (2003, 15).

45. Lad (2001, 15).

46. Tiwari (1995, 11) and Lad (2001, 56).

47. Wujastyk (2003, 273).

48. Lad (2001, 67).

49. Pole (2013, 20).

50. Tiwari (1995, 14). Lad (2001, 71) adds the spine.

51. See Kutumbiah (1969, 60–67).

52. Wujastyk (2003, 272)

53. Kutumbiah (1969, 70)

Chapter 3

1. Vitalism posits an imbalance in vital forces associated with the four humors as the cause of disease, akin to ayurveda's imbalance in the gunas.

2. Farmer (2003). The field of medical anthropology also offers insight into social inequality and health. To explore further, see Nichter (2008).

3. The *Edwin Smith Papyrus* is an Egyptian medical text from around 1600 BCE that offers the earliest known rational and scientific approach to medicine. See Ghalioungui (1965), James Allen (2005), and Nunn (1996).

4. The term *humor* is from the Greek *chymos*, meaning "juice." The four humors are closely related to the four elements of earth (black bile), fire (yellow bile), water (phlegm), and air (blood). Note the similarities with Samkhya's and ayurveda's categories of qualities.

5. On teleology in biology, see Beckner (1969), Brandon (1981), Mayr (1988), and Wimsatt (1972).

6. De Vos (2010, 28–47).

7. See Potter and Mattingly (2002, 63).

8. Majno (1975, 395).

9. Bynum (2008, 15).

10. See Hankinson (1991, 197–233) for a discussion of Galen's *On the Diagnosis and Cure of the Soul's Passion.*

11. Kohn (2008, 245).

12. Tuchman (1978, 116–125). Lucretius (2007), writing just before the dawn of the Common Era (around 50 BCE), lays bare many of the ill-founded assumptions underlying antiscientific thinking and mystification in his radical poem, *On the*

Nature of Things. Lost for fifteen hundred years, its discovery by the fifteenth-century papal emissary Poggio Bracciolini is considered a major factor sparking the Renaissance. See Greenblatt (2011).

13. Infusino et al. (1965), Olmi (2006), and Siraisi (1990).

14. See T. K. Stewart (1995, 389–397) and Ferrari (2015). India was by no means alone in its superstitious response to smallpox. In China, one pleased the goddess T'ou-Shen Niang-Niang, who was said to prey mostly on attractive children, thus the prescription of wearing a mask to appear ugly. Many in Europe believed in a smallpox demon that was afraid of the color red, which lead to victims being placed in rooms painted red. Such mystified reactions were found across all regions and cultures of the world. There is a vast array of sources on superstition and smallpox. A good starting place for further exploration is McNeill (1977).

15. As of this writing, we find a growing number of such studies, including several with results published in the *Journal of Yoga Therapy*.

16. See Good (1994) for a discussion of medical belief, experience, and practice across cultures.

Chapter 4

1. Max Roser (2017). Anecdotal claims of incredibly long lifespans (150–300 years) among certain individuals in India and China should be considered myth or incredulous exceptions for which there is no evidence.

2. Again, it is important to note that average life expectancy worldwide in 1500 CE was around thirty years. Coincident with the rise of scientific medicine, we find clear evidence that life expectancy rose in countries where it was applied, while countries that relied primarily on traditional forms of medicine began to see significant rises in life expectancy only after they adopted scientific medicine (in what is known as the *health transition*). This casts some pallor over claims of efficacy with many traditional approaches, even as some aspects of these approaches show promise.

3. Clearly, social inequality and injustice are still widespread and remain evident in the propensity to develop certain diseases and relative life expectancy by race and social class. On how social class mattered in the rise of scientific medicine, see Starr (1982).

4. Risk-factor reduction and medical efficacy both get credit in explaining advances in health and life expectancy. How to balance that credit remains unclear. Regarding coronary disease, see Ford et al. (2007).

5. See Bonah (2005, 669–721) on the BCG vaccine. Sledzik and Bellantoni (1994, 269–274) discuss vampire folk belief in New England. The recent emergence of drug-resistant strains of TB led WHO to declare a global health emergency, with greatest concern in India, which had the highest total number of cases worldwide in 2010 due to poor disease management. On TB in India today, see Mishra (2013, 71–78).

6. PAHO.org (2017).

7. Flexner (1910).

8. Cooke et al. (2006, 1339–1344) weigh the effects of Flexner's impact a century after his influential report, including the growing tendency of medical school faculty to be concerned about such things as market share, units of service, and capitation.

9. Ironically, many yoga teacher and yoga therapy training programs are notoriously demanding and stressful, as if by intention and design.

10. Recent evidence is found in The Leapfrog Group's (2015) Spring 2015 Hospital Safety Score, which reports that forty-one percent of 2,523 U.S. hospitals surveyed in 2014–15 received a C, D, or F grade on patient safety due to medical errors, injuries, accidents, and infections.

11. Weil (1998, 51).

12. Hurley (2006, 182).

13. Ibid., 184.

14. Ibid., 184.

15. Ibid., 184.

16. Ibid., 189.

17. NCCIH (2017).

18. Ibid.

19. See Tindle et al. (2005) on baby boomers and others going to alternative medical providers.

20. Snyderman and Weil (2002). To explore further, see Chopra (2000; 2015) and Weil (1985; 1998; 2004; 2007).

21. Although this is purely anecdotal evidence, the public yoga classes I teach in Santa Cruz, California, are filled with a variety of scientists associated with our local University of California campus—astronomers, astrophysicists, molecular biologists, marine scientists, anthropologists, chemists, and others, from graduate students to all ranks of faculty and pure scientific researchers. Most do not believe

in magic or miracles yet are fascinated by mysteries, and all seem to find in yoga something that adds ease and meaning to their lives.

22. Lerner (1996, 15).

23. Also see Buchholz (2012) and Siegel (1986) on hope.

24. Siegel (1986).

25. Psychoneuroimmunologists are producing a growing body of scientific evidence on the relationship between psychological stress and the immune system. See Vedhara and Irwin (2005) for a general overview of the field. Zorilla et al. (2001) look at mental state and immunological assays. See Elenkov (2005) for more on stress and cytokine dysregulation.

26. Although we also find some free and reduced-cost services offered by many providers in the yoga and alternative health communities, most of the best and brightest providers charge hefty prices for their services while offering little to nothing on a pro bono or sliding scale basis. Meanwhile, it is not uncommon to find yoga classes in most major U.S. cities priced at $20 and more, and 200-hour teacher training programs that charge over $5,000, despite having inexperienced trainers, poorly developed curricula, and minimal adherence to the Yoga Alliance's extremely anemic standards—for which there is no accountability.

27. St. Sauver et al. (2013) identifies the most common reasons people sought primary care in the U.S. in 2013 as skin disorders (42.7%), arthritis and other joint disorders (33.6%), back problems (23.9%), disorders of lipid metabolism (22.4%), and upper respiratory tract disease (22.1%), all of which invite a wide range of treatment options.

28. Dossey and Keegan (2016). The great nest of being consists of successively greater wholes, from the whole of an atom to the whole of molecules, to the whole of a cell, and so on, to the whole of one's being, ecosystems, and the world, with each successive whole comprised of the multiple wholes that constitute it and, ultimately, the whole of the universe, which Wilber then distills into an elegant four-quadrant model. Wilber's model is an expression of spiritual evolution, a wide tradition that proposes a higher level of evolution connected to a cosmological pattern and it is typically presented as a teleological process. Wilber, tapping Plato and Aristotle's "great chain of being" concept, expands it to cover how we get from matter to body to mind to soul to spirit. See Wilber (2007) for a succinct introduction to his thinking.

29. Dalen (1998, 2216).

30. Mohan and Mohan (2004, 38).

31. Lerner (1996).

32. American Psychological Association (2002).

Part II

1. For a discussion of touch, somatics, and the awakening of conscious awareness, see Stephens (2014, 15–19).

Chapter 5

1. Between two and three million people worldwide contract skin cancer annually. See WHO (2016).

2. Squamous means "flattened," referring to the tissue cells that in their layered combination give us the outermost layer of the skin as well as the inner lining of the mouth, esophagus, and vagina.

3. For more on skin cancer, see Gloster and Brodland (1996, 217–26), Armstrong and Kricker (2001, 8–18), Roewert-Huber et al. (2007, 47–51), Madan et al. (2006, 5–7), Stang and Jöckel (2003, 436–442), Madea and Rothschild (2010, 575–586), and Polsky and Wang (2011).

4. Stiles (2012).

Chapter 6

1. See Lee et al. (2007, 456–469).

2. Later in life there is a tendency toward osteoporosis, in which bone density diminishes and the bone resilience weakens. For a discussion of age- and developmentally appropriate asana practices, see Stephens (2012b). For a more general discussion of growing bones and bone mechanics, see Caine and Lindner (1985, 51–64), Micheli (1986, 359–74), Mirbey et al. (1988, 336–340), and Ryan and Salciccioli (1976, 26–27).

3. Indeed, there is only one bone—the hyoid at the base of the tongue, which is significant in jalandhara bandha—that is not connected to at least one other bone.

4. These are structural classifications. Joints can also be classified functionally as amphiarthrodial (slightly moveable), diarthrodial (freely moveable), or synarthrodial (immovable). There are several other ways of classifying a joint: its number of axes of movement, its range of motion, and the shape of its articular surfaces.

5. See Floyd (2014) for range of motion (ROM) by angular degree in the spine, upper extremities, and lower extremities.

6. Shulman (1949).

7. See Tiwari (1995, 9, 17, 125–128, 230–232) and Lad (2001, 52, 132, 145–149).

Chapter 7

1. Netter (1997, plates 488–499).

2. Todd (1937).

3. Hately (2004, 30).

4. Tiwari (1995, 25, 192, 317–18).

5. Lad (2001, 130–2).

Chapter 8

1. See Höfle et al. (2010).

2. Barboi (2014).

3. McCorry (2007, 78).

4. Berthoud and Neuhuber (2000, 1–17).

5. Gomez-Pinilla and Gomez (2011, 111–116).

6. Vedhara and Irwin (2005).

7. Fox et al. (2014, 48–73), Jao et al. (2016, 9–24), Luders (2014, 82–88), and Simkin and Black (2014, 487–534).

8. Tiwari (1995, 112–3, 173–6).

Chapter 9

1. Schiffmann (1996).

2. Many books on yoga anatomy contribute to our understanding of yoga asanas, yet none provide information on biomechanics or neuromuscular relationships. See Coulter (2010), Kaminoff and Matthews (2012), Lasater (2009), and Long (2009; 2010). Curiously, Lasater notes innervation without discussing movement. Calais-Germain (1991) addresses movement but without reference to innervation. The author dreams of these sources collaborating in producing a yoga kinesiology

textbook and in partnering with Pixar to depict neuromuscular forces for each of at least 108 asanas, including the movement in and out of each asana.

3. Abernathy et al. (2013).

4. Here we are discussing kinesiology as the scientific study of human movement and its applications to biomechanics, yoga, and other activities. We are decidedly not considering the diagnostic medical methodology called applied kinesiology.

5. Doidge (2007, 256–266), Pascual-Leone (2005, 377–401), and Young (2011, 70–80).

6. For basic study of biomechanics, see Abernethy et al. (2013),Cowin (2008), Hatze (1974, 189–190), Mow and Huiskes (2005), and Peterson and Bronzino (2008).

7. This point might make one wonder about those who call themselves yoga masters (almost all are self-anointed). What have they mastered? All 840,000 asanas? Even one? What does it even mean to master an asana? Is it no longer your teacher? Does one know it all, having mastered all the superpowers Patanjali presents in Chapter 3 of his *Yoga Sutra*, and thus is one able to move through space, time, bodies, minds (including yours and mine) and anything and everything along the way? This writer thinks not. Another view is that in yoga there is no end, nothing to master, only a practice that allows us to live in greater balance, with clearer awareness, and healthier tissues for the rest of our lives.

8. Wolff (1986), Frost (1994), Duncan and Turner (1995), and Liedert et al. (2005).

9. Muscular deformation or injury is strain; ligamentous deformation or injury is sprain.

10. Electromyography (EMG) measures the functional conduction of nerves by recording the electrical activity produced by skeletal muscles. See Kamen (2004). See Behm et al. (2002) for variation in intermuscle activation.

11. There are many different fiber-typing methods, including the commonly confused histochemical and immunohistochemical staining, and others that give direct metabolic measures. See MacIntosh et al. (2006) and Pette and Staron (2000) for further exploration.

12. There is evidence that an external source of warming (such as being in a hot room) gives quicker release of tension in muscles around the hips only. However, vigorous activity in a hot environment is contraindicated for many conditions, including young age, pregnancy, and low or high blood pressure. Doing yoga in a hot room can also create a false sense of flexibility, leading to excessive ROM given the normal condition of one's muscles and ligaments. Heat stress also reduces the ability to achieve maximal metabolic rates during exercise and can increase difficulty

with cardiac output. To explore, see Adolph (1947), Brouha et al. (1961, 133–140), Daanen et al. (2006), Dimri et al.(1980, 43–50), King et al. (1985,1350–1354), Nadel (1983, 134–143), Sawka(1992, 657–70), and Young (1990, 65–70).

13. Proprioceptors function with other sense organs to also give us conscious awareness of the position of our body in space, a perceptual quality called *kinesthesis*.

14. See Collins (2009, 3311–15) for evidence of the role of cutaneous receptors in proprioception.

15. The literal meaning of *hatha*, as first recorded in the *Rigveda*, is "a blow, stroke," a masculine gender term implying with force. See Monier-Williams (1899, 1287).

Chapter 10

1. For general background, see Katz (2010), Sherwood (2011), and Patwardhan (2012, 77–82).

2. For more on this circulation, see Caro et al. (2012).

3. Klabunde (2005, 93–4).

4. Physiologists debate whether the Frank–Starling Law best explains venous return because it posits response to increased volumes of blood filling the heart as the mechanism that determines stroke volume (the volume of blood pumped from a ventricle with each beat) rather than other measures such as effects on cardiac output (diastolic pressure, for example). See Reddi and Carpenter (2005). Regarding Mercury in retrograde, the planet does not actually reverse its orbital path but merely appears to. Nonetheless, among astrologers this illusion is the source of much theorizing and prediction about disturbed human communication, a curious notion given that the celestial bodies are moving as they always do.

Chapter 11

1. On the history of lymphatics, see Ambrose (2006, 1–8).

2. The deeper origin of lymphocytes are lymphocytic stem cells in bone marrow, some of which remain in the bone marrow to mature into B cells and NK cells while most migrate to the thymus to become T cells. See Abbas et al. (2003, 115–137).

Chapter 12

1. Taylor (1949).

2. Kirk et al. (1984, 196).

3. For a thorough primer on respiratory physiology, see West (2000).

4. French (2003).

5. Barrett (2016) and Standring (2008).

6. Although most pranayama practices are done through the nose, the mouth offers a shorter and more direct pathway to the lungs and thus greater ease in inhaling and exhaling large quantities of air (as we will see with bastrika pranayama and sitali pranayama); complete exhalations through the mouth also stretch the diaphragm more, as we discuss in detail later.

7. On the number of alveoli in the human lung, see Ochs et al. (2004), who put the mean at 480 million.

8. Netter (1997, plates 180–181).

9. Calais-Germain (2005, 101).

10. Thiara and Goldman (2012, 165–66).

Chapter 13

1. Cawadis (1941, 303–308), Zrenner (1985).

2. Barrett et al. (2016) and Standring (2008).

3. Nussey and Whitehead (2013).

4. We will survey the exocrine pancreas in Chapter 14.

Chapter 14

1. Bagchi and Swaroop (2017).

2. Iio et al. (2014, 72), Galley (2014, 748–760), Chuang et al. (2010, 1344–1353), Maunder and Levenstein (2008, 247–52), and Farhadi et al. (2005, 1796-804).

3. Kong and Singh (2008, 80), Mishellany (2006, 87–94), Jalabert-Malbos (2007, 803–12), Jiffry (1981, 113–19), and Peyron (2004, 578–82).

4. We appreciate that the vegetarian diet is taken as a given among some in the yoga community, a lifestyle choice supported in some of the yoga literature, including in B.K.S. Iyengar's *Light on Yoga*, where Iyengar makes two arguments: First, relating to *ahimsa*, he writes (1966, 32) that "... a vegetarian diet is a necessity for the practice of yoga" because one is otherwise involved in killing "a thing or a being." He does not explain why killing a plant is morally different from killing a single-cell amoeba. Second, relating to *saucha*, he argues that eventually the yogi

must be a vegetarian to attain "one-pointed attention and spiritual evolution" (1966, 37), adding that the yogi should "avoid foods that are sour, bitter, salty, pungent, burning, stale, tasteless, heavy, and unclean."

Chapter 15

1. To explore, see Calais-German (2003).

Chapter 16

1. Kucinshas and Just (2004), Siiteri and Wilson (1974), and Wilson and Reiner (1998).

Part III

Chapter 17

1. See Nichala Joy Devi (2014) and Kraftsow (2014).

2. See Desikachar (1995; 1998), Mohan (1993), Payne and Usatine (2002), Mohan and Mohan (2004), Kraftsow (1999; 2002), Khalsa et al. (2016), and Payne et al. (2016).

3. Cohen and Nelson (2011).

4. Seitz (2010, 36).

5. Laurence (2010, 65–71).

6. Forbes et al. (2011, 7)

7. Ibid, 7–8.8. There are many other contrasting definitions of yoga therapy offered by contributors to Larry Payne et al. (2016).

9. Respiratory Care Board of California (2017).

10. IAYT (2016).

11. Broad (2012b).

Chapter 18

1. Nichala Joy Devi (2014).

2. These paths correspond to the "path of method" and "path of practice" as given by Patanjali in Chapters 1 and 2, respectively, of the *Yoga Sutra*.

3. Various extremes of self-mortification practice are found across the ancient to modern yoga landscape.

4. See Monier-Williams (1899, 1275–80). Most commentaries on the *Yoga Sutra of Patanjali* emphasize the study of sacred texts, which is not in Patanjali's aphorism. The entire point is self-reflection, not reflection on printed or spoken words or other external objects!

5. Others give us "profound longing," "meditation," even "vow." See David G. White (2014, 172–84). On the what—*ishvara*—see White's discussion and conclusion that "it is unlikely that there will ever be a final word on what Patanjali meant by ishvara-pranidhana."

6. There is a rich literature on cognitive dissonance that builds on Festinger's (1957) original work, including how it plays out in irrational insistence (Elster, 1983), how it can be reinforced in neural correlates (Qin et al. 2011, 240–6; Monroe and Read, 2008, 733–59), and models for resolving it (Van Harreveld et al. 2009).

7. B. K. S. Iyengar (2001, 35).

8. Prabhavananda and Isherwood (1944, 64–65).

9. See Baldwin et al. (2007), Kuutman and Hilsenroth (2012), and Høglend (2014) on how therapist-client dynamics are a factor in the therapeutic process.

10. Frymoyer and Frymoyer (2002, 995–96).

11. See Institute of Medicine (2001, 48–51) on patient-centered care as one of the six main elements of high-quality care. Also, cf. Beckman and Frankel (1984), Roter et al. (1997), and Gerteis et al. (1993).

12. See Byock (1998) and Cassell (1991) on these and other emotional and spiritual dimensions of fear and anxiety.

13. IAYT (2016, 7).

14. American Association of Medical Colleges (1999).

15. See Tongue et al. (2005) on the joint initiative between Bayer and AAOS.

16. Weintraub (2012).

17. Some yoga therapy schools teach students how to take pulse, monitor heart rate with a stethoscope, measure range of motion with a goniometer, and test breath capacity with a spirometer. Used conservatively in support of a client's healing, these tools can provide helpful insight; applied liberally or for medical diagnostics,

these practices can create ethical and even legal problems, or worse—misdiagnosis that causes harm.

18. Mindful listening is akin to active listening, a specific communication skill rooted in the work of humanistic psychologist Carl Rogers (1951; 1980) on client-centered therapy, which is of growing interest in all health professions. See Rogers and Farson (1987) for a concise discussion of active listening in effecting personal transformation. See Fassaert et al. (2007, 258–64) on development and testing of the Active Listening Observation Scale and how active listening differentiates between health professionals. Lang et al. (2000) call for active listening to better gain clues to patients' explanations and concerns about their illness.

19. Weintraub (2012).

20. Stephens (2014), Field (2001; 2003), and Montagu (1986).

21. Kabat-Zinn (1994) and Kornfield (1993; 2009).

22. Krishnamurti (1987; 1996) and Tolle (1999).

23. Kramer and Alstad (2009, 201) also emphasize that only being in the present tends to cause dismissal of the historicity of one's being, thereby slighting the importance of both reflection and imagination as one exists in the inexorable movement of time.

24. See Thorne (1948) on the origins and principles of directive counseling and psychotherapy.

25. Rogers (1951; 1961) and Maslow (1954).

Chapter 19

1. This may lead you to wonder why it is important for yoga teachers to learn as much as we can about functional anatomy and physiology. In guiding asana practices, we invite students to move into a variety of postures that have various effects on joints, muscles, nerves, and other tissues. To the extent that you have a practical grasp of functional anatomy, you will have better insight into the physical risks, contraindications, and related modifications or alternative postures for the asanas you are teaching. Add knowledge of physiology and you will have better insight into the deeper effects of the asanas, including on respiration, digestion, and circulation. In the absence of such knowledge and insight, we might instead wonder why there are not considerably higher standards of competency for all yoga teachers, the vast preponderance of whom teach complex asanas with little understanding of how the body works and how it does not work.

2. Cope (2012).

3. IAYT (2016, 9).

4. Stephens (2010).

5. The fascinating modern history of muscle testing was profoundly affected by the polio pandemic in the early twentieth century, starting with the work of Lovett (and his assistant, Wilhemene Wright) (1917). For more on the history, see Wright (1912), Stewart (1925), Kendall and Kendall (1949), Lilienfield (1954), Bohannon (1986), and Zimney and Kirk (1987).

6. Kendall and Kendall (1949, 26).

7. Harry Eaton Stewart (1929, 125 *passim*).

8. Bohannon and Schaubert (2005), Dvir (1997), and Jepsen et al. (2004) discuss variability and reliability.

9. Lamb (1985, 47–55).

10. Originally developed by Silver (1923), this is the method adopted by the American Academy of Orthopaedic Surgeons, as described in Heckman and Greene (1994).

11. See Boone and Azen (1979), Bell and Hoshizaki (1981), and Kalsheur et al. (2003).

12. See Whipple and Wolfson (1989) and Lizardi et al. (1989) on the neurology of aging and balance.

13. Goebel (2008, 1).

14. On vestibular disorders, see Black and Pesznecker (2006, 252–270), Vouriot et al. (2004, 239–247), and Meli et al. (2006, 259–66). On orthopedic disorders, see della Volpe et al. (2006, 349–55) and Popa et al. (2006). On the effects of medications, see Fife (2006, 103–9) and Fujisawa et al. (2006, 1–4).

15. Marchetti and Whitney (2006, 1653–58).

16. Shumway-Cook and Woollacott (1995, 323–4).

17. Many group studies support the healthy outcomes of meditation (Orme-Johnson 2006; Benson 1974; Kabat-Zinn et al. 1987; Rosenzweig et al. 2010; Witek-Janusek et al. 2008; Ornish 1990). With respect to yoga therapy assessment, we are interested in individual outcomes over time.

18. Cope (2012).

19. Merton (1997, 332).

20. Cope (2012, xv-xvi).

21. See Stephens (2012a).

22. As noted elsewhere, we do not assume that ayurveda is the necessary starting point in considering health and well-being or in practicing yoga, let alone that

it provides universally efficacious treatments. Rather, we consider it as we do a variety of approaches to health, looking for how and where its treatments might promote curing or healing.

23. Burns (1785) and Steinbeck ([1937] 1994).

24. Quoted in Osterberg and Blaschke (2005, 487–97).

Part IV

Chapter 20

1. Many of these studies are cited in Part V.

2. The Ashtanga Vinyasa practice developed by Krishnamacharya and his student K. Pattabhi Jois beginning in the 1930s is also considered a form of yoga therapy, with the first of its six set sequences called *yoga chikitsa*. However, it is less an adaptive practice than a prescriptive practice in which all students are taught to do the same asanas in the same ways, with only the exceptional teacher offering modifications to the sequences, asanas, and actions within them. In recent years—in the wake of Jois's death in 2009—more and more senior Ashtanga Vinyasa teachers are following the lead of David Swenson (2007) and others who encourage individualized modification of asanas—omitting certain asanas from the set sequences, allowing modification of asanas, even encouraging the use of props—so that it can be safely and beneficially explored by students who might lack the strong athleticism required in this approach.

3. The branding of a Viniyoga style of yoga therapy in the 1990s led Desikachar to dissociate himself and his father from that name. See Harvey (2015).

4. Desikachar (1995, 13).

5. We use the neologism *bodymind* in keeping with the view that the body and mind are not separate but rather a whole—and that sensing this whole is at the heart of yoga practice. This view stands in contrast to the dominant dualist views found in both Eastern and Western philosophy and forms a central theme of this book, which is primarily concerned with offering guidance to students that might help them more easily cultivate clear awareness of the wholeness of their being while keeping with whatever intention motivates their yoga practice.

6. Yoga originated in a culture rich in diverse spiritual and cultural practices and most significantly in Hindu-related belief, including Samkhya philosophy, but it is neither reducible to nor necessarily bound to any belief system or religion.

Such ties are a matter of choice. To explore further, see Indra Devi (1960), Eliade (1969), Feuerstein (2001), Freeman (2010), Gates (2006), B. K. S. Iyengar (1966), Kempton (2013), Kramer and Alstad (1993), Rosen (2012), Scaravelli (1991), Stephens (2010, 2012a; 2014), David G. White (2000; 2012; 2014), and Ganga White (2007).

7. See Dorandi (2013, 91, 95).

8. James (1952, 306–311 *passim*).

9. McDermott (1981, 29–30).

10. Ibid., 21–22.

11. See Shusterman (2008) for a critical analysis of how Dewey's work rescues analytical philosophy and phenomenology from dualism through the principles of mindfulness and somaesthetics. For a brilliant discussion of embodied habit and its effects upon and expression in posture, emotion, and thought, see the pioneering work of Todd and Brackett (1920).

12. Mark Johnson (1989, 10).

13. Ibid., 271–278. Csikszentmihalyi (1990 and 1997) offers insights into how these qualities of being in everyday engagement in the flow of life generate deeper happiness through mindful challenge.

14. For a general introduction to somatics, see Hanna (2004). For practices of embodiment, see Mark Johnson (1995) and Don Johnson (1995). For an anthology on body, breath, and consciousness, see Macnaughton (2004); for deeper exploration, see Lakoff and Johnson (1999) and Schusterman (2008 and 2012). For an essential work on embodied trauma and its release, see Levine (2010).

15. The *Yoga Sutra of Patanjali* is from around 325 CE. There are numerous and often contradictory translations and transliterations. The earliest writings on Hatha yoga date to a little over a thousand years later. Compare Bouanchaud (1999), Remski (2012), and Satchidananda (1978) for highly contrasting interpretations.

16. For a deep exploration of the nature of the senses, see Ackerman (1990).

17. Bikram Choudhury leads the way with competitive yoga, including current efforts to establish yoga as an Olympic sport. This is a curious phenomenon only if one ignores the origin of his yoga style in India's competitive bodybuilding culture rather than believing his assertion that his style—and only his style—is the true expression of Patanjali's synthesis of yoga philosophy and method, which he either fails to understand or willfully distorts. See Choudhury (2000). On oxymoronic competitive yoga, see Lorr (2012) and the IYSF (2014). On the proliferation of injuries when approaching yoga competitively, see Broad (2012a and 2012b).

18. Muktibodhananda(1985, 54, 67, 132).

19. Kramer (1977).

20. Stephens (2012a and 2014).

21. Stephens (2012a, 2015).

22. Stephens (2014).

23. For detailed guidance on sequencing, see Stephens (2012a, 2015, and 2017.).

Chapter 21

1. Many traditional spiritual perspectives give primacy to "being present," yet some also appreciate the natural human capacity for reflection and imagination, sensing context, and thinking of alternative possibilities. While opening ourselves to what Eckhart Tolle describes as the "power of now" as part of conscious awareness, we need not limit ourselves to a belief or sense of the "now" being all there is. For further exploration, see Kramer and Alstad (2009).

2. Differing definitions are found in the Vedas, Upanishads, *Yoga Sutra of Patanjali*, tantric literature, and the classical Hatha yoga literature from the fourteenth to seventeenth centuries. See Chapter 3 for a discussion of prana. To explore more recent interpretations, see Rosen (2002), Rosen (2006), and B. K. S. Iyengar (1985).

3. Various translations use the terms *perfected, accomplished*, or *mastery*. There is wide debate over when and under what conditions pranayama can be safely practiced. Although B. K. S. Iyengar states that asanas must first be perfected, in other commentary regarding inhalation, exhalation, and retention, he states that "all are to be performed, prolonged, and refined according to the capacity of the aspirant" (2001, 165).

4. Holleman and Sen-Gupta (1999, 266–268).

5. Ibid., 268.

6. Rosen (2002, 19).

7. Ramaswami (2005, 95–96).

8. B.K.S. Iyengar (1985, 10).

9. Bouanchaud (1999, 1.31).

10. On breathing patterns, see Farhi (1996).

11. Ibid., 72–73.

12. Rosen (2002, 72).

13. These exercises are adapted from the detailed anatomical practices discussed in Calais-Germain (2005, 176–203). See Netter (1997, plate 183) for muscles of inspiration and expiration.

14. B. K. S. Iyengar (1985, 99).

15. Ibid.

16. See Ganga White (2007, 66–67) for a succinct discussion of this debate.

17. Breath retention practice is found in the *Yoga Sutra*, where the cessation of breath is associated with *chitta vritti nirodha*, calming the fluctuations of the mind (*Yoga Sutra*, II.49–52). The term *kumbhaka* appears in the *Hatha Yoga Pradipika* (II.43–46) along with a more elaborate description of its practice. Here we focus on forms of *sahita kumbhakas*, those that concern the threefold practices of inhalation, exhalation, and retention. A fourth form, *kevala-kumbhaka*, spontaneously arises from these practices and transcends the phases of breathing; beyond technique, in kevala-kumbhaka the body-breath-mind are in effortless suspension. According to the *Hatha Yoga Pradipika*, there are eight kumbhaka practices (all sahita): suryabheda, ujjayi, seetkari, sitali, bhastrika, bhramari, morchha, and plavini.

18. Beyond inhalation, exhalation, and retention.

19. Regarding both kapalabhati and bastrika, Iyengar (1985, 180) tells us: "If people perform them because they believe that they awaken the kundalini, disaster to body, nerves, and brain may result." In contrast, the *Hatha Yoga Pradipika* (II.66), Iyengar's primary source, says that this pranayama "quickly arouses kundalini. It is pleasant and beneficial, and removes obstruction due to excess mucus accumulated at the entrance to brahma nadi."

20. Satyadharma (2003, 258, 230–231). Also see Powell (1996).

21. The approach here draws primarily from the *Hatha Yoga Pradipika* (II.7–9) while informed by Farhi (1996), Levine and MacNaughton (2004), and Rosen (2002 and 2006).

22. B.K.S. Iyengar (1985, 210).

23. Muktibodhananda (1985, 166).

Chapter 22

1. Watts (1980, 5–6).

2. Chödron (2007, 29).

3. For a practical modern-day treatment, see Cope (1999).

4. There is a tendency for many spiritual practices to offer promised outcomes in exchange for commitment to a specific practice, guru, or religion. It is no different in much of yoga. For a fascinating discussion, see Kramer and Alstad (2009).

5. Bouanchaud (1999, 142).

6. Watts (1980, 8).

7. Kempton (2011, 61).

8. Ibid., 67.

9. For a discussion of how dharana can be experienced amid a variety of activities, see Cope (2006, 68–71).

10. Kempton (2011, 72).

11. Bouanchaud (1999, 144). See Eliade's (1969, 69–73) discussion.

12. Bouanchaud (1999, 187).

13. Ibid., 216.

14. See Fischer-Schreiber et al. (1994).

15. There are infinite mudra possibilities. For guidance, see Hirschi (2000).

16. See Kempton (2011) for a variety of approaches to using the breath in meditation.

17. Watts (1980, 6).

18. This is a modified version of the counting meditation technique I learned from Erich Schiffmann starting in 1991. For more on his approach, see Schiffmann (1996).

19. This perspective blends my separate conversations with Sally Kempton and Daniel Odier. For more on Odier's approach and his translation of the *Vijnana Bhairava*, see Odier (2004). On the concept of paradigms and shifts in how we think of basic ideas, see Kuhn (1996).

Chapter 23

1. See Tahirian et al. (2012, 799–804) and Yin et al. (2014, 1585–1593).

2. Beeson (2014, 160–65).

3. Weak arches are sometimes reduced to weakness in the tibialis posterior. Although the tibialis posterior is an essential part of arch support, it is misguided to emphasize only this muscle rather than the combined set of muscles, the collective action of which gives balanced awakening of the arches. For an approach that focuses narrowly on the tibialis posterior, see Keller (2013).

4. It is quite a stretch—no pun intended—to relate "heel" and "heal" as they mostly have separate etymological roots, although the proto-Germanic *haila*, "undamaged,"

and *hanhilon*, the source of the Old English *hele*, "back of the foot," offers one possible link.

5. Irwin (2014) provides a clear description of different Achilles tendon injuries.

6. See Gollwitzer et al. (2007) for a study of extracorporeal shock wave therapy for Achilles tendon injuries.

7. Wilder and Sethi (2004, 55–81) and Beck (1998, 265–79).

8. Mark W. Anderson (1997, 177–80), Michael Fredericson (1996, 49–72), and Detmer (1986, 436–46).

9. Yates and White (2004, 772–80) and Niemuth et al. (2005, 15–21).

10. Korkola and Amendola (2001, 35–50).

11. Couture and Karlson (2002, 29–36).

12. Orava (1978), McNicol et al. (1981), Fredericson et al. (2000), and Linenger and Christensen (1992).

13. Devan et al. (2004).

14. Gajdosik et al. (2003) tested IT band tightness in relation to ITBS using the Ober method and found no correlation.

15. Fairclough et al. (2007) and Hariri et al. (2009).

16. Linenger and Christensen (1992, 98–108), McNicol et al. (1981, 76–80), Orava (1978, 69–73), Fairclough et al. (2007, 74–76), Fredericson et al. (2000, 169–175), and Gajdosik et al. (2003, 77–79).

17. Valle et al. (2015) cite seven recent studies of hamstring injuries in different sports. See Opar et al. (2012) on factors leading to hamstring tears in these and other sports.

18. De Visser et al. (2012).

19. Opar et al. (2012) discuss injury and reinjury. See also Freckleton et al. (2012).

20. Alter (1998).

21. See Järvinen et al. (2005) on general treatment strategies for muscles tears. On the question of ice in treating hamstring tears, see Bleakley et al. (2012). On the benefits of compression, see Kwak et al. (2006).

22. Ziltener et al. (2010).

23. Lu et al. (2013, 130) and Evans (1994, 158–59).

24. Zeni (2000, 929–47).

25. Er (2014, 117–21), Ly and Swiontkowski (2008, 2254–66), and Waters and Millis (1988, 513–26).

26. Ernst (1964, 71–83).

27. Muldoon et al. (2001, 181–85).

28. Cosman et al. (2013, 359–66) and De Paulis et al. (1998, 49–59).

29. Muldoon et al. (2001, 181–85).

30. Davis et al. (2012).

31. Estwanik and Rosenberg (1990, 59–65). See Ziprin and Foster (1999, 56–68) on referred pain.

32. Falvey et al. (2015).

33. Hrysomallis (2009, 1514–17).

34. Weir et al. (2010, 99–103), Schlegel et al. (2009, 139–49), and Wiktorsson-Moller et al. (1983, 249–52).

35. CDC (2016).

36. Woo and Morrey (1982, 1295–306), Weeden et al. (2003, 709–13), and Howell et al. (2004, 153–62).

37. Sköldenberg et al. (2010, 583–87) and Zhang et al. (2008, 1358–63).

38. Kennon et al. (2004, 91–97).

39. Goosen et al. (2011, 200–8).

40. Windisch et al. (2007, 37–45).

41. Guvencer et al. (2009, 8–17).

42. Fishman and Zybert (1992, 358–64) and Fishman et al. (2002, 295–301).

43. Yeoman (1928, 1119–22).

44. Judith Lasater (2012) asserts that there is no objective measure of SIJ misalignment, referencing her own orthopedist as one who does debate the significance of the SIJ in low back pain. Yet there is a wide array of sources on measuring SIJ alignment. To explore, start with Kirkaldy Willis and Bernard, Jr. (1999, 206–26). On low back pain associated with SIJ dysfunction, see Schwarzer et al. (1995, 31–37) and Arnbak et al. (2016, 237).

45. Foley and Buschbacher (2006, 997–1006) and Lippitt (1995, 369–90).

46. Lippitt (1995, 369–90) and Heller (2006).

47. MacLennan and MacLennan (1997, 760–764).

48. There is some confusion over the term *lordosis*, which is often used to describe the normal lordotic curvature of the lumbar and cervical spine segments *and* their

excessive anterior curvature, which is also called *hyperlordosis*. Hyperlordosis is often employed only when referring to a painful condition.

49. Esola et al. (1996, 71–78), Manniche et al. (1994, 317–26), and Porter (1997, 1508–13).

50. Coventry et al. (1945, 105).

51. Haefeli et al. (2006, 15–22).

52. Zander, et al. (2010, 551–57).

53. Adams et al. (2009, 384), Adams et al. (1996, 965), and Buckwalter (1976, 130–37), Backwater (1995).

54. Urban(2000, 53) and Podichetty (2006, 4).

55. Hadjipavlou et al. (2008, 1261).

56. For a literature review, see Moriguchi et al. (2016, 497–518).

57. Fon et al. (1980, 979–83).

58. Keleman (1985).

59. Goh et al. (1999, 439–48).

60. Renno et al. (2005, 113–118), Greendale et al. (2002, 1611–14), Greendale et al, (2009, 1569–79), and Itoi and Sinaki (1994, 1054–59).

61. Brocklehurst et al. (1982, 534–38).

62. The earliest coinage of this euphemism was in 1908. By 1934 the expression became less socially polite in making reference to an anatomically inferior location.

63. Over two-thirds of the population experiences neck pain. See Najera et al. (2015, Ch. 6) and Binder (2007, 527–31).

64. March et al. (2014, 353–66) and Mattu et al. (2007, 46).

65. Brezinschek (2008, 653–54, 656–57) and Simons (2008, 157–59).

66. Cohen (2015, 284–299) and Garra et al. (2010, 484–89).

67. Dubousset (1999, 699–704) and Kouwenhoven and Castelein (2008, 2898–2908).

68. It is also called "adolescent idiopathic scoliosis," which can continue into adulthood, in which case it is called "adult idiopathic scoliosis." Weinstein et al. (2008, 1527–37), Fong et al. (2010, 1061–1071), and Haumont et al. (2011, 847–54).

69. Pehrsson (1992, 109–16).

70. Recent research is finding some evidence of etiology. See Gorman et al. (2012, 1905–19), Ogilvie et al. (2012, 679–81), and Montanaro, et al. (2006, 21).

71. Lambert et al. (2009, 12477–83); Čakrt et al. (2011, 161–65), and Guo et al. (2006, 437–40)

72. Bettany-Saltikov et al.(2014, 111–21), Weiss, Goodall (2008, 177–93), and Romano et al. (2012, 8).

73. Fishman et al. (2014, 16–21). Miller (2003), Krentzman (2016), and Monroe (2011) describe various yoga practices that they have found in their personal practices to be beneficial.

74. W. S. Moore (1993, 600–3).

75. J.E. Kuhn et al. (2015, 222–32), Sanders and Hag (1991), and Sadat et al. (2008, 260–63).

76. Cuetter and Bartoszek (1989, 410–19), Roos (1999, 126–29), and Wilbourn (1999, 130–37).

77. Upton and McComas (1973, 359–62).

78. Roos (1976, 771–78) and Huang and Zager (2004, 897–903).

79. Esposito et al. (1997, 598–99) and Al-Shekhlee and Katirji (2003, 383–85).

80. Povlsen et al. (2014) and Orlando et al. (2015, 934–39).

81. Kenny et al.(1993, 282–84).

82. Wadsworth (1986, 1878–83).

83. Milgrom et al. (2008, 361–64).

84. Ewald (2011, 417–422) and Van der Windt et al. (1995, 959–64).

85. Craik et al. (2014, 547–552) and Robert Miller et al. (2013).

86. Yamamoto et al. (2010, 116–120).

87. Brasseur et al. (2004, 857–864), Tempelhof et al. (1999, 296–299), Abate et al. (2014, 275–280), Baumgarten et al. (2010, 1534–1541), Bishop et al. (2015, 1598–1605), Carbone et al. (2012, 56–60),Yamamoto et al. (2015, 446–452), and Gumina et al. (2008, 93–96).

88. Ellman et al. (1986, 1136–1144), Gartsman (1990, 169–180), and Bartolozzi et al. (1994, 890–97).

89. Moosmayer et al. (2010, 83–91), Kim et al. (2009, 289–296), Zingg, et al. (2007, 11928—1934), and Rudzki and Shaffer (2008, 691–717).

90. Ainsworth and Lewis (2007, 200–210).

91. John E. Kuhn (2009, 138–60) and Maman et al. (2009, 1898–906).

92. Bigliani and Levine (1997, 1854–1868) and Koester et al. (2005, 452–55).

93. Kibler (1998, 325–337).

94. Pitzer et al. (2014, 833–49) and Walker-Bone et al. (2004, 642–651).

95. Kraushaar and Nirschl (1999, 259–278), Nirschl (1992, 851–870), and Regan et al. (1992, 74–76).

96. Herquelot et al. (2013, 578–88) and Hong et al. (2004, 369–373).

97. Roetert et al. (1995, 47–57) and Loftice et al. (2004, 519–530).

98. Boyer and Hastings (1999, 481–491) and Rak et al. (2004, 461–464).

99. Borkholder et al. (2004, 181–199), Strujis et al. (2001, 924–929), and Strujis et al. (2004, 462–469).

100. Brosseau et al. (2002, 4), Fink et al. (2002, 205–209), and Trinh et al. (2004, 1085–1090).

101. Smidt et al. (2002, 23–40) and Kaleli et al. (2004, 131–133).

102. Daniels et al. (2004, 1941–1948) and Ingari (2009).

103. Bickel (2010, 147–52) and Lazaro (1997, 115–17).

104. Elhassan and Steinmann (2007, 672–681) and Husarik et al. (2009, 148–156).

105. Ekenstam et al. (1984, 363–5), Dobyns et al. (1982), and Grover (1996, 341–343).

106. S. E. Anderson et al. (2004, 719–724).

107. Husarik et al.(2009, 148–156).

108. Diop et al. (2008, 1081–1084) and Wolf et al. (2009, 112–115).

Chapter 24

1. Lao-Tzu ([1891] 1995).

2. To explore Jung's interest in yoga, see Jung (1953).

3. American Psychiatric Association (2015). There are many controversies with the DSM, including over the classification and definition of certain disorders as well as the treatments prescribed for them, which some critics note are heavily influenced by powerful pharmaceutical interests on the DSM task forces. See Cosgrove et al. (2006, 154–160).

4. American Psychiatric Association (2015).

5. DeNoon (2011).

6. To explore this perspective, see Keedwell (2008).

7. Vinters (2015, 291–319).

8. Storandt et al. (2006, 467–473) and Knopman et al. (2012, 1576–82).

9. Hulette et al. (1998, 1168–1274) and Sperling et al. (2011, 280–92).

10. Johnson et al. (2009, 1254–1559) and Wadley et al. (2009, 87–94).

11. Sabat (2001).

12. Ashford et al. (2015).

13. Waelde et al. (2004) and Danucalov et al. (2015).

14. Eyre et al. (2016).

15. McCaffrey et al. (2014).

16. Kleinman and Kleinman (2011, 275–301).

17. Walitza et al. (2012, 467–73).

18. Thapar et al. (2013, 3–16).

19. Barkley (2000, 1064–68) and Rowland et al. (2002, 162–70).

20. Burt (2009, 608–37), Gilbert-Diamond et al. (2014, 427–34), Lo et al. (2015, 1–3), and Jeffrey G. Johnson et al. (2007, 480–86).

21. Bidwell et al. (2011, 262–74).

22. Kamp et al. (2014, 709–14).

23. Burke et al.(2005, 7770–76).

24. Lowinson et al. (2005).

25. Stahre et al. (2004, 866–70).

26. United Nations (2016).

27. Despite the U.S. government classification of cannabis as a Schedule 1 narcotic (the same as heroin), which severely restricts research into its effects, there is abundant emerging scientific literature on what is popularly called medical marijuana. To explore, see The National Academies of Sciences, Engineering, and Medicine (2017), Carlini (2004, 461–67), Baker et al. (2003, 291–98), Voth (2001, 305–306), Pertwee (2006, 163–71), Ben Amar (2006, 1–25), Zuardi (2006, 153–57), Ashton (1999, 637–49), Elikkottil et al. (2009, 341–57), O'Connell and Bou-Matar (2007, 16), Wilkins (2006, 16–18), Crippa et al. (2009, 515–23), Furler (2004, 215–28), Raphael et al. (2005,161–76), and Reiman (2009, 35–39).

28. Jenkins (1999).

29. Carter et al. (2013, 3), (Smith et al. (2007, 16), Reddy et al. (2014, 750–56), Jacobson et al. (2009, 613–622), and White et al. (2011, 27).

30. Bock et al. (2012, 240–48), Shaffer et al. (1997, 57–66), and Vedamurthachar et al. (2006, 249–253).

31. Akiskal (1983, 11–20), Chu et al. (2010, 624–645), and Qualter et al. (2010, 493–501).

32. Blazer et al. (1994, 979–986), Cole and Dendukuri (2003, 1147–1156), Jackson et al. (2004, 196–207), Jacobi et al. (2004, 597–611), Lorant et al. (2003, 98–112), Nolen-Hoeksema and Morrow (1991, 115–121), and D. R. Williams et al. (2007, 305–15).

33. Thase et al. (1997, 1009–15).

34. Hofmann et al. (2010, 169–83), Kessler, et al. (2001, 289–94), Payne and Crane-Godreau (2015, 71), and Walsh and Shapiro (2006, 227–39).

35. Kabat-Zinn (1982, 33–47), Barnhofer et al. (2009, 366–73), and Dobkin (2008, 8–16), Kenny and Williams (2007, 617–25), and Kingston et al. (2007, 193–203).

36. Weissman and Weissman (1996).

37. Rama (1976), Weintraub (2004), Forbes (2011), Emerson (2015), Emerson and Hopper (2011), and Emerson et al. (2009).

38. Bershadsky et al. (2014, 106–13), Gard et al. (2014, 770), Kinser et al. (2012, 118–26), Kinser et al. (2014, 377–83), Balasubramaniam et al. (2012, 117), and Telles et al. (2015, 260–65).

39. Stephens (2014).

40. Roth (2007, 7–10).

41. Rosa and Bonnet (2000, 97–111).

42. Alholaand Polo-Kantola (2007, 553–67), Carney et al. (2013, 567–75), and Morin et al. (2009, 447–53).

43. Carney et al. (2013, 567–75).

44. Riemann et al. (2009, 1754–60), Spiegel et al. (1999, 1435–39), Alhola and Polo-Kantola (2007, 553–67), and Joo (2013, 1552-68).

45. Staner (2010, 35–46), Jansson and Linton (2006, 383–97), and Vollrath et al. (1989, 113–24).

46. Riemann et al. (2010, 19–31), Drake et al. (2011, 1179–88), and Pillai and Drake (2014).

47. Shaver and Woods (2015, 899–915).

48. Qaseem et al. (2016, 125–33).

49. Smith et al. (2002, 5–11).

50. Mustian et al. (2014, 164–68), Balasubramaniam et al. (2012, 117), Ray et al. (2011, 241–294), and Bertisch et al. (2012, 681–91).

Chapter 25

1. Gates (2006) goes on to discuss the powerful emergence of women in yoga that continues today as the leading source of creativity in yoga.

2. Geeta Iyengar (2002).

3. Clennell (2007).

4. Menstrual egress can be blocked by endometriosis, primary dysmenorrhea (menstrual cramps), cervical stenosis (scarring around the cervical opening), congenital anomalies of the reproductive tract, or adenomyosis (the growth of glands in the uterine muscles that, when the tissue is sloughed, has nowhere to go). In the early years of women's participation in NASA's space programs, NASA's male-dominated medical research staff first questioned women's emotional fitness while menstruating. After a generation of women in space since Sally Ride's inaugural flight in 1983, the issue is settled. See articles in National Geographic (http://phenomena.nationalgeographic.com/2016/04/22/how-do-women-deal-with-having-a-period-in-space/), The Atlantic (http://www.theatlantic.com/health/archive/2016/04/menstruating-in-space/479229/), and other popular publications relating the experience of a generation of female astronauts. For further exploration, see Porth and Martin (2008, 1056–65) and Moore and Dalley (2006, 105–12 and 410–42).

5. Many yoga teachers make a further case against inverting during menstruation based on the movement of and effects of prana, specifically the idea that apana-vayu's role in expelling unneeded materials from the body (urine, feces, menses) is disrupted. This is a curious proposition given that all prana-vayus manifest as part of subtle energetics that are generally posited as functioning beyond material forces such as gravity.

6. Benagh (2003).

7. Mittlemark et al. (1991).

8. Vaughan (1951).

9. For fascinating stories of how fear can limit a woman's cervical dilation in labor, see Gaskin (2003, 133–42).

10. For specific exercises, see Calais-Germain (2003). This book should be required reading for all prenatal and postnatal yoga teachers; all women should be encouraged to read it as well.

11. For specific modifications of asanas in working with these two classes of students, there are excellent prenatal and postnatal books that closely correspond to the

two groups: for more basic prenatal and postnatal classes, see Balaskas (1994); for regular yoga classes and experienced students, see Freedman (2004).

12. The term *menopause* is often used interchangeably to describe the very different conditions and phases of perimenopause and postmenopause, the former marking the onset of hormonal shifts that will eventually lead to postmenopause, when there is no longer a menstrual cycle. The distinction is vitally important as there are different symptoms and treatment protocols that, if confused, can create a variety of problems. For an excellent source on menopause in general, see Edelman (2009). For a more holistic perspective, see Boice (2007).

13. For a wonderful resource on yoga and menopause written from the Iyengar perspective, see Francina (2003).

14. Boivin et al. (2007, 1506–12) and Greil et al. (1988, 172–99).

15. Olive and Pritts (2006, 529–53) and WHO (2017).

16. Livshits and Seidman (2009, 701–7), Lis et al. (2015, 418–26), Zenzes (2000, 122–31), and Tersigni et al. (2014, 582–93).

17. Meng et al. (2005, 1926–31), Jain et al. (2002, 661–66), and Bitler and Schmidt (2012, 125–49).

18. Kolettis and Sabanegh (2001, 178–80), T. J. Walsh et al. (2010, 2140–47), and Jensen et al. (2009, 559–65).

19. See Calais-Germain (2003) for specific exercises designed to heighten awareness, control, and release in the muscles that affect the lower pelvic organs.

20. Eisenberg et al. (2013, 1030–34).

21. Cramer et al. (2002, 11–22, 34–36, 396–406).

22. For examples, see Giangarra et al. (1987, 290–92) and Wang et al. (2016, 497–503).

23. Pearce et al. (2012, 385–94).

24. van der Linden (1996, 53–65).

25. Johnson and Hummelsho (2013, 1552–68), Dunselman et al. (2014, 400–12), and Burney and Giudice (2012, 511–19).

26. Warren and Perlroth (2001, 3–11), Dhillon and Holt (2003, 156–164), Carpenter et al. (1995, 299–304), and Bergström et al. (2005, 380–83).

27. Calais-Germain (2003).

28. *Yoga Journal* (2017).

29. Anderson et al. (2011, 1294–99).

30. Sandman et al. (2000).

31. Pereira (2011, 53–58), Rubio-Aurioles et al. (2009, 1314–23), and Wagner et al. (2000, 144–46).

32. Selvin et al. (2007, 151–57).

33. Mannino et al. (1994, 1003–08), Shabsigh et al. (1991, 227–31), and Hirshkowitz et al. (1992, 101–7).

34. Selvin et al. (2007, 151–57), Nicolosi (2004, 235–43), and Perelman (2011, 1125–39).

Bibliography

Abate, M., C. Schivone, L. Di Carlo, and V. Salini. 2014. "Prevalence of and Risk Factors for Asymptomatic Rotator Cuff Tears in Postmenopausal Women." *Menopause* 21 (3): 275–280.

Abbas, Abul K., Andrew H. Lichtman, and J. S. Pober. 2003. "Antigen Processing and Presentation to T Lymphocytes." In *Cellular and Molecular Immunology*, 115–137. 5th ed. Philadelphia: Elsevier Saunders.

Abernathy, Bruce, Vaughn Kippers, Stephanie Hanrahan, Marcus Pandy, Ali McManus, and Laurel Mackinnon. 2013. *Biophysical Foundations of Human Movement*. 3rd ed. Champaign, IL: Human Kinetics.

Ackerman, Diane. 1990. *A Natural History of the Senses*. New York: Random House.

Adams, M. A., P. Dolan, and D. S. McNally. 2009. "The Internal Mechanical Functioning of Intervertebral Discs and Articular Cartilage, and Its Relevance to Matrix Biology." *Matrix Biology* 28: 384.

Adams, M. A., D. S. McNally, and P. Dolan. 1996. "'Stress' Distributions Inside Intervertebral Discs. The Effects of Age and Degeneration." *Journal of Bone and Joint Surgery* (Britain) 78: 965.

Adolph, Edward Frederick. 1947. *Physiology of Man in the Desert*. New York: Interscience Publishers, Inc.

Ainsworth, Roberta, and Jeremy S. Lewis. 2007. "Exercise Therapy for the Conservative Management of Full Thickness Tears of the Rotator Cuff: A Systematic Review." *British Journal of Sports Medicine* 41 (4): 200–210.

Aiyar, K. Narayanasvami, trans. (1914) 2009. *Thirty Minor Upanishads*. Santa Cruz, CA: Evinity Publishing.

Akiskal, H. S. 1983. "Dysthymic Disorder: Psychopathology of Proposed Chronic Depressive Subtypes." *American Journal of Psychiatry* 140: 11–20.

Alhola, Paula, and Päivi Polo-Kantola. 2007. "Sleep Deprivation: Impact on Cognitive Performance." *Neuropsychiatric Disease and Treatment* 3(5): 553–567.

Allen, Colin, Marc Bekoff, and George Lauder. 1998. *Nature's Purposes: Analyses of Function and Design in Biology*. Cambridge, MA: The MIT Press.

Allen, James. 2005. *The Art of Medicine in Ancient Egypt*. New Haven, CT: Yoga University Press.

Al-Shekhlee, Amer, and Bashar Katirji. 2003. "Spinal Accessory Neuropathy, Droopy Shoulder, and Thoracic Outlet Syndrome." *Muscle & Nerve* 28 (3): 383–385.

Alter, Michael J. 1998. *Science of Flexibility*. 2nd ed. Champaign, IL: Human Kinetics.

Ambrose, Charles T. 2006. "Immunology's First Priority Dispute—An Account of the 17th-Century Rudbeck–Bartholin Feud." *Cellular Immunology* 242 (1).

American Association of Medical Colleges. 1999. *Annual Report: Closing the Gaps—A Resolution for the New Millennium*. Washington, D.C.: American Association of Medical Colleges.

American Psychiatric Association. 2015. *Diagnostic and Statistical Manual of Mental Disorders*. 5th ed. Arlington, Virginia: American Psychiatric Publishing.

American Psychological Association. 2002. "Criteria for Evaluating Treatment Guidelines." *American Psychology* 57 (12): 1052–59.

———. "Stress in America 2009." 2009. American Psychological Association. www.apa.org/news/press/releases/stress/2009/stress-exec-summary.pdf.

Anderson, Mark W., Viviane Ugalde, Mark Batt, and Jose Gacayan. 1997. "Shin Splints: MRI Appearance in a Preliminary Study." *Radiology* 204 (1): 177–180.

Anderson, R. U., D. Wise, T. Sawyer, P. Glowe, and E. K. Orenberg. 2011. "6-Day Intensive Treatment Protocol for Refractory Chronic Prostatitis/Chronic Pelvic Pain Syndrome Using Myofascial Release and Paradoxical Relaxation Training." *Journal of Urology* 185 (4): 1294–99.

Anderson, S. E., L. S. Steinbach, D. De Monaco, H. M. Bonel, Y. Hurtienne, and E. Voegelin. 2004. "'Baby Wrist': MRI of an Overuse Syndrome in Mothers." *AJR American Journal of Roentgenology* 182 (3): 719–24.

Armstrong B. K., and A. Kricker. 2001. "The Epidemiology of UV Induced Skin Cancer." *Journal of Photochemistry and Photobiology* 63: 8–18.

Arnbak, Bodil, Rikke Krüger Jensen, Claus Manniche, Ilover Hendricks, Peter Kent, Anne Grehe Jurik, and Tue Secher Jensen. 2016. "Identification of Subgroups of Inflammatory and Degenerative MRI Findings in the Spine and Sacroiliac Joints: A Latent Class Analysis of 1037 Patients with Persistent Low Back Pain." *Arthritis Research & Therapy* 18 (1): 237.

Ashford, J. W., L. Mahoney, and T. Burkett. 2015. "A Role for Complementary and Integrative Medicine in Alzheimer's Disease Prevention."*Journal of Alzheimer's Disease* 487 (1): 13–14.

Ashton, C. H. 1999. "Adverse Effects of Cannabis and Cannabinoids." *British Journal of Anaesthesia* 83: 637–649.

Backwater, J. A. 1995. "Aging and Degeneration of the Human Intervertebral Disc." *Spine* 20: 1307.

Bagchi, Debasis, and Anand Swaroop, eds.. 2017. *Food Toxicology*. Boca Raton, FL: CRC Press.

Baker, D., G. Pryce, G. Giovannoni, and A. J. Thompson. 2003. "The Therapeutic Potential of Cannabis." *Lancet: Neurology* 2: 291–298.

Balaskas, Janet. 1994. *Preparing for Birth with Yoga: Exercises for Pregnancy and Childbirth*. Shaftesbury, CT: Element Books.

Balasubramaniam, M., S. Telles, and P. M. Doraiswamy. 2012. "Yoga on Our Minds: A Systematic Review of Yoga for Neuropsychiatric Disorders." *Frontiers in Psychiatry* 3: 117.

Baldwin, Scott A., Bruce E. Wampold, and Zac E. Imel. 2007. "Untangling the Alliance-Outcome Correlation: Exploring the Relative Importance of Therapist and Patient Variability in the Alliance." *Journal of Consulting and Clinical Psychology* 75 (6): 842.

Barboi, Alexandru, and Vivialyn Cadell. 2014. "Blood Pressure Dipping During the Deep Breathing Maneuver (BPDB) While Supine May Be a Marker of Severe Sympathetic Denervation." *Neurology* 82 (10) Suppl: 6–90.

Barkley, Russell A., and Paul J. Lombroso. 2000. "Genetics of Childhood Disorders: XVII. ADHD, Part 1: The Executive Functions and ADHD." *Journal of the American Academy of Child & Adolescent Psychiatry* 39 (8): 1064–68.

Barnhofer, T., C. Crane, E. Hargus, M. Amarasinghe, R. Winder, J. M. G. Williams. 2009. "Mindfulness-Based Cognitive Therapy as a Treatment for Chronic Depression: A Preliminary Study." *Behaviour Research and Therapy* 47: 366–373.

Barrett, Kim E., Susan M. Barman, Scott Boitano, and Heddwen L. Brooks. 2016. *Ganong's Review of Medical Physiology*. 25th ed. New York: McGraw Hill Education.

Bartolozzi, A., D. Andreychik, and S. Ahmad. 1994. "Determinants of Outcome in the Treatment of Rotator Cuff Disease." *Clinical Orthopaedics and Related Research* 308: 90–97.

Baumgarten, K. M., D. Gerlach, L. M. Galatz, S. A. Teefey, W. D. Middleton, K. Ditsios, and K. Yamaguchi. 2010. "Cigarette Smoking Increases the Risk for Rotator Cuff Tears." *Clinical Orthopaedics and Related Research* 468 (6): 1534–41.

Beck, B. R. 1998. "Tibial Stress Injuries: An Aetiological Review for the Purposes of Guiding Management." *Sports Medicine* 26 (4): 265–279.

Beckman, Howard B., and Richard M. Frankel. 1984. "The Effect of Physician Behavior on the Collection of Data." *Annals of Internal Medicine* 101 (5): 692–96.

Beckner, Morton. 1969. "Function and Teleology." *Journal of History of Biology* 2: 151–164.

Beeson, Paul. 2014. "Plantar Fasciopathy: Revisiting the Risk Factors." *The Journal of Foot and Ankle Surgery* 20 (3): 160–165.

Behm, David G., Kenneth Anderson, and Robert S. Curnew. 2002. "Muscle Force and Activation Under Stable and Unstable Conditions." *Journal of Strength & Conditioning Research* 16 (3): 416–422.

Bell, R. D., and T. B. Hoshizaki. 1981. "Relationships of Age and Sex with Range of Motion of Seventeen Joint Actions in Humans." *Journal Canadien des Sciences Appliquees au Sport* [*Canadian Journal of Applied Sport Sciences*] 6 (4): 202–6.

Ben Amar, M. 2006. "Cannabinoids in Medicine: A Review of Their Therapeutic Potential." *Journal of Ethnopharmacology* 105: 1–25.

Benagh, Barbara. 2003. "Inversions and Menstruation." *Yoga Journal*, http://yoga-journal.com/practice/546_I.cfm.

Benson, Herbert. 1974. "Decreased Alcohol Intake Associated with the Practice of Meditation: A Retrospective Investigation." *Annals of the New York Academy of Sciences* 233 (1): 174–77.

Bergström, I., B. Freyschuss, H. Jacobsson, and B. M. Landgren. 2005. "The Effect of Physical Training on Bone Mineral Density in Women with Endometriosis Treated with GnRH Analogs: A Pilot Study." *Acta Obstetrics et Gynecologica Scandanavia* 84 (4): 380–83.

Bershadsky, S., L. Trumpfheller, H. B. Kimble, D. Pipaloff, and I. S. Yim. 2014. "The Effect of Prenatal Hatha Yoga on Affect, Cortisol and Depressive Symptoms." *Complementary Therapies in Clinical Practice* 20 (2), 106–113.

Berthoud, Hans-Rudolf, and Winfried L. Neuhuber. 2000. "Functional and Chemical Anatomy of the Afferent Vagal System." *Autonomic Neuroscience* 85 (1): 1–17.

Bertisch, S. M., R. E. Wells, M. T. Smith, and E. P. McCarthy. 2012. "Use of Relaxation Techniques and Complementary and Alternative Medicine by American Adults with Insomnia Symptoms: Results from a National Survey." *Journal of Clinical Sleep Medicine* 8 (6): 681–691.

Bettany-Saltikov, Josette, Eric Parent, Michele Romano, Monica Villagrasa, and S. Negrini. 2014. "Physiotherapeutic Scoliosis—Specific Exercises for Adolescents with Idiopathic Scoliosis." *European Journal of Physical Rehabilitation Medicine* 50 (1): 111–21.

Bickel, K. D. 2010. "Carpal Tunnel Syndrome." *The Journal of Hand Surgery* 35 (1): 147–52.

Bidwell, L. C., F. J. McClernon, and S. H. Kollins. 2011. "Cognitive Enhancers for the Treatment of ADHD." *Pharmacology, Biochemistry, and Behavior* 99 (2): 262–74.

Bigliani, Louis U., and William N. Levine. 1997. "Current Concepts Review—Subacromial Impingement Syndrome." *Journal of Bone and Joint Surgery* (American) 79 (12): 1854–68.

Binder, Allan I. 2007. "Cervical Spondylosis and Neck Pain." *BMJ: British Medical Journal* 334 (7592): 527–31.

Bishop, J. Y., J. E. Santiago-Torres, N. Rimmke, and D. C. Flanigan. 2015. "Smoking Predisposes to Rotator Cuff Pathology and Shoulder Dysfunction: A Systematic Review." *Arthroscopy: The Journal of Arthroscopic and Related Surgery* 31 (8): 1598–1605.

Bitler, M. P., and L. Schmidt. 2012. "Utilization of Infertility Treatments: The Effects of Insurance Mandates." *Demography* 49: 125–49.

Black, F. O., and S. Pesznecker. 2006. "Chapter 17: Vestibular Ototoxicity." In *Pharmacology and Ototoxicity for Audiologists*, edited by K. C. M. Campbell, 252–70. Independence, KY: Delmar Cengage Learning.

Blavatsky, H.P. 1888. *The Secret Doctrine*. 2 vols. London: The Theosophical Publishing Company.

Blazer D. G., R. C. Kessler, K. A. McGonagle, and M. S. Swartz. 1994. "The Prevalence and Distribution of Major Depression in a National Community Sample: The National Comorbidity Survey." *American Journal of Psychiatry* 151: 979–86.

Bleakley, C. M., J. T. Costello, and P. D. Glasgow. 2012. "Should Athletes Return to Sport After Applying Ice?" *Sports Medicine* 42 (1): 69–87.

Bock, B. C., J. L. Fava, and R. Gaskins. 2012. "Yoga as a Complementary Treatment for Smoking Cessation in Women." *Journal of Women's Health* 21: 240–48.

Bohannon, Richard. 1986. "Manual Muscle Test Scores and Dynamometer Test Scores of Knee Extension Strength." *Archives of Physical Medicine and Rehabilitation* 67 (6): 390–92.

Bohannon, Richard, and Karen Schaubert. 2005. "Reliability and Validity of Three Strength Measures Obtained from Community-Dwelling Elderly Persons." *The Journal of Strength & Conditioning Research* 19 (3): 717–20.

Boice, Judith. 2007. *Menopause with Science and Soul: A Guidebook for Navigating the Journey*. Berkeley, CA: Celestial Arts.

Boivin J., L. Bunting, J. A. Collins, and K. G. Nygren. 2007. "International Estimates of Infertility Prevalence and Treatment Seeking: Potential Need and Demand for Infertility Medical Care." *Human Reproduction* 22: 1506–12.

Bolling, G. M. 1962. "Disease and Medicine (Vedic)." In *Encyclopaedia of Religion and Ethics*, edited by James Hastings, 762–72 Vol. 4. New York: Scribner.

Bonah, Christian. 2005. "The 'Experimental Stable' of the BCG Vaccine: Safety, Efficacy, Proof, and Standards, 1921–1933." *Studies in History and Philosophy of Science Part C: Studies in History and Philosophy of Biological and Biomedical Sciences* 36 (4): 669–721.

Boone, Donna C., and Stanley P. Azen. 1979. "Normal Range of Motion of Joints in Male Subjects." *The Journal of Bone and Joint Surgery* (American) 61 (5): 756–59.

Borkholder, C. D., V. A. Hill, and E. E. Fess. 2004. "The Efficacy of Splinting for Lateral Epicondylitis: A Systematic Review." *Journal of Hand Therapy* 17 (2): 181–99.

Bouanchaud, Bernard. 1999. *The Essence of Yoga: Reflections on the Yoga Sutras of Patanjali*. New York: Sterling.

Boudry, G., C. I. Cheeseman, and M. H. Perdue. 2007. "Psychological Stress Impairs Na+-Dependent Glucose Absorption and Increases GLUT2 Expression in the Rat Jejunal Brush-Border Membrane." *American Journal of Physiology-Regulatory, Integrative and Comparative Physiology* 292: 862–67.

Boyer, Martin I., and Hill Hastings. 1999. "'Lateral Tennis Elbow:' Is There Any Science Out There?" *Journal of Shoulder and Elbow Surgery* 8 (5): 481–91.

Brandon, R. N. 1981. "Biological Teleology: Questions and Explanations." *Studies in the History and Philosophy of Science* 12: 91–105.

Brasseur, J. L., O. Lucidarme, M. Tardieu, M. Tordeur, B. Montalvan, J. Pariet, P. Le Goux, A. Gires, and P. Grenier. 2004. "Ultrasonographic Rotator-Cuff Changes in Veteran Tennis Players: The Effect of Hand Dominance and Comparison with Clinical Findings." *European Radiology* 14 (5): 857–64.

Brezinschek, H. P. 2008. "Mechanismen des Muskelschmerzes: Bedeutung von Trigger Points und Tender Points." [Mechanisms of Muscle Pain: Significance of Trigger Points and Tender Points]. *Zeitschrift für Rheumatologie* (in German) 67 (8): 653–54, 656–57.

Brinker, M. R., and M. D. Miller. 1999. "The Adult Hip." In *Fundamentals of Orthopedics*, 269–85. Philadelphia: W. B. Saunders,.

Broad, William J. 2012a. "How Yoga Can Wreck Your Body." *New York Times*, January 5.

———. 2012b. *The Science of Yoga: The Risks and Rewards*. London: Simon & Schuster.

Brocklehurst, J. C., Duncan Robertson, and Pauline James-Groom. 1982. "Skeletal Deformities in the Elderly and Their Effect on Postural Sway." *Journal of the American Geriatrics Society* 30: 534–38.

Bronzino, Joseph D., ed. 2008. *Biomechanics: Principles and Applications* 2nd rev. ed. Boca Raton: CRC Press.

Brosseau, L., L. Casimiro, S. Milne, B. Shea, P. Tugwell, and G. Wells. 2002. "Deep Transverse Friction Massage for Treating Tendinitis." *The Cochrane Database of Systematic Reviews* 4: CD003528.

Brouha, Lucien, P. E. Smith, R. De Lanne, and Mary E. Maxfield. 1961. "Physiological Reactions of Men and Women During Muscular Activity and Recovery in Various Environments." *Journal of Applied Physiology* 16(1): 133–40.

Buchholz, William. 2012. *Living Beyond Expectations: Stories Patients Have Taught Me About Living Longer and Better Lives*. Bloomington, IN: Xlibris Corporation.

Buckwalter. 1976. 130–37.

Burgin, Timothy. 2014. "History of Yoga." *Yoga Basics*. www.yogabasics.com/learn/history-of-yoga/.

Burke, P. J., J. O'Sullivan, and B. L. Vaughan. 2005. "Adolescent Substance Use: Brief Interventions by Emergency Care Providers." *Pediatric Emergency Care* 21 (11): 770–76.

Burney, R. O., and L. C. Giudice. 2012. "Pathogenesis and Pathophysiology of Endometriosis." *Fertility and Sterility* 98: 511–19.

Burns, Robert. 1785. "To a Mouse, On Turning Up in Her Nest with the Plough." www.robertburns.org/works/75.shtml.

Burt, S. Alexandra. 2009. "Rethinking Environmental Contributions to Child and Adolescent Psychopathology: A Meta-analysis of Shared Environmental Influences." *Psychological Bulletin* 135 (4): 608.

Bynum, W. F. 2008. *History of Medicine: A Very Short Introduction.* Oxford: Oxford University Press.

Byock, Ira. 1998. *Dying Well: Peace and Possibilities at the End of Life.* New York: Riverhead Books.

Caine, Dennis J., and Koenraad J. Lindner. 1985. "Overuse Injuries of Growing Bones: The Young Female Gymnast at Risk?" *Physician and Sportsmedicine* 13 (12): 51–64.

Čakrt, Ondřej, Kryštof Slabý, Lucie Viktorinová, Pavel Kolář, and Jaroslav Jeřábek. 2015. "Subjective Visual Vertical in Patients with Idiopathic Scoliosis." *Journal of Vestibular Research* 25 (5–6): 195–99.

Calais-Germain, Blandine. 1991. *Anatomy of Movement.* Seattle: Eastland.

———. 2003. *The Female Pelvis: Anatomy and Exercises.* Seattle: Eastland.

———. 2005. *Anatomy of Breathing.* Seattle: Eastland.

Carbone, S., S. Gumina, V. Arceri, V. Campagna, C. Fagnani, and F. Postacchini. 2012. "The Impact of Preoperative Smoking Habit on Rotator Cuff Tear: Cigarette Smoking Influences Rotator Cuff Tear Sizes." *Journal of Shoulder and Elbow Surgery* 21 (1): 56–60.

Carlini, E. A. 2004. "The Good and the Bad Effects of (–) Trans-Delta-9-Tetrahydrocannabinol (Δ9-THC) on Humans." *Toxicon* 44 (4): 461–67.

Carney, C. E., A. L. Harris, A. Falco, J. D. Edinger. 2013. "The Relation Between Insomnia Symptoms, Mood, and Rumination About Insomnia Symptoms." *Journal of Clinical Sleep Medicine* 9: 567–75.

Caro, C. G., T. J. Pedley, R. C. Schroter, and W. A. Seed. 2012. *The Mechanics of the Circulation.* 2nd ed. Cambridge: Cambridge University Press.

Carpenter, S. E., B. Tjaden, J. A. Rock, and A. Kimball. 1995. "The Effect of Regular Exercise on Women Receiving Danazol for Treatment of Endometriosis." *International Journal of Gynaecology and Obstetrics* 49: 299–304.

Carter J. J., P. L. Gerbarg, and R. P. Brown. 2013. "Multi-component Yoga Breath Program for Vietnam Veteran Post Traumatic Stress Disorder: Randomized Controlled Trial." *Journal of Traumatic Stress Disorders and Treatment* 2 (3).

Cassell, Eric J. 1991. *The Nature of Suffering: And the Goals of Medicine.* New York: Oxford University Press.

Cawadis, A. P. 1941. "The Story of Endocrinology." *Proceedings of the Royal Society of Medicine* 34 (6): 303–8.

CDC (Centers for Disease Control and Prevention). 2016. "Alcohol Use and Your Health." www.cdc.gov/alcohol/fact-sheets/alcohol-use.htm.

Chattopadhyaya, Debiprasad. 1979. *Lenin, the Philosopher*. New Delhi: Sterling.

Chödron, Pema. 2007. *Always Maintain a Joyful Mind: And Other Lojong Teachings on Awakening Compassion and Fearlessness*. Boston: Shambhala Publications. 29.

Chopra, Deepak. 2000. *Perfect Health: The Complete Mind/Body Guide*. New York: Random House.

———. 2015. *Quantum Healing: Exploring the Frontier of Mind/Body Medicine*. Revised and Updated. New York: Bantam Books.

Choudhury, Bikram, and Bonnie Jones Reynolds. 2000. *Bikram's Beginning Yoga Class*. New York: Tarcher.

Chu P. S., D. A. Saucier, and E. Hafner. 2010. "Meta-analysis of the Relationships Between Social Support and Well-Being in Children and Adolescents." *Journal of Social and Clinical Psychology* 29: 624–45.

Chuang, J. C., H. Cui, B. L. Mason, M. Mahgoub, A. L. Bookout, H. G. Yu, M. Perello, et al. 2010. "Chronic Social Defeat Stress Disrupts Regulation of Lipid Synthesis." *Journal of Lipid Research* 51: 1344–53.

Clennell, Bobby. 2007. *The Woman's Yoga Book: Asana and Pranayama for All Phases of the Menstrual Cycle*. Berkeley, CA: Rodmell.

Cohen, M. H., H. Nelson. 2011. "Licensure of Complementary and Alternative Practitioners." Policy forum. *Virtual Mentor* 13 (6): 374–378.

Cohen, S. P. 2015. "Epidemiology, Diagnosis, and Treatment of Neck Pain." *Mayo Clinic Proceedings* 90 (2): 284–99.

Cole, M. G., and N. Dendukuri. 2003. "Risk Factors for Depression Among Elderly Community Subjects: A Systematic Review and Meta-analysis." *American Journal of Psychiatry* 160: 1147–56.

Collins, Amber T., J. Troy Blackburn, Chris W. Olcott, Douglas R. Dirschl, and Paul S. Weinhold. 2009. "The Effects of Stochastic Resonance Electrical Stimulation and Neoprene Sleeve on Knee Proprioception." *Journal of Orthopaedic Surgery and Research* 4 (1): 3311–15.

Cooke, Molly, David M. Irby, William Sullivan, and Kenneth M. Ludmerer. 2006. "American Medical Education 100 Years After the Flexner Report." *New England Journal of Medicine* 355 (1): 1339–44.

Cope, Stephen. 1999. *Yoga and the Quest for the True Self*. New York: Bantam.

———. 2006 *The Wisdom of Yoga: A Seeker's Guide to Extraordinary Living*. New York: Bantam-Bell.

———. 2012. *The Great Work of Your Life: A Guide for the Journey to Your True Calling*. New York: Bantam.

Cosgrove, Lisa, Sheldon Krimsky, Manisha Vijayaraghavan, and Lisa Schneider. 2006. "Financial Ties Between DSM-IV Panel Members and the Pharmaceutical Industry." *Psychotherapy and Psychosomatics* 75 (3): 154–60.

Cosman, F., J. Ruffing, M. Zio, J. Uhorchak, S. Ralston, S. Tendy, F. E. McGuigan, R. Lindsay, and J. Nieves. 2013. "Determinants of Stress Fracture Risk in United States Military Academy Cadets." *Bone* 55 (2): 359–66.

Coulter, H. David. 2010. *Anatomy of Hatha Yoga: A Manual for Students, Teachers, and Practitioners.* Honesdale, PA: Body and Breath.

Couture, Christopher J., and Kristine A. Karlson. 2002. "Tibial Stress Injuries: Decisive Diagnosis and Treatment of 'Shin Splints.'" *The Physician and Sports Medicine* 30 (6): 29–36.

Coventry, Mark B., Ralph K. Ghormley, and James W. Kernohan. 1945. "The Intervertebral Disc: Its Microscopic Anatomy and Pathology: Part I Anatomy, Development, and Physiology." *Journal of Bone and Joint Surgery* (American) 27: 105.

Cowin, Stephen C., ed. 2008. *Bone Mechanics Handbook.* 2nd ed. New York: Informa Healthcare.

Craik, Johnathan D., Ravi Mallina, Vijayraj Ramasamy, and Nick J. Little. 2014. "Human Evolution and Tears of the Rotator Cuff." *International Orthopaedics* 38 (3): 547–52.

Cramer, Daniel W., and Stacey A. Missmer. 2002. "The Epidemiology of Endometriosis." *Annals of the New York Academy of Science.* 955: 11–22, 34–36, 396–406.

Crangle, Edward Fitzpatrick. 1994. *The Origin and Development of Early Indian Contemplative Practices.* Wiesbaden, Germany: Harrassowitz Verlag.

Crippa, J. A., A. W. Zuardi, and R. Martin-Santos. 2009. "Cannabis and Anxiety: A Critical Review of the Evidence." *Human Psychopharmacology* 24: 515–23.

Csikszentmihalyi, Mihaly. 1990. *Flow. The Psychology of Optimal Experience.* New York: HarperPerennial.

———. 1997. *Finding Flow: The Psychology of Engagement with Everyday Life.* New York: Basic Books.

Cuetter, Albert C., and David M. Bartoszek. 1989. "The Thoracic Outlet Syndrome: Controversies, Overdiagnosis, Overtreatment, and Recommendations for Management." *Muscle & Nerve* 12 (5): 410–19.

Cushman, Anne. 2007. "New Pieces of Yoga History Shed More Light on the Practice." *Yoga Journal.* www.yogajournal.com/article/philosophy/new-light-on-yoga/.

Daanen, H. A., E. M. Van Es, and J. L. De Graaf. 2006. "Heat Strain and Gross Efficiency During Endurance Exercise After Lower, Upper, or Whole Body Precooling in the Heat." *International Journal of Sports Medicine* 27 (5): 379–88.

Dalen, James E. 1998. "Conventional and Unconventional Medicine: Can They Be Integrated?" *Archives of Internal Medicine* 158 (20): 2215–24.

Daniels, J. M. II, E. G. Zook, and J. M. Lynch. 2004. "Hand and Wrist Injuries: Part I. Non-emergent Evaluation." *American Family Physician* 69 (8): 1941–48.

Danucalov, Marcelo, Elisa Kozasa, Rui Afonso, Jose Galduroz, and Jose Leite. 2015. "Yoga and Compassion Meditation Program Improve Quality of Life and Self-Compassion in Family Caregivers of Alzheimer's Disease Patients: A Randomized Controlled Trial." *Geriatrics and Gerontology International*. Accessed Dec. 21. doi:10.1111/ggi.12675.

Davidson, Ronald M. 2003. *Indian Esoteric Buddhism: A Social History of the Tantric Movement*. New York: Oxford University Press.

Davis, J. A., M. D. Stringer, and S. J. Woodley. 2012. "New Insights into the Proximal Tendons of Adductor Longus, Adductor Brevis and Gracilis." *British Journal of Sports Medicine* 46 (12): 871–76.

della Volpe, R., T. Popa, F. Ginanneschi, R. Spidalieri, R. Mazzocchio, and A. Rossi. 2006. "Changes in Coordination of Postural Control During Dynamic Stance in Chronic Low Back Pain Patients." *Gait Posture* 24 (3): 349–55.

De Michelis, Elizabeth. 2004. *A History of Modern Yoga*. New York: Continuum.

DeNoon, Daniel J. 2011. "The 10 Most Prescribed Drugs." WebMD. www.webmd.com/drug-medication/news/20110420/the-10-most-prescribed-drugs#1.

Dent v. West Virginia. 129 U.S. (1889). https://supreme.justia.com/cases/federal/us/129/114/case.html.

De Paulis, F., A. Cacchio, O. Michelini, A. Damiani, and R. Saggini. 1998. "Sports Injuries in the Pelvis and Hip: Diagnostic Imaging." *European Journal of Radiology* 27: 49–59.

Desikachar, T. K. V. 1995. *The Heart of Yoga: Developing a Personal Practice*. Rochester, Vermont: Inner Traditions International.

———. 1998. *Health, Healing, and Beyond: Yoga and the Living Tradition of T. Krishnamacharya*. New York: North Point Press.

Detmer, Don E. 1986. "Chronic Shin Splints: Classification and Management of Medial Tibial Stress Syndrome." *Sports Medicine* 3 (6): 436–46.

Devan, Michelle R., Linda S. Pescatello, Pouran Faghri, and Jeffrey Anderson. 2004. "A Prospective Study of Overuse Knee Injuries Among Female Athletes with Muscle Imbalances and Structural Abnormalities." *Journal of Athletic Training* 39 (3): 263.

Devi, Indra. 1960. *Yoga for You: A Complete 6 Weeks' Course for Home Practice*. Preston, Great Britain: A. Thomas & Co.

———. 1969. *Renew Your Life Through Yoga*. New York: Warner Books.

Devi, Nichala Joy. 2000. *The Healing Path of Yoga: Time-Honored Wisdom and Scientifically Proven Methods that Alleviate Stress, Open Your Heart, and Enrich Your Life*. CreateSpace Independent Publishing Platform.

————2014. "Yoga Teaching or Yoga Therapy." *International Journal of Yoga Therapy* (24): 9–10.

De Visser, H. M., M. Reijman, M. P. Heijboer, and P. K. Bos. 2012. "Risk Factors of Recurrent Hamstring Injuries: A Systematic Review." *British Journal of Sports Medicine* 46 (2): 124–30.

De Vos, Paula. 2010. "European Materia Medica in Historical Texts: Longevity of a Tradition and Implications for Future Use." *Journal of Ethnopharmacology* 132 (1): 28–47.

Dhillon, P. K., and V. L. Holt. 2003. "Recreational Physical Activity and Endometrioma Risk." *American Journal of Epidemiology* 158: 156–64.

Dimri, G. P., M. S. Malhotra, J. Sen Gupta, T. Sampath Kumar, and B. S. Arora. 1980. "Alterations in Aerobic-Anaerobic Proportions of Metabolism During Work in Heat." *European Journal of Applied Physiology and Occupational Physiology* 45 (1): 43–50.

Diop, A. N., S. Ba-Diop, J. C. Sane, Alfidya A. Tomolet, M. H. Sy, L. Boyer, and M. Badiane. 2008. "Role of US in the Management of de Quervain's Tenosynovitis: Review of 22 Cases." *Journal de Radioligie* 89 (9, part 1): 1081–84.

Dobkin P. L. 2008. "Mindfulness-based Stress Reduction: What Processes Are at Work?" *Complementary Therapies in Clinical Practice* 14: 8–16.

Dobyns, J. H., R. D. Beckerball, and F. S. Bryon. 1982. "Fractures of the Hand and Wrist." In *Hand Surgery*, edited by J. E. Flynn. 3rd ed. Baltimore, MD: Williams and Wilkins.

Doidge, Norman. 2007. *The Brain That Changes Itself: Stories of Personal Triumph from the Frontiers of Brain Science*. London: Penguin.

Dorandi, Tiziano, ed. 2013. *Diogenes Laertius: Lives of Eminent Philosophers*. Vol. 50. Paris: Cambridge University Press.

Dossey, Barbara. 2008. *Florence Nightingale: Mystic, Visionary, Healer*. Philadelphia: F. A. Davis Company.

Dossey, Barbara, and Lynn Keegan, eds. 2016. *Holistic Nursing: A Handbook for Practice*. Burlington, MA: Jones and Bartlett Learning.

Drake, C. L., N. P. Friedman, K. P. Wright Jr., and T. Roth. 2011. "Sleep Reactivity and Insomnia: Genetic and Environmental Influences." *Sleep* 34 (9): 1179–88.

Dubousset, J. 1999. "Idiopathic Scoliosis. Definition—Pathology—Classification—Etiology." *Bulletin de l'Académie Nationale Médecine* 183 (4): 699–704.

Duncan, R. L., and C. H. Turner. 1995. "Mechanotransduction and the Functional Response of Bone to Mechanical Strain." *Calcified Tissue International* 57 (5): 344–58.

Dunselman, G. A., N. Vermeulen, and C. Becker. 2014. "ESHRE Guideline: Management of Women with Endometriosis." *Human Reproduction* 29: 400–12.

Dvir, Zeevi. 1997. "Grade 4 in Manual Muscle Testing: The Problem with Submaximal Strength Assessment." *Clinical Rehabilitation* 11 (1).

Edelman, Julia Schlam. 2009. *Menopause Matters: Your Guide to a Long and Healthy Life*. Baltimore: Johns Hopkins University Press.

Eisenberg, M. L., R. B. Lathi, V. L. Baker, L. M. Westphal, and A. A. Milki. 2013. "Frequency of the Male Infertility Evaluation: Data from the National Survey of Family Growth." *Journal of Urology* 189: 1030–34.

Ekenstam, F. W., A. K. Palmer, and R. R. Glisson. 1984. "The Load on the Radius and Ulna in Different Positions of the Wrist and Forearm. A Cadaver Study." *Acta Orthopaedica Scandinavica* 55 (3): 363–65.

Elenkov, I. J., D. G. Iessoni, A. Daly, A. G. Harris, and G. P. Chrousos. 2005. Cytokine Dysregulation, Inflammation and Well-Being." *Neuroimmunomodulation* 12 (5): 255–69.

Eliade, Mircea. 1969. *Yoga: Immortality and Freedom*. New York: Pantheon.

Elhassan, B., and S. P. Steinmann. 2007. "Entrapment Neuropathy of the Ulnar Nerve." *Journal of the American Academy of Orthopedic Surgeons* 15 (11): 672–81.

Elikkottil, J., P. Gupta, and K. Gupta. 2009. "The Analgesic Potential of Cannabinoids." *Journal of Opioid Management* 5: 341–57.

Ellman, Harvard, Gregory Hanker, and Michael Bayer. 1986. "Repair of the Rotator Cuff. End-Result Study of Factors Influencing Reconstruction." *Journal of Bone and Joint Surgery* (American) 68 (8): 1136–44.

Elster, Jon. 1983. *Explaining Technical Change: A Case Study in the Philosophy of Science*. Cambridge: Cambridge University Press.

Emerson, David. 2015. *Trauma-Sensitive Yoga: Bringing the Body into Treatment*. New York: W. W. Norton and Company.

Emerson, David, and Elizabeth Hopper. 2011. *Overcoming Trauma Through Yoga: Reclaiming Your Body*. Berkeley, CA: North Atlantic Books.

Emerson, David, R. Sharma, S. Chaudhry, and J. Turner. 2009. "Trauma-Sensitive Yoga: Principles, Practice, and Research." *International Journal of Yoga Therapy* 19: 123–28.

Er, Mehmet S., Mehmet Eroglu, and Levent Altinel. 2014. "Femoral Neck Stress Fracture in Children: A Case Report, Up-to-Date Review, and Diagnostic Algorithm." *Journal of Pediatric Orthopaedics B* 23 (2): 117–21.

Ernst, J. 1964. "Stress Fracture of the Neck of the Femur." *Journal of Trauma and Acute Care Surgery* 4 (1): 71–83.

Esola, M. A., P. W. McClure, G. K. Fitzpatrick, and S. Siegler. 1996. "Analysis of Lumbar Spine and Hip Motion During Forward Bending in Subjects with and Without a History of Low Back Pain." *Spine* 21 (1): 71–78.

Esposito, M. D., John A. Arrington, M. N. Blackshear, F. R. Murtagh, and M. L. Silbiger. 1997. "Thoracic Outlet Syndrome in a Throwing Athlete Diagnosed with MRI and MRA." *Journal of Magnetic Resonance Imaging* 7 (3): 598–99.

Estwanik, Joseph J., Beth Sloane, and Michael A. Rosenberg. 1990. "Groin Strain and Other Possible Causes of Groin Pain." *The Physician and Sports Medicine* 18 (2): 54–65.

Evans, P. D., C. Wilson, and K. Lyons. 1994. "Comparison of MRI with Bone Scanning for Suspected Hip Fracture in Elderly Patients." *Bone & Joint Journal* 76 (1): 158–59.

Ewald, Anthony. 2011. "Adhesive Capsulitis: A Review." *American Family Physician* 83 (4).

Eyre, H. A., B. Acevedo, H. Yang, P. Siddarth, K. Van Dyk, L. Ercoli, A. M. Leaver, et al. 2016. "Changes in Neural Connectivity and Memory Following a Yoga Intervention for Older Adults: A Pilot Study." *Journal of Alzheimer's Disease* 52 (2): 673–84.

Fairclough, J., K. Hayashi, H. Toumi, K. Lyons, G. Bydder, N. Phillips, T. M. Best, and M. Benjamin. 2007. "Is Band Syndrome Really a Friction Syndrome?" *Journal of Science and Medicine in Sport* 10 (2): 74–76.

Falvey, É. C., E. King, S. Kinsella, and A. Franklyn-Miller. 2015. "Athletic Groin Pain (Part 1): A Prospective Anatomical Diagnosis of 382 Patients—Clinical Findings, MRI Findings and Patient-Reported Outcome Measures at Baseline." *British Journal of Sports Medicine*. doi:10.1136/bjsports-2015-094912.

Farhadi, A., A. Keshavarzian, L. D. Van de Kar, S. Jakate, A. Domm, and L. Zhang. 2005. "Heightened Responses to Stressors in Patients with Inflammatory Bowel Disease." *American Journal of Gastroenterology* 100: 1796–804.

Farhi, Donna. 1996. *The Breathing Book: Good Health and Vitality Through Essential Breath Work*. New York: Henry Holt.

———. 2006. *Teaching Yoga: Exploring the Teacher-Student Relationship*. Berkeley, CA: Rodmell Press.

Farmer, Paul. 2003. *Pathologies of Power: Health, Human Rights, and the New War on the Poor*. Berkeley: University of California Press.

Fassaert, Thijs, Sandra van Dulmen, François Schellevis, and Jozien Bensing. 2007. "Active Listening in Medical Consultations: Development of the Active Listening Observation Scale (ALOS-global)." *Patient Education and Counseling* 68 (3): 258–64.

Ferrari, Fabrizio M. 2015. *Religion, Devotion and Medicine in North India. The Healing Power of Śītalā*. London: Bloomsbury.

Festinger, Leon. 1957. *A Theory of Cognitive Dissonance*. Stanford, CA: Stanford University Press.

Feuerstein, Georg. 2001. The *Yoga Tradition: Its History, Literature, Philosophy, and Practice*. Prescott, AZ: Hohm Press.

Field, Tiffany. 2001. *Touch*. Cambridge, MA: MIT Press.

———. 2003. *Touch Therapy*. Philadelphia: Churchill Livingstone.

Fife, T. D., D. Blum, and R. S. Fisher. 2006. "Measuring the Effects of Antiepileptic Medications on Balance in Older People." *Epilepsy Research* 70 (2–3): 103–9.

Fink, M., E. Wolkenstein, M. Karst, and A. Gehrke. 2002. "Acupuncture in Chronic Epicondylitis: A Randomized Controlled Trial." *Rheumatology* 41 (2): 205–9.

Fischer-Schreiber and Franz-Karl Ehrhard, Kurt Friedrichs, and Michael S. Diener. *Encyclopedia of Eastern Philosophy and Religion*. Boston: Shambhala, 1994.

Fishman, Loren M. 2014. *Healing Yoga: Proven Postures to Treat Twenty Common Ailments*. New York: W. W. Norton.

Fishman, Loren M., George W. Dombi, Christopher Michaelsen, Stephen Ringel, Jacob Rozbruch, Bernard Rosner, and Cheryl Weber. 2002. "Piriformis Syndrome: Diagnosis, Treatment, and Outcome—A 10-Year Study." *Archives of Physical Medicine and Rehabilitation* 83 (3): 295–301.

Fishman, Loren M., Erik J. Groessl, and Karen J. Sherman. 2014. "Serial Case Reporting Yoga for Idiopathic and Degenerative Scoliosis." *Global Advances in Health and Medicine* 3 (5): 16–21.

Fishman, Loren M., and Patricia A. Zybert. 1992. "Electrophysiologic Evidence of Piriformis Syndrome." *Archives of Physical Medicine and Rehabilitation* 73 (4): 359–64.

Flexner, Abraham. 1910. *Medical Education in the United States and Canada: A Report to the Carnegie Foundation for the Advancement of Teaching*. New York: The Carnegie Foundation for the Advancement of Teaching.

Floyd, R. T., and Clem W. Thompson. 2014. *Manual of Structural Kinesiology*. New York: McGraw-Hill Education.

Foley, Brian S., and Ralph M. Buschbacher. 2006. "Sacroiliac Joint Pain: Anatomy, Biomechanics, Diagnosis, and Treatment." *American Journal of Physical Medicine & Rehabilitation* 85 (12): 997–1006.

Fon, G. T., M. J. Pitt, and A. C. Thies Jr. 1980. "Thoracic Kyphosis: Range in Normal Subjects." *American Journal of Roentgenology* 134 (5): 979–83.

Fong, D. Y., C. F. Lee, K. M. Cheung, J. C. Cheng, B. K. Ng, T. P. Lam, K. H. Mak, P. S. Yip, and K. D. Luk. 2010. "A Meta-analysis of the Clinical Effectiveness of School Scoliosis Screening." *Spine* 35: 1061–71.

Forbes, Bo. 2011. *Yoga for Emotional Balance: Simple Practices to Help Relieve Anxiety and Depression*. Boston: Shambhala Publications.

Forbes, Bo, Fiona Akhtar, and Laura Douglass. 2011. "Training Issues in Yoga Therapy and Mental Health Treatment." *International Journal of Yoga Therapy* 21 (1): 7–11.

Ford, Earl S., Umed A. Ajani, Janet B. Croft, Julia A. Critchley, Darwin R. Labarthe, Thomas E. Kottke, Wayne H. Giles, and Simon Capewell. 2007. "Explaining the Decrease in U.S. Deaths from Coronary Disease, 1980–2000." *The New England Journal of Medicine* 356: 2388–98.

Fox, Kieran C., Savannah Nijeboer, Matthew L. Dixon, James L. Floman, Melissa Ellamil, Samuel P. Rumak, Peter Sedlmeier, and Kalina Christoff. 2014. "Is Meditation Associated with Altered Brain Structure? A Systematic Review and Meta-analysis of Morphometric Neuroimaging in Meditation Practitioners." *Neuroscience Biobehavioral Reviews* 43: 48–73.

Francina, Suzi. 2003. *Yoga and the Wisdom of Menopause: A Guide to Physical, Emotional, and Spiritual Health at Midlife and Beyond.* Deerfield Beach, FL: Health Communications.

Frawley, David. 1999. *Yoga and Ayurveda: Self-Healing and Self-Realization.* Twin Lakes, WI: Lotus Light Publishing.

Freckleton, Grant, and Tania Pizzari. 2012. "Risk Factors for Hamstring Muscle Strain Injury in Sport: A Systematic Review and Meta-analysis." *British Journal of Sports Medicine.* doi:10.1136/bjsports-2011-090664.

Fredericson, M., C. L. Cookingham, A. M. Chaudhari, B. C. Dowdell, N. Oestreicher, and S. A. Sahrmann. 2000. "Hip Abductor Weakness in Distance Runners with Iliotibial Band Syndrome." *Clinical Journal of Sport Medicine* 10 (3): 169–75.

Fredericson, Michael. 1996. "Common Injuries in Runners: Diagnosis, Rehabilitation and Prevention." *Sports Medicine* 21 (1): 49–72.

Freedman, Françoise Barbira. 2004. *Yoga for Pregnancy, Birth and Beyond.* London: Dorling Kindersley Ltd.

Freeman, Richard. 2010. *The Mirror of Yoga Awakening the Intelligence of Body and Mind.* 2nd ed. Boulder, CO: Shambhala Publications.

French, Roger Kenneth. 2003. *Medicine Before Science: The Rational and Learned Doctor from the Middle Ages to the Enlightenment.* Cambridge, UK: Cambridge University Press.

Frost, Harold M. 1994. "Wolff's Law and Bone's Structural Adaptations to Mechanical Usage: An Overview for Clinicians." *The Angle Orthodontist* 64 (3): 175–88.

Frymoyer, John W., and Nan P. Frymoyer. 2002. "Physician Patient Communication: A Lost Art?" *Journal of the American Academy of Orthopaedic Surgeons* 10 (2): 95–105.

Fujisawa, T., S. Takuma, H. Koseki, and K. Kimura. 2006. "Recovery of Intentional Dynamic Balance Function After Intravenous Sedation with Midazolam in Young and Elderly Subjects." *European Journal of Anaesthesiology* 23 (5): 1–4.

Furler, M. D., T. R. Einarson, M. Millson, S. Walmsley, and R. Bendayan. 2004. "Medicinal and Recreational Marijuana Use by Patients Infected with HIV." *AIDS Patient Care and STDs* 18: 215–28.

Gajdosik, R. L., M. M. Sandler, and H. L. Marr. 2003. "Influence of Knee Positions and Gender on the Ober Test for Length of the Iliotibial Band." *Clinical Biomechanics* 18 (1): 77–79.

Galley, J. D., and M. T. Bailey. 2014. "Impact of Stressor Exposure on the Interplay Between Commensal Microbiota and Host Inflammation." *Gut Microbe* 5: 748–60.

Gard T., J. J. Noggle, C. L. Park, D. R. Vago, and A. Wilson. 2014. "Potential Self-Regulatory Mechanisms of Yoga for Psychological Health." *Frontiers in Human Neuroscience* 8: 770.

Garra, G., A. J. Singer, R. Leno, B. R. Taira, N. Gupta, B. Mathaikutty, and H. J. Thode. 2010. "Heat or Cold Packs for Neck and Back Strain: A Randomized Controlled Trial of Efficacy." *Academic Emergency Medicine* 17 (5): 484–89.

Gartsman, Gary M. 1990. "Arthroscopic Acromioplasty for Lesions of the Rotator Cuff." *Journal of Bone and Joint Surgery* (American) 72 (2): 169–80.

Gaskin, Ina May. 2003. *Ina May's Guide to Childbirth*. New York: Bantam.

Gates, Janice. 2006. *Yogini: The Power of Women in Yoga*. San Rafael, CA: Mandala Publications.

Gerteis, Margaret, Susan Edgman-Levitan, Jennifer Daley, and Thomas L. Delbanco, eds. 1993. *Through the Patient's Eyes: Understanding and Promoting Patient-Centered Care*. San Francisco: Jossey-Bass.

Ghalioungui, Paul. 1965. *Magic and Medical Science in Ancient Egypt*. New York: Barnes and Noble.

Giangarra, C., G. Gallo, and R. Newman. 1987. "Endometriosis in the Biceps Femoris. A Case Report and Review of the Literature." *Journal of Bone and Joint Surgery* (American) 69 (2): 290–92.

Gilbert-Diamond, Diane, Li Zhigang, Anna M. Adachi-Mejia, Auden C. McClure, and James D. Sargent. 2014. "Association of a Television in the Bedroom with Increased Adiposity Gain in a Nationally Representative Sample of Children and Adolescents." *JAMA Pediatrics* 168 (5): 427–34.

Gloster H. M. Jr., and D. G. Brodland. 1996. "The Epidemiology of Skin Cancer." *Dermatological Surgery* 22: 217–26.

Goebel, Joel A., ed. 2008. *Practical Management of the Dizzy Patient*. Philadelphia: Lippincott Williams and Wilkins.

Goh, S., R. I. Price, P. J. Leedman, and K. P. Singer. 1999. "The Relative Influence of Vertebral Body and Intervertebral Disc Shape on Thoracic Kyphosis." *Clinical Biomechanics* 14: 439–48.

Gollwitzer, H., P. Diehl, A. von Korff, V. W. Rahlfs, and L. Gerdesmeyer. 2007. "Extra-corporeal Shock Wave Therapy for Chronic Painful Heel Syndrome: A Prospective, Double Blind, Randomized Trial Assessing the Efficacy of a New Electromagnetic Shock Wave Device." *Journal of Foot and Ankle Surgery* 46 (5): 348–57.

Gomez-Pinilla, F., and A. G. Gomez. 2011. "The Influence of Dietary Factors in Central Nervous System Plasticity and Injury Recovery." *American Academy of Physical Medicine and Rehabilitation* 3 (6 0 1): 111–16.

Good, Byron J. 1994. *Medicine, Rationality and Experience: An Anthropological Perspective.* New York: Cambridge University Press.

Goosen, Jon H. M., Boudewijn J. Kollen, René M. Castelein, Bart M. Kuipers, and Cees C. Verheyen. 2011. "Minimally Invasive Versus Classic Procedures in Total Hip Arthroplasty: A Double-Blind Randomized Controlled Trial." *Clinical Orthopaedics and Related Research* 469 (1): 200–8.

Gorman, Kristen Fay, Cédric Julien, and Alain Moreau. 2012. "The Genetic Epidemiology of Idiopathic Scoliosis." *European Spine Journal* 21 (10): 1905–19.

Grad, Frank P. 2002. "The Preamble of the Constitution of the World Health Organization." *Bulletin of the World Health Organization* 80 (12).

Greenblatt, Stephen. 2011. *The Swerve: How the World Became Modern.* New York: W. W. Norton and Company.

Greendale, G.A., M. H. Huang, A. S. Karlamangla, L. Seeger, and S. Crawford. 2009. "Yoga Decreases Kyphosis in Senior Women and Men with Adult-Onset Hyperkyphosis: Results of a Randomized Controlled Trial." *Journal of the American Geriatrics Society* 57: 1569–79.

Greendale, Gail A., Anna McDivit, Leanne Seeger, and Mai-Hua Huang. 2002. "Yoga for Women with Hyperkyphosis: Results of a Pilot Study." *American Journal of Public Health* 92: 1611–14.

Greil A. L., T. A. Leitko, and K. L. Porter. 1988. "Infertility: His and Hers." *Gender and Society* 2: 172–99.

Grover R. 1996. "Clinical Assessment of Scaphoid Injuries and the Detection of Fractures." *Journal of Hand Surgery* (Britain) 21 (3): 341–43.

Gumina, Stefano, Giantony Di Giorgio, Franco Postacchini, and Roberto Postacchini. 2008. "Subacromial Space in Adult Patients with Thoracic Hyperkyphosis and in Healthy Volunteers." *La Chirurgia Degli Organi di Movimento* 91 (2): 93–96.

Guo, X., W. W. Chau, C. W. Hui-Chan, C. S. Cheung, W. W. Tsang, and J. C. Cheng. 2006. "Balance Control in Adolescents with Idiopathic Scoliosis and Disturbed Somatosensory Function." *Spine* 31 (14): E437–40.

Guvencer, M., C. Iyem, P. Akyer, S. Tetik, and S. Naderi. 2009. "Variations in the High Division of the Sciatic Nerve and Relationship Between the Sciatic Nerve and the Piriformis." *Turkish Neurosurgery* 2: 139–44.

Hadjipavlou, A. G., M. N. Tzermiadianos, N. Bogduk, and M. R. Zindrick. 2008. "The Pathophysiology of Disc Degeneration: A Critical Review." *Journal of Bone and Joint Surgery* (American) 90: 1261.

Haefeli et al. 2006. 15–22.

Hankinson, R. James. 1991. "Galen's Anatomy of the Soul." *Phronesis* 36 (2): 197–233.

Hanna, Thomas. 2004. *Somatics: Reawakening the Mind's Control of Movement, Flexibility, and Health.* Cambridge, MA: Da Capo Press.

Hariri, Sanaz, Edgar T. Savidge, Michael M. Reinold, James Zachazewski, and Thomas J. Gill. 2009. "Treatment of Recalcitrant Iliotibial Band Friction Syndrome with Open Iliotibial Band Bursectomy Indications, Technique, and Clinical Outcomes." *American Journal of Sports Medicine* 37 (7): 1417–24.

Harvey, Paul. 2015. "What Is the Yoga of Viniyoga?" www.yogastudies.org/art-personal-sadhana-overview/personal-lessons/viniyoga/.

Hately, Susi Aldous. 2004. *Anatomy and Asana: Preventing Yoga Injuries.* Calgary, Canada: Functional Synergy.

Hatze, Herbert. 1974. "The Meaning of the Term 'Biomechanics.'" *Journal of Biomechanics* 7 (2): 189–90.

Haumont, T., G. C. Gauchard, P. Lascombes, and P. P. Perrin. 2011. "Postural Instability in Early-Stage Idiopathic Scoliosis in Adolescent Girls." *Spine* 36: 847–54.

2017. "Health." *Wiktionary: The Free Dictionary.* https://en.wiktionary.org/wiki/health.

Wiktorsson-Moller, Margareta, Birgitta Öberg, Jan Ekstrand, and Jan Gillquist. 1983.

Heckman, James D., and Walter D. Greene, eds. 1994. *The Clinical Measurement of Joint Motion.* Resonant, IL: American Academy of Orthopaedic Surgeons.

Heller, M. 2006. "Sacroiliac Instability: An Overview." *Dynamic Chiropractic* 24 (21).

Herquelot, E., A. Guéguen, Y. Roquelaure, J. Bodin, C. Sérazin, C. Ha, A. Leclrec, M. Goldberg, M. Zins, and A. Descatha. 2013. "Work-Related Risk Factors for Incidence of Lateral Epicondylitis in a Large Working Population." *Scandinavian Journal of Work, Environment & Health.* 39 (6): 578–88.

Hirschi, Gertrud. 2000. *Mudras: Yoga in Your Hands.* Newburyport, MA: Weiser Books.

Hirshkowitz, M. I. Karacan, J. W. Howell, M. O. Arcasoy, and R. L. Williams. 1992. "Nocturnal Penile Tumescence in Cigarette Smokers with Erectile Dysfunction." *Urology* 34: 101–7.

Hoernle, A. F. Rudolf. 1987. *The Bower Manuscript.* Facsimile leaves, Nagari transcript, Romanized transliteration and English translation with notes (Calcutta: Supt., Govt. Print., India, 1908–1912). Reprint, New Delhi: Aditya Prakashan.

Höfle, Dipl-Psych Marion, Michael Hauck, Andreas K. Engel, and Daniel Senkowski. 2010. "Pain Processing in Multisensory Environments." *e-Neuroforum* 1 (2): 23–28.

Hofmann, S. G., A. T. Sawyer, A. A. Witt, D. Oh. 2010. "The Effect of Mindfulness-Based Therapy on Anxiety and Depression: A Meta-analytic Review." *Journal of Consulting and Clinical Psychology* 78 (2): 169–83.

Høglend, Randi, Svein Amlo, Anne Grete Hersoug, Hanne-Sofia Johnsen Dahl, and Per Høglend. 2014. "The Effects of the Therapist's Disengaged Feelings on the In-Session Process in Psychodynamic Psychotherapy." *Journal of Clinical Psychology* 70 (5): 440–51.

Holleman, Dona, and Orit Sen-Gupta. 1999. *Dancing the Body Light: The Future of Yoga*. New York: Pegasus.

Hong, Quan Nha, Marie-José Durand, and Patrick Loisel. 2004. "Treatment of Lateral Epicondylitis: Where Is the Evidence?" *Joint Bone Spine* 71 (5): 369–73.

Howell, Jonathan R., Bassam A. Masri, and Clive P. Duncan. 2004. "Minimally Invasive Versus Standard Incision Anterolateral Hip Replacement: A Comparative Study." *Orthopedic Clinics of North America* 35 (2): 153–62.

Hrysomallis, Con. 2009. "Hip Adductors' Strength, Flexibility, and Injury Risk." *Journal of Strength and Conditioning Research* 23 (5): 1514–17.

Huang, Jason H., and Eric L. Zager. 2004. "Thoracic Outlet Syndrome." *Neurosurgery* 55 (4): 897–903.

Hulette, C., K. Welsh-Bohmer, M. Murray, A. Saunders, D. Mash, and L. Mcintyre. 1998. "Neuropathological and Neuropsychological Changes in 'Normal' Aging: Evidence for Preclinical Alzheimer Disease in Cognitively Normal Individuals." *Journal of Neuropathology Experimental Neurology* 57: 1168–74.

Hurley, Dan. 2006. *Natural Causes: Death, Lies, and Politics in America's Vitamin and Herbal Supplement Industry*. New York: Broadway Books.

Husarik, D.B., Nadja Saupe, Christian W. A. Pfirrmann, Bernhard Jost, Juerg Hodler, and Marco Zanetti. 2009. "Elbow Nerves: MR Findings in 60 Asymptomatic Subjects—Normal Anatomy, Variants, and Pitfalls." *Radiology* 252 (1): 148–56.

IAYT. 2012. "Educational Standards for the Training of Yoga Therapists," *Journal of the International Association of Yoga Therapists*, July 1, 4.

———. 2016. "Educational Standards for the Training of Yoga Therapists," *Journal of the International Association of Yoga Therapists*, August 1, 7.

Iio, Wataru, Haruyoshi Takagi, Yasuki Ogawa, Takamitsu Tsukahara, Shigeru Chohnan, and Atsushi Toyoda. 2014. "Effects of Chronic Social Defeat Stress on Peripheral Leptin and Its Hypothalamic Actions." *BMC Neuroscience* 15: 72.

Infusino, M. H., D. Win, and Y. V. O'Neill. 1965. "Mondino's Book and the Human Body." *Vesalius* 1 (2): 71–76.

Ingari, J. V. 2009. "The Adult Wrist." In *DeLee and Drez's Orthopaedic Sports Medicine*, edited by J. C. DeLee, D. Drez, and M. D. Miller. 3rd ed. Philadelphia: Saunders.

Institute of Medicine (U. S.) Committee on Quality Health Care in America. 2001. *Crossing the Quality Chasm: A New Health System for the 21st Century.* Washington, D. C.: National Academies Press.

Irwin, T. A. 2014. "Tendon Injuries of the Foot and Ankle." In *DeLee and Drez's Orthopaedic Sports Medicine*, edited by M. D. Miller and S. R. Thompson. 4th ed. Philadelphia: Elsevier Saunders.

Itoi, E., and M. Sinaki. 1994. "Effect of Back-Strengthening Exercise on Posture in Healthy Women 49 to 65 Years of Age." *Mayo Clinic Proceedings* 69: 1054–59.

Iyengar, B. K. S. 1966. *Light on Yoga.* New York: Schockten.

———. 1985. *Light on Pranayama: The Yogic Art of Breathing.* New York: Crossroad.

———. 2001. *Yoga: The Path to Holistic Health.* London: Dorling Kindersley.

———. 2009. *Yoga Wisdom and Practice.* London: Dorling Kindersley.

Iyengar, Geeta S. 2002. *Yoga: A Gem for Women.* Kootenay, BC: Timeless Books.

IYSF. 2014. International Yoga Sports Federation. www.iysf.org.

Jackson J. S., M. Torres, C. H. Caldwell, H. W. Neighbors, R. M. Nesse, R. J. Taylor, S. J. Trierweiler, and D. R. Williams. 2004. "The National Survey of American Life: A Study of Racial, Ethnic and Cultural Influences on Mental Disorders and Mental Health." *International Journal of Methods in Psychiatric Research* 13: 196–207.

Jacobi F., H. U. Wittchen, C. Holting, M. Hofler, H. Pfister, N. Muller, R. Lieb. 2004. "Prevalence, Co-morbidity and Correlates of Mental Disorders in the General Population: Results from the German Health Interview and Examination Survey (GHS)." *Psychological Medicine* 34: 597–611.

Jacobson, I. G., M. R. White, and T. C. Smith. 2009. "Self-Reported Health Symptoms and Conditions Among Complementary and Alternative Medicine Users in a Large Military Cohort." *Annals of Epidemiology* 19: 613–22.

Jain, T. et al. 2002. "Insurance Coverage and Outcomes of in vitro Fertilization." *New England Journal of Medicine* 347: 661–66.

Jalabert-Malbos, M. L., A. Mishellany-Dutour, A. Woda, and M. A. Peyton. 2007. "Particle Size Distribution in the Food Bolus After Mastication of Natural Foods." *Food Quality Preferences* 18: 803–12.

James, William. *The Principles of Psychology.* (1890) 1952. New York: Dover Publications.

Jansson, M., and S. J. Linton. 2006. "The Role of Anxiety and Depression in the Development of Insomnia: Cross-Sectional and Prospective Analyses." *Psychological Health* 21: 383–97.

Jao T., C. W. Li, P. E. Vértes, C. W. Wu, S. Achard, C. H. Hsieh, C. H. Liou, J. H. Chen, and E. T. Bullmore. 2016. "Large-Scale Functional Brain Network Reorganization During Taoist Meditation." *Brain Connectivity* 6 (1): 9–24.

Järvinen, T. A., T. L. Järvinen, M. Kääriänen, H. Kalimo, and M. Järvinen. 2005. "Muscle Injuries Biology and Treatment." *The American Journal of Sports Medicine* 33 (5): 745–64.

Jenkins, Philip. 1999. *Synthetic Panics: The Symbolic Politics of Designer Drugs.* New York: NYU Press.

Jensen, T. K., R. Jacobsen, K. Christensen, N. C. Nielsen, and E. Bostofte. 2009. "Good Semen Quality and Life Expectancy: A Cohort Study of 43,277 Men." *American Journal of Epidemiology* 170: 559–65.

Jepsen, J., L. Laursen, A. Larsen, and C. G. Hagert. 2004. "Manual Strength Testing in 14 Upper Limb Muscles: A Study of Inter-rater Reliability." *Acta Orthopaedica Scandinavica* 75 (4).

Jiffry, M. T. 1981. "Analysis of Particles Produced at the End of Mastication in Subjects with Normal Dentition." *Journal of Oral Rehabilitation* 8: 113–19.

Johnson, D. K., M. Storandt, J. C. Morris, and J. E. Galvin. 2009. "Longitudinal Study of the Transition from Healthy Aging to Alzheimer's Disease." *Archives of Neurology* 66 (10): 1254–59.

Johnson, Don, ed. 1995. *Bone, Breath & Gesture: Practices of Embodiment.* Vol. 1. Berkeley, CA: North Atlantic Books.

Johnson, Jeffrey G., Patricia Cohen, Stephanie Kasen, and Judith S. Brook. 2007. "Extensive Television Viewing and the Development of Attention and Learning Difficulties During Adolescence." *Archives of Pediatrics and Adolescent Medicine* 161 (5): 480–86.

Johnson, Mark. 1989. *The Meaning of the Body: Aesthetics of Human Understanding.* Chicago: University of Chicago Press.

———. 1995. *The Body in the Mind: The Bodily Basis of Meaning, Imagination, and Reason.* Chicago: University of Chicago Press.

Johnson, N. P., and L. Hummelshoj. 2013. "Consensus on Current Management of Endometriosis." *Human Reproduction* 28: 1552–68.

Joo, E. Y., H. J. Noh, and J. S. Kim. 2013. "Brain Gray Matter Deficits in Patients with Chronic Primary Insomnia." *Sleep* 36 (7): 999–1007.

Jung, Carl. 1953. "Yoga and the West." In *The Collected Works of Carl Jung*, edited by Herbert Read, Michael Fordham, and Gerard Adler. Vol 1. New York: Bollingen.

Kabat-Zinn, Jon. 1982. "An Outpatient Program in Behavioral Medicine for Chronic Pain Patients Based on the Practice of Mindfulness Meditation: Theoretical Considerations and Preliminary Results." *General Hospital Psychiatry* 4: 33–47.

———. 1994. *Wherever You Go, There You Are.* New York: Hyperion.

Kabat-Zinn, Jon, L. Lipworth, R. Burney, and W. Sellers. 1987. "Four-Year Follow-Up of a Meditation-Based Program for the Self-Regulation of Chronic Pain: Treatment Outcomes and Compliance." *The Clinical Journal of Pain* 3 (1): 60.

Kaleli, Tufan, Cagatay Ozturk, Aytun Temiz, and Onur Tirelioglu. 2004. "Surgical Treatment of Tennis Elbow: Percutaneous Release of the Common Extensor Origin." *Acta Orthopaedica Belgica* 70 (2): 131–33.

Kalscheur, Jean A., Patricia S. Costello, and Lynnda J. Emery. 2003. "Gender Differences in Range of Motion in Older Adults." *Physical and Occupational Therapy in Geriatrics* 22 (1).

Kamen, Gary. 2004. "Electromyographic Kinesiology." In *Research Methods in Biomechanics*, edited by Gordon Robertson, Graham Caldwell, Joseph Hamill, Gary Kamen, and Saunders Whittlesey. Champaign, IL: Human Kinetics Publications.

Kaminoff, Leslie, and Amy Matthews. 2012. *Yoga Anatomy*. 2nd ed. Champaign, IL: Human Kinetics.

Kamp, Carolin Friederike, Billy Sperlich, and Hans Christer Holmberg. 2014. "Exercise Reduces the Symptoms of Attention Deficit/Hyperactivity Disorder and Improves Social Behaviour, Motor Skills, Strength and Neuropsychological Parameters." *Acta Paediatrica* 103 (7): 709–14.

Katz, A. M. 2010. *Physiology of the Heart*. 5th ed. Philadephia: Lippincott Williams & Wilkins.

Katzman, W. B., L. Wanek, J. A. Shepherd, and D. E. Sellmeyer. 2010. "Age-Related Hyperkyphosis: Its Causes, Consequences, and Management." *Journal of Orthopaedic and Sports Physical Therapy* 40 (6): 352–60.

Keedwell, Paul. 2008. *How Sadness Survived: The Evolutionary Basis of Depression*. London: Radcliffe Publishing.

Keleman, Stanley. 1985. *Emotional Anatomy: The Structure of Experience*. Berkeley, CA: Center Press.

Keller, Doug. 2013. "Yoga for Your Aching Feet." *Yoga International*, June. https://yogainternational.com/article/view/yoga-for-your-aching-feet.

Keller, Timothy A., and Marcel Adam Just. 2016. "Structural and Functional Neuroplasticity in Human Learning of Spatial Routes." *NeuroImage* 125: 256–66.

Kempton, Sally. 2011. *Meditation for the Love of It: Enjoying Your Own Deepest Experience*. Boulder, CO: Sounds True.

———. 2013. *Awakening Shakti: The Transformative Power of the Goddesses of Yoga*. Louisville, CO: Sounds True.

Kendall, H. O., and F. M. P. Kendall. 1949. *Muscles: Testing and Function*. Baltimore: Williams and Wilkins.

Kennon, Robert, John Keggi, Laurine E. Zatorski, and Kristaps J. Keggi. 2004. "Anterior Approach for Total Hip Arthroplasty: Beyond the Minimally Invasive Technique." *Journal of Bone and Joint Surgery* (American) 86 (2): 91–97.

Kenny, M. A., and J. M. G. Williams. 2007. "Treatment-Resistant Depressed Patients Show a Good Response to Mindfulness-Based Cognitive Therapy." *Behaviour Research and Therapy* 45: 617–25.

Kenny, R. A., G. B. Traynor, D. Withington, and D. J. Keegan. 1993. "Thoracic Outlet Syndrome: A Useful Exercise Treatment Option." *American Journal of Surgery* 165 (2): 282–84.

Kessler, R. C., J. Soukup, and R. B. Davi. 2001. "The Use of Complementary and Alternative Therapies to Treat Anxiety and Depression in the United States." American Journal of Psychiatry 158 (2): 289–94.

Khalsa, Sat Bir, Lorenzo Cohen, Timothy McCall, and Shirley Telles. 2016. *Principles and Practice of Yoga in Health Care*. Scotland, UK: Handspring Publishing.

Kibler, W. Ben. 1998. "The Role of the Scapula in Athletic Shoulder Function." *American Journal of Sports Medicine* 26 (2): 325–37.

Kim, H. Mike, Sharlene A. Teefey, Ari Zelig, Leesa M. Galatz, Jay D. Keener, and Ken Yamaguchi. 2009. "Shoulder Strength in Asymptomatic Individuals with Intact Compared with Torn Rotator Cuffs." *Journal of Bone and Joint Surgery* (American) 91 (2): 289–96.

King, Douglas S., David L. Costill, William J. Fink, Mark Hargreaves, and Roger A. Fielding. 1985. "Muscle Metabolism During Exercise in the Heat in Unacclimatized and Acclimatized Humans." *Journal of Applied Physiology* 59 (5): 1350–54.

Kingston T., B. Dooley, A. Bates, E. Lawlor, K. Malone. 2007. "Mindfulness-Based Cognitive Therapy for Residual Depressive Symptoms." *Psychology and Psychotherapy: Theory, Research and Practice* 80: 193–203.

Kinser, P. A., R. K. Elswick, and S. Kornstein. 2014. "Potential Long-Term Effects of a Mind-Body Intervention for Women with Major Depressive Disorder: Sustained Mental Health Improvements with a Pilot Yoga Intervention." *Archives of Psychiatric Nursing* 28 (6): 377–83.

Kinser, P. A., L. Goehler, and A. G. Taylor. 2012. "How Might Yoga Help Depression? A Neurobiological Perspective." *Explore* 8 (2), 118–26.

Kirk, G. S., J. E. Raven, and M. Schofield. 1984. "Anaximenes of Miletus." *The Presocratic Philosophers*. Cambridge: Cambridge University Press.

Kirkaldy-Willis, H. William, and Thomas N. Bernard Jr., eds. 1999. "Making a Specific Diagnosis" In *Managing Low Back Pain*, 206–26. Philadelphia: Churchill Livingstone.

Klabunde, Richard E. 2005. *Cardiovascular Physiology Concepts*. Philadelphia: Lippincott Williams and Wilkins.

Kleinman, Arthur, and Joan Kleinman. 2011. "Suffering and Its Professional Transformation: Toward an Ethnography of Interpersonal Experience." *Culture, Medicine and Psychiatry* 15: 275–301.

Koester, M. C., M. S. George, and J. E. Kuhn. 2005. "Shoulder Impingement Syndrome." *American Journal of Medicine* 118 (5): 452–55.

Kohn, George C. 2008. *Encyclopedia of Plague and Pestilence: From Ancient Times to the Present*. New York: Facts on File.

Kolettis, P. N., and E. S. Sabanegh. 2001. "Significant Medical Pathology Discovered During a Male Infertility Evaluation." *Journal of Urology* 166: 178–80.

Kong, F., and R. P. Singh. 2008. "Disintegration of Solid Foods in Human Stomach." *Journal of Food Science* 73: R67–80.

Korkola, Michael, and Annunziato Amendola. 2001. "Exercise-Induced Leg Pain: Sifting Through a Broad Differential." *The Physician and Sportsmedicine* 29 (6): 35–50.

Kornfield, Jack. 1993. *The Path with Heart: A Guide Through the Perils and Promises of Spiritual Life.* New York: Bantam Books.

———. 2009. *The Wise Heart: A Guide to the Universal Teachings of Buddhist Psychology.* New York: Bantam Books.

Kouwenhoven, J. W., and R. M. Castelein. 2008. "The Pathogenesis of Adolescent Idiopathic Scoliosis: Review of the Literature." *Spine* 33: 2898–2908.

Knopman, D. S., et al. "Short-Term Clinical Outcomes for Stages of NIA-AA Preclinical Alzheimer Disease." *Neurology* 78 (20): 1576–82.

Kraftsow, Gary. 1999. *Yoga for Wellness: Healing with the Timeless Teachings of Viniyoga.* New York: The Penguin Group.

———. 2002. *Yoga for Transformation: Ancient Teachings and Practices for Healing the Body, Mind, and Heart.* New York: The Penguin Group.

———. 2014. "The Differences Between Yoga Teacher Training Programs and Yoga Therapist Training Programs." *International Journal of Yoga Therapy* 24 (1): 15–16.

Kramer, Joel. 1977. "A New Look at Yoga: Playing the Edge of Mind and Body." *Yoga Journal*, January.

———. 1980. "Yoga as Self-Transformation." *Yoga Journal*, May/June.

Kramer, Joel, and Diana Alstad. 1993. *The Guru Papers: Masks of Authoritarian Power.* Mumbai: Frog Books.

———. 2009. *The Passionate Mind Revisited: Expanding Personal and Social Awareness.* Berkeley, CA: North Atlantic Books.

Kraushaar, Barry S., and Robert P. Nirschl. 1999. "Tendinosis of the Elbow (Tennis Elbow): Clinical Features and Findings of Histological, Immunohistochemical, and Electron Microscopy Studies." *Journal of Bone and Joint Surgery* (American) 81 (2): 259.

Krentzman, Rachel. 2016. *Scoliosis, Yoga Therapy, and the Art of Letting Go.* Philadelphia: Singing Dragon.

Krishnamurti, Jiddu. *Total Freedom: The Essential Krishnamurti.* New York: HarperCollins, 1996.

———. *The Awakening of Intelligence.* New York: HarperCollins, 1987.

Kucinskas, L., and Walter Just. 2004. "Human Male Sex Determination and Sexual Differentiation: Pathways, Molecular Interactions and Genetic Disorders." *Medicina* 41 (8): 633–40.

Kuhn, John E. 2009. "Exercise in the Treatment of Rotator Cuff Impingement: A Systematic Review and a Synthesized Evidence-Based Rehabilitation Protocol." *Journal of Shoulder and Elbow Surgery* 18 (1): 138–60.

Kuhn, John E., George F. Lebus, and Jesse E. Bible. 2015. "Thoracic Outlet Syndrome." *Journal of the American Academy of Orthopaedic Surgeons* 23 (4): 222–32.

Kuhn, Thomas. 1996. *The Structure of Scientific Revolutions.* Chicago: University of Chicago Press.

Kutumbiah, P. 1969. *Ancient Indian Medicine.* Bombay: Orient Longmans.

Kuutmann, Klara, and Mark J. Hilsenroth. 2012. "Exploring In-Session Focus on the Patient–Therapist Relationship: Patient Characteristics, Process and Outcome." *Clinical Psychology & Psychotherapy* 19 (3): 187–202.

Kwak, Hyo-Sung, Kwang-Bok Lee, and Young-Min Han. 2006. "Ruptures of the Medial Head of the Gastrocnemius ('Tennis Leg'): Clinical Outcome and Compression Effect." *Clinical Imaging* 30 (1): 48–53.

Lad, Vasant. 1985. *Ayurveda: The Science of Self-healing.* Twin Lakes, WI: Lotus.

———. 2001. *Textbook of Ayurveda. Volume 1: Fundamental Principles of Ayurveda.* Albuquerque, NM: The Ayurvedic Press.

Lakoff, George, and Mark Johnson. 1999. *Philosophy in the Flesh: The Embodied Mind and Its Challenge to Western Thought.* New York: Basic Books.

Lamb, R. I. 1985. "Manual Muscle Testing." In *Measurement in Physical Therapy*, edited by J. M. Rothstein. New York: Churchill Livingstone.

Lambert, Francios M., David Malinvaud, Joan Glaunès, Catherine Bergot, Hans Straka, and Pierre-Paul Vidal. 2009. "Vestibular Asymmetry as the Cause of Idiopathic Scoliosis: A Possible Answer from Xenopus." *Journal of Neuroscience* 29 (40): 12477–83.

Lang, F., M. R. Floyd, and K. L. Beine. 2000. "Clues to Patients' Explanations and Concerns About Their Illnesses: A Call for Active Listening." *Archives of Family Medicine* 9 (3): 222–27.

Lao-Tzu. *Tao Te Ching.* New York: Dover Publications, 1995 (1891).

Lappe, Francis Moore. 1971. *Diet for a Small Planet.* New York: Random House.

Larson, G. J., and Ram Shankar Bhattacharya, eds. 2008. "Yoga: India's Philosophy of Meditation." In *Encyclopedia of Indian Philosophy*, series edited by Karl Potter. Vol. 12. Delhi: Motilal Banarsidass Publishers.

Lasater, Judith. 2009. *Yoga Body: Anatomy, Kinesiology, and Asana.* Berkeley, CA: Rodmell.

———. 2012. "How to Deal with SI Joint Discomfort." *Yoga Journal.* www.yogajournal.com/article/practice-section/out-of-joint-2/.

Laurence, Scott. 2010. "The Role of Outcome-Based Standards in Yoga Therapy." *International Journal of Yoga Therapy* 20: 65–71.

Lazaro, R. 1997. "Neuropathic Symptoms and Musculoskeletal Pain in Carpal Tunnel Syndrome: Prognostic and Therapeutic Implications." *Surgical Neurology* 47 (2): 115–17.

The Leapfrog Group. 2015. "Enhanced Hospital Safety Score Helps Patients Track U.S. Hospitals' Consistency in Preventing Harm." *Leapfrog Hospital Safety Grade.* www.hospitalsafetyscore.org/about-us/newsroom/display/46972.

Lee, Na Kyung, Hideaki Sowa, Eiichi Hinoi, Mathieu Ferron, Jong Deok Ahn, Cyrille Confavreux, and Romain Dacquin. 2007. "Endocrine Regulation of Energy Metabolism by the Skeleton." *Cell* 130 (3): 456–469.

Lerner, Aaron B., James D. Case, and Yoshiyata Takahashi. 1960. "Isolation of Melatonin and 5-Methoxyindole-3-acetic Acid from Bovine Pineal Glands." *The Journal of Biological Chemistry* 235 (7)

Lerner, Michael. 1996. *Choices in Healing: Integrating the Best of Conventional and Complementary Approaches to Cancer.* Boston: MIT Press.

Levine, Peter. 2010. *In an Unspoken Voice: How the Body Releases Trauma and Restores Goodness.* Berkeley, CA: North Atlantic Books.

Levine, Peter, and Ian Macnaughton. 2004. "Breath and Consciousness: Reconsidering the Viability of Breathwork in Psychological and Spiritual Interventions in Human Development." In *Body, Breath, and Consciousness: A Somatics Anthology*, edited by Ian Macnaughton. Berkeley: North Atlantic Books.

Liedert, Astrid, Daniela Kaspar, Peter Augat, Anita Ignatius, and Lutz Claes. 2005. *Mechanobiology of Bone Tissue and Bone Cells.* Moscow: Academia.

Lilienfeld, Abraham M., Miriam Jacobs, and Myron Willis. 1954. "A Study of the Reproducibility of Muscle Testing and Certain Other Aspects of Muscle Scoring." *Physical Therapy Review* 34 (6): 279–89.

Linenger, J. M., and C. P. Christensen. 1992. "Is Iliotibial Band Syndrome Often Overlooked?" *Physician and Sportsmedicine* 20 (2): 98–108.

Lippitt, A. B. 1995. "Percutaneous Fixation of the Sacroiliac Joint." In *The Integrated Function of the Lumbar Spine and Sacroiliac Joint.* Vleeming, A. et al. Rotterdam: European Conference Organizers: 369–90.

Lis, R., A. Rowhani-Rahba, and L. E. Manhart. 2015. "Mycoplasma Genitalium Infection and Female Reproductive Tract Disease: A Meta-Analysis." *Clinical Infectious Diseases* 61: 418–26.

Livshits, A., and D. S. Seidman. 2009. "Fertility Issues in Women with Diabetes." *Womens Health* (British) 5 (6): 701–7.

Lizardi, J. Enrique, Leslie I. Wolfson, and Robert H. Whipple. 1989. "Review Article: Neurological Dysfunction in the Elderly Prone to Fall." *Neurorehabilitation and Neural Repair* 3 (3): 113–6.

Lo, Charmaine B., Molly E. Waring, Sherry L. Pagoto, and Stephanie C. Lemon. 2015. "A Television in the Bedroom Is Associated with Higher Weekday Screen Time Among Youth with Attention Deficit Hyperactivity Disorder (ADD/ADHD)." *Preventive Medicine Reports* 2: 1–3.

Loftice, J., G. S. Fleisig, N. Zheng, and J. R. Andrews. 2004. "Biomechanics of the Elbow in Sports." *Clinics in Sports Medicine* 23 (4): 519–30.

Long, Ray. 2009. *The Key Muscles of Yoga: Scientific Keys.* Vol. I. Plattsburgh, NY: Bandha Yoga.

———. 2010. *The Key Poses of Yoga: Scientific Keys.* Vol. II. Plattsburgh, NY: Bandha Yoga.

Lorant V., D. Deliege, W. Eaton, A. Robert, P. Philippot, and M. Ansseau. 2003. "Socioeconomic Inequalities in Depression: A Meta-analysis." *American Journal of Epidemiology* 157: 98–112.

Lorr, Benjamin. 2012. *Hell-Bent: Obsession, Pain, and the Search for Something Like Transcendence in Competitive Yoga.* London: Macmillan Publishers.

Lovett, Robert Williamson. 1917. *The Treatment of Infantile Paralysis.* Philadelphia: P. Blakiston's Son & Company.

Lowinson, Joyce H., Pedro Ruiz, Robert B. Millman, and John G. Langrod, eds. 2005. *Substance Abuse: A Comprehensive Textbook.* 4th ed. Philadelphia: Lippincott Williams and Wilkins.

Lu, Yaogang, Lei Wang, Yongqiang Hao, Ziping Wang, Minghui Wang, and Shengfang Ge. 2013. "Analysis of Trabecular Distribution of the Proximal Femur in Patients with Fragility Fractures." *BMC Musculoskeletal Disorders* 14 (1): 130.

Lucretius, Titus Carus. 2007. *On the Nature of Things.* Translated by A. E. Stallings. London: Penguin.

Luders, Ellen. 2014. "Exploring Age-Related Brain Degeneration in Meditation Practitioners." *Annals of the New York Academy of Science* 1307: 82–88.

Ly, Thuan V., and Marc F. Swiontkowski. 2008. "Treatment of Femoral Neck Fractures in Young Adults." *Journal of Bone and Joint Surgery* (American) 90 (10): 2254–66.

MacIntosh, Brian R., Phillip F. Gardiner, and Alan J. McComas. 2006. *Skeletal Muscle: Form and Function.* Champaign, IL: Human Kinetics.

Mackenzie, Elizabeth R., and Birgit Rakel. 2006. *Complementary and Alternative Medicine for Older Adults: A Guide to Holistic Approaches to Healthy Aging.* New York: Springer Pub.

MacLennan, A. H., and S. C. MacLenna. 1997. "Symptom-Giving Pelvic Girdle Relaxation of Pregnancy, Postnatal Pelvic Joint Syndrome and Developmental Dysplasia of Hip." *Acta Obstetrica et Gynecoligica Scandanavica* 76 (8): 760–64.

Macnaughton, Ian. 2004. *Body, Breath, and Consciousness: A Somatics Anthology*. Berkeley: North Atlantic Books.

Madan V., P. Hoban, R. C. Strange, A. A. Fryer, and J. T. Lear. 2006. "Genetics and Risk Factors for Basal Cell Carcinoma." *British Journal of Dermatology* 154 (Suppl 1): 5–7.

Madea B., and M. Rothschild. 2010. "The Post Mortem External Examination: Determination of the Cause and Manner of Death." *Deutsches Ärzteblatt* 107: 575–86.

Majno, Guido. 1975. *The Healing Hand: Man and Wound in the Ancient World*. Boston: Harvard University Press.

Malinar, Angelika, trans. 2008. *The Bhagavadgita: Doctrines and Contexts*. Cambridge: Cambridge University Press.

Maman, E., C. Harris, L. White, G. Tomlinson, M. Shashank, and Boynton. 2009. "Outcome of Nonoperative Treatment of Symptomatic Rotator Cuff Tears Monitored by Magnetic Resonance Imaging." *Journal of Bone and Joint Surgery* (American) 91 (8): 1898–1906.

Manniche, C., K. Asmussen, B. Lauritsen, and A. Jordan. 1994. "Low Back Pain Rating Scale: Validation of a Tool for Assessment of Low Back Pain." *Pain* 57 (3): 317–26.

Mannino, D. M., R. M. Klevens, and W. D. Flanders. 1994. "Cigarette Smoking: An Independent Risk Factor for Impotence?" *American Journal of Epidemiology* 140: 1003–8.

March, Lyn, Emma U. R. Smith, Damian G. Hoy, Marita J. Cross, Lidia Sanchez-Riera, Fiona Blyth, Rachelle Buchbinder, Theos Vos, and Anthony D. Woolf. 2014. "Burden of Disability Due to Musculoskeletal (MSK) Disorders." *Best Practice and Research Clinical Rheumatology* 28 (3): 353–66.

Marchetti, Gregory F., and Susan L Whitney. 2006. "Construction and Validation of the 4-Item Dynamic Gait Index." *Physical Therapy* (86) 12: 1651–59.

Maslow, Abraham. 1954. *Motivation and Personality*. New York: Harper.

Mattu, Amal, and Deepi G. Goyal, eds. 2007. *Emergency Medicine: Avoiding the Pitfalls and Improving the Outcomes*. Malden, MA: Blackwell Pub./BMJ Books.

Maunder, R. G., and S. Levenstein. 2008. "The Role of Stress in the Development and Clinical Course of Inflammatory Bowel Disease: Epidemiological Evidence." *Current Molecular Medicine* 8: 247–52.

Mayr, E. 1988. "The Multiple Meanings of Teleological." In *Towards a New Philosophy of Biology*, 38–66. Cambridge, MA: Harvard University Press.

McCaffrey, R., J. Park, D. Newman, and D. Hagen. 2014. "The Effect of Chair Yoga in Older Adults with Moderate and Severe Alzheimer's Disease." *Research in Gerontological Nursing* 7 (4): 171–77.

McCall, Timothy. 2007. *Yoga as Medicine: A Yogic Prescription for Health and Healing.* New York: Bantam Dell.

McCorry, Laurie Kelly. 2007. "Physiology of the Autonomic Nervous System." *American Journal of Pharmaceutical Education* 71 (4): 78.

McDermott, John J., ed. 1981. *The Philosophy of John Dewey.* Chicago: University of Chicago Press.

McNicol, K., J. E. Taunton, and D. B. Clement. 1981. "Iliotibial Tract Friction Syndrome in Athletes." *Journal Canadien des Sciences Appliquees au Sport* [*Canadian Journal of Applied Sport Sciences*] 6 (2): 76–80.

McNeill, William Hardy. 1977. *Plagues and Peoples.* Oxford: Basil Blackwell.

Mead, Margaret. 1935. *Sex and Temperament in Three Primitive Societies.* New York: Harper.

Mehta, Miro. 2002. *Health Through Yoga: Simple Practice Routines and a Guide to the Ancient Teachings.* London: Thorsons.

Meli, A., G. Zimatore, C. Badaracco, E. De Angelis, and D. Tufarelli. 2006. "Vestibular Rehabilitation and 6-Month Follow-Up Using Objective and Subjective Measures." *Acta Otolaryngologica* 126 (3): 259–66.

Meng, M. V., K. L. Greene, and P. J. Turek. 2005. "Surgery or Assisted Reproduction? A Decision Analysis of Treatment Costs in Male Infertility." *Journal of Urology* 174: 1926–31.

Merleau-Ponty, Maurice. 1958. *Phenomenology of Perception.* London: Routledge.

Merriam-Webster. 2017. "Vocabulary." www.merriam-webster.com/dictionary/vocabulary.

Merton, Thomas. 1997. *Learning to Love. The Journals of Thomas Merton, Volume Six 1966–1967.* San Francisco: Harper.

Michaels, Axel. 2004. *Hinduism: Past and Present.* Princeton, NJ: Princeton University Press.

Micheli, Lyle J., 1986. "12 Pediatric and Adolescent Sports Injuries: Recent Trends." *Exercise and Sport Sciences Reviews* 14 (1): 359–74.

Michigan Board of Medicine. 2016. Department of Licensing and Regulatory Affairs. State of Michigan. www.michigan.gov/lara/0,4601,7-154-72600_72603_27529_27541-58914--,00.html.

Milgrom, Charles, Victor Novack, Yoram Weil, Saleh Jaber, Denitsa R. Radeva-Petrova, and Aharon Finestone. 2008. "Risk Factors for Idiopathic Frozen Shoulder." *Israel Medical Association Journal* 10 (5): 361.

Miller, Elise Browning. 2003. *Yoga for Scoliosis.* Atlanta: Shanti Productions.

Miller, Robert, Frederick Azar, and Thomas Throckmorton. 2013. "Shoulder and Elbow Injuries." In *Campbell's Operative Orthopedics*, edited by S. T. Canale and J. H. Beaty. 12th ed. Philadelphia: Elsevier Mosby.

Mirbey, J., J. Besancenot, R. T. Chambers, A. Durey, and P. Vichard. 1988. "Avulsion Fractures of the Tibial Tuberosity in the Adolescent Athlete: Risk Factors, Mechanism of Injury, and Treatment." *American Journal of Sports Medicine* 16 (4): 336–40.

Mishellany, A., A. Woda, R. Labas, and M. A. Peyton. 2006. "The Challenge of Mastication: Preparing a Bolus Suitable for Deglutition." *Dysphagia* 21: 87–94.

Mishra, Gyanshankar, and Jasmin Mulani. 2013. "Tuberculosis Prescription Practices in Private and Public Sector in India." *National Journal of Integrated Research in Medicine* 4, 71–78.

Mittlemark, Raul Artal, Robert A. Wiswell, and Barbara L. Drinkwater, eds. 1991. *Exercise in Pregnancy*, 2nd edition. Baltimore: Williams and Wilkins.

Mohan, A. G. 1993. *Yoga for Body, Breath, and Mind: A Guide to Personal Reintegration*. Boston: Shambhala Publications.

Mohan, A. G., and Indra Mohan. 2004. *Yoga Therapy: A Guide to the Therapeutic Use of Yoga and Ayurveda for Health and Fitness*. Boston: Shambhala Publications.

Monier Williams, Monier. 1899. *A Sanskrit-English Dictionary: Etymologically and Philologically Arranged with Special Reference to Cognate Indo-European Languages*. Oxford: Clarendon Press.

Monroe, Brian M., and Stephen J. Read. 2008. "A General Connectionist Model of Attitude Structure and Change: The ACS (Attitudes as Constraint Satisfaction) Model." *Psychological Review* 115 (3): 733.

Monroe, Marcia P. 2011. *Yoga and Scoliosis: A Journey to Health and Healing*. New York: Demos Medical Publishing.

Montagu, Ashley. 1986. *Touching: The Human Significance of Skin*. New York: William Morrow.

Montanaro, L., P. Parisini, T. Greggi, M. Di Silvestre, D. Campoccia, S. Rizzi, and C. R. Arciola. 2006. "Evidence of a Linkage Between Matrilin-1 Gene (MATN1) and Idiopathic Scoliosis." *Scoliosis and Spinal Disorders* 1 (1): 1.

Moore, Keith L., Arthur F. Dalley, and Anne M. R. Agur. 2006. *Clinically Oriented Anatomy*. 5th ed. Philadephia: Lippincott Williams and Wilkins.

Moore, W. S., ed. 1993. *Vascular Surgery: A Comprehensive Review*. 4th ed. Philadelphia: W. B. Saunders Co.

Moosmayer, S., G. Lund, U. Seljom, I. Svege, T. Hennig, R. Tariq, and H. J. Smith. 2010. "Comparison Between Surgery and Physiotherapy in the Treatment of Small and Medium-Sized Tears of the Rotator Cuff." *Journal of Bone and Joint Surgery* (British) 92 (1): 83–91.

Moriguchi, Yu, Marjan Alimi, Thamina Khair, George Manolarakis, Connnon Berlin, Lawrence J. Bonasssar, and Roger Härtl. 2016. "Biological Treatment Approaches to Degenerative Disk Disease: A Literature Review of In Vivo Animal and Clinical Data." *Global Spine* 6 (5): 497–518.

Morin C. M., L. Belanger, and M. LeBlanc. 2009. "The Natural History of Insomnia: A Population-Based 3-Year Longitudinal Study." *Archives of Internal Medicine* 169: 447–53.

Mow, Van C., and Rik Huiskes, eds. 2005. *Basic Orthopaedic Biomechanics and Mechano-biology*. 3rd ed. Philadelphia: Lippincott Williams and Wilkins.

Muktibodhananda, Saraswati, trans. 1985. *Hatha Yoga Pradipika: The Light on Hatha Yoga*. Munger, India: Bihar School of Yoga.

Muldoon, M. P., D. E. Padgett, D. E. Sweet, P. A. Deuster, and G. R. Mack. 2001. "Femoral Neck Stress Fractures and Metabolic Bone Disease." *Journal of Orthopedic Trauma* 15 (3): 181–185.

Mustian, K. M., M. Janelsins, L. J. Peppone, and C. Kamen. 2014. "Yoga for the Treatment of Insomnia Among Cancer Patients: Evidence, Mechanisms of Action, and Clinical Recommendations." *Oncology and Hematology Review* 10 (2): 164–168.

Nadel, E. R. 1983. "Effects of Temperature on Muscle Metabolism." In *Biochemistry of Exercise*, edited by J. A. Vogel. Champaign: Human Kinetics Publishers.

Najera et al. 2015. "Cervical Sprain or Strain." Chapter 6 in *Essentials of Physical Medicine and Rehabilitation*. 3rd ed. Philadelphia: Elsevier Saunders.

National Academies of Sciences, Engineering, and Medicine. 2017. *The Health Effects of Cannabis and Cannabinoids: The Current State of Evidence and Recommendations for Research*. Washington, D.C.: National Academies Press.

NCCIH (National Center for Complementary and Integrative Health). 2017. "NCCIH Facts-at-a-Glance and Mission." NCCIH. https://nccih.nih.gov/about/ataglance.

Netter, Frank H. 1997. *Atlas of Human Anatomy*. 2nd ed. East Hanover, NJ: Novartis.

Nichter, Mark. 2008. *Global Health: Why Cultural Perceptions, Social Representations, and Biopolitics Matter*. Tucson: The University of Arizona Press.

Nicolosi, A. 2004. "A Population Study of the Association Between Sexual Function, Sexual Satisfaction and Depressive Symptoms in Men." *Journal of Affective Disorders* 82 (2): 235–243.

Niemuth, P. E., R. J. Johnson, M. J. Myers, and T. J. Thieman. 2005. "Hip Muscle Weakness and Overuse Injuries in Recreational Runners." *Clinical Journal of Sport Medicine* 15 (1): 14–21.

Nirschl, R. P. 1992. "Elbow Tendonosis/Tennis Elbow." *Clinical Sports Medicine* 11: 851–870.

Nolen-Hoeksema S., and Morrow J. A. 1991. "A Prospective Study of Depression and Posttraumatic Stress Symptoms After a Natural Disaster: The 1989 Loma Prieta Earthquake." *Journal of Personality and Social Psychology* 61: 115–121.

Nunn, John. 1996. *Ancient Egyptian Medicine*. Norman, OK: Oklahoma University Press.

Nurkovic, Jasmine, Ljubisa Jovasevic, Admira Konicanin, Zoran Bajin, Katarina Parezanovic Ilic, Vesna Grbovic, Aleksandra Jurisic Skevin, and Zana Dolicanin. 2016. "Treatment of Trochanteric Bursitis: Our Experience." *Journal of Physical Therapy Science* 28 (7): 2078–81.

Nussey, Stephen S., and Saffron A. Whitehead. 2013. *Endocrinology: An Integrated Approach*. Boca Raton: CRC Press.

Ochs, Mathias, Jens R. Nyengaard, Anja Jung, Lars Knudsen, Marion Voigt, Thorsten Wahlers, Joachin Richter, and Jørgen G. Gundersen. 2004. "The Number of Alveoli in the Human Lung." *American Journal of Respiratory and Critical Care Medicine* 169 (1): 120–24.

O'Connell, Thomas, J., and Ché. B. Bou-Matar. 2007. "Long Term Marijuana Users Seeking Medical Cannabis in California (2001–2007): Demographics, Social Characteristics, Patterns of Cannabis and Other Drug Use of 4117 Applicants." *Harm Reduction Journal* 4: 16.

Odier, Daniel. 2004. *Yoga Spandakarika: The Sacred Texts at the Origins of Tantra*. Rochester, Vermont: Inner Traditions.

Ogilvie, James W., John Braun, VeeAnn Argyle, Lesa Nelson, Mary Meade, and Kenneth Ward. 2012. "The Search for Idiopathic Scoliosis Genes." *Spine* 31 (6): 679–81.

Olive, David. L., and Elizabeth A. Pritts. 2006. "Estimating Infertility: The Devil Is in the Details." *Fertility and Sterility* 86 (3): 529–530.

Olmi, Giuseppe. 2006. *Representing the Body: Art and Anatomy from Leonardo to the Enlightenment*. Bologna: Bologna University Press.

Opar, D. A., M. D. Williams, and A. J. Shield. 2012. "Hamstring Strain Injuries: Factors That Lead to Injury and Reinjury." *Sports Medicine* 42 (3): 209–26.

Orava, S. 1978. "Iliotibial Tract Friction Syndrome in Athletes—An Uncommon Exertion Syndrome on the Lateral Side of the Knee." *British Journal of Sports Medicine* 12 (2): 69–73.

Orlando, M. S., K. C. Likes, S. Mizra, Y. Cao, Y. W. Lum, T. Reifsnyder, and J. A. Freischlag. 2015. "A Decade of Excellent Outcomes After Surgical Intervention in 538 Patients with Thoracic Outlet Syndrome." *Journal of the American College of Surgeons* 220 (5): 934–39.

Orme-Johnson, David. 2006. "Evidence That the Transcendental Meditation Program Prevents or Decreases Diseases of the Nervous System and Is Specifically Beneficial for Epilepsy." *Medical Hypotheses* 67 (2): 240–46.

Ornish, Dean. 1990. *Dr. Dean Ornish's Program for Reversing Heart Disease: The Only System Scientifically Proven to Reverse Heart Disease*. New York: Ballentine Books.

Osterberg, Lars, and Terrence Blaschke. 2005. "Adherence to Medication." *New England Journal of Medicine* 353 (5): 487–97.

PAHO (Pan American Health Organization). 2017. PAHO.org. www.paho.org/hq/.

Pascual-Leone, A., A. Amedi, F. Fregni, and L. B. Merabet. 2005. "The Plastic Human Brain Cortex." *Annual Review of Neuroscience* 28: 377–401.

Patwardhan, Kishor. 2012. "The History of the Discovery of Blood Circulation: Unrecognized Contributions of Ayurveda Masters." *Advances in Physiology Education* 36 (2): 77–82.

Payne, Larry, and Richard Usatine. 2002. *Yoga Rx: A Step-by-Step Program to Promote Health, Wellness, and Healing for Common Ailments*. New York: Broadway Books.

Payne, Larry, Terra Gold, and Eden Goldman. 2016. *Yoga Therapy and Integrative Medicine: Where Ancient Science Meets Modern Medicine*. Laguna Beach, CA: Basic Health Publications.

Payne, Peter, and Mardi A. Crane-Godreau. 2015. "Meditative Movement for Depression and Anxiety." *Frontiers in Psychiatry* 4: 71.

Pearce, C. L., C. Templeman, and M. A. Rossing. 2012. "Association Between Endometriosis and Risk of Histological Subtypes of Ovarian Cancer: A Pooled Analysis of Case-Control Studies." *Lancet Oncology* 133 (4): 385–94.

Pehrsson, K., S. Larsson, A. Oden, and A. Nachemson. 1992. "Long-Term Follow-Up of Patients with Untreated Scoliosis: A Study of Mortality, Causes of Death, and Symptoms." *Spine* 17 (9): 1091–96.

Pereira, R. F. 2011. "Quality of Life, Behavioral Problems, and Marital Adjustment in the First Year After Radical Prostatectomy." *Clinical Genitourinary Cancer* 9 (1): 53–58.

Perelman, M. A. 2011. "Erectile Dysfunction and Depression: Screening and Treatment." *Urologic Clinics of North America* 38 (2): 125–39.

Pertwee, R. G. 2006. "Cannabinoid Pharmacology: The First 66 Years." *British Journal of Pharmacology* 147: S163–71.

Peterson, Donald R., and Joseph D. Bronzino, eds. 2008. *Biomechanics: Principles and Applications*. 2nd rev. ed. Boca Raton: CRC Press.

Pette, Dirk, and Robert S. Staron. 2000. "Myosin Isoforms, Muscle Fiber Types, and Transitions." *Microscopy Research and Technique* 50 (6): 500–9.

Peyron M. A., A. Mishellany, and A. Woda. 2004. "Particle Size Distribution of Food Boluses After Mastication of Six Natural Foods." *Journal of Dental Research* 83: 578–82.

Pillai, V., and C. L. Drake. 2014. "Sleep and Repetitive Thought: The Role of Rumination and Worry in Sleep Disturbance." In *Sleep and Affect: Assessment, Theory, and Clinical Implications*, edited by K. A. Babson and M. T. Feldner. Amsterdam: Elsevier.

Pitzer, Michael E., Peter H. Seidenberg, and Dov A. Bader. 2014. "Elbow Tendinopathy." *Medical Clinics of North America* 98 (4): 833–49.

Podichetty, Vinod K. 2006. "The Aging Spine: The Role of Inflammatory Mediators in Intervertebral Disc Degeneration." *Cellular and Molecular Biology* (Noisy-le-Grand, France) 53 (5): 4–18.

Pole, Sebastian. 2013. *Ayurvedic Medicine: The Principles of Traditional Practice.* London: Singing Dragon.

Pollan, Michael. 2006. *The Omnivore's Dilemma: The Search for a Perfect Meal in a Fast-Food World.* London: Penguin Press.

Polsky D., and S. Q. Wang. 2011. *Skin Cancer Facts.* New York: The Skin Cancer Foundation. www.skincancer.org.

Popa, T., M. Bonifazi, R. Della Volpe, A. Rossi, and R. Mazzocchio. 2006. "Adaptive Changes in Postural Strategy Selection in Chronic Low Back Pain." *Experimental Brain Research* 177 (3): 411–18.

Porter J. L. and A. Wilkinson. 1997. "Lumbar-Hip Flexion Motion. A Comparative Study Between Asymptomatic and Chronic Low Back Pain in 18- to 36-Year-Old Men." *Spine* 22 (13): 1508–13.

Porth, Carol Mattson, and Genn Martin. 2008. *Pathophysiology: Concepts of Altered Health States.* 8th ed. Philadelphia: Lippincott Williams and Wilkins.

Potter, D. S., and D. J. Mattingly. 2010. *Life, Death, and Entertainment in the Roman Empire.* Ann Arbor, MI: University of Michigan Press.

Povlsen, Bo, Thomas Hansson, and Sebastian D. Povlsen. 2014. "Treatment for Thoracic Outlet Syndrome." *Cochrane Database System Review* 11.

Powell, Barbara. 1996. *Windows into the Infinite: A Guide to Hindu Scriptures.* Fremont, CA: Jain Publishing.

Prabhavananda, S., and C. Isherwood, trans. 1944. *Bhagavad-Gita: The Song of God.* Hollywood: The Marcel Rodd Co.

Qaseem, A., D. Kansagara, M. A. Forciea, M. Cooke, and T. D. Denberg. 2016. "Management of Chronic Insomnia Disorder in Adults: A Clinical Practice Guideline from the American College of Physicians." *Annals of Internal Medicine* 165 (2): 125–33.

Qin, J., S. Kimel, S. Kitayama, X. Wang, X. Yang, and S. Han. 2011. "How Choice Modifies Preference: Neural Correlates of Choice Justification." *NeuroImage* 55 (1): 240–46.

Qualter P., S. L. Brown, P. Munn, and K. J. Rotenberg. 2010. "Childhood Loneliness as a Predictor of Adolescent Depressive Symptoms: An 8-Year Longitudinal Study." *European Child Adolescent Psychiatry* 19: 493–501.

Rak, S., R. Day, and A. Wang. 2004. "The Role of the Supinator in the Pathogenesis of Chronic Lateral Elbow Pain: A Biomechanical Study." *Journal of Hand Surgery* (British) 29 (5): 461–64.

Rama, Swami, Swami Ajaya, and Rudolpy Ballentine. 1976. *Yoga and Psychotherapy: The Evolution of Consciousness.* Honesdale, PA: The Himalayan Institute.

Ramaswami, Srivatsu. 2005. *The Complete Book of Vinyasa Yoga*. Cambridge: Da Capo Press.

Raphael, B., S. Wooding, G. Stevens, and J. Connor. 2005. "Comorbidity: Cannabis and Complexity." *Journal of Psychiatric Practice* 11: 161–76.

Ray, U. S., A. Pathak, O. S.Tomer. 2011. "Hatha Yoga Practices: Energy Expenditure, Respiratory Changes and Intensity of Exercise." *Evidence-based Complementary and Alternative Medicine: eCAM*. doi:10.1093/ecam/neq046.

Reddi, B. A. J., and R. H. S. Carpenter. 2005. "Venous Excess: A New Approach to Cardiovascular Control and Its Teaching." *Journal of Applied Physiology* 98 (1): 356–64.

Reddy S., A. M. Dick, and K. Mitchell. 2014. "The Effect of a Yoga Intervention on Alcohol and Drug Abuse Risk in Veteran and Civilian Women with Posttraumatic Stress Disorder." *Journal of Alternative Complementary Medicine* 20 (10): 750–56.

Regan, W., L. E. Wold, R. Coonrad, and B. F. Morrey. 1992. "Microscopic Histopathology of Chronic Refractory Lateral Epicondylitis." *American Journal of Sports Medicine* 20 (6): 746–49.

Reiman, A. 2009. "Cannabis as a Substitute for Alcohol and Other Drugs." *Harm Reduction Journal* 6: 35–39.

Remski, Matthew. 2012. *Threads of Yoga: A Remix of Patanjali's Sutras, with Commentary and Reverie*. CreateSpace Independent Publishing Platform.

Renno, A., R. Granito, P. Driusso, D. Costa, and J. Oishi. 2005. "Effects of an Exercise Program on Respiratory Function, Posture, and on Quality of Life in Osteoporotic Women: A Pilot Study." *Physiotherapy* 91 (1): 113–18.

Respiratory Care Board of California. 2017. "Scope of Practice Defined: Business and Professions Code Section 3702." www.rcb.ca.gov/licensees/forms/scope_of_practice.pdf.

Riemann D., C. Kloepfer, and M. Berger. 2009. "Functional and Structural Brain Alterations in Insomnia: Implications for Pathophysiology." *European Journal of Neuroscience* 29 (9): 1754–60.

Riemann D., K. Spiegelhalder, B. Feige, U. Voderholzer, M. Berger, M. Perlis, and C. Nissen. 2010. "The Hyperarousal Model of Insomnia: A Review of the Concept and Its Evidence." *Sleep Medicine Review* 14 (1): 19–31.

Roebuck, Valerie J. 2000. *The Upaniṣhads*. New Delhi: Penguin Books.

Roetert, E. P., H. Brody, C. J. Dillman, J. L. Groppel, and J. M. Schultheis. 1995. "The Biomechanics of Tennis Elbow. An Integrated Approach." *Clinics in Sports Medicine* 14 (1): 47–57.

Roewert-Huber, J., B. Lange-Asschenfeldt, E. Stockfleth, and H. Kerl. 2007. "Epidemiology and Aetiology of Basal Cell Carcinoma." *British Journal of Dermatology* 157 (Suppl 2): 47–51.

Rogers, Carl R. 1951. *Client-Centered Therapy: Its Current Practice, Implications, and Theory*. Cambridge, MA: The Riverside Press.

———. 1961. *On Becoming a Person: A Therapist's View of Psychotherapy.* Boston: Houghton Mifflin.

———. 1980. *A Way of Being.* Boston: Houghton Mifflin.

Rogers, C. R., and R. E. Farson. 1987. "Active Listening." In *Communicating in Business Today*, edited by R. G. Newman, M. A. Danzinger, and M. Cohen. Washington, D. C.: Heath and Company.

Romano, M., S. Minozzi, F. Zaina, J. B. Saltikov, N. Chockalingam, T. Kotwicki, A. M. Hennes, and S. Negrini. 2012. "Exercises for Adolescent Idiopathic Scoliosis." *The Cochrane Library* 38 (14): 883–93.

Roos, David B. 1976. "Congenital Anomalies Associated with Thoracic Outlet Syndrome: Anatomy, Symptoms, Diagnosis, and Treatment." *American Journal of Surgery* 132 (6): 771–78.

Roos, David B. 1999. "Thoracic Outlet Syndrome Is Underdiagnosed." *Muscle and Nerve* 22 (1): 126–29.

Rosa, R. R., and M. H. Bonnet. 2000. "Reported Chronic Insomnia Is Independent of Poor Sleep as Measured by Electroencephalography." *Psychosomatic Medicine* 62 (4): 474–82.

Rosen, Richard. 2002. *The Yoga of Breath: A Step-by-Step Guide to Pranayama.* Boulder: Shambhala Publications.

———. 2006. *Pranayama Beyond the Fundamentals: An In-Depth Guide to Yogic Breathing.* Boulder: Shambhala Publications.

———. 2012. *Original Yoga: Rediscovering Traditional Practices of Hatha Yoga.* Boulder: Shambhala Publications.

Rosenzweig, S., J. M. Greeson, D. K. Reibel, J. S. Green, S. A. Jasser, and D. Beasley. 2010. "Mindfulness-based Stress Reduction for Chronic Pain Conditions: Variation in Treatment Outcomes and Role of Home Meditation Practice." *Journal of Psychosomatic Research* 68 (1): 29–36.

Roser, Max. 2017. "Life Expectancy." OurWorldInData.org. https://ourworldindata.org/life-expectancy/.

Roter, D. L., M. Stewart, S. M. Putnam, M. Lipkin Jr., W. Stiles, and T. S. Inui. 1997. "Communication Patterns of Primary Care Physicians." *Journal of the American Medical Association* 277 (4).

Roth, T. 2007. "Insomnia: Definition, Prevalence, Etiology, and Consequences." *Journal of Clinical Sleep Medicine* 3 (Suppl 5): 7–10.

Rowland, Andrew S., Catherine A. Lesesne, and Ann J. Abramowitz. 2002. "The Epidemiology of Attention Deficit/Hyperactivity Disorder (ADHD): A Public Health View." *Mental Retardation and Developmental Disabilities Research Reviews* 8 (3): 162–70.

Rubio-Aurioles, E., E. D. Kim, R. C. Rosen, H. Porst, and P. Burns. 2009. "Impact on Erectile Function and Sexual Quality of Life of Couples: A Double-Blind, Randomized, Placebo-Controlled Trial of Tadalafil Taken Once Daily." *Journal of Sex Medicine* 6: 1314–23.

Rudzki, J. R., and Benjamin Shaffer. 2008. "New Approaches to Diagnosis and Arthroscopic Management of Partial-Thickness Cuff Tears." *Clinics in Sports Medicine* 27 (4): 691–717.

Ryan, James R., and Gino G. Salciccioli. 1976. "Fractures of the Distal Radial Epiphysis in Adolescent Weight Lifters." *American Journal of Sports Medicine* 4 (1): 26–42.

Sabat, Steven. 2001. *The Experience of Alzheimer's Disease: Life Through a Tangled Veil.* Hoboken, NJ: Wiley-Blackwell.

Sadat, Umar, Ruwan Weerakkody, and Kevin Varty. 2008. "Thoracic Outlet Syndrome: An Overview." *British Journal of Hospital Medicine* 69 (5): 260–63.

Samuel, Goeffrey. 2008. *The Origins of Yoga and Tantra: Indic Religions to the Thirteenth Century.* Cambridge: Cambridge University Press.

Sanders, R. J. and C. E. Haug. 1991. *Thoracic Outlet Syndrome: A Common Sequela of Neck Injuries.* Philadelphia: Lipppincott.

Sandman, David, Elizabeth Simantov, Christina An. 2000. *Out of Touch: American Men and the Health Care System.* New York: Commonwealth Fund.

Satchidananda, Sri Swami. 1978. *Integral Yoga: The Yoga Sutras of Patanjali.* 1st ed. Yogaville, VA: Integral Yoga Publications.

Sawka, Michael N. "Physiological Consequences of Hypohydration: Exercise Performance and Thermoregulation." *Medicine and Science in Sports and Exercise* 24 (6): 657–70.

Satyadharma, Swami. 2003. *Yoga Chudamani Upanishad: Crown Jewel of Yoga.* Bihar, India: Yoga Publications Trust.

Scaravelli, Vanda. 1991. *Awakening the Spine: The Stress Free Yoga That Works with the Body to Restore Health, Vitality, and Energy.* New York: Harper Collins Publishers.

Schiffmann, Erich. 1996. *Yoga: The Spirit and Practice of Moving into Stillness.* New York: Pocket Books.

Schlegel, T. F., B. D. Bushnell, J. Godfrey, and M. Boublik. 2009. "Success of Nonoperative Management of Adductor Longus Tendon Ruptures in National Football League Athletes." *The American Journal of Sports Medicine* 37 (7): 1394–39.

Schwarzer, A. C., C. N. Aprill, and N. Bogduk. 1995. "The Sacroiliac Joint in Chronic Low Back Pain." *Spine* 20 (1): 31–37.

Seitz, Daniel D. 2010. "An Overview of Regulatory Issues for Yoga, Yoga Therapy, and Ayurveda. "*International Journal of Yoga Therapy* 20: 34–39.

Selvin, E., A. L. Burnett, and E. A. Platz. 2007. "Prevalence and Risk Factors for Erectile Dysfunction in the US." *American Journal of Medicine* 120 (2): 151–57.

Shabsigh, R., I. J. Fishman, C. Schum, and J. K. Dunn. 1991. "Cigarette Smoking and Other Vascular Risk Factors in Vasculogenic Impotence." *Urology* 38: 227–231.

Shaffer, H. J., T. A. LaSalvia, and J. P. Stein. 1997. "Comparing Hatha Yoga with Dynamic Group Psychotherapy for Enhancing Methadone Maintenance Treatment: A Randomized Clinical Trial." *Alternative Therapies in Health and Medicine* 3: 57–66.

Sharma, Arvind. 1997. *The Philosophy of Religion and Advaita Vedānta: A Comparative Study in Religion and Reason*. New Delhi, India: Sri Satguru.

Sharma, P. V., trans. 1992. *Caraka-Sa. V.,trans.,1992. and Advaita Vedānta: A Comparative Study in Religion and Reasbala* (text with English translation).Varanasi, India: Chaukhambha Orientalia.

———, trans. 2001. *Suśruta-Sa01. dia: Chaukhambha Orientalia.ānta: A Comparative Study in Religion and Reasbala* (text w. Haridas Ayurveda Series 9. 3 volumes.) Varanasi, India: Chaukhambha Visvabharati.

Shaver, J. L., and N. F. Woods. 2015. "Sleep and Menopause: A Narrative Review." *Menopause* 22 (8): 899–915.

Sherwood, Lauralee. 2011. *Fundamentals of Human Physiology*. Boston: Cengage Learning.

Shulman, Samuel B. 1949. "Survey in China and India of Feet That Have Never Worn Shoes." *Journal of the National Association of Chiropodists* 49: 26–30.

Shumway-Cook, Anne, and Marjorie H. Woollacott. 1995. *Motor Control: Translating Research into Clinical Practice*. 4th edition. Philadelphia: Lippincott Williams and Wilkins.

Shusterman, Richard. 2008. *Body Consciousness: A Philosophy of Mindfulness and Somaesthetics*. Cambridge, UK: Cambridge University Press.

———. 2012. *Thinking Through the Body: Essays in Somaesthetics*. New York: Cambridge University Press.

Siegel, Bernie. 1986. *Love, Medicine, and Miracles: Lessons Learned about Self-Healing from a Surgeon's Experience with Exceptional Patients*. New York: Harper Collins.

Siiteri, Pentii K., and Jean D. Wilson. 1974. "Testosterone Formation and Metabolism During Male Sexual Differentiation in the Human Embryo." *The Journal of Clinical Endocrinology and Metabolism* 38 (1).

Silver, David. 1923. "Measurement of the Range of Motion in Joints." *Journal of Bone and Joint Surgery* (American) 5 (3): 569–78.

Simkin, D. R., and N. B. Black. 2014. "Meditation and Mindfulness in Clinical Practice." *Child and Adolescent Psychiatric Clinics of North America*, 23 (3): 487–534.

Simons, D. G. 2008. "New Views of Myofascial Trigger Points: Etiology and Diagnosis." *Archives of Physical Medicine and Rehabilitation* 89 (1): 157–59.

Singer, Charles Joseph. 1957. *A Short History of Anatomy and Physiology from the Greeks to Harvey.* Mineola, NY: Dover Publications.

Singh, S., V. Malhotra, K. P. Singh, P. Guppta, S. B. Sharma, S. V. Madhu, and O. P. Tandon. 2002. "Study of Yoga Asanas in Assessment of Pulmonary Function in NIDDM Patients." *Indian Journal of Physiology and Pharmacology* 46 (3): 313–20.

Singleton, Mark. 2010. *Yoga Body: The Origins of Modern Posture Practice.* Oxford, UK: Oxford University Press.

Siraisi, N. 1990. *Medieval and Early Renaissance Medicine: An Introduction to Knowledge and Practice.* Chicago: University of Chicago Press.

Sjoman, Norman E. 1999. *The Yoga Tradition of the Mysore Palace.* New Delhi, India: Abhinav Publications.

Sköldenberg, Olaf, Anna Ekman, Mats Salemyr, and Henrik Bodén. 2010. "Reduced Dislocation Rate After Hip Arthroplasty for Femoral Neck Fractures When Changing from Posterolateral to Anterolateral Approach: A Prospective Study of 372 Hips." *Acta Orthopaedica* 81 (5): 583–87.

Sledzik, Paul S., and Nicholas Bellantoni. 1994. "Bioarcheological and Biocultural Evidence for the New England Vampire Folk Belief." *American Journal of Physical Anthropology* 94 (2): 269–74.

Smidt, N., W. J. Assendelft, D. A. van der Windt, E. M. Hay, R. Buchbinder, and L. M. Bouter. 2002. "Corticosteroid Injections for Lateral Epicondylitis: A Systematic Review." *Pain* 96 (1): 23–40.

Smith, M. T., M. L. Perlis, A. Park, M. S. Smith, J. Pennington, D. E. Giles. 2002. "Comparative Meta-analysis of Pharmacotherapy and Behavior Therapy for Persistent Insomnia." *American Journal of Psychiatry* 159: 5–11.

Smith, T. C., M. A. Ryan, and B. Smith. 2007. "Complementary and Alternative Medicine Use Among US Navy and Marine Corps Personnel." *BMC Complementary and Alternative Medicine* 7: 16.

Snyderman, Ralph, and Andrew Weil. 2002. "Integrative Medicine: Bringing Medicine Back to Its Roots." *Archives of Internal Medicine* 162 (4): 395–97.

Sperling, R. A. et al. 2011. "Toward Defining the Preclinical Stages of Alzheimer's Disease: Recommendations from the National Institute on Aging and the Alzheimer's Association Workgroup." *Alzheimer's and Dementia* 7 (3): 280–92.

Spiegel, K., R. Leproult, and E. Van Cauter. 1999. "Impact of Sleep Debt on Metabolic and Endocrine Function." *Lancet* 354 (9188): 1435–39.

Stahre, M., R. Brewer, T. Naimi, and J. Miller. 2004. "Alcohol-Attributable Deaths and Years of Potential Life Lost Due to Excessive Alcohol Use in the U.S." *Morbidity and Mortality Weekly Report* 53: 866–70.

Standring, Susan. 2008. "Azygos Vein." *Gray's Anatomy: The Anatomical Basis of Clinical Practice*. 40th ed. London: Churchill Livingstone Elsevier.

Staner L. 2010. "Comorbidity of Insomnia and Depression." *Sleep Medicine Review* 14: 35–46.

Stang, A., and K. H. Jöckel. 2003. "Changing Patterns of Skin Melanoma Mortality in West Germany from 1968 through 1999." *Annals of Epidemiology* 13: 436–442.

Starr, Paul. 1982. *The Social Transformation of American Medicine*. New York: Basic Books.

Steinbeck, John (1937). 1994. *Of Mice and Men*. 6th edition. New York: Penguin Books.

Stephens, Mark. 2010. *Teaching Yoga: Essential Foundations and Techniques*. Berkeley: North Atlantic Books.

———. 2012a. *Yoga Sequencing: Designing Transformative Yoga Classes*. Berkeley: North Atlantic Books.

———. 2012b. "How Yoga Will Not Wreck Your Body." *Elephant Journal*. www.elephantjournal.com/2012/01/how-yoga-will-not-wreck-your-body-mark-stephens.

———. 2014. *Yoga Adjustments: Philosophy, Principles, and Techniques*. Berkeley: North Atlantic Books.

———. 2015. "Tricky Transitions." *Yoga Journal*, October 2015.

———. 2017. "Der Lehrer im Inneren." *Yoga Journal Deutschland*, February 2017.

Stewart, Harry Eaton. 1929. *Physiotherapy: Theory and Clinical Application*. New York: Paul B. Hoeber.

Stewart, T. K. 1995. "Encountering the Smallpox Goddess: The Auspicious Song of Śītalā." In *Religions of India in Practice*, edited by D. S. Lopez, Jr., Princeton, NJ: Princeton University Press.

Stiles, Tara. 2012. *Yoga Cures: Simple Routines to Conquer More Than 50 Ailments and Live Pain Free*. New York: Random House.

Storandt, Matha, Elizabeth A.Grant, J. Phillip Miller, and John C. Morris. 2006. "Longitudinal Course and Neuropathologic Outcomes in Original vs. Revised MCI and in Pre-MCI." *Neurology* 67 (3): 467–73.

Struijs, P. A., G. M. Kerkhoffs, W. J. Assendelft, and C. N. Van Dijk. 2004. "Conservative Treatment of Lateral Epicondylitis Brace Versus Physical Therapy or a Combination of Both: A Randomized Clinical Trial." *American Journal of Sports Medicine* 32 (2): 462–69.

Struijs, P. A., N. Schmidt, H. Arola, C. N. Van Dijk, and W. J. Assendelft. 2001. "Orthotic Devices for Tennis Elbow: A Systematic Review." *British Journal of General Practice* 51 (472): 924–29.

St. Suaver, J. L., D. O. Warner, B. P. Yawn, D. J. Jacobson, M. E. McGree, J. J. Pankratz, L. J. Meton III, V. L. Roger, J. O. Ebbert, and W. A. Rocca. 2013. "Why Patients

Visit Their Doctors: Assessing the Most Prevalent Conditions in a Defined American Population." *Mayo Clinic Proceedings* 88 (1): 56–67.

Svoboda, Robert. 1988. *Prakriti: Your Ayurvedic Constitution*. Bellingham, WA: Sadhanaa, 1988.

Svoboda, Robert, and Arnie Lade. 1995. *Tao and Dharma: Chinese Medicine and Ayurveda*. Twin Lakes, WI: Lotus.

Swenson, David. 2007. *Ashtanga Yoga: The Practice Manual*. Houston: Ashtanga Yoga Productions.

Tahirian, M. A., M. Motififard, M. N. Tahmasebi, and B. Siavashi. 2012. "Plantar Fasciitis." *Journal of Research in Medical Sciences* 17 (8): 799–804.

Taylor, F. Sherwood. 1949. *A Short History of Science and Scientific Thought*. New York: Norton.

Telles, S., S. Pathak, A. Kumar, P. Mishra, A. Balkrishna. 2015. "Influence of Intensity and Duration of Yoga on Anxiety and Depression Scores Associated with Chronic Illness." *Annals of Medical and Health Sciences Research* 5 (4): 260–65.

Tempelhof, S., S. Rupp, and R. Seil. 1999. "Age-Related Prevalence of Rotator Cuff Tears in Asymptomatic Shoulders." *Journal of Shoulder and Elbow Surgery* 8 (4): 296–99.

Tersigni, C., R. Castellani, C. de Waure, A. Fattorossi, M. De Spirito, A. Gasbarrini, G. Scambia, N. Di Simone. 2014. "Celiac Disease and Reproductive Disorders: Meta-analysis of Epidemiologic Associations and Potential Pathogenic Mechanisms." *Human Reproduction Update* 20 (4): 582–93.

Thapar, Anita, Miriam Cooper, Olga Eyre, and Kate Langley. 2013. "Practitioner Review: What Have We Learnt About the Causes of ADHD?" *Journal of Child Psychology and Psychiatry* 54 (1): 3–16.

Thase M. E., J. B. Greenhouse, and E. Frank. 1997. "Treatment of Major Depression with Psychotherapy or Psychotherapy-Pharmacotherapy Combinations." *Archives of General Psychiatry* 54 (11): 1009–15.

Thiara, Gurkaran, and Ran D. Goldman. 2012. "Milk Consumption and Mucus Production in Children with Asthma." *Canadian Family Physician* 58 (2): 165–166.

Thorne, Frederick C. 1948. "Further Critique of Nondirective Methods of Psychotherapy." *Journal of Clinical Psychology* 4 (3): 256–63.

Tigunait, Rajmani. 1999. *Tantra Unveiled: Seducing the Forces of Matter and Spirit*. Honesdale, PA: Himalayan Institute Press.

Tindle, Hilary A., Roger B. Davis, Russell S. Phillips, and David M. Eisenberg. 2005. "Trends in Use of Complementary and Alternative Medicine by US Adults: 1997–2002." *Alternative Therapies in Health and Medicine* 11 (1): 42.

Tiwari, Maya. 1995. *Ayurveda: Secrets of Healing*. Twin Lakes, WI: Lotus.

Todd, Mabel. 1937. *The Thinking Body: Study of the Balancing Forces of Dynamic Man*. Princeton, NJ: Princeton Book Company.

Todd, Mabel, and E. G. Brackett. 1920. "Principles of Posture." *Boston Medical and Surgical Journal* 182 (26): 645–49.

Tolle, Eckhart. 1999. *The Power of Now: A Guide to Spiritual Enlightenment.* Novato, CA: New World Library.

Tongue, John R., Howard R. Epps, and Laura L. Foresee. 2005. "Communication Skills for Patient-Centered Care." *Journal of Bone and Joint Surgery* 87 (3): 652–58.

Trinh, K. V., S. D. Phillips, E. Ho, and K. Damsma. 2004. "Acupuncture for the Alleviation of Lateral Epicondyle Pain: A Systematic Review." *Rheumatology* 43 (9): 1085–90.

Tuchman, Barbara. 1978. *The Distant Mirror: The Calamitous 14th Century.* New York: Random House.

United Nations. 2016. "World Drug Report 2016." United Nations Office on Drugs and Crime. www.unodc.org/wdr2016.

Upton, A. R., and A. J. McComas. 1973. "The Double Crush in Nerve-Entrapment Syndromes." *Lancet* 302 (7825): 359–62.

Urban, J. P. G., S. Roberts, and J. R. Ralphs. 2000. "The Nucleus of the Intervertebral Disc from Development to Degeneration." *American Zoology* 40 (1): 53–61.

Vagbhata. 1999. *Vagbhata's Astanga Samgraha: The Compendium of Eight Branches of Ayurveda.* Text and English translation with illustrations. New Delhi: Sri Satguru Publications.

Valle, Xavier, L. Tol Johannes, Bruce Hamilton, Gil Rodas, Peter Milliaras, Nikos Malliaropoulos, Vicenc Rizo, Marcel Moreno, and Jaume Jardi. 2015. "Hamstring Muscle Injuries: A Rehabilitation Protocol Purpose." *Asian Journal of Sports Medicine* 6 (4): E25411.

van der Linden, Paul. J. Q. 1996. "Theories on the Pathogenesis of Endometriosis." *Human Reproduction* (British) 11 (Suppl 3): 53–65.

van der Windt, D. A., Bart W. Koes, Bareld A. de Jong, and Lex M. Bouter. 1995. "Shoulder Disorders in General Practice: Incidence, Patient Characteristics, and Management." *Annals of the Rheumatic Diseases* 54 (12): 959–64.

Van Harreveld, F., B. Rutjens, M. Rotteveel, L. Nordgren, and J. van der Plight. 2009. "Ambivalence and Decisional Conflict as a Cause of Psychological Discomfort: Feeling Tense Before Jumping Off the Fence." *Journal of Experimental Social Psychology* 45 (1): 167–73.

Vaughan, Kathleen. 1951. *Exercise Before Childbirth.* London: Faber.

Vedamurthachar, A., N. Janakiramaiah, and J. M. Hegde. 2006. "Antidepressant Efficacy and Hormonal Effects of Sudarshana Kriya Yoga (SKY) in Alcohol Dependent Individuals." *Journal of Affective Disorders* 94: 249–53.

Vedhara, Kavita, and Michael Irwin. 2005. *Human Psychoneuroimmunology.* Oxford University Press on Demand.

Vinters. 2015. "Emerging Concepts in Alzheimer's Disease." *Annual Review of Pathology*. 10: 291–319.

Vivekananda, Swami. 1956. *Raja Yoga*. New York: Ramakrishna-Vivekananda Center.

Vollrath M., W. Wicki, and J. Angst. 1989. "The Zurich Study. VIII. Insomnia: Association with Depression, Anxiety, Somatic Syndromes, and Course of Insomnia." *European Archives of Psychiatry and Neurological Science* 239: 113–24.

Voth, E. A. 2001. "Guidelines for Prescribing Medical Marijuana." *The Western Journal of Medicine* 175: 305–6.

Vouriot A., G. C. Gauchard, N. Chau, L. Benamghar, M. L. Lepori, J. M. Mur, and P. P. Perrin. 2004. "Sensorial Organization Favouring Higher Visual Contribution Is a Risk Factor of Falls in an Occupational Setting." *Neuroscience Research* 48: 239–47.

Wadley, V. G., O. Okonkwo, and M. Crowe. 2009. "Mild Cognitive Impairment and Everyday Function: An Investigation of Driving Performance." *Journal of Geriatric Psychiatry and Neurology* 22: 87–94.

Wadsworth, Carolyn T. 1986. "Frozen Shoulder." *Physical Therapy* 66 (12): 1878–83.

Waelde, L. C., L. Thompson, and D. Gallagher-Thompson. 2004. "A Pilot Study of a Yoga and Meditation Intervention for Dementia Caregiver Stress."*Journal of Clinical Psychology* 60 (6): 677–87.

Wagner, G., K. S. Fugl-Meyer, and A. R. Fugl-Meyer. 2000. "Impact of Erectile Dysfunction on Quality of Life: Patient and Partner Perspectives." *International Journal of Impotence Research* 12 (Suppl 4): S144–46.

Walitza, S., R. Drechsle, and J. Ball. 2012. "Das Schulkind Mit ADHS." *Therapeitiche Umschau Journal* 69 (8): 467–73.

Walker Bone, K., K. T. Palmer, I. Reading, D. Coggon, and C. Cooper. 2004. "Prevalence and Impact of Musculoskeletal Disorders of the Upper Limb in the General Population." *Arthritis Care and Research* 51 (4): 642–51.

Walsh R., and S. L. Shapiro. 2006. "The Meeting of Meditative Disciplines and Western Psychology: A Mutually Enriching Dialogue." *American Psychologist* 61 (3): 227–39.

Walsh, T. J., M. Schembri, P. J. Turek, J. M. Chan, and P. R. Carroll. 2010. "Increased Risk of High-Grade Prostate Cancer Among Infertile Men." *Cancer* 116: 2140–47.

Wang, J., D. C. Strauss, and C. Messiou. 2016. "Endometriosis of Extraabdominal Soft Tissues: A Tertiary Center Experience." *International Journal of Surgery and Pathology* 24 (6): 497–503.

Warren, M. P., and N. E. Perlroth. 2001. "The Effects of Intense Exercise on the Female Reproductive System." *Journal of Endocrinology* 170: 3–11.

Waters, P. M., and M. B. Millis. 1988. "Hip and Pelvic Injuries in the Young Athlete." *Clinics in Sports Medicine* 7 (3): 513–26.

Watts, Alan. 1980. *Om: Creative Meditations*. Berkeley, CA: Crystal Arts.

Webster's Third New International Dictionary of the English Language, Unabridged. 1993. Springfield, MA: Merriam-Webster.

Weeden, Steven, Wayne Paprosky, and Jack Bowling. 2003. "The Early Dislocation Rate in Primary Total Hip Arthroplasty Following the Posterior Approach with Posterior Soft-Tissue Repair." *The Journal of Arthroplasty* 18 (6): 709–13.

Weil, Andrew T. 1995. *Spontaneous Healing: How to Discover and Enhance Your Body's Natural Ability to Maintain and Heal Itself*. Boston: Houghton Mifflin.

———. 1998. *The Marriage of the Sun and the Moon*. Boston: Houghton Mifflin Harcourt.

———. 2004. *Natural Health, Natural Medicine: The Complete Guide to Wellness and Self-Care for Optimum Health*. Boston: Houghton Mifflin.

———. 2007. *Healthy Aging: A Lifelong Guide to Your Well-being*. New York: Random House.

Weintraub, Amy. 2004. *Yoga for Depression: A Compassionate Guide to Relieve Suffering Through Yoga*. New York: Broadway.

———. 2012. *Yoga Skills for Therapists: Effective Practices for Mood Management*. New York: W. W. Norton and Company.

Weinstein, S. L., L. A. Dolan, J. C. Cheng, A. Danielsson, and J. A. Morcuende. 2008. "Adolescent Idiopathic Scoliosis." *Lancet* 371: 1527–37.

Weir, A., J. Jansen, J. van Keulen, J. Mens, F. Backx, and H. Stam. 2010. "Short and Mid-term Results of a Comprehensive Treatment Program for Longstanding Adductor-Related Groin Pain in Athletes: A Case Series." *Physical Therapy in Sport* 11 (3): 99–103.

Weiss, H. R., and D. Goodall. 2008. "The Treatment of Adolescent Idiopathic Scoliosis (AIS) According to Present Evidence. A Systematic Review." *European Journal of Physical and Rehabilitation Medicine* 44 (2): 177–93.

Weissman, S., and R. Weissman. 1996. *Meditation, Compassion and Loving Kindness. An Approach to Vipassana Practice*. York Beach, ME: Weiser.

West, John B. 2000. *Respiratory Physiology: The Essentials*. Philadelphia: Lippincott Williams and Wilkins.

Whipple, R., and L. I. Wolfson. 1989. "Abnormalities of Balance, Gait and Sensorimotor Function in the Elderly Population." *Proceedings of the APTA Forum*, American Physical Therapy Association, Alexandria, VA, 61–86.

White, David Gordon. 1996. *The Alchemical Body: Siddha Traditions in Medieval India*. Chicago: University of Chicago Press.

———, ed. 2000. *Tantra in Practice*. Princeton, NJ: Princeton University Press.

———. 2003. *Kiss of the Yogini: "Tantric Sex" in its South Asian Contexts*. Chicago: University of Chicago Press.

———. 2009. *Sinister Yogis*. Chicago: University of Chicago Press.

———, ed. 2012. *Yoga in Practice*. Princeton, NJ: Princeton University Press.

———. 2014. *The Yoga Sutra of Patanjali: A Biography*. Princeton, NJ: Princeton University Press.

White, Ganga. 2007. *Yoga Beyond Belief: Insights to Awaken and Deepen Your Practice*. Berkeley: North Atlantic Books.

White, Martin R., Isabel G. Jacobson, Besa Smith, Timothy S. Wells, Gary D. Gackstetter, Edward J. Boyko, Tyler C, Smith, et al. 2011. "Health Care Utilization Among Complementary and Alternative Medicine Users in a Large Military Cohort." *BMC Complementary and Alternative Medicine* 11: 27.

WHO (Word Health Organization). 2017. "Infertility Is a Global Public Health Issue." WHO. www.who.int/reproductivehealth/topics/infertility/perspective/en.

———. 2003. "International Classification of Primary Care (ICPC)." WHO. www.who.int/classifications/icd/adaptations/icpc2/en.

———. 2016. *World Health Statistics 2016: Monitoring the SDGs, Sustainable Development Goals*. Geneva: WHO Press.

"Effects of Warming Up, Massage, and Stretching on Range of Motion and Muscle Strength in the Lower Extremity." *American Journal of Sports Medicine* 11 (4): 249–52.

Wilber, Ken. 2007. *Integral Spirituality*. Boston: Shambhala Publications.

Wilbourn, A. J. 1999. "The Thoracic Outlet Syndrome Is Overdiagnosed." *Muscle Nerve* 22 (1): 130–37.

Wilder, Robert P., and Shikha Sethi. 2004. "Overuse Injuries: Tendinopathies, Stress Fractures, Compartment Syndrome, and Shin Splints." *Clinics in Sports Medicine* 23 (1): 55–81.

Wilkins, M. R. 2006. "Cannabis and Cannabis-based Medicines: Potential Benefits and Risks to Health." *Clinical Medicine* 6: 16–18.

Williams D. R., H. M. Gonzalez, H. Neighbors, R. Nesse, J. M. Abelson, J. Sweetman, J. S. Jackson. 2007. "Prevalence and Distribution of Major Depressive Disorder in African Americans, Caribbean Blacks, and Non-Hispanic Whites: Results from the National Survey of American Life." *Archives of General Psychiatry* 64: 305–15.

Wilson, Bruce E., and William G. Reiner. 1998. "Management of Intersex: A Shifting Paradigm." *Journal of Clinical Ethics* 9 (4): 360.

Wimsatt, W. C. 1972. "Teleology and the Logical Structure of Function Statements." *Studies in the History and Philosophy of Science* 3 (1): 1–80.

Windisch, Gunther, Eva Maria Braun, and Friedrich Anderhuber. 2007. "Piriformis Muscle: Clinical Anatomy and Consideration of the Piriformis Syndrome." *Surgical and Radiologic Anatomy* 29 (1): 37–45.

Witek-Janusek, L., K. Albuquerque, K. Chroniak, C. Chroniak, R. Durazo, and H. Mathews. 2008. "Effect of Mindfulness Based Stress Reduction on Immune

Function, Quality of Life and Coping in Women Newly Diagnosed with Early Stage Breast Cancer." *Brain, Behavior, and Immunity* 22 (6): 969–81.

Witzel, Michael. 1997. "The Development of the Vedic Canon and Its Schools: The Social and Political Milieu." (materials on Vedic Sakhas 8). In *Inside the Texts, Beyond the Texts. New Approaches to the Study of the Vedas.* Harvard Oriental Series. Opera Minora. Vol. 2. Cambridge, MA. http://michaelwitzel.org/wp-content/uploads/2014/06/canon.pdf.

Wolf, J. M., R. X. Sturdivant, B. D. Owens. 2009. "Incidence of de Quervain's Tenosynovitis in a Young, Active Population." *Journal of Hand Surgery* (American) 34 (1): 112–115.

Wolff, Julius. 1986. *The Law of Bone Remodelling.* Heidelberg/Berlin, Germany: Springer-Verlag.

Woo, Ronald Y., and Bernard F. Morrey. 1982. "Dislocations After Total Hip Arthroplasty." *Journal of Bone and Joint Surgery* (American) 64 (9): 1295–1306.

Wright, Wilhelmine G. 1912. "Muscle Training in the Treatment of Infantile Paralysis." *Boston Medical and Surgical Journal* 167 (17).

Wujastyk, D. 2003. *The Roots of Ayurveda: Selections from Sankskrit Medical Writings.* London: Penguin Books.

———. 2012. "The Path to Mindfulness Through Yoga Mindfulness in Early Ayurveda." In *Yoga in Practice*, edited by D. G. White. Princeton, NJ: Princeton University Press.

Yamamoto, A., K. Takagishi, T. Kobayashi, H. Shitara, T. Ichonose, E. Takasawa, D. Shimoyama, and T. Osawa. 2015. "The Impact of Faulty Posture on Rotator Cuff Tears with and Without Symptoms." *Journal of Shoulder and Elbow Surgery* 24 (3): 446–52.

Yamamoto, A., K. Takagishi, T. Osawa, T. Yanagawa, D. Nakajima, H. Shitara, and T. Kobayashi. 2010. "Prevalence and Risk Factors of a Rotator Cuff Tear in the General Population." *Journal of Shoulder and Elbow Surgery* 19 (1): 116–20.

Yates, Ben, and Shaun White. 2004. "The Incidence and Risk Factors in the Development of Medial Tibial Stress Syndrome Among Naval Recruits." *American Journal of Sports Medicine* 32 (3): 772–80.

Yeoman, W. 1928. "The Relation of Arthritis of the Sacroiliac Joint to Sciatica." *Lancet* 2: 1119–22.

Yin, M., J. Ye, M. Yao, X. Cui, Y. Xia, Q. Shen, Z. Tong, X. Wu, J. Ma, and W. Mo. 2014. "Is Extracorporeal Shock Wave Therapy Clinical Efficacy for Relief of Chronic, Recalcitrant Plantar Fasciitis?" *Archives of Physical Medicine and Rehabilitation* 95 (8): 1585–93.

Yoga Journal. 2015. "Annual Survey." Boulder, CO: Active Interest Media.

———. 2017. "Poses for Your Prostate." www.yogajournal.com/category/poses/anatomy/prostate/.

Young, Andrew J. 1990. "Energy Substrate Utilization During Exercise in Extreme Environments." *Exercise and Sport Sciences Reviews* 18 (1): 65–118.

Young, James A., and Margarita Tolentino. 2011. "Neuroplasticity and Its Applications for Rehabilitation." *American Journal of Therapeutics* 18 (1): 70–80.

Zander, T., P. Krishnakanth, G. Bergmann, and A. Rohlman. 2010. "Diurnal Variations in Intervertebral Disk Height Affect Spine Flexibility, Intradiscal Pressure and Contact Compressive Forces in the Facet Joints." *Computer Methods in Biomechanics and Biomedical Engineering* 13 (5): 551–57.

Zeni, Anne I., Carole C. Street, Rania L. Dempsey, and Megan Staton. 2000. "Stress Injury to the Bone Among Women Athletes." *Physical Medicine and Rehabilitation Clinics of North America* 11 (4): 929–47.

Zenzes, M. T. 2000. "Smoking and Reproduction: Gene Damage to Human Gametes and Embryos." *Human Reproduction Update* 6 (2): 122–31.

Zhang X. L., H. Shen, X. L. Qin, and Q. Wang. 2008. "Anterolateral Muscle Sparing Approach to Total Hip Arthroplasty: An Anatomic and Clinical Study." *Chinese Medicine Journal* 121 (15): 1358–63.

Ziltener, J. L., Sandra Leal, and P. E. Fournier. 2010. "Non-steroidal Anti-inflammatory Drugs for Athletes: An Update." *Annals of Physical and Rehabilitation Medicine* 53 (4): 278–88.

Zimmer, H. R. 1948. *Hindu Medicine.* Baltimore: Johns Hopkins Press.

———. 1951. *Philosophies of India*, edited by Joseph Campbell. New York: Pantheon Books.

Zimny, N., and Kirk C. 1987. "A Comparison of Methods of Manual Muscle Testing." *Clinical Management* 7: 6–11.

Zingg, P. O., B. Jost, A. Sukthankar, M. Buhler, C. W. A. Pfirrmann, and C. Gerber. 2007. "Clinical and Structural Outcomes of Nonoperative Management of Massive Rotator Cuff Tears." *Journal of Bone and Joint Surgery* (American) 89 (9): 1928–34.

Ziprin, P., P. Williams, and M. E. Foster. 1999. "External Oblique Aponeurosis Nerve Entrapment as a Cause of Groin Pain in the Athlete." *British Journal of Surgery* 86 (4): 566–68.

Zorrilla, E. P., L. Luborsky, J. R. Mckay, R. Rosenthal, A. Houdlin, A. Tax, R. McCorkle, D. A. Seligman, and K. Schmidt. 2001. "The Relationship of Depression and Stressors to Immunological Assays: A Meta-analytic Review." *Brain, Behavior, and Immunity* 15 (3): 199–226.

Zrenner, C. 1985. "Theories of Pineal Function from Classical Antiquity to 1900: A History." *Pineal Research Reviews* 3: 1–40.

Zuardi, A. W. 2006. "History of Cannabis as a Medicine: A Review." *Revista Brasiliera Psiquiatria (RBP)* 28: 153–157.

Zysk, Kenneth G. 1991. *Asceticism and Healing in Ancient India: Medicine in the Buddhist Monastery.* New York: Oxford University Press.

———.1998. *Medicine in the Veda: Religious Healing in the Veda: With Translations and Annotations of Medical Hymns from the Rgveda and the Atharvaveda and Renderings from the Corresponding Ritual Texts.* Delhi: Motilal Banarsidass.

Index

Ornish, Dean, 150, 205
Osgood-Schlatter disease, 136
Osteology, 83
Osteoporosis, 97, 98, 587–88, 607
Ovaries, 170, 175–76, 198–99
Oxytocin, 171, 174

P

Pachaka pitta, 33
Pada bandha, 332–33
Panca kosha, 213
Pancreas, 170, 175, 185
Pancreatic disease, 186
Parasympathetic nervous system (PN), 130
Paratenonitis, 335
Parathyroid gland, 174
Parathyroid hormone (PTH), 174
Parinamavada, 264
Particulate pollutants, 165
Pasteur, Louis, 46, 47
Pasteur, Marie, 47
Patanjali, 5, 8–9, 11, 15, 22, 69, 207, 219, 275, 278,
    280, 282, 289, 310–13, 552, 556, 565, 609, 613, 617
PCL (posterior cruciate ligament), 109–10, 351
Pee-blocking, 193
Pelvis, anatomy of, 111–14
Penis, 198
Peripheral artery disease, 149
Peripheral nervous system (PNS), 128–29, 138, 140
Peripheral neuropathy (PN), 131
Phagocytes, 154
Phalanges, 124
Pharynx, 160
Pineal gland, 169, 172–73
Piriformis, 113, 417–18
Piriformis syndrome, 417–28
Pitta, 29, 32–33, 253–55
Pituitary gland, 169, 170, 173–74
Pivot joints, 88, 89
Plane joints, 88, 89
Plantar aponeurosis, 324
Plantar fasciitis, 324–29
Plantar flexion, 95, 108
Plasticity, 136
Plato, 276, 606
"Playing the edge," 134, 135, 281
Pleural effusion, 166
PN. *See* Parasympathetic nervous system; Peripheral
    neuropathy
Pneumonia, 165
PNF (proprioceptive neuromuscular facilitation), 141
PNS (peripheral nervous system), 128–29, 138, 140
Posterior, as anatomical direction, 92
Posterior cruciate ligament (PCL), 109–10, 351
Postpartum reintegration, 584–86
Postural kyphosis, 463–71
Pradipika. See Hatha Yoga Pradipika

Prakriti, 23, 24, 27, 30, 601
Prana
    cultivation of, 6
    definition of, 6
    history of, 8
Prana-vayu, 31
Pranayama
    asana practices and, 282, 287, 289, 294–95
    assessment, 255–58
    benefits of, 289–90
    etymology of, 287
    history of, 14, 288–90
    techniques, 295–307
Pranidhana, 219
Prasna Upanishad, 289
Pratiloma pranayama, 302, 307
Pratyahara, 276, 311, 313, 551–52
Prayatna, 289
Pregnancy, 573–84
Presence, attentive, 227–28
Primary care, 62–63
Prolactin, 173
Pronation, 95
Prone, as anatomical direction, 92
Proprioception, 139–42, 610
Proprioceptive neuromuscular facilitation (PNF), 141
Prostate gland, 197
Prostatitis, 192–93, 591–92
Protraction, 95, 96
Proximal, as anatomical direction, 90, 92
Pseudosciatica, 418
Pseudoscience, 21, 172
Psoas, 113, 119–20
Psoriasis, 79
Psychosis, 551
PTH (parathyroid hormone), 174
Puja, 10
Pulmonary edema, 166
Pulmonary embolism, 166
Pulmonary hypertension, 166
Punya mandala, 219, 222, 223
Puraka, 290–93
Purusha, 23, 27, 601
Pyelonephritis, 192

Q

Quadratus lumborum (QL), 120, 439
    stretching, 442–44
Quadriceps, 110, 352

R

RA (rectus abdominus), 115, 116
Rajas, 24
Rajastic state, 554
Raja yoga, 5, 8
Rakta dhatu, 36

About the Author

MARK STEPHENS is a dedicated yoga student whose personal experience of yoga's promise to make life better inspires him to share the practice through teaching and scholarly writing.

Described by *Yoga Journal* as "the teacher's teacher," Stephens, a certified yoga therapist and member of the International Association of Yoga Therapists, is the author of the international best sellers *Teaching Yoga*, *Yoga Sequencing*, and *Yoga Adjustments*, which have been published in nine languages.

From deep study of yoga history and philosophy, human anatomy and physiology, social and interpersonal dynamics, and Eastern and Western theories of being and consciousness, Stephens brings a nondogmatic, accessible, and integrated perspective to yoga therapy that makes yoga a more refined resource for healthy living.

Practicing yoga daily for more than twenty-five years and teaching for more than twenty years, Stephens draws from his prior years in academia, as an education consultant, and as a progressive social change activist to create practical resources for yoga teachers and therapists. In 1997 he founded Yoga Inside Foundation—establishing therapeutic yoga programs in more than 300 schools, treatment centers, and prisons across North America—for which he received *Yoga Journal's* first annual Karma Yoga Award.

Stephens lives in Santa Cruz, California, and teaches globally.

For additional resources and to learn more, visit www.markstephensyoga.com.

ALSO BY MARK STEPHENS

available from North Atlantic Books

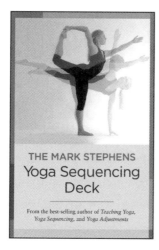

*The Mark Stephens Yoga
Sequencing Deck*
978-1-62317-061-5

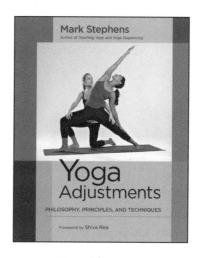

Yoga Adjustments
978-1-58394-770-8

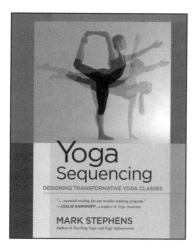

Yoga Sequencing
978-1-58394-497-4

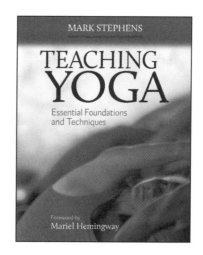

Teaching Yoga
978-1-55643-885-1

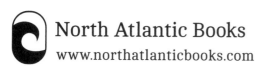
North Atlantic Books
www.northatlanticbooks.com

North Atlantic Books is an independent,
nonprofit publisher committed to a bold
exploration of the relationships between
mind, body, spirit, and nature.

About North Atlantic Books

North Atlantic Books (NAB) is an independent, nonprofit publisher committed to a bold exploration of the relationships between mind, body, spirit, and nature. Founded in 1974, NAB aims to nurture a holistic view of the arts, sciences, humanities, and healing. To make a donation or to learn more about our books, authors, events, and newsletter, please visit www.northatlanticbooks.com.

North Atlantic Books is the publishing arm of the Society for the Study of Native Arts and Sciences, a 501(c)(3) nonprofit educational organization that promotes cross-cultural perspectives linking scientific, social, and artistic fields. To learn how you can support us, please visit our website.